MARIJUANA
AND MEDICINE
Assessing the Science Base

Janet E. Joy, Stanley J. Watson, Jr., and
John A. Benson, Jr., *Editors*

Division of Neuroscience and Behavioral Health

INSTITUTE OF MEDICINE

NATIONAL ACADEMY PRESS
Washington, D.C.

NATIONAL ACADEMY PRESS • 2101 Constitution Avenue, N.W. • Washington, D.C. 20418

NOTICE: The project that is the subject of this report was approved by the Governing Board of the National Research Council, whose members are drawn from the councils of the National Academy of Sciences, the National Academy of Engineering, and the Institute of Medicine. The principal investigators responsible for the report were chosen for their special competences and with regard for appropriate balance.

The Institute of Medicine was chartered in 1970 by the National Academy of Sciences to enlist distinguished members of the appropriate professions in the examination of policy matters pertaining to the health of the public. In this, the Institute acts under both the Academy's 1863 congressional charter responsibility to be an adviser to the federal government and its own initiative in identifying issues of medical care, research, and education. Dr. Kenneth I. Shine is president of the Institute of Medicine.

This study was supported under Contract No. DC7C02 from the Executive Office of the President, Office of National Drug Control Policy.

Library of Congress Cataloging-in-Publication Data

Marijuana and medicine : assessing the science base / Janet E. Joy,
Stanley J. Watson, Jr., and John A. Benson, Jr., editors ; Division
of Neuroscience and Behavioral Health, Institute of Medicine.
        p. cm.
    Includes bibliographical references and index.
    ISBN 0-309-07155-0 (hardcover)
    1. Marijuana—Therapeutic use. 2. Cannabinoids—Therapeutic use.
I. Joy, Janet E. (Janet Elizabeth), 1953- II. Watson, Stanley J.,
1943- III. Benson, John A. IV. Institute of Medicine (U.S.).
Division of Neuroscience and Behavioral Health.
    RM666.C266 M365 1999
    615'.32345—dc21
                        99-6484

Cover: Illustration from *Marijuana Botany* by Robert Connell Clarke, Ronin Publishing, 1981.

The serpent has been a symbol of long life, healing, and knowledge among almost all cultures and religions since the beginning of recorded history. The image adopted as a logotype by the Institute of Medicine is based on a relief carving from ancient Greece, now held by the Staatliche Museen in Berlin.

PRINCIPAL INVESTIGATORS AND ADVISORY PANEL

JOHN A. BENSON, JR. (*Co-Principal Investigator*), Dean and Professor of Medicine, Emeritus, Oregon Health Sciences University School of Medicine

STANLEY J. WATSON, JR. (*Co-Principal Investigator*), Co-Director and Research Scientist, Mental Health Research Institute, University of Michigan

STEVEN R. CHILDERS, Professor of Physiology and Pharmacology, Center for Neuroscience, Bowman Gray School of Medicine, Wake Forest University

J. RICHARD CROUT, President of Crout Consulting, Drug Development and Regulation, Bethesda, Maryland

THOMAS J. CROWLEY, Professor, Department of Psychiatry, and Executive Director, Addiction Research and Treatment Services, University of Colorado Health Sciences Center

JUDITH FEINBERG, Professor, Department of Internal Medicine, and Associate Director, Division of Infectious Diseases, University of Cincinnati School of Medicine

HOWARD L. FIELDS, Professor of Neurology and Physiology, University of California at San Francisco

DOROTHY HATSUKAMI, Professor of Psychiatry, University of Minnesota

ERIC B. LARSON, Medical Director, University of Washington Medical Center, and Associate Dean for Clinical Affairs, University of Washington

BILLY R. MARTIN, Professor of Pharmacology and Toxicology, and Director of National Institute on Drug Abuse Center on Drug Abuse, Medical College of Virginia, Virginia Commonwealth University

TIMOTHY L. VOLLMER, Professor of Medicine, Multiple Sclerosis Research Center, Yale University School of Medicine

Study Staff

JANET E. JOY, Study Director
DEBORAH O. YARNELL, Research Associate
AMELIA B. MATHIS, Project Assistant
CHERYL MITCHELL, Administrative Assistant (until September 1998)
THOMAS J. WETTERHAN, Research Assistant (until September 1998)
CONSTANCE M. PECHURA, Division Director (until April 1998)
NORMAN GROSSBLATT, Manuscript Editor

Consultant

MIRIAM DAVIS

Section Staff

CHARLES H. EVANS, JR., Head, Health Sciences Section
LINDA DEPUGH, Administrative Assistant
CARLOS GABRIEL, Financial Associate

Reviewers

This report has been reviewed in draft form by individuals chosen for their diverse perspectives and technical expertise, in accordance with procedures approved by the National Research Council's Report Review Committee. The purpose of this independent review is to provide candid and critical comments that will assist the Institute of Medicine in making the published report as sound as possible and to ensure that the report meets institutional standards for objectivity, evidence, and responsiveness to the study charge. The review comments and draft manuscript remain confidential to protect the integrity of the deliberative process. The committee wishes to thank the following individuals for their participation in the review of this report:

JAMES C. ANTHONY, Johns Hopkins University
JACK D. BARCHAS, Cornell University Medical College
SUMNER H. BURSTEIN, University of Massachusetts Medical School
AVRAM GOLDSTEIN, Stanford University
LESTER GRINSPOON, Harvard Medical School
MILES HERKENHAM, National Institute of Mental Health, National
    Institutes of Health, Bethesda, Maryland
HERBERT D. KLEBER, Columbia University
GEOFFREY M. LEVITT, Venable Attorneys at Law, Washington, D.C.
KENNETH P. MACKIE, University of Washington
RAPHAEL MECHOULAM, The Hebrew University of Jerusalem
CHARLES P. O'BRIEN, University of Pennsylvania
JUDITH G. RABKIN, Columbia University

ERIC G. VOTH, International Drug Strategy Institute, Topeka, Kansas
VIRGINIA V. WELDON, Washington University

While the individuals listed above provided constructive comments and suggestions, it must be emphasized that responsibility for the final content of this report rests entirely with the authoring committee and the Institute of Medicine.

Preface

Public opinion on the medical value of marijuana has been sharply divided. Some dismiss medical marijuana as a hoax that exploits our natural compassion for the sick; others claim it is a uniquely soothing medicine that has been withheld from patients through regulations based on false claims. Proponents of both views cite "scientific evidence" to support their views and have expressed those views at the ballot box in recent state elections. In January 1997, the White House Office of National Drug Control Policy (ONDCP) asked the Institute of Medicine to conduct a review of the scientific evidence to assess the potential health benefits and risks of marijuana and its constituent cannabinoids. That review began in August 1997 and culminates with this report.

The ONDCP request came in the wake of state "medical marijuana" initiatives. In November 1996, voters in California and Arizona passed referenda designed to permit the use of marijuana as medicine. Although Arizona's referendum was invalidated five months later, the referenda galvanized a national response. In November 1998, voters in six states (Alaska, Arizona, Colorado, Nevada, Oregon, and Washington) passed ballot initiatives in support of medical marijuana. (The Colorado vote will not count, however, because after the vote was taken a court ruling determined there had not been enough valid signatures to place the initiative on the ballot.)

Information for this study was gathered through scientific workshops, site visits to cannabis buyers' clubs and HIV/AIDS clinics, analysis of the relevant scientific literature, and extensive consultation with biomedical and social scientists. The three 2-day workshops—in Irvine, California; New Orleans, Louisiana; and Washington, D.C.—were open to the public and included scientific presentations and individual reports, mostly from patients and their families, about experiences with and perspectives on the medical use of marijuana. Scientific experts in various fields were selected to talk about the latest research on marijuana, cannabinoids, and related topics. (Cannabinoids are drugs with actions similar to THC, the primary psychoactive ingredient in marijuana.) In addition, advocates for and against the medical use of marijuana were invited to present scientific evidence in support of their positions. Finally, the Institute of Medicine appointed a panel of nine experts to advise the study team on technical issues.

Public outreach included setting up a Web site that provided information about the study and asked for input from the public. The Web site was open for comment from November 1997 until November 1998. Some 130 organizations were invited to participate in the public workshops. Many people in the organizations—particularly those opposed to the medical use of marijuana—felt that a public forum was not conducive to expressing their views; they were invited to communicate their opinions (and reasons for holding them) by mail or telephone. As a result, roughly equal numbers of persons and organizations opposed to and in favor of the medical use of marijuana were heard from.

Advances in cannabinoid science over the past 16 years have given rise to a wealth of new opportunities for the development of medically useful cannabinoid-based drugs. The accumulated data suggest a variety of indications, particularly for pain relief, antiemesis, and appetite stimulation. For patients who suffer simultaneously from severe pain, nausea, and appetite loss, such as those with AIDS or who are undergoing chemotherapy, cannabinoid drugs might offer broad-spectrum relief not found in any other single medication.

Marijuana is not a completely benign substance. It is a powerful drug with a variety of effects. However, the harmful effects to individuals from the perspective of possible medical use of marijuana are not necessarily the same as the harmful physical effects of drug abuse.

Although marijuana smoke delivers THC and other cannabinoids to the body, it also delivers harmful substances, including most of those found in tobacco smoke. In addition, plants contain a variable mixture of biologically active compounds and cannot be expected to provide a precisely defined drug effect. For those reasons, the report concludes that the future of cannabinoid drugs lies not in smoked marijuana but in chemically defined drugs that act on the cannabinoid systems that are a natural component of human physiology. Until such drugs can be developed and made available for medical use, the report recommends interim solutions.

John A. Benson, Jr.
Stanley J. Watson, Jr.
Co-Principal Investigators

Acknowledgments

This report covers such a broad range of disciplines—neuroscience, pharmacology, immunology, drug abuse, drug laws, and a variety of medical specialties, including neurology, oncology, infectious diseases, and ophthalmology—that it would not have been complete without the generous support of many people. Our goal in preparing this report was to identify the solid ground of scientific consensus and to steer clear of the muddy distractions of opinions that are inconsistent with careful scientific analysis. To this end we consulted extensively with experts in each of the disciplines covered in this report. We are deeply indebted to each of them.

Members of the Advisory Panel, selected because each is recognized as among the most accomplished in their respective disciplines (see page iii), provided guidance to the study team throughout the study—from helping to lay the intellectual framework to reviewing early drafts of the report.

The following people wrote invaluable background papers for the report: Steven R. Childers, Paul Consroe, Howard Fields, Richard J. Gralla, Norbert Kaminski, Paul Kaufman, Thomas Klein, Donald Kotler, Richard Musty, Clara Sanudo-Peña, C. Robert Schuster, Stephen Sidney, Donald P. Tashkin, and J. Michael Walker. Others provided expert technical commentary on draft sections of the report: Richard Bonnie, Keith Green, Frederick Fraunfelder, Andrea Hohmann, John McAnulty, Craig Nichols, John Nutt, and Robert Pandina. Still others responded to many inquiries, provided expert counsel, or shared their unpublished data: Paul Consroe, Geoffrey Levitt, Raphael Mechoulam, Richard Musty, David Pate, Roger

Pertwee, Clara Sanudo-Peña, Carl Soderstrom, J. Michael Walker, and Scott Yarnell. Miriam Davis, consultant to the study team, provided excellent written material for the chapter on cannabinoid drug development.

The reviewers for the report (see page iv) provided extensive, constructive suggestions for improving the report. It was greatly enhanced by their thoughtful attention. Many of these people assisted us through many iterations of the report. All of them made contributions that were essential to the strength of the report. At the same time, it must be emphasized that responsibility for the final content of report rests entirely with the authors and the Institute of Medicine.

We would also like to thank the people who hosted our visits to their organizations. They were unfailingly helpful and generous with their time. Jeffrey Jones and members of the Oakland Cannabis Buyers' Cooperative, Denis Peron of the San Francisco Cannabis Cultivators Club, Scott Imler and staff at the Los Angeles Cannabis Resource Center, Victor Hernandez and members of Californians Helping Alleviate Medical Problems (CHAMPS), Michael Weinstein of the AIDS Health Care Foundation, and Marsha Bennett of the Louisiana State University Medical Center. We also appreciate the many people who spoke at the public workshops or wrote to share their views on the medical use of marijuana (see Appendix A).

Jane Sanville, project officer for the study sponsor, was consistently helpful during the many negotiations and discussion held throughout the study process. Many Institute of Medicine staff members provided greatly appreciated administrative, research, and intellectual support during the study. Robert Cook-Deegan, Marilyn Field, Constance Pechura, Daniel Quinn, and Michael Stoto provided thoughtful and insightful comments on draft sections of the report. Others provided advice and consultation on many other aspects of the study process: Clyde Behney, Susan Fourt, Carolyn Fulco, Carlos Gabriel, Linda Kilroy, Catharyn Liverman, Dev Mani, and Kathleen Stratton. As project assistant throughout the study, Amelia Mathis was tireless, gracious, and reliable.

Deborah Yarnell's contribution as research associate for this study was outstanding. She organized site visits, researched and drafted technical material for the report, and consulted extensively with relevant experts to ensure the technical accuracy of the text. The quality of her contributions throughout this study was exemplary.

Finally, the principal investigators on this study wish to personally thank Janet Joy for her deep commitment to the science and shape of this report. In addition, her help in integrating the entire data gathering and information organization of this report was nothing short of essential. Her knowledge of neurobiology, her sense of quality control, and her unflagging spirit over the 18 months illuminated the subjects and were indispensable to the study's successful completion.

Contents

EXECUTIVE SUMMARY   1

1   INTRODUCTION   13
How This Study Was Conducted, 15
Marijuana Today, 16
Marijuana and Medicine, 19
Who Uses Medical Marijuana? 20
Cannabis and the Cannabinoids, 24
Organization of the Report, 30

2   CANNABINOIDS AND ANIMAL PHYSIOLOGY   33
Introduction, 33
Cannabinoid Receptors, 39
The Endogenous Cannabinoid System, 43
Sites of Action, 48
Cannabinoid Receptors and Brain Functions, 51
Chronic Effects of THC, 56
Cannabinoids and the Immune System, 59
Conclusions and Recommendations, 69

**3   FIRST, DO NO HARM: CONSEQUENCES OF
      MARIJUANA USE AND ABUSE**   83
The Marijuana "High," 83
Drug Dynamics, 84

Marijuana Use and Dependence, 92
Link Between Medical Use and Drug Abuse, 101
Psychological Harms, 104
Physiological Harms: Tissue and Organ Damage, 109
Summary and Conclusions, 125

4   THE MEDICAL VALUE OF MARIJUANA AND
    RELATED SUBSTANCES   137
    Standards for Evaluating Clinical Trials, 138
    Analgesia, 139
    Nausea and Vomiting, 145
    Wasting Syndrome and Appetite Stimulation, 154
    Neurological Disorders, 159
    Glaucoma, 173
    Summary, 177
    Other Reports on Marijuana as Medicine, 180

5   DEVELOPMENT OF CANNABINOID DRUGS   193
    Federal Drug Development Policy, 194
    Development and Marketing of Marinol, 202
    Market Outlook for Cannabinoids, 208
    Regulation of and Market Outlook for Marijuana, 213
    Conclusions, 218

APPENDIXES
A   Individuals and Organizations That Spoke or Wrote to the
    Institute of Medicine About Marijuana and Medicine   225
B   Workshop Agendas   232
C   Scheduling Definitions   240
D   Statement of Task   242
E   Recommendations Made in Recent Reports on the
    Medical Use of Marijuana   244
F   Rescheduling Criteria   256

INDEX   259

List of Tables and Figures

TABLES

1.1 Self-Reported Disorders Treated with Marijuana by Members of San Francisco Cannabis Cultivators Club, 21

1.2 Self-Reported Disorders Treated with Marijuana by Members of Los Angeles Cannabis Resource Center (LACRC), According to Center Staff, 22

1.3 Summary of Reports to IOM Study Team by 43 Individuals, 23

1.4 Primary Symptoms of 43 Individuals Who Reported to IOM Study Team, 24

1.5 Cannabinoids Identified in Marijuana, 25

2.1 Landmark Discoveries Since the 1982 IOM Report, 34

2.2 Compounds That Bind to Cannabinoid Receptors, 44

2.3 Comparison of Cannabinoid Receptor Agonists, 46

2.4 Cellular Processes That Can Be Targeted for Drug Development, 48

2.5 Brain Regions in Which Cannabinoid Receptors Are Abundant, 49

2.6 Cannabinoid Receptors, 51

2.7 Effects of Cannabinoids on the Immune System, 60

2.8 Historical Comparisons Between Cannabinoids and Opiates, 69

3.1 Psychoactive Doses of THC in Humans, 85

3.2 Drug Withdrawal Symptoms, 90

3.3 Factors That Are Correlated with Drug Dependence, 94

xv

3.4   Prevalence of Drug Use and Dependence in the General Population, 95

3.5   Relative Prevalence of Diagnoses of Psychiatric Disorders Associated with Drug Use Among Children, 96

3.6   Effect of Decriminalization on Marijuana Use in Emergency Room (ER) Cases, 103

4.1   Studies on the Effects of Marijuana and Cannabinoids in Multiple Sclerosis, 163

4.2   Classes of Antispasticity Drugs, 164

4.3   Drugs Used to Treat Movement Disorders, 168

4.4   Clinical Trials of Cannabidiol (CBD) in Epileptics, 171

4.5   Anticonvulsant Drugs for Various Types of Seizures, 172

4.6   Classes of Drugs Used to Treat Glaucoma, 176

5.1   Cannabinoids and Related Compounds Commonly Used in Research, 201

5.2   Cannabinoids Under Development for Human Use, 209

FIGURES

1.1   Cannabinoid biosynthesis, 26

2.1   Diagram of neuron with synapse, 38

2.2   Cannabinoid receptors, 40

2.3   Cannabinoid agonists trigger a series of reactions within cells, 41

2.4   Chemical structures of selected cannabinoid agonists, 45

2.5   Locations of brain regions in which cannabinoid receptors are abundant, 50

2.6   Diagrams showing motor regions of the brain, 52

3.1   Age distribution of marijuana users among the general population, 93

4.1   Emesis-stimulating pathways, 146

4.2   Effect of nabilone on multiple sclerosis symptoms, 162

5.1   Stages of clinical testing, 196

MARIJUANA
AND MEDICINE

Executive Summary

 Public opinion on the medical value of marijuana has been sharply divided. Some dismiss medical marijuana as a hoax that exploits our natural compassion for the sick; others claim it is a uniquely soothing medicine that has been withheld from patients through regulations based on false claims. Proponents of both views cite "scientific evidence" to support their views and have expressed those views at the ballot box in recent state elections. In January 1997, the White House Office of National Drug Control Policy (ONDCP) asked the Institute of Medicine (IOM) to conduct a review of the scientific evidence to assess the potential health benefits and risks of marijuana and its constituent cannabinoids (see the Statement of Task on page 9). That review began in August 1997 and culminates with this report.

The ONDCP request came in the wake of state "medical marijuana" initiatives. In November 1996, voters in California and Arizona passed referenda designed to permit the use of marijuana as medicine. Although Arizona's referendum was invalidated five months later, the referenda galvanized a national response. In November 1998, voters in six states (Alaska, Arizona, Colorado, Nevada, Oregon, and Washington) passed ballot initiatives in support of medical marijuana. (The Colorado vote will not count, however, because after the vote was taken a court ruling determined there had not been enough valid signatures to place the initiative on the ballot.)

Can marijuana relieve health problems? Is it safe for medical use?

Those straightforward questions are embedded in a web of social concerns, most of which lie outside the scope of this report. Controversies concerning the nonmedical use of marijuana spill over into the medical marijuana debate and obscure the real state of scientific knowledge. In contrast with the many disagreements bearing on social issues, the study team found substantial consensus among experts in the relevant disciplines on the scientific evidence about potential medical uses of marijuana.

This report summarizes and analyzes what is known about the medical use of marijuana; it emphasizes evidence-based medicine (derived from knowledge and experience informed by rigorous scientific analysis), as opposed to belief-based medicine (derived from judgment, intuition, and beliefs untested by rigorous science).

Throughout this report, *marijuana* refers to unpurified plant substances, including leaves or flower tops whether consumed by ingestion or smoking. References to the "effects of marijuana" should be understood to include the composite effects of its various components; that is, the effects of tetrahydrocannabinol (THC), which is the primary psychoactive ingredient in marijuana, are included among its effects, but not all the effects of marijuana are necessarily due to THC. *Cannabinoids* are the group of compounds related to THC, whether found in the marijuana plant, in animals, or synthesized in chemistry laboratories.

Three focal concerns in evaluating the medical use of marijuana are:

1. Evaluation of the effects of isolated cannabinoids;
2. Evaluation of the risks associated with the medical use of marijuana; and
3. Evaluation of the use of smoked marijuana.

EFFECTS OF ISOLATED CANNABINOIDS

Cannabinoid Biology

Much has been learned since the 1982 IOM report *Marijuana and Health*. Although it was clear then that most of the effects of marijuana were due to its actions on the brain, there was little information about how THC acted on brain cells (neurons), which cells were affected by THC, or even what general areas of the brain were most affected by THC. In addition, too little was known about cannabinoid physiology to offer any scientific insights into the harmful or therapeutic effects of marijuana. That all changed with the identification and characterization of cannabinoid receptors in the 1980s and 1990s. During the past 16 years, science has advanced greatly and can tell us much more about the potential medical benefits of cannabinoids.

CONCLUSION: At this point, our knowledge about the biology of marijuana and cannabinoids allows us to make some general conclusions:

- Cannabinoids likely have a natural role in pain modulation, control of movement, and memory.
- The natural role of cannabinoids in immune systems is likely multi-faceted and remains unclear.
- The brain develops tolerance to cannabinoids.
- Animal research demonstrates the potential for dependence, but this potential is observed under a narrower range of conditions than with benzodiazepines, opiates, cocaine, or nicotine.
- Withdrawal symptoms can be observed in animals but appear to be mild compared to opiates or benzodiazepines, such as diazepam (Valium).

CONCLUSION: The different cannabinoid receptor types found in the body appear to play different roles in normal human physiology. In addition, some effects of cannabinoids appear to be independent of those receptors. The variety of mechanisms through which cannabinoids can influence human physiology underlies the variety of potential therapeutic uses for drugs that might act selectively on different cannabinoid systems.

RECOMMENDATION 1: **Research should continue into the physiological effects of synthetic and plant-derived cannabinoids and the natural function of cannabinoids found in the body. Because different cannabinoids appear to have different effects, cannabinoid research should include, but not be restricted to, effects attributable to THC alone.**

Efficacy of Cannabinoid Drugs

The accumulated data indicate a potential therapeutic value for cannabinoid drugs, particularly for symptoms such as pain relief, control of nausea and vomiting, and appetite stimulation. The therapeutic effects of cannabinoids are best established for THC, which is generally one of the two most abundant of the cannabinoids in marijuana. (Cannabidiol is generally the other most abundant cannabinoid.)

The effects of cannabinoids on the symptoms studied are generally modest, and in most cases there are more effective medications. However, people vary in their responses to medications, and there will likely always be a subpopulation of patients who do not respond well to other medications. The combination of cannabinoid drug effects (anxiety reduction, appetite stimulation, nausea reduction, and pain relief) suggests that cannabinoids would be moderately well suited for particular conditions, such as chemotherapy-induced nausea and vomiting and AIDS wasting.

Defined substances, such as purified cannabinoid compounds, are preferable to plant products, which are of variable and uncertain composition. Use of defined cannabinoids permits a more precise evaluation of their effects, whether in combination or alone. Medications that can maximize the desired effects of cannabinoids and minimize the undesired effects can very likely be identified.

Although most scientists who study cannabinoids agree that the pathways to cannabinoid drug development are clearly marked, there is no guarantee that the fruits of scientific research will be made available to the public for medical use. Cannabinoid-based drugs will only become available if public investment in cannabinoid drug research is sustained and if there is enough incentive for private enterprise to develop and market such drugs.

CONCLUSION: Scientific data indicate the potential therapeutic value of cannabinoid drugs, primarily THC, for pain relief, control of nausea and vomiting, and appetite stimulation; smoked marijuana, however, is a crude THC delivery system that also delivers harmful substances.

RECOMMENDATION 2: **Clinical trials of cannabinoid drugs for symptom management should be conducted with the goal of developing rapid-onset, reliable, and safe delivery systems.**

Influence of Psychological Effects on Therapeutic Effects

The psychological effects of THC and similar cannabinoids pose three issues for the therapeutic use of cannabinoid drugs. First, for some patients—particularly older patients with no previous marijuana experience—the psychological effects are disturbing. Those patients report experiencing unpleasant feelings and disorientation after being treated with THC, generally more severe for oral THC than for smoked marijuana. Second, for conditions such as movement disorders or nausea, in which anxiety exacerbates the symptoms, the antianxiety effects of cannabinoid drugs can influence symptoms indirectly. This can be beneficial or can create false impressions of the drug effect. Third, for cases in which symptoms are multifaceted, the combination of THC effects might provide a form of adjunctive therapy; for example, AIDS wasting patients would likely benefit from a medication that simultaneously reduces anxiety, pain, and nausea while stimulating appetite.

CONCLUSION: The psychological effects of cannabinoids, such as anxiety reduction, sedation, and euphoria can influence their potential therapeutic value. Those effects are potentially undesirable for certain patients and situations and beneficial for others. In addition, psychological effects can complicate the interpretation of other aspects of the drug's effect.

RECOMMENDATION 3: **Psychological effects of cannabinoids such as anxiety reduction and sedation, which can influence medical benefits, should be evaluated in clinical trials.**

RISKS ASSOCIATED WITH MEDICAL USE OF MARIJUANA

Physiological Risks

Marijuana is not a completely benign substance. It is a powerful drug with a variety of effects. However, except for the harms associated with smoking, the adverse effects of marijuana use are within the range of effects tolerated for other medications. The harmful effects to individuals from the perspective of possible medical use of marijuana are not necessarily the same as the harmful physical effects of drug abuse. When interpreting studies purporting to show the harmful effects of marijuana, it is important to keep in mind that the majority of those studies are based on *smoked* marijuana, and cannabinoid effects cannot be separated from the effects of inhaling smoke from burning plant material and contaminants.

For most people the primary adverse effect of *acute* marijuana use is diminished psychomotor performance. It is, therefore, inadvisable to operate any vehicle or potentially dangerous equipment while under the influence of marijuana, THC, or any cannabinoid drug with comparable effects. In addition, a minority of marijuana users experience dysphoria, or unpleasant feelings. Finally, the short-term immunosuppressive effects are not well established but, if they exist, are not likely great enough to preclude a legitimate medical use.

The *chronic* effects of marijuana are of greater concern for medical use and fall into two categories: the effects of chronic smoking and the effects of THC. Marijuana smoking is associated with abnormalities of cells lining the human respiratory tract. Marijuana smoke, like tobacco smoke, is associated with increased risk of cancer, lung damage, and poor pregnancy outcomes. Although cellular, genetic, and human studies all suggest that marijuana smoke is an important risk factor for the development of respiratory cancer, proof that habitual marijuana smoking does or does not cause cancer awaits the results of well-designed studies.

CONCLUSION: Numerous studies suggest that marijuana smoke is an important risk factor in the development of respiratory disease.

RECOMMENDATION 4: **Studies to define the individual health risks of smoking marijuana should be conducted, particularly among populations in which marijuana use is prevalent.**

Marijuana Dependence and Withdrawal

A second concern associated with chronic marijuana use is dependence on the psychoactive effects of THC. Although few marijuana users develop dependence, some do. Risk factors for marijuana dependence are similar to those for other forms of substance abuse. In particular, antisocial personality and conduct disorders are closely associated with substance abuse.

CONCLUSION: A distinctive marijuana withdrawal syndrome has been identified, but it is mild and short lived. The syndrome includes restlessness, irritability, mild agitation, insomnia, sleep disturbance, nausea, and cramping.

Marijuana as a "Gateway" Drug

Patterns in progression of drug use from adolescence to adulthood are strikingly regular. Because it is the most widely used illicit drug, marijuana is predictably the first illicit drug most people encounter. Not surprisingly, most users of other illicit drugs have used marijuana first. In fact, most drug users begin with alcohol and nicotine before marijuana— usually before they are of legal age.

In the sense that marijuana use typically precedes rather than follows initiation of other illicit drug use, it is indeed a "gateway" drug. But because underage smoking and alcohol use typically precede marijuana use, marijuana is not the most common, and is rarely the first, "gateway" to illicit drug use. There is no conclusive evidence that the drug effects of marijuana are causally linked to the subsequent abuse of other illicit drugs. An important caution is that data on drug use progression cannot be assumed to apply to the use of drugs for medical purposes. It does not follow from those data that if marijuana were available by prescription for medical use, the pattern of drug use would remain the same as seen in illicit use.

Finally, there is a broad social concern that sanctioning the medical use of marijuana might increase its use among the general population. At this point there are no convincing data to support this concern. The existing data are consistent with the idea that this would not be a problem if the medical use of marijuana were as closely regulated as other medications with abuse potential.

CONCLUSION: Present data on drug use progression neither support nor refute the suggestion that medical availability would increase drug abuse. However, this question is beyond the issues normally considered for medical uses of drugs and should not be a factor in evaluating the therapeutic potential of marijuana or cannabinoids.

USE OF SMOKED MARIJUANA

Because of the health risks associated with smoking, smoked marijuana should generally not be recommended for long-term medical use. Nonetheless, for certain patients, such as the terminally ill or those with debilitating symptoms, the long-term risks are not of great concern. Further, despite the legal, social, and health problems associated with smoking marijuana, it is widely used by certain patient groups.

RECOMMENDATION 5: Clinical trials of marijuana use for medical purposes should be conducted under the following limited circumstances: trials should involve only short-term marijuana use (less than six months), should be conducted in patients with conditions for which there is reasonable expectation of efficacy, should be approved by institutional review boards, and should collect data about efficacy.

The goal of clinical trials of smoked marijuana would not be to develop marijuana as a licensed drug but rather to serve as a first step toward the possible development of nonsmoked rapid-onset cannabinoid delivery systems. However, it will likely be many years before a safe and effective cannabinoid delivery system, such as an inhaler, is available for patients. In the meantime there are patients with debilitating symptoms for whom smoked marijuana might provide relief. The use of smoked marijuana for those patients should weigh both the expected efficacy of marijuana and ethical issues in patient care, including providing information about the known and suspected risks of smoked marijuana use.

RECOMMENDATION 6: Short-term use of smoked marijuana (less than six months) for patients with debilitating symptoms (such as intractable pain or vomiting) must meet the following conditions:

- failure of all approved medications to provide relief has been documented,
- the symptoms can reasonably be expected to be relieved by rapid-onset cannabinoid drugs,
- such treatment is administered under medical supervision in a manner that allows for assessment of treatment effectiveness, and
- involves an oversight strategy comparable to an institutional review board process that could provide guidance within 24 hours of a submission by a physician to provide marijuana to a patient for a specified use.

Until a nonsmoked rapid-onset cannabinoid drug delivery system becomes available, we acknowledge that there is no clear alternative for people suffering from *chronic* conditions that might be relieved by smoking marijuana, such as pain or AIDS wasting. One possible approach is to treat patients as *n*-of-1 clinical trials (single-patient trials), in which patients are fully informed of their status as experimental subjects using a harmful drug delivery system and in which their condition is closely monitored and documented under medical supervision, thereby increasing the knowledge base of the risks and benefits of marijuana use under such conditions.

STATEMENT OF TASK

The study will assess what is currently known and not known about the medical use of marijuana. It will include a review of the science base regarding the mechanism of action of marijuana, an examination of the peer-reviewed scientific literature on the efficacy of therapeutic uses of marijuana, and the costs of using various forms of marijuana versus approved drugs for specific medical conditions (e.g., glaucoma, multiple sclerosis, wasting diseases, nausea, and pain).

The study will also include an evaluation of the acute and chronic effects of marijuana on health and behavior; a consideration of the adverse effects of marijuana use compared with approved drugs; an evaluation of the efficacy of different delivery systems for marijuana (e.g., inhalation vs. oral); an analysis of the data concerning marijuana as a gateway drug; and an examination of the possible differences in the effects of marijuana due to age and type of medical condition.

Specific Issues

Specific issues to be addressed fall under three broad categories: science base, therapeutic use, and economics.

Science Base

- Review of the neuroscience related to marijuana, particularly the relevance of new studies on addiction and craving
- Review of the behavioral and social science base of marijuana use, particularly an assessment of the relative risk of progression to other drugs following marijuana use
- Review of the literature determining which chemical components of crude marijuana are responsible for possible therapeutic effects and for side effects

Therapeutic Use

- Evaluation of any conclusions on the medical use of marijuana drawn by other groups
- Efficacy and side effects of various delivery systems for marijuana compared to existing medications for glaucoma, wasting syndrome, pain, nausea, or other symptoms
- Differential effects of various forms of marijuana that relate to age or type of disease

Economics

- Costs of various forms of marijuana compared with costs of existing medications for glaucoma, wasting syndrome, pain, nausea, or other symptoms
- Assessment of differences between marijuana and existing medications in terms of access and availability

RECOMMENDATIONS

RECOMMENDATION 1: **Research should continue into the physiological effects of synthetic and plant-derived cannabinoids and the natural function of cannabinoids found in the body. Because different cannabinoids appear to have different effects, cannabinoid research should include, but not be restricted to, effects attributable to THC alone.**

Scientific data indicate the potential therapeutic value of cannabinoid drugs for pain relief, control of nausea and vomiting, and appetite stimulation. This value would be enhanced by a rapid onset of drug effect.

RECOMMENDATION 2: **Clinical trials of cannabinoid drugs for symptom management should be conducted with the goal of developing rapid-onset, reliable, and safe delivery systems.**

The psychological effects of cannabinoids are probably important determinants of their potential therapeutic value. They can influence symptoms indirectly which could create false impressions of the drug effect or be beneficial as a form of adjunctive therapy.

RECOMMENDATION 3: **Psychological effects of cannabinoids such as anxiety reduction and sedation, which can influence medical benefits, should be evaluated in clinical trials.**

Numerous studies suggest that marijuana smoke is an important risk factor in the development of respiratory diseases, but the data that could conclusively establish or refute this suspected link have not been collected.

RECOMMENDATION 4: **Studies to define the individual health risks of smoking marijuana should be conducted, particularly among populations in which marijuana use is prevalent.**

Because marijuana is a crude THC delivery system that also delivers harmful substances, smoked marijuana should generally not be recommended for medical use. Nonetheless, marijuana is widely used by certain patient groups, which raises both safety and efficacy issues.

RECOMMENDATION 5: Clinical trials of marijuana use for medical purposes should be conducted under the following limited circumstances: trials should involve only short-term marijuana use (less than six months), should be conducted in patients with conditions for which there is reasonable expectation of efficacy, should be approved by institutional review boards, and should collect data about efficacy.

If there is any future for marijuana as a medicine, it lies in its isolated components, the cannabinoids and their synthetic derivatives. Isolated cannabinoids will provide more reliable effects than crude plant mixtures. Therefore, the purpose of clinical trials of smoked marijuana would not be to develop marijuana as a licensed drug but rather to serve as a first step toward the development of nonsmoked rapid-onset cannabinoid delivery systems.

RECOMMENDATION 6: Short-term use of smoked marijuana (less than six months) for patients with debilitating symptoms (such as intractable pain or vomiting) must meet the following conditions:

- **failure of all approved medications to provide relief has been documented,**
- **the symptoms can reasonably be expected to be relieved by rapid-onset cannabinoid drugs,**
- **such treatment is administered under medical supervision in a manner that allows for assessment of treatment effectiveness, and**
- **involves an oversight strategy comparable to an institutional review board process that could provide guidance within 24 hours of a submission by a physician to provide marijuana to a patient for a specified use.**

1

Introduction

 This report summarizes and analyzes what is known about the medical use of marijuana; it emphasizes evidence-based medicine (derived from knowledge and experience informed by rigorous scientific analysis), as opposed to belief-based medicine (derived from judgment, intuition, and beliefs untested by rigorous science). Scientific data on controversial subjects are commonly misinterpreted, overinterpreted, and misrepresented, and the medical marijuana debate is no exception. We have tried to present the scientific studies in such a way as to reveal their strengths and limitations. One of the goals of this report is to help people to understand the scientific data, including the logic behind the scientific conclusions, so it goes into greater detail than previous reports on the subject. In many cases, we have explained why particular studies are inconclusive and what sort of evidence is needed to support particular claims about the harms or benefits attributed to marijuana. Ideally, this report will enable the thoughtful reader to interpret new information about marijuana that will continue to emerge rapidly well after this report is published.

Can marijuana relieve health problems? Is it safe for medical use? Those straightforward questions are embedded in a web of social concerns, which lie outside the scope of this report. Controversies concerning nonmedical use of marijuana spill over onto the medical marijuana debate and tend to obscure the real state of scientific knowledge. In contrast with the many disagreements bearing on the social issues, the study team found substantial consensus, among experts in the relevant disciplines, on the scientific evidence bearing on potential medical use. This report analyzes science, not the law. As in any policy debate, the value of scientific analysis is that it can provide a foundation for further discussion. Distilling scientific evidence does not in itself solve a policy problem. What it can do is illuminate the common ground, bringing to light fundamental differences out of the shadows of misunderstanding and misinformation that currently prevail. Scientific analysis cannot be the end of the debate, but it should at least provide the basis for an honest and informed discussion.

Our analysis of the evidence and arguments concerning the medical use of marijuana focuses on the strength of the supporting evidence and does not refer to the motivations of people who put forth the evidence and arguments. That is, it is not relevant to scientific validity whether an argument is put forth by someone who believes that all marijuana use should be legal or by someone who believes that any marijuana use is highly damaging to individual users and to society as a whole. Nor does this report comment on the degree to which scientific analysis is compatible with current regulatory policy. Although many have argued that current drug laws pertaining to marijuana are inconsistent with scientific data, it is important to understand that decisions about drug regulation are based on a variety of moral and social considerations, as well as on medical and scientific ones.

Even when a drug is used only for medical purposes, value judgments affect policy decisions concerning its medical use. For example, the magnitude of a drug's expected medical benefit affects regulatory judgments about the acceptability of risks associated with its use. Also, although a drug is normally approved for medical use only on proof of its "safety and efficacy," patients with life-threatening conditions are sometimes (under protocols for "compassionate use") allowed access to unapproved drugs whose benefits and risks are uncertain. Value judgments play an even more substantial role in regulatory decisions concerning drugs, such as marijuana, that are sought and used for nonmedical purposes. Then policymakers must take into account not only the risks and benefits associated with medical use but also possible interactions between the regulatory arrangements governing medical use and the integrity of the legal controls set up to restrict nonmedical use.

It should be clear that many elements of drug control policy lie outside the realm of biology and medicine. Ultimately, the complex moral and social judgments that underlie drug control policy must be made by the American people and their elected officials. A goal of this report is to evaluate the biological and medical factors that should be taken into account in making those judgments.

HOW THIS STUDY WAS CONDUCTED

Information was gathered through scientific workshops, site visits, analysis of the relevant scientific literature, and extensive consultation with biomedical and social scientists. The three 2-day workshops—in Irvine, California; New Orleans, Louisiana; and Washington, D.C.—were open to the public and included scientific presentations and reports, mostly from patients and their families, about their experiences with and perspectives on the medical use of marijuana. Scientific experts in various fields were selected to talk about the latest research on marijuana, cannabinoids, and related topics (listed in Appendix B). Selection of the experts was based on recommendations by their peers, who ranked them among the most accomplished scientists and the most knowledgeable about marijuana and cannabinoids in their own fields. In addition, advocates for (John Morgan) and against (Eric A. Voth) the medical use of marijuana were invited to present scientific evidence in support of their positions.

Information presented at the scientific workshops was supplemented by analysis of the scientific literature and evaluating the methods used in various studies and the validity of the authors' conclusions. Different kinds of clinical studies are useful in different ways: results of a controlled double-blind study with adequate sample sizes can be expected to apply to the general population from which study subjects were drawn; an isolated case report can suggest further studies but cannot be presumed to be broadly applicable; and survey data can be highly informative but are generally limited by the need to rely on self-reports of drug use and on unconfirmed medical diagnoses. This report relies mainly on the most relevant and methodologically rigorous studies available and treats the results of more limited studies cautiously. In addition, study results are presented in such a way as to allow thoughtful readers to judge the results themselves.

The Institute of Medicine (IOM) appointed a panel of nine experts to advise the study team on technical issues. These included neurology and the treatment of pain (Howard Fields); regulation of prescription drugs (J. Richard Crout); AIDS wasting and clinical trials (Judith Feinberg); treatment and pathology of multiple sclerosis (Timothy Vollmer); drug dependence among adolescents (Thomas Crowley); varieties of drug dependence (Dorothy Hatsukami); internal medicine, health care delivery, and clinical epidemiology (Eric B. Larson); cannabinoids and marijuana pharmacology (Billy R. Martin); and cannabinoid neuroscience (Steven R. Childers).

Public outreach included setting up a Web site that provided information about the study and asked for input from the public. The Web site was open for comment from November 1997 until November 1998. Some 130 organizations were invited to participate in the public workshops. Many people in the organizations—particularly those opposed to the medical use of marijuana—felt that a public forum was not conducive to expressing their views; they were invited to communicate their opinions (and reasons for holding them) by mail or telephone. As a result, roughly equal numbers of persons and organizations opposed to and in favor of the medical use of marijuana were heard from.

The study team visited four cannabis buyers' clubs in California (the Oakland Cannabis Buyers' Cooperative, the San Francisco Cannabis Cultivators Club, the Los Angeles Cannabis Resource Center, and Californians Helping Alleviate Medical Problems, or CHAMPS) and two HIV/AIDS clinics (AIDS Health Care Foundation in Los Angeles and Louisiana State University Medical Center in New Orleans). We listened to many individual stories from the buyers' clubs about using marijuana to treat a variety of symptoms and heard clinical observations on the use of Marinol to treat AIDS patients. Marinol is the brand name for dronabinol, which is Δ^9-tetrahydrocannabinol (THC) in pill form and is available by prescription for the treatment of nausea associated with chemotherapy and AIDS wasting.

MARIJUANA TODAY

The Changing Legal Landscape

In the 20th century, marijuana has been used more for its euphoric effects than as a medicine. Its psychological and behavioral effects have concerned public officials since the drug first appeared in the southwestern and southern states during the first two decades of the century. By 1931, at least 29 states had prohibited use of the drug for nonmedical purposes.[3] Marijuana was first regulated at the federal level by the Marijuana Tax Act of 1937, which required anyone producing, distributing, or using marijuana for medical purposes to register and pay a tax and which effectively prohibited nonmedical use of the drug. Although the act did not make medical use of marijuana illegal, it did make it expensive and inconvenient. In 1942, marijuana was removed from the U.S. Pharmacopoeia because it was believed to be a harmful and addictive drug that caused psychoses, mental deterioration, and violent behavior.

In the late 1960s and early 1970s, there was a sharp increase in marijuana use among adolescents and young adults. The current legal status of marijuana was established in 1970 with the passage of the Controlled

Medical Marijuana Legislation Among the States

The 1996 California referendum known as Proposition 215 allowed seriously ill Californians to obtain and use marijuana for medical purposes without criminal prosecution or sanction. A physician's recommendation is needed. Under the law, physicians cannot be punished or denied any right or privilege for recommending marijuana to patients who suffer from any illness for which marijuana will provide relief.

The 1996 Arizona referendum known as Proposition 200 was largely about prison reform but also gave physicians the option to prescribe controlled substances, including those in Schedule I (e.g., marijuana), to treat the disease or relieve the suffering of seriously or terminally ill patients. Five months after the referendum was passed, it was stalled whenArizona legislators voted that all prescription medications must be approved by the Food and Drug Administration, and marijuana is not so approved. In November 1998, Arizona voters passed a second referendum designed to allow physician's to prescribe marijuana as medicine, but this is still at odds with federal law.[8]

As of summer 1998, eight states—California, Connecticut, Louisiana, New Hampshire, Ohio, Vermont, Virginia, and Wisconsin—had laws that permit physicians to prescribe marijuana for medical purposes or to allow a medical necessity defense.[8] In November 1998, five states—Arizona, Alaska, Oregon, Nevada, and Washington—passed medical marijuana ballot initiatives. The District of Columbia also voted on a medical marijuana initiative, but was barred from counting the votes because an amendment designed to prohibit them from doing so was added to the federal appropriations bill; however, exit polls suggested that a majority of voters had approved the measure.

Substances Act, which divided drugs into five schedules and placed marijuana in Schedule I, the category for drugs with high potential for abuse and no accepted medical use (see Appendix C, Scheduling Definitions). In 1972, the National Organization for the Reform of Marijuana Legislation (NORML), an organization that supports decriminalization of marijuana, unsuccessfully petitioned the Bureau of Narcotics and Dangerous Drugs to move marijuana from Schedule I to Schedule II. NORML argued that marijuana is therapeutic in numerous serious ailments, less toxic, and in many cases more effective than conventional medicines.[13] Thus, for 25 years the medical marijuana movement has been closely linked with the marijuana decriminalization movement, which has colored the debate. Many people criticized that association in their letters to IOM and during the public workshops of this study. The argument against the medical use of marijuana presented most often to the IOM study team was that "the medical marijuana movement is a Trojan horse"; that is, it is a deceptive tactic used by advocates of marijuana decriminalization who would exploit the public's sympathy for seriously ill patients.

Since NORML's petition in 1972, there have been a variety of legal decisions concerning marijuana. From 1973 to 1978, 11 states adopted statutes that decriminalized use of marijuana, although some of them recriminalized marijuana use in the 1980s and 1990s. During the 1970s, reports of the medical value of marijuana began to appear, particularly claims that marijuana relieved the nausea associated with chemotherapy. Health departments in six states conducted small studies to investigate the reports. When the AIDS epidemic spread in the 1980s, patients found that marijuana sometimes relieved their symptoms, most dramatically those associated with AIDS wasting. Over this period a number of defendants charged with unlawful possession of marijuana claimed that they were using the drug to treat medical conditions and that violation of the law was therefore justified (the so-called medical necessity defense). Although most courts rejected these claims, some accepted them.[8]

Against that backdrop, voters in California and Arizona in 1996 passed two referenda that attempted to legalize the medical use of marijuana under particular conditions. Public support for patient access to marijuana for medical use appears substantial; public opinion polls taken during 1997 and 1998 generally reported 60–70 percent of respondents in favor of allowing medical uses of marijuana.[15] However, those referenda are at odds with federal laws regulating marijuana, and their implementation raises complex legal questions.

Despite the current level of interest, referenda and public discussions have not been well informed by carefully reasoned scientific debate. Although previous reports have all called for more research, the nature of the research that will be most helpful depends greatly on the specific health conditions to be addressed. And while there have been important recent advances in our understanding of the physiological effects of marijuana, few of the recent investigators have had the time or resources to permit detailed analysis. The results of those advances, only now beginning to be explored, have significant implications for the medical marijuana debate.

Several months after the passage of the California and Arizona medical marijuana referendums, the Office of National Drug Control Policy (ONDCP) asked whether IOM would conduct a scientific review of the medical value of marijuana and its constituent compounds. In August 1997, IOM formally began the study and appointed John A. Benson Jr. and Stanley J. Watson Jr. to serve as principal investigators for the study.

The charge to IOM was to review the medical use of marijuana and the harms and benefits attributed to it (details are given in Appendix D).

MARIJUANA AND MEDICINE

Marijuana plants have been used since antiquity for both herbal medication and intoxication. The current debate over the medical use of marijuana is essentially a debate over the value of its medicinal properties relative to the risk posed by its use.

Marijuana's use as an herbal remedy before the 20th century is well documented.[1,10,11] However, modern medicine adheres to different standards from those used in the past. The question is not whether marijuana can be used as an herbal remedy but rather how well this remedy meets today's standards of efficacy and safety. We understand much more than previous generations about medical risks. Our society generally expects its licensed medications to be safe, reliable, and of proven efficacy; contaminants and inconsistent ingredients in our health treatments are not tolerated. That refers not only to prescription and over-the-counter drugs but also to vitamin supplements and herbal remedies purchased at the grocery store. For example, the essential amino acid *l*-tryptophan was widely sold in health food stores as a natural remedy for insomnia until early 1990 when it became linked to an epidemic of a new and potentially fatal illness (eosinophilia-myalgia syndrome).[9,12] When it was removed from the market shortly thereafter, there was little protest, despite the fact that it was safe for the vast majority of the population. The 1,536 cases and 27 deaths were later traced to contaminants in a batch produced by a single Japanese manufacturer.

Although few herbal medicines meet today's standards, they have provided the foundation for modern Western pharmaceuticals. Most current prescriptions have their roots either directly or indirectly in plant remedies.[7] At the same time, most current prescriptions are synthetic compounds that are only distantly related to the natural compounds that led to their development. Digitalis was discovered in foxglove, morphine in poppies, and taxol in the yew tree. Even aspirin (acetylsalicylic acid) has its counterpart in herbal medicine: for many generations, American Indians relieved headaches by chewing the bark of the willow tree, which is rich in a related form of salicylic acid.

Although plants continue to be valuable resources for medical advances, drug development is likely to be less and less reliant on plants and more reliant on the tools of modern science. Molecular biology, bioinformatics software, and DNA array-based analyses of genes and chemistry are all beginning to yield great advances in drug discovery and development. Until recently, drugs could only be *discovered*; now they can be *designed*. Even the discovery process has been accelerated through the use of modern drug-screening techniques. It is increasingly possible to identify or isolate the chemical compounds in a plant, determine which compounds are responsible for the plant's effects, and select the most effective and safe compounds—either for use as purified substances or as tools to develop even more effective, safer, or less expensive compounds.

Yet even as the modern pharmacological toolbox becomes more sophisticated and biotechnology yields an ever greater abundance of therapeutic drugs, people increasingly seek alternative, low-technology therapies.[4,5] In 1997, 46 percent of Americans sought nontraditional medicines and spent over 27 billion unreimbursed dollars; the total number of visits to alternative medicine practitioners appears to have exceeded the number of visits to primary care physicians.[5,6] Recent interest in the medical use of marijuana coincides with this trend toward self-help and a search for "natural" therapies. Indeed, several people who spoke at the IOM public hearings in support of the medical use of marijuana said that they generally preferred herbal medicines to standard pharmaceuticals. However, few alternative therapies have been carefully and systematically tested for safety and efficacy, as is required for medications approved by the FDA (Food and Drug Administration).[2]

WHO USES MEDICAL MARIJUANA?

There have been no comprehensive surveys of the demographics and medical conditions of medical marijuana users, but a few reports provide some indication. In each case, survey results should be understood to reflect the situation in which they were conducted and are not necessarily characteristic of medical marijuana users as a whole. Respondents to surveys reported to the IOM study team were all members of "buyers' clubs," organizations that provide their members with marijuana, although not necessarily through direct cash transactions. The atmosphere of the marijuana buyers' clubs ranges from that of the comparatively formal and closely regulated Oakland Cannabis Buyers' Cooperative to that of a "country club for the indigent," as Denis Peron described the San Francisco Cannabis Cultivators Club (SFCCC), which he directed.

John Mendelson, an internist and pharmacologist at the University of California, San Francisco (UCSF) Pain Management Center, surveyed 100 members of the SFCCC who were using marijuana at least weekly. Most of the respondents were unemployed men in their forties. Subjects were paid $50 to participate in the survey; this might have encouraged a greater representation of unemployed subjects. All subjects were tested for drug use. About half tested positive for marijuana only; the other half tested positive for drugs in addition to marijuana (23% for cocaine and 13% for

TABLE 1.1 Self-Reported Disorders Treated with Marijuana by Members of San Francisco Cannabis Cultivators Club

Disorder	No. of Subjects
HIV	60
Musculoskeletal disorders and arthritis	39
Psychiatric disorders (primarily depression)	27
Neurological disorders and nonmusculoskeletal pain syndromes	9
Gastrointestinal disorders (most often nausea)	7
Other disorders	
Glaucoma, allergies, nephrolithiasis, and the skin manifestations of Reiter syndrome	7
Total disorders	149
Total number of respondents	100

amphetamines). The predominant disorder was AIDS, followed by roughly equal numbers of members who reported chronic pain, mood disorders, and musculoskeletal disorders (Table 1.1).

The membership profile of the San Francisco club was similar to that of the Los Angeles Cannabis Resource Center (LACRC), where 83% of the 739 patients were men, 45% were 36–45 years old, and 71% were HIV positive. Table 1.2 shows a distribution of conditions somewhat different from that in SFCCC respondents, probably because of a different membership profile. For example, cancer is generally a disease that occurs late in life; 34 (4.7%) of LACRC members were over 55 years old; only 2% of survey respondents in the SFCCC study were over 55 years old.

Jeffrey Jones, executive director of the Oakland Cannabis Buyers' Cooperative, reported that its largest group of patients is HIV-positive men in their forties. The second-largest group is patients with chronic pain.

Among the 42 people who spoke at the public workshops or wrote to the study team, only six identified themselves as members of marijuana buyers' clubs. Nonetheless, they presented a similar profile: HIV/AIDS was the predominant disorder, followed by chronic pain (Tables 1.3 and 1.4). All HIV/AIDS patients reported that marijuana relieved nausea and vomiting and improved their appetite. About half the patients who reported using marijuana for chronic pain also reported that it reduced nausea and vomiting.

Note that the medical conditions referred to are only those reported to the study team or to interviewers; they cannot be assumed to represent complete or accurate diagnoses. Michael Rowbotham, a neurologist at the UCSF Pain Management Center, noted that many pain patients referred

TABLE 1.2 Self-Reported Disorders Treated with Marijuana by Members of Los Angeles Cannabis Resource Center (LACRC), According to Center Staff[a]

Treated Disorder	No. of Subjects	% of Subjects
HIV[b]	528	71
Cancer	40	5.4
Terminal cancer	10	1.4
Mood disorders (depression)	4	0.5
Musculoskeletal (multiple sclerosis, arthritis)	30	4.1
Chronic pain and back pain	33	4.5
Gastrointestinal	7	2.3
Neurological disorders (epilepsy, Tourette syndrome, brain trauma)	7	0.9
Seizures or migraines[c]	13	1.8
Glaucoma	15	2.0
Miscellaneous	42	5.7
Total number	739	100

[a]Results are based on a review of 739 individual records by LACRC staff members. In contrast with Mendelson's survey of San Francisco Cannabis Cultivators Club (Table 1.1), only the primary disorder is indicated here. Membership in LACRC is contingent on a doctor's letter of acknowledgment, but diagnoses are not independently confirmed.

[b]HIV patients use marijuana to control nausea, increase appetite (to combat wasting), and relieve gastrointestinal distress caused by AIDS medications. These uses are not indicated separately.

[c]As described by LACRC staff, some of these cases might also be neurological disorders.

to that center arrive with incorrect diagnoses or with pain of unknown origin. At that center the patients who report medical benefit from marijuana say that it does not reduce their pain but enables them to cope with it.

Most—not all—people who use marijuana to relieve medical conditions have previously used it recreationally. An estimated 95% of the LACRC members had used marijuana before joining the club. It is important to emphasize the absence of comprehensive information on marijuana use before its use for medical conditions. Frequency of prior use almost certainly depends on many factors, including membership in a buyers' club, membership in a population sector that uses marijuana more often than others (for example, men 20–30 years old), and the medical condition being treated with marijuana (for example, there are probably relatively fewer recreational marijuana users among cancer patients than among AIDS patients).

TABLE 1.3 Summary of Reports to IOM Study Team by 43 Individuals

Symptoms	Dominant Disease	Symptoms	Dominant Disease
Anorexia, nausea, vomiting	AIDS	Pain	Migraine
	AIDS		Injury
	AIDS		Injury
	AIDS		Epilepsy and postpolio syndrome
	AIDS		Trauma and epilepsy
	AIDS		Degenerative disk disease
	AIDS		Rheumatoid arthritis
	AIDS and cancer		Nail-patella syndrome
	Cancer		Reflex sympathetic dystrophy
	Testicular cancer		Gulf War chemical exposure
	Cancer and multiple sclerosis		Multiple congenital cartilaginous exostosis
	Thyroid condition[a]		Histiocytosis X
	Migraine		
	Wilson's disease	Muscle spasticity	Spasticity[a]
Mood disorders	Depression		Multiple sclerosis
	Depression		Multiple sclerosis
	Depression and anxiety		Multiple sclerosis
	Depression and anxiety		Paralysis
	Manic depression		Spinal-cord injury
			Spasmodic torticollis
	Manic depression	Intraocular pressure	Glaucoma
	Posttraumatic stress		
	Premenstrual syndrome		
		Diarrhea	Crohn's disease

[a]Not specified.

NOTE: This table lists the people who reported to the IOM study team during the public workshops, or through letters, that they use marijuana as medicine; it should not be interpreted as a representative sample of the full spectrum of people who use marijuana as medicine. Each dominant disease represents an individual report.

Patients who reported their experience with marijuana at the public workshops said that marijuana provided them with great relief from symptoms associated with disparate diseases and ailments, including AIDS wasting, spasticity from multiple sclerosis, depression, chronic pain, and nausea associated with chemotherapy. Their circumstances and symptoms were varied, and the IOM study team was not in a position to make medical evaluations or confirm diagnoses. Three representative cases presented to the IOM study team are presented in Box 1.1; the stories have been edited for brevity, but each case is presented in the patient's words and with the patient's permission.

TABLE 1.4 Primary Symptoms of 43 Individuals Who Reported to IOM Study Team

	Symptom Frequency		Multiple Symptoms	
Primary Symptom	No. of Reports[a]	% of Total Symptoms Reported	No. Who Reported (primary) Additional Symptoms	% of Those Who Reported Primary Symptoms
Anorexia, nausea, vomiting	21	31	13	62
Diarrhea	4	6	3	75
Intraocular pressure	2	3	1	50
Mood disorders	12	18	7	58
Muscle spasticity	12	18	7	58
Pain	16	24	13	81
Total	67		44	66

[a]Forty-three persons reporting; 20 reported relief from more than one symptom.

The variety of stories presented left the study team with a clear view of people's beliefs about how marijuana had helped them. But this collection of anecdotal data, although useful, is limited. We heard many positive stories but no stories from people who had tried marijuana but found it ineffective. This is a fraction with an unknown denominator. For the numerator we have a sample of positive responses; for the denominator we have no idea of the total number of people who have tried marijuana for medical purposes. Hence, it is impossible to estimate the clinical value of marijuana or cannabinoids in the general population based on anecdotal reports. Marijuana clearly seems to relieve some symptoms for some people—even if only as a placebo effect. But what is the balance of harmful and beneficial effects? That is the essential medical question that can be answered only by careful analysis of data collected under controlled conditions.

CANNABIS AND THE CANNABINOIDS

Marijuana is the common name for *Cannabis sativa*, a hemp plant that grows throughout temperate and tropical climates. The most recent review of the constituents of marijuana lists 66 cannabinoids (Table 1.5).[16] But that does not mean there are 66 different cannabinoid effects or interactions. Most of the cannabinoids are closely related; they fall into only 10

TABLE 1.5 Cannabinoids Identified in Marijuana

Cannabinoid Group	Common Abbreviation	No. of Known Variants in Each Group
Δ^9-Tetrahydrocannabinol	Δ^9-THC	9
Δ^8-Tetrahydrocannabinol	Δ^8-THC	2
Cannabichromene	CBC	5
Cannabicyclol	CBL	3
Cannabidiol	CBD	7
Cannabielsoin	CBE	5
Cannabigerol	CBG	6
Cannabinidiol	CBND	2
Cannabinol	CBN	7
Cannabitriol	CBT	9
Miscellaneous types		11
Total		66

groups of closely related cannabinoids, many of which differ by only a single chemical moiety and might be midpoints along biochemical pathways—that is, degradation products, precursors, or byproducts.[16,18] Δ^9-tetrahydrocannabinol (Δ^9-THC) is the primary psychoactive ingredient; depending on the particular plant, either THC or cannabidiol is the most abundant cannabinoid in marijuana (Figure 1.1). Throughout this report, THC is used to indicate Δ^9-THC. In the few cases where variants of THC are discussed, the full names are used. All the cannabinoids are lipophilic—they are highly soluble in fatty fluids and tissues but not in water. Indeed, THC is so lipophilic that it is aptly described as "greasy."

Throughout this report, *marijuana* refers to unpurified plant extracts, including leaves and flower tops, regardless of how they are consumed—whether by ingestion or by smoking. References to the effects of marijuana should be understood to include the composite effects of its various components; that is, the effects of THC are included among the effects of marijuana, but not all the effects of marijuana are necessarily due to THC. Discussions concerning *cannabinoids* refer only to those particular compounds and not to the plant extract. This distinction is important; it is often blurred or exaggerated.

Cannabinoids are produced in epidermal glands on the leaves (especially the upper ones), stems, and the bracts that support the flowers of the marijuana plant. Although the flower itself has no epidermal glands, it has the highest cannabinoid content anywhere on the plant, probably because of the accumulation of resin secreted by the supporting bracteole

FIGURE 1.1 Cannabinoid biosynthesis. Arrows indicate cannabinoid biosynthesis pathway; dark arrows indicate established pathways; the light gray arrow indicates a probable but not well-established pathway (R. Mechoulam, Hebrew University, personal communication, 1999).[11] The great majority of studies reporting on the effects of cannabinoids refer to THC; most of the rest are about CBD and CBN. Other cannabinoids found in marijuana do not appear to play an important role in the drug's effects.

(the small leaf-like part below the flower). The amounts of cannabinoids and their relative abundance in a marijuana plant vary with growing conditions, including humidity, temperature, and soil nutrients (reviewed in Pate, 1994[14]). The chemical stability of cannabinoids in harvested plant material is also affected by moisture, temperature, sunlight, and storage. They degrade under any storage condition.

BOX 1.1 Selected Cases from the Public Sessions

G.S. spoke at the IOM workshop in Louisiana about his use of marijuana first to combat AIDS wasting syndrome and later for relief from the side effects of AIDS medications.

Skin rashes, dry mouth, foul metallic aftertaste, numbness of the face, swelling of the limbs, fever spikes, headaches, dizziness, anemia, clinical depression, neuropathy so crippling that I could not type, so painful that the bed sheets felt like sandpaper, nausea so severe that I sometimes had to leave the dinner table to vomit, and diarrhea so unpredictable that I dared not leave the house without diapers.

These are some of the horrors that I have endured in the past 10 years during my fight for life against the human immunodeficiency virus. But these ravages were not caused by HIV itself, or by any of the opportunistic infections that mark the steady progression of AIDS. Each of these nightmares was a side effect of one of the hundreds of medications I have taken to fight one infection after another on my way to a seemingly certain early grave.

Had you known me three years ago, you would not recognize me now. After years of final-stage AIDS, I had wasted to 130 lb. The purple Kaposi's sarcoma lesions were spreading. The dark circles under my eyes told of sleepless nights and half-waking days. I encountered passages of time marked by medication schedules, nausea, and diarrhea. I knew that I was dying. Every reflection shimmered with death, my ghost-like pallor in the mirror, the contained terror on the face of a bus passenger beside me, and most of all the resigned sadness in my mother's eyes.

But still I was fortunate because along the way I rediscovered the ancient understanding of marijuana's medicinal benefit. So I smoked pot. Every day. The pot calmed my stomach against handfuls of pills. The pot made me hungry so that I could eat without a tube. The pot eased the pain of crippling neural side effects so that I could dial the phone by myself. The pot calmed my soul and allowed me to accept that I would probably die soon. Because I smoked pot I lived long enough to see the development of the first truly effective HIV therapies. I lived to gain 50 lb., regain my vigor, and celebrate my 35th birthday. I lived to sit on the bus without frightening the passenger beside me.

Even at this stage of my recovery I take a handful of pills almost every day and will probably continue to do so for the rest of my life. While I am grateful for the life-saving protease inhibitor therapies, they bring with them a host of adverse reactions and undesirable side effects. Different patients experience different reactions, of course, but almost all patients experience some. Smoking marijuana relieves many of these side effects.

I am not one of the exceptional eight patients in the United States with

Continued

legal permission to smoke marijuana. Every day I risk arrest, property forfeiture, fines, and imprisonment. But I have no choice, you see, just as I have no choice but to endure the side effects of these toxic medications. So, many patients like me are breaking the law to enjoy relief that no other therapy provides.

I sit here, I believe, as living proof that marijuana can have a beneficial effect in staving off wasting. Every pound was a day. I figured that for every pound of body weight I could maintain, that was another day that I could live in hopes that some effective therapy would emerge.

* * *

B.D. spoke at the IOM workshop in Louisiana. She is one of eight patients who are legally allowed to smoke marijuana under a Compassionate Use Protocol. She uses marijuana to relieve nausea, muscle spasticity, and pain associated with multiple sclerosis.

I was diagnosed with multiple sclerosis in 1988. Prior to that, I was an active person with ballet and swimming. I now have a swimming pool, so I swim each and every day, and I smoke marijuana. The government has given me the marijuana to smoke. Each month I pick up a can filled with the marijuana cigarettes rolled by the government.

At one time I weighed 85 lb. and I now weigh 105. Twenty pounds is quite a bit to put on. I could not walk. I did not have the appetite. I use a scooter now for distance. I can get around the house. I have a standard poodle who is kind of like an assistant dog. She is good at it. She helps me.

When I found out that there was a program to get marijuana from the government, I decided that was the answer. I was not a marijuana smoker before that. In fact, I used to consider the people I knew who smoked the marijuana as undesirables. Now, I myself am an undesirable.

But it works. It takes away the backache. With multiple sclerosis, you can get spasms, and your leg will just go straight out and you cannot stop that leg. You may have danced all of your life and put the leg where you wanted it to be, but the MS takes that from you. So I use the swimming pool, and that helps a lot. The kicks are much less when I have smoked a marijuana cigarette. Since 1991, I've smoked 10 cigarettes a day. I do not take any other drugs. Marijuana seems to have been my helper. At one time, I did not think much of the people who smoke it. But when it comes to your health, it makes a big difference.

* * *

J.H. spoke at the IOM workshop in Washington, D.C. He was seriously injured in an accident, suffers from a form of arthritis associated with abnormal activity of the sympathetic nervous system known as reflex sympathetic dystrophy, and has hepatitis C. He uses marijuana to relieve nausea from liver disease, pain, and muscle spasms.

I am 48 years old, married with two children. I am a veteran who served during the Vietnam war. I was exposed to hepatitis C in 1972 by a blood transfusion, which I needed because of a motor vehicle accident that broke my back; ruined my right shoulder, my left thumb, and hand; and almost amputated my right leg at the knee. My hepatitis C was not diagnosed until 1997—after the disease had destroyed my pancreas* and I had four heart attacks, one angioplasty, and a minor stroke. In 1989, while at work, I was involved in an accident with a large soil survey auger. My pelvis was crushed, and serious nerve damage was the result. I also have reflex sympathetic dystrophy, which is a neurological disease that has a tremendous amount of pain and muscle spasms.

I have reached what the doctors call end-stage liver disease from the hepatitis C. I have lost 85 lbs. due to the severe bouts of nausea and vomiting. Every time I come home from a hospital stay, my 7 year old asks if I got the liver transplant. I am on a transplant list, but I am not a candidate until I am seven days from death.

In October 1997, after trying four different antinausea medications, four of the doctors that I see told me to go to Europe and see a doctor and try medicinal cannabis. My primary care doctor wrote me a letter to carry with my medical records asking that the doctor help me in any way that he could to alleviate the symptoms of the hepatitis C and the reflex sympathetic dystrophy. Those symptoms are severe nausea and pain from the hepatitis C and pain and muscle spasms from the neurological disease.

I went to Europe in November 1997, where I saw a doctor of internal medicine. He prescribed me cannabis, 1–2 g a day. I got the medicine and a pipe and tried it. Within two minutes of taking two puffs from the pipe, the nausea was gone. I don't think that I felt the high, although I was quite elated. In about 45 min. I was starving. Normally, I have a fear of eating because I vomit almost always after I eat or take a pill. I forgot about that, and I think I ate more that night than I had eaten in months. I did feel a little nauseated after about four hours, but I smoked two more puffs, and in about two hours I went to bed. The next morning I felt hungry. During my nine-day stay in Europe, I was able to stay free of vomiting and the waves of nausea became less frequent.

I had experienced four years of pain control using Tegretol, a drug used by epileptics to control seizures. Now I can't use that medication because of the damage that it causes my cirrhotic liver. When I smoked about 2 g of marijuana a day, the nausea was gone and I was no longer losing weight. The pain was at an acceptable level. Sometimes I still find it necessary to use an opiate painkiller, but only when the pain is at its worst. Surprisingly, I lost an associated high within a few days. I also think the cannabis has an antidepressant effect on me, as I no longer have what I call the "poor me" feelings that I experienced after learning about the hepatitis C.

---

*This is an unlikely consequence of hepatitis C; it is more likely that the patient's liver was damaged.

ORGANIZATION OF THE REPORT

Throughout the report, steps that might be taken to fill the gaps in understanding both the potential harms and benefits of marijuana and cannabinoid use are identified. Those steps include identifying knowledge gaps, promising research directions, and potential therapies based on scientific advances in cannabinoid biology.

Chapter 2 reviews basic cannabinoid biology and provides a foundation to understand the medical value of marijuana or its constituent cannabinoids. In consideration of the physician's first rule, "first, do no harm," the potential harms attributed to the medical use of marijuana are reviewed before the potential medical benefits. Chapter 3 reviews the risks posed by marijuana use, with emphasis on medical use.

Chapter 4 analyzes the most credible clinical data relevant to the medical use of marijuana. It reviews what is known about the physiological mechanisms underlying particular conditions (for example, chronic pain, vomiting, anorexia, and muscle spasticity), what is known about the cellular actions of cannabinoids, and the levels of proof needed to show that marijuana is an effective treatment for specific symptoms. It does not analyze the historical literature; history is informative in enumerating uses of marijuana, but it does not provide the sort of information needed for a scientifically sound evaluation of the efficacy and safety of marijuana for clinical use. Because marijuana is advocated primarily as affording relief from the symptoms of disease rather than as a cure, this chapter is organized largely by symptoms as opposed to disease categories. Finally, chapter 4 compares the conclusions of this report with those of other recent reports on the medical use of marijuana.

Chapter 5 describes the process of and analyzes the prospects for cannabinoid drug development.

REFERENCES

1. Abel EL. 1980. *Marijuana: The First Twelve Thousand Years*. New York: Plenum Press.
2. Angell M, Kassirer JP. 1998. Alternative medicine—The risks of untested and unregulated remedies. *New England Journal of Medicine* 339:839–841.
3. Bonnie RJ, Whitebread II CH. 1974. *The Marihuana Conviction: A History of Marihuana Prohibition in the United States*. Charlottesville, VA: University Press of Virginia.
4. Eisenberg DM. 1997. Advising patients who seek alternative medical therapies. *Annals of Internal Medicine* 127:61–69.
5. Eisenberg DM, Davis RB, Ettner SL, Appel S, Wilkey S, Van Rompay M, Kessler RC. 1998. Trends in alternative medicine use in the United States, 1990–1997: Results of a follow-up national survey. *Journal of the American Medical Association* 280:1569–1575.
6. Eisenberg DM, Kessler RC, Foster C, Norlock FE, Calkins DR, Delbanco TL. 1993. Unconventional medicine in the United States: Prevalence, costs, and patterns of use. *New England Journal of Medicine* 328:246–252.

7. Grifo F, Newman D, Fairfield A, Bhattacharya B, Grupenhoff JT. 1997. The origins of prescription drugs. In: Grifo F, Rosenthal J, Editors. *Biodiversity and Human Health.* Washington, DC: Island Press. Pp. 131–163.

8. Herstek J. 1998. *Behavioral Health Issue Briefs. Medical Marijuana.* Washington, DC: Health Policy Tracking Service, National Conference of State Legislatures.

9. Kilbourne EM, Philen RM, Kamb ML, Falk H. 1996. Tryptophan produced by Showa Denko and epidemic eosinophilia-myalgia syndrome. *Journal of Rheumatology Supplement* 46:81–88. Comment on: *Journal of Rheumatology Supplement* 1996 46:44–58 and 60–72; discussion 58–59.

10. Mathre ML, Editor. 1997. *Cannabis in Medical Practice.* Jefferson, NC: MacFarland and Co.

11. Mechoulam R. 1986. The pharmacohistory of *Cannabis Sativa.* In: Mechoulam R , Editor. *Cannabinoids as Therapeutic Agents.* Boca Raton, FL: CRC Press. Pp. 1–19.

12. Milburn DS, Myers CW. 1991. Tryptophan toxicity: A pharmacoepidemiologic review of eosinophilia-myalgia syndrome. *DICP* 25:1259–1262.

13. NORML. The Medical Use of Marijuana [WWW document]. URL http://norml.org/medical/index.html (accessed July 9, 1998).

14. Pate DW. 1994. Chemical ecology of cannabis. *Journal of the International Hemp Association* 1:29, 32–37.

15. Peterson K. 15 January 1997. Notes: Weighing in on a medical controversy; *USA Today's* Baby Boomer Panel. *USA Today,* p. 12D.

16. Ross SA, Elsohly MA. 1995. Constituents of *Cannabis sativa* L. XXVIII. A review of the natural constituents: 1980–1994. *Zagazig Journal for Pharmaceutical Sciences* 4:1–10.

17. Taura F, Morimoto S, Shoyama Y. 1995. First direct evidence for the mechanism of delta 1-tetrahydrocannabinolic acid biosysnthesis. *Journal of the American Chemical Society* 117:9766–9767.

18. Turner CE, Elsohly MA, Boeren EG. 1980. Constituents of *Cannabis sativa* L. XVII. A review of the natural constituents. *Journal of Natural Products* 43:169–234.

2

Cannabinoids and Animal Physiology

INTRODUCTION

Much has been learned since the publication of the 1982 Institute of Medicine (IOM) report *Marijuana and Health*.* Although it was clear then that most of the effects of marijuana were due to its actions on the brain, there was little information about how THC acted on brain cells (neurons), which cells were affected by THC, or even what general areas of the brain were most affected by THC. Too little was known about cannabinoid physiology to offer any scientific insights into the harmful or therapeutic effects of marijuana. That is no longer true. During the past 16 years, there have been major advances in what basic science discloses about the potential medical benefits of cannabinoids, the group of compounds related to THC. Many variants are found in the marijuana plant, and other cannabinoids not found in the plant have been chemically synthesized. Sixteen years ago it was still a matter of debate as to whether THC acted nonspecifically by affecting the fluidity of cell membranes or whether a specific pathway of action was mediated by a receptor that responded selectively to THC (Table 2.1).

---

*The field of neuroscience has grown substantially since the publication of the 1982 IOM report. The number of members in the Society for Neuroscience provides a rough measure of the growth in research and knowledge about the brain: as of the middle of 1998, there were over 27,000 members, more than triple the number in 1982.

TABLE 2.1   Landmark Discoveries Since the 1982 IOM Report

Year	Discovery	Primary Investigators
1986	Potent cannabinoid agonists are developed; they are the key to discovering the receptor.	M. R. Johnson and L. S. Melvin[75]
1988	First conclusive evidence of specific cannabinoid receptors.	A. Howlett and W. Devane[36]
1990	The cannabinoid brain receptor (CB_1) is cloned, its DNA sequence is identified, and its location in the brain is determined.	L. Matsuda[107] and M. Herkenham et al.[60]
1992	Anandamide is discovered—a naturally occurring substance in the brain that acts on cannabinoid receptors.	R. Mechoulam and W. Devane[37]
1993	A cannabinoid receptor is discovered outside the brain; this receptor (CB_2) is related to the brain receptor but is distinct.	S. Munro[112]
1994	The first specific cannabinoid antagonist, SR 141716A, is developed.	M. Rinaldi-Carmona[132]
1998	The first cannabinoid antagonist, SR144528, that can distinguish between CB_1 and CB_2 receptors discovered.	M. Rinaldi-Carmona[133]

Basic science is the wellspring for developing new medications and is particularly important for understanding a drug that has as many effects as marijuana. Even committed advocates of the medical use of marijuana do not claim that all the effects of marijuana are desirable for every medical use. But they do claim that the combination of specific effects of marijuana enhances its medical value. An understanding of those specific effects is what basic science can provide. The multiple effects of marijuana can be singled out and studied with the goals of evaluating the medical value of marijuana and cannabinoids in specific medical conditions, as well as minimizing unwanted side effects. An understanding of the basic mechanisms through which cannabinoids affect physiology permits more strategic development of new drugs and designs for clinical trials that are most likely to yield conclusive results.

Research on cannabinoid biology offers new insights into clinical use, especially given the scarcity of clinical studies that adequately evaluate the medical value of marijuana. For example, despite the scarcity of substantive clinical data, basic science has made it clear that cannabinoids can affect pain transmission and, specifically, that cannabinoids interact with the brain's endogenous opioid system, an important system for the medical treatment of pain (see chapter 4).

The cellular machinery that underlies the response of the body and brain to cannabinoids involves an intricate interplay of different systems. This chapter reviews the components of that machinery with enough detail to permit the reader to compare what is known about basic biology with the medical uses proposed for marijuana. For some readers that will be too much detail. Those readers who do not wish to read the entire chapter should, nonetheless, be mindful of the following key points in this chapter:

- The most far reaching of the recent advances in cannabinoid biology are the identification of two types of cannabinoid receptors (CB$_1$ and CB$_2$) and of anandamide, a substance naturally produced by the body that acts at the cannabinoid receptor and has effects similar to those of THC. The CB$_1$ receptor is found primarily in the brain and mediates the psychological effects of THC. The CB$_2$ receptor is associated with the immune system; its role remains unclear.

- The physiological roles of the brain cannabinoid system in humans are the subject of much active research and are not fully known; however, cannabinoids likely have a natural role in pain modulation, control of movement, and memory.

- Animal research has shown that the potential for cannabinoid dependence exists, and cannabinoid withdrawal symptoms can be observed. However, both appear to be mild compared to dependence and withdrawal seen with other drugs.

- Basic research in cannabinoid biology has revealed a variety of cellular pathways through which potentially therapeutic drugs could act on the cannabinoid system. In addition to the known cannabinoids, such drugs might include chemical derivatives of plant-derived cannabinoids or of endogenous cannabinoids such as anandamide but would also include noncannabinoid drugs that act on the cannabinoid system.

This chapter summarizes the basics of cannabinoid biology—as known today. It thus provides a scientific basis for interpreting claims founded on anecdotes and for evaluating the clinical studies of marijuana presented in chapter 4.

The Value of Animal Studies

Much of the research into the effects of cannabinoids on the brain is based on animal studies. Many speakers at the public workshops associated with this study argued that animal studies of marijuana are not relevant to humans. Animal studies are not a substitute for clinical trials, but they are a necessary complement. Ultimately, every biologically active substance exerts its effects at the cellular and molecular levels, and the evidence has shown that this is remarkably consistent among mammals, even those as different in body and mind as rats and humans. Animal studies typically provide information about how drugs work that would not be obtainable in clinical studies. At the same time, animal studies can never inform us completely about the full range of psychological and physiological effects of marijuana or cannabinoids on humans.

The Active Constituents of Marijuana

Δ^9-THC and Δ^8-THC are the only compounds in the marijuana plant that produce all the psychoactive effects of marijuana. Because Δ^9-THC is much more abundant than Δ^8-THC, the psychoactivity of marijuana has been attributed largely to the effects of Δ^9-THC. 11-OH-Δ^9-THC is the primary product of Δ^9-THC metabolism by the liver and is about three times as potent as Δ^9-THC.[128]

There have been considerably fewer experiments with cannabinoids other than Δ^9-THC, although a few studies have been done to examine whether other cannabinoids modulate the effects of THC or mediate the nonpsychological effects of marijuana. Cannabidiol (CBD) does not have the same psychoactivity as THC, but it was initially reported to attenuate the psychological response to THC in humans;[81,177] however, later studies reported that CBD did not attenuate the psychological effects of THC.[11,69] One double-blind study of eight volunteers reported that CBD can block the anxiety induced by high doses of THC (0.5 mg/kg).[177] There are numerous anecdotal reports claiming that marijuana with relatively higher ratios of THC:CBD is less likely to induce anxiety in the user than marijuana with low THC:CBD ratios; but, taken together, the results published thus far are inconclusive.

The most important effect of CBD seems to be its interference with drug metabolism, including Δ^9-THC metabolism in the liver.[14,114] It exerts that effect by inactivating cytochrome P450s, which are the most important class of enzymes that metabolize drugs. Like many P450 inactivators, CBD can also induce P450s after repeated doses.[13] Experiments in which mice were treated with CBD followed by THC showed that CBD treatment was associated with a substantial increase in brain concentrations of

THC and its major metabolites, most likely because it decreased the rate of clearance of THC from the body.[15]

In mice, THC inhibits the release of luteinizing hormone, the pituitary hormone that triggers the release of testosterone from the testes; this effect is increased when THC is given with cannabinol or CBD.[113]

Cannabinol also lowers body temperature and increases sleep duration in mice.[175] It is considerably less active than THC in the brain, but studies of immune cells have shown that it can modulate immune function (see "Cannabinoids and the Immune System" later in this chapter).

The Pharmacological Toolbox

A researcher needs certain key tools in order to understand how a drug acts on the brain. To appreciate the importance of these tools, one must first understand some basic principles of drug action. All recent studies have indicated that the behavioral effects of THC are receptor mediated.[27] Neurons in the brain are activated when a compound binds to its receptor, which is a protein typically located on the cell surface. Thus, THC will exert its effects only after binding to its receptor. In general, a given receptor will accept only particular classes of compounds and will be unaffected by other compounds.

Compounds that activate receptors are called *agonists*. Binding to a receptor triggers an event or a series of events in the cell that results in a change in the cell's activity, its gene regulation, or the signals that it sends to neighboring cells (Figure 2.1). This agonist-induced process is called signal transduction.

Another set of tools for drug research, which became available only recently for cannabinoid research, are the *receptor antagonists*, so-called because they selectively bind to a receptor that would have otherwise been available for binding to some other compound or drug. Antagonists block the effects of agonists and are tools to identify the functions of a receptor by showing what happens when its normal functions are blocked. Agonists and antagonists are both *ligands*; that is, they bind to receptors. Hormones, neurotransmitters, and drugs can all act as ligands. Morphine and naloxone provide a good example of how agonists and antagonists interact. A large dose of morphine acts as an agonist at opioid receptors in the brain and interferes with, or even arrests, breathing. Naloxone, a powerful opioid antagonist, blocks morphine's effects on opiate receptors, thereby allowing an overdose victim to resume breathing normally. Naloxone itself has no effect on breathing.

Another key tool involves identifying the receptor protein and determining how it works. That makes it possible to locate where a drug activates its receptor in the brain—both the general region of the brain and

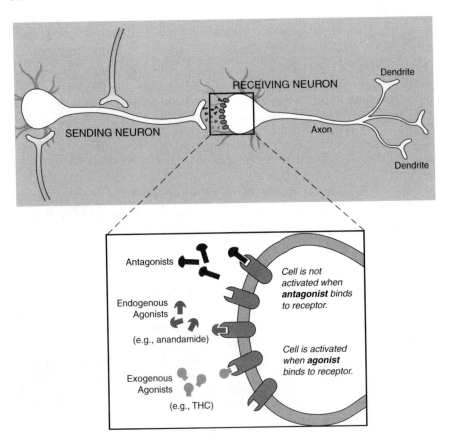

FIGURE 2.1 Diagram of neuron with synapse. Individual nerve cells, or neurons, both send and receive cellular signals to and from neighboring neurons, but for the purposes of this diagram only one activity is indicated for each cell. Neurotransmitter molecules are released from the neuron terminal and move across the gap between the "sending" and "receiving" neurons. A signal is transmitted to the receiving neuron when the neurotransmitters have bound to the receptor on its surface. The effects of a transmitted signal include:

- Changing the cell's permeability to ions, such as calcium and potassium.
- Turning a particular gene on or off.
- Sending a signal to another neuron.
- Increasing or decreasing the responsiveness of the cell to other cellular signals.

Those effects can lead to cognitive, behavioral, or physiological changes, depending on which neuronal system is activated.

Continued on bottom of p. 39

the cell type where the receptor is located. The way to find a receptor for a drug in the brain is to make the receptor "visible" by attaching a radioactive or fluorescent marker to the drug. Such markers show where in the brain a drug binds to the receptor, although this is not necessarily the part of the brain where the drug ultimately has its greatest effects.

Because drugs injected into animals must be dissolved in a water-based solution, it is easier to deliver water-soluble molecules than to deliver fat-soluble (lipophilic) molecules such as THC. THC is so lipophilic that it can stick to glass and plastic syringes used for injection. Because it is lipophilic, it readily enters cell membranes and thus can cross the blood brain barrier easily. (This barrier insulates the brain from many blood-borne substances.) Early cannabinoid research was hindered by the lack of potent cannabinoid ligands (THC binds to its cannabinoid receptors rather weakly) and because they were not readily water soluble. The synthetic agonist CP 55,940, which is more water soluble than THC, was the first useful research tool for studying cannabinoid receptors because of its high potency and ability to be labeled with a radioactive molecule, which enabled researchers to trace its activity.

CANNABINOID RECEPTORS

The cannabinoid receptor is a typical member of the largest known family of receptors: the G protein-coupled receptors with their distinctive pattern in which the receptor molecule spans the cell membrane seven times (Figure 2.2). For excellent recent reviews of cannabinoid receptor biology, see Childers and Breivogel,[27] Abood and Martin,[1] Felder and Glass,[43] and Pertwee.[124] Cannabinoid receptor ligands bind *reversibly* (they bind to the receptor briefly and then dissociate) and *stereoselectively* (when there are molecules that are mirror images of each other, only one

---

The expanded view of the synapse illustrates a variety of *ligands*, that is, molecules that bind to receptors. Anandamide is a substance produced by the body that binds to and activates cannabinoid receptors; it is an *endogenous agonist*. THC can also bind to and activate cannabinoid receptors but is not naturally found in the body; it is an *exogenous agonist*. SR 141716A binds to but does not activate cannabinoid receptors. In this way it prevents agonists, such as anandamide and THC, from activating cannabinoid receptors by binding to the receptors without activating them; SR 141716A is an *antagonist*, but it is not normally produced in the body. Endogenous antagonists, that is, those normally produced in the body, might also exist, but none has been identified.

H_2N

Extracellular

Cell Membrane

Intracellular

CB-1 receptors ●
CB-2 receptors ◐

COOH

FIGURE 2.2 Cannabinoid receptors. Receptors are proteins, and proteins are made up of strings of amino acids. Each circle in the diagram represents one amino acid. The shaded bar represents the cell membrane, which like all cell membranes in animals is composed largely of phospholipids. Like many receptors, the cannabinoid receptors span the cell membrane; some sections of the receptor protein are outside the cell membrane (extracellular); some are inside (intracellular). THC, anandamide, and other known cannabinoid receptor agonists bind to the extracellular portion of the receptor, thereby activating the signal pathway inside the cell. The CB_1 molecule is larger than CB_2. The receptor molecules are most similar in four of the seven regions where they are embedded in the cell membrane (known as the transmembrane regions). The intracellular loops of the two receptor subtypes are quite different, which might affect the cellular response to the ligand because these loops are known to mediate G protein signaling, the next step in the cell signaling pathway after the receptor. Receptor homology between the two receptor subtypes is 44% for the full-length protein and 68% within the seven transmembrane regions. The ligand binding sites are typically defined by the extracellular loops and the transmembrane regions.

version activates the receptor). Thus far, two cannabinoid receptor subtypes (CB_1 and CB_2) have been identified, of which only CB_1 is found in the brain.

The cell responds in a variety of ways when a ligand binds to the cannabinoid receptor (Figure 2.3). The first step is activation of G proteins, the first components of the signal transduction pathway. That leads to changes in several intracellular components—such as cyclic AMP and calcium and potassium ions—which ultimately produce the changes in cell functions. The final result of cannabinoid receptor stimulation de-

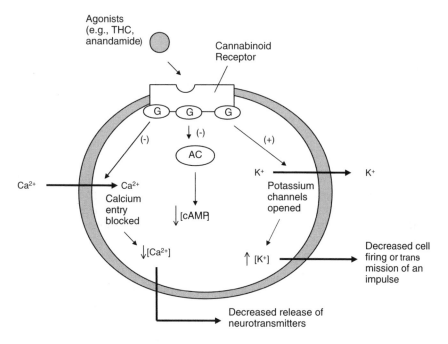

FIGURE 2.3 Cannabinoid agonists trigger a series of reactions within cells. Cannabinoid receptors are embedded in the cell membrane, where they are coupled to G proteins (G) and the enzyme adenylyl cyclase (AC). Receptors are activated when they bind to ligands, such as anandamide or THC in this case. This triggers a variety of reactions, including inhibition (–) of AC, which decreases the production of cAMP and cellular activities dependent on cAMP; opening of potassium (K^+) channels, which decreases cell firing; and closing of calcium (Ca^{2+}) channels, which decreases the release of neurotransmitters. Each of those changes can influence cellular communication.

pends on the particular type of cell, the particular ligand, and the other molecules that might be competing for receptor binding sites. Different agonists vary in binding *potency*, which determines the effective dose of the drug, and *efficacy*, which determines the maximal strength of the signal that they transmit to the cell. The potency and efficacy of THC are both relatively lower than those of some synthetic cannabinoids; in fact, synthetic compounds are generally more potent and efficacious than endogenous agonists.

CB$_1$ receptors are extraordinarily abundant in the brain. They are more abundant than most other G protein-coupled receptors and 10 times more abundant than *mu* opioid receptors, the receptors responsible for the effects of morphine.[148]

The cannabinoid receptor in the brain is a protein referred to as CB_1. The peripheral receptor (outside the nervous system), CB_2, is most abundant on cells of the immune system and is not generally found in the brain.[43,124] Although no other receptor subtypes have been identified, there is a genetic variant known as CB_1A (such variants are somewhat different proteins that have been produced by the same genes via alternative processing). In some cases, proteins produced via alternative splicing have different effects on cells. It is not yet known whether there are any functional differences between the two, but the structural differences raise the possibility.

CB_1 and CB_2 are similar, but not as similar as members of many other receptor families are to each other. On the basis of a comparison of the sequence of amino acids that make up the receptor protein, the similarity of the CB_1 and CB_2 receptors is 44% (Figure 2.2). The differences between the two receptors indicate that it should be possible to design therapeutic drugs that would act only on one or the other receptor and thus would activate or attenuate (block) the appropriate cannabinoid receptors. This offers a powerful method for producing biologically selective effects. In spite of the difference between the receptor subtypes, most cannabinoid compounds bind with similar affinity* to both CB_1 and CB_2 receptors. One exception is the plant-derived compound CBD, which appears to have greater binding affinity for CB_2 than for CB_1,[112] although another research group has failed to substantiate that observation.[129] Other exceptions include the synthetic compound WIN 55,212-2, which shows greater affinity for CB_2 than CB_1, and the endogenous ligands, anandamide and 2-AG, which show greater affinity for CB_1 than CB_2.[43] The search for compounds that bind to only one or the other of the cannabinoid receptor types has been under way for several years and has yielded a number of compounds that are useful research tools and have potential for medical use.

Cannabinoid receptors have been studied most in vertebrates, such as rats and mice. However, they are also found in invertebrates, such as leeches and mollusks.[156] The evolutionary history of vertebrates and invertebrates diverged more than 500 million years ago, so cannabinoid receptors appear to have been conserved throughout evolution at least this long. This suggests that they serve an important and basic function in animal physiology. In general, cannabinoid receptor molecules are similar among different species.[124] Thus, cannabinoid receptors likely fill many similar functions in a broad range of animals, including humans.

Affinity is a measure of how avidly a compound binds to a receptor. The higher the affinity of a compound, the higher its potency; that is, lower doses are needed to produce its effects.

THE ENDOGENOUS CANNABINOID SYSTEM

For any drug for which there is a receptor, the logical question is, "Why does this receptor exist?" The short answer is that there is probably an endogenous agonist (that is, a compound that is naturally produced in the brain) that acts on that receptor. The long answer begins with a search for such compounds in the area of the body that produces the receptors and ends with a determination of the natural function of those compounds. So far, the search has yielded several endogenous compounds that bind selectively to cannabinoid receptors. The best studied of them are anandamide[37] and arachidonyl glycerol (2-AG).[108] However, their physiological roles are not yet known.

Initially, the search for an endogenous cannabinoid was based on the premise that its chemical structure would be similar to that of THC; that was reasonable, in that it was really a search for another "key" that would fit into the cannabinoid receptor "keyhole," thereby activating the cellular message system. One of the intriguing discoveries in cannabinoid biology was how chemically different THC and anandamide are. A similar search for endogenous opioids (endorphins) also revealed that their chemical structure is very different from the plant-derived opioids, opium and morphine.

Further research has uncovered a variety of compounds with quite different chemical structures that can activate cannabinoid receptors (Table 2.2 and Figure 2.4). It is not yet known exactly how anandamide and THC bind to cannabinoid receptors. Knowing this should permit more precise design of drugs that selectively activate the endogenous cannabinoid systems.

Anandamide

The first endogenous cannabinoid to be discovered was arachidonyl-ethanolamine, named anandamide from the Sanskrit word *ananda*, meaning "bliss."[37] Compared with THC, anandamide has only moderate affinity for CB_1 receptor and is rapidly metabolized by amidases (enzymes that remove amide groups). Despite its short duration of action, anand-amide shares most of the pharmacological effects of THC.[37,152] Rapid degradation of active molecules is a feature of neurotransmitter systems that allows them control of signal timing by regulating the abundance of signaling molecules. It creates problems for interpreting the results of many experiments and might explain why *in vivo* studies with anandamide injected into the brain have yielded conflicting results.

Anandamide appears to have both central (in the brain) and peripheral (in the rest of the body) effects. The precise neuroanatomical localiza-

TABLE 2.2 Compounds That Bind to Cannabinoid Receptors

Compound	Properties
Agonists (receptor activators)	
Plant-derived compounds	
Δ^9-THC	Main psychoactive cannabinoid in marijuana plant; largely responsible for psychological and physiological effects (except in discussions of the different forms of THC, THC is used as a synonym for Δ^9-THC).
Δ^8-THC	Slightly less potent than Δ^9-THC and much less abundant in marijuana plant but otherwise similar.
11-OH-Δ^9-THC	Bioactive compound formed when body breaks down Δ^9-THC; presumed to be responsible for some effects of marijuana.
Cannabinoid agonists found in animals	
Anandamide (arachidonyl-ethanolamide)	Found in animals ranging from mollusks to mammals; appears to be primary endogenous cannabinoid agonist in mammals; chemical structure very different from plant cannabinoids and related to prostaglandins.
2-AG (arachidonyl glycerol)	Endogenous agonist; structurally similar to anandamide; more abundant but less potent than anandamide.
THC analogues	
Dronabinol	Synthetic THC; marketed in the United States as Marinol for nausea associated with chemotherapy and for AIDS-related wasting.
Nabilone	THC analogue; marketed in the United Kingdom as Cesamet for same indications as dronabionol.
CP 55,940	Synthetic cannabinoid; THC analogue; that is, it is structurally similar to THC.
Levonantradol	THC analogue.
HU-210	THC analogue, 100- to 800-fold greater potency than THC[97].
Chemical structure unlike THC or anandamide	
WIN-55,212-2	Chemical structure different from known cannabinoids, but binds to both cannabinoid receptors; chemically related to cyclo-oxygenase inhibitors, which include antiinflammatory drugs.
Antagonists (receptor blockers)	
SR 141716A	Synthetic CB_1 antagonist; developed in 1994[132].
SR 144528	Synthetic CB_2 antagonist; developed in 1997[133].

SOURCES: Mechoulam et al., 1998;[109] Felder and Glass, 1998;[43] and British Medical Association.[17]

FIGURE 2.4 Chemical structures of selected cannabinoid agonists or molecules that bind to and activate cannabinoid receptors. **THC** is the primary psychoactive molecule found in marijuana. **CP 55,940** is a THC analogue; that is, its chemical structure is related to THC. **Anandamide** and **2-arachidonyl glycerol (2-AG)** are endogenous molecules, meaning they are naturally produced in the body. Although the chemical structure of **WIN 55,212** is very different from either THC or anandamide, it is also a canabinoid agonist.

tion of anandamide and the enzymes that synthesize it are not yet known. This information will provide essential clues to the natural role of anandamide and an understanding of the brain circuits in which it is a neurotransmitter. The importance of knowing specific brain circuits that involve anandamide (and other endogenous cannabinoid ligands) is that such circuits are the pivotal elements for regulating specific brain functions, such as mood, memory, and cognition. Anandamide has been found in numerous regions of the human brain: hippocampus (and

TABLE 2.3   Comparison of Cannabinoid Receptor Agonists

Potency can be measured in a variety of ways, from behavioral to physiological to cellular. This table shows potency in terms of receptor binding, which is the most broadly applicable to the many possible actions of cannabinoids. For example, anandamide binds to the cannabinoid receptor only about half as avidly as does THC. Measures of potency might include effects on activity (behavior) or hypothermia (physiologic).

The apparently low potency of 2-AG may, however, be misleading. A study published late in 1998 reports that 2-AG is found with two other closely related compounds that by themselves are biologically inactive; but in the presence of those two compounds, 2-AG is only three times less active than THC.[9] Further, 2-AG is much more abundant than anandamide, although the biological significance of this remains to be determined.

Receptor Binding in Brain Tissue[124]

Compound	Potency Relative to Δ^9-THC
CP 55,940	59
Δ^9-THC	1
Anandamide	0.47
2-AG	0.08

parahippocampic cortex), striatum, and cerebellum; but it has not been precisely identified with specific neuronal circuits. CB_1 receptors are abundant in these regions, and this further implies a physiological role for endogenous cannabinoids in the brain functions controlled by these areas. But substantial concentrations of anandamide are also found in the thalamus, an area of the brain that has relatively few CB_1 receptors.[124]

Anandamide has also been found outside the brain. It has been found in spleen tissue, which also has high concentrations of CB_2 receptors, and small amounts have been detected in heart tissue.[44]

In general, the affinity of anandamide for cannabinoid receptors is only one-fourth to one-half that of THC (see Table 2.3). The differences depend on the cells or tissue that are tested and on the experimental conditions, such as the binding assay used (reviewed by Pertwee[124]).

The molecular structure of anandamide is relatively simple, and it can be formed from arachidonic acid and ethanolamine. Arachidonic acid is a common precursor of a group of biologically active molecules known as eicosanoids, including prostaglandins.* Although anandamide can be synthesized in a variety of ways, the physiologically relevant pathway

---

*Eicosanoids all contain a chain of 20 carbon atoms and are named after *eikosi*, the Greek word for 20.

seems to be through enzymatic cleavage of N-arachidonyl-phosphatidyl-ethanolamine (NAPE), which yields anandamide and phosphatidic acid (reviewed by Childers and Breivogel[27]).

Anandamide can be inactivated in the brain via two mechanisms. In one it is enzymatically cleaved to yield arachidonic acid and ethanolamine—the reverse of what was initially proposed as its primary mode of synthesis. In the other it is inactivated through neuronal uptake—that is, by being transported into the neuron, which prevents its continuing activation of neighboring neurons.

Other Endogenous Agonists

Several other endogenous compounds that are chemically related to anandamide and that bind to cannabinoid receptors have been discovered, one of which is 2-AG.[108] 2-AG is closely related to anandamide and is even more abundant in the brain. At the time of this writing, all known endogenous cannabinoid receptor agonists (including anandamide) were eicosanoids, which are arachidonic acid metabolites. Arachidonic acid (a free fatty acid) is released via hydrolysis of membrane phospholipids.

Other, noneicosanoid, compounds that bind cannabinoid receptors have recently been isolated from brain tissue, but they have not been identified, and their biological effects are under investigation. This is a fast-moving field of research, and no review over six months old will be fully up to date.

The endogenous compounds that bind to cannabinoid receptors probably perform a broad range of natural functions in the brain. This neural signaling system is rich and complex and has many subtle variations, many of which await discovery. In the next few years much more will probably be known about these naturally occurring cannabinoids.

Some effects of cannabinoid agonists are receptor independent. For example, both THC and CBD can be neuroprotective through their antioxidative activity; that is, they can reduce the toxic forms of oxygen that are released when cells are under stress.[54] Other likely examples of receptor-independent cannabinoid activity are modulation of activation of membrane-bound enzymes (such as ATPase), arachidonic acid release, and perturbation of membrane lipids. An important caution in interpreting those reports is that concentrations of THC or CBD used in cellular studies, such as these, are generally much higher than the concentrations of THC or CBD in the body that would likely be achieved by smoking marijuana.

TABLE 2.4   Cellular Processes That Can Be Targeted for Drug Development

Drug Action		Biological Result
Block synthesis	Synthesis of bioactive compounds is a continuous process and is one means by which concentrations of that compound are regulated.	*Weaker signal*, due to decreased agonist concentration.
Inhibit degradation	Chemical breakdown is one method the body uses to inactivate endogenous substances.	*Stronger signal*, due to increased agonist concentration.
Facilitate neuronal uptake	Neuronal uptake is one of the natural ways in which a receptor agonist is inactivated.	*Stronger signal*, due to increased amount of time during which agonist is present in the synapse where it can stimulate the receptor.

NOTE: Endogenous cannabinoids are part of a cellular signaling system. This table lists categories of natural processes that regulate such systems and shows the results of altering those processes.

Novel Targets for Therapeutic Drugs

Drugs that alter the natural biology of anandamide or other endogenous cannabinoids might have therapeutic uses (Table 2.4). For example, drugs that selectively inhibit neuronal uptake of anandamide would increase the brain's own natural cannabinoids, thereby mimicking some of the effects of THC. A number of important psychotherapeutic drugs act by inhibiting neurotransmitter uptake. For example, antidepressants like fluoxetine (Prozac) inhibit serotonin uptake and are known as selective serotonin reuptake inhibitors, or SSRIs. Another way to alter levels of endogenous cannabinoids would be to develop drugs that act on the enzymes involved in anandamide synthesis. Some antihypertensive drugs work by inhibiting enzymes involved in the synthesis of endogenous hypertensive agents. For example, anti-converting enzyme (ACE) inhibitors are used in hypertensive patients to interfere with the conversion of angiotensin I, which is inactive, to the active hormone, angiotensin II.

SITES OF ACTION

Cannabinoid receptors are particularly abundant in some areas of the brain. The normal biology and behavior associated with these brain areas

TABLE 2.5   Brain Regions in Which Cannabinoid Receptors Are Abundant

Brain Region	Functions Associated with Region
Brain regions in which cannabinoid receptors are abundant	
Basal ganglia	Movement control
Substantia nigra pars reticulata	
Entopeduncular nucleus	
Globus pallidus	
Putamen	
Cerebellum	Body movement coordination
Hippocampus	Learning and memory, stress
Cerebral cortex, especially cingulate, frontal, and parietal regions	Higher cognitive functions
Nucleus accumbens	Reward center
Brain regions in which cannabinoid brain receptors are moderately concentrated	
Hypothalamus	Body housekeeping functions (body temperature regulation, salt and water balance, reproductive function)
Amygdala	Emotional response, fear
Spinal cord	Peripheral sensation, including pain
Brain stem	Sleep and arousal, temperature regulation, motor control
Central gray	Analgesia
Nucleus of the solitary tract	Visceral sensation, nausea and vomiting

SOURCES: Based on reviews by Pertwee (1997b)[124] and Herkenham (1995).[57]

are consistent with the behavioral effects produced by cannabinoids (Table 2.5 and Figure 2.5). The highest receptor density is found in cells of the basal ganglia that project locally and to other brain regions. These cells include the substantia nigra pars reticulata, entopeduncular nucleus, and globus pallidus, regions that are generally involved in coordinating body movements. Patients with Parkinson's or Huntington's disease tend to have impaired functions in these regions.

CB_1 receptors are also abundant in the putamen, part of the relay system within the basal ganglia that regulates body movements; the cerebellum, which coordinates body movements; the hippocampus, which is involved in learning, memory, and response to stress; and the cerebral cortex, which is concerned with the integration of higher cognitive functions.

CB_1 receptors are found on various parts of neurons, including the

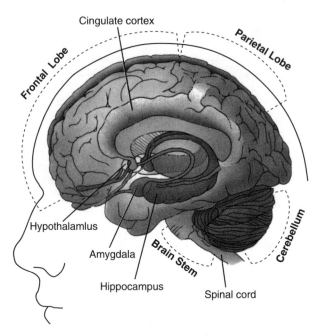

Cingulate cortex

Frontal Lobe

Parietal Lobe

Hypothalamlus

Amygdala

Brain Stem

Cerebellum

Hippocampus

Spinal cord

FIGURE 2.5   Locations of brain regions in which cannabinoid receptors are abundant. See Table 2.5 for a summary of functions associated with those regions.

axon, cell bodies, terminals, and dendrites.[57,165] Dendrites are generally the "receiving" part of a neuron, and receptors on axons or cell bodies generally modulate other signals. Axon terminals are the "sending" part of the neuron.

Cannabinoids tend to inhibit neurotransmission, although the results are somewhat variable. In some cases, cannabinoids diminish the effects of the inhibitory neurotransmitter, g-aminobutyric acid (GABA);[144] in other cases, cannabinoids can augment the effects of GABA.[120] The effect of activating a receptor depends on where it is found on the neuron: if cannabinoid receptors are presynaptic (on the "sending" side of the synapse) and inhibit the release of GABA, cannabinoids would diminish GABA effects; the net effect would be stimulation. However, if cannabinoid receptors are postsynaptic (on the "receiving" side of the synapse) and on the same cell as GABA receptors, they will probably mimic the effects of GABA; in that case, the net effect would be inhibition.[120,144,160]

CB_1 is the predominant brain cannabinoid receptor. CB_2 receptors have not generally been found in the brain, but there is one isolated report suggesting some in mouse cerebellum.[150] CB_2 is found primarily on cells

TABLE 2.6   Cannabinoid Receptors

	CB_1	CB_2
Effects of various cannabinoids		
Δ^9-THC	Agonist	Weak antagonist
Anandamide	Agonist	Agonist
Cannabinol	Weak agonist	Agonist; greater affinity for CB_2 than for CB_1
Cannabidiol	Does not bind to receptor	Does not bind to receptor
Receptor distribution		
Areas of greatest abundance	Brain	Immune system, especially B cells and natural killer cells

of the immune system. CB_1 receptors are also found in immune cells, but CB_2 is considerably more abundant there (Table 2.6) (reviewed by Kaminski[80] in 1998).

As can be appreciated in the next section, the presence of cannabinoid systems in key brain regions is strongly tied to the functions and pathology associated with those regions. The clinical value of cannabinoid systems is best understood in the context of the biology of these brain regions.

CANNABINOID RECEPTORS AND BRAIN FUNCTIONS

Motor Effects

Marijuana affects psychomotor performance in humans. The effects depend both on the nature of the task and the experience with marijuana. In general, effects are clearest in steadiness (body sway and hand steadiness) and in motor tasks that require attention. The results of testing cannabinoids in rodents are much clearer.

Cannabinoids clearly affect movement in rodents, but the effects depend on the dose: low doses stimulate and higher doses inhibit locomotion.[111,159] Cannabinoids mainly inhibit the transmission of neural signals, and they inhibit movement through their actions on the basal ganglia and cerebellum, where cannabinoid receptors are particularly abundant (Figure 2.6). Cannabinoid receptors are also found in the neurons that project from the striatum and subthalamic nucleus, which inhibit and stimulate movement, respectively.[58,101]

Cannabinoids decrease both the inhibitory and stimulatory inputs to the substantia nigra and therefore might provide dual regulation of move-

a.

Globus pallidus
and putamen

Caudate
nucleus

Cerebellum

b.

Caudate
nucleus

Putamen
Thalamus
Globus pallidus

Subthalamic
nucleus
Substantia
nigra

FIGURE 2.6 Diagrams showing motor regions of the brain. Basal ganglia are a group of three brain regions, or nuclei—**caudate**, **putamen**, and **globus pallidus**. Figure 2.6a is a three-dimensional view showing the location of those nuclei in the brain. Figure 2.6b shows those structures in a vertical cross-sectional view. The major output pathways of the basal ganglia arise from the globus pallidus and pars reticulata of the **substantia nigra**. Their main target is the **thalamus**. SOURCE: Figure 2.6a is reprinted from *Principles of Neural Science*, 2nd ed., 1985 (E.R. Kandel and J.H. Schwartz, eds.), with permission from the copyright holder, Appleton and Lange.

ment at this nucleus. In the substantia nigra, cannabinoids decrease transmission from both the striatum and the subthalamic nucleus.[141] The globus pallidus has been implicated in mediating the cataleptic effects of large doses of cannabinoids in rats.[126] (Catalepsy is a condition of diminished responsiveness usually characterized by trancelike states and waxy rigidity of the muscles.) Several other brain regions—the cortex, the cerebellum, and the neural pathway from cortex to striatum—are also involved in the control of movement and contain abundant cannabinoid receptors.[52,59,101] They are therefore possible additional sites that might underlie the effects of cannabinoids on movement.

Memory Effects

One of the primary effects of marijuana in humans is disruption of short-term memory.[68] That is consistent with the abundance of CB_1 receptors in the hippocampus, the brain region most closely associated with memory. The effects of THC resemble a temporary hippocampal lesion.[63] Deadwyler and colleagues have demonstrated that cannabinoids decrease neuronal activity in the hippocampus and its inputs.[23,24,83] *In vitro*, several cannabinoid ligands and endogenous cannabinoids can block the cellular processes associated with memory formation.[29,30,116,157,163] Furthermore, cannabinoid agonists inhibit release of several neurotransmitters: acetylcholine from the hippocampus,[49-51] norepinephrine from human and guinea pig (but not rat or mouse) hippocampal slices,[143] and glutamate in cultured hippocampal cells.[144] Cholinergic and noradrenergic neurons project into the hippocampus, but circuits within the hippocampus are glutamatergic.* Thus, cannabinoids could block transmission both into and within the hippocampus by blocking presynaptic neurotransmitter release.

Pain

After nausea and vomiting, chronic pain was the condition cited most often to the IOM study team as a medical use for marijuana. Recent research presented below has shown intriguing parallels with anecdotal reports of the modulating effects of cannabinoids on pain—both the effects of cannabinoids acting alone and the effects of their interaction with opioids.

---

*Neurons are often defined by the primary neurotransmitter released at their terminals. Thus, *cholinergic* neurons release acetylcholine, *noradrenergic* neurons release noradrenalin (also known as norepinephrine), and *glutamergic* neurons release glutamate.

Behavioral Studies

Cannabinoids reduce reactivity to acute painful stimuli in laboratory animals. In rodents, cannabinoids reduced the responsiveness to pain induced through various stimuli, including thermal, mechanical, and chemical stimuli.[12,19,46,72,96,154,174] Cannabinoids were comparable with opiates in potency and efficacy in these experiments.[12,72]

Cannabinoids are also effective in rodent models of chronic pain. Herzberg and co-workers found that cannabinoids can block allodynia and hyperalgesia associated with neuropathic pain in rats.[62] This is an important advance because chronic pain frequently results in a series of neural changes that increase suffering due to allodynia (pain elicited by stimuli that are normally innocuous), hyperalgesia (abnormally increased reactivity to pain), and spontaneous pain; furthermore, some chronic pain syndromes are not amenable to therapy, even with the most powerful narcotic analgesics.[10]

Pain perception is controlled mainly by neurotransmitter systems within the central nervous system, and cannabinoids clearly play a role in the control of pain in those systems.[45] However, pain-relieving and pain-preventing mechanisms also occur in peripheral tissues, and endogenous cannabinoids appear to play a role in peripheral tissues. Thus, the different cannabinoid receptor subtypes might act synergistically. Experiments in which pain is induced by injecting dilute formalin into a mouse's paw have shown that anandamide and palmitylethanolamide (PEA) can block peripheral pain.[22,73] Anandamide acts primarily at the CB_1 receptor, whereas PEA has been proposed as a possible CB_2 agonist; in short, there might be a biochemical basis for their independent effects. When injected together, the analgesic effect is stronger than that of either alone. That suggests an important strategy for the development of a new class of analgesic drug: a mixture of CB_1 and CB_2 agonists. Because there are few, if any, CB_2 receptors in the brain, it might be possible to develop drugs that enhance the peripheral analgesic effect while minimizing the psychological effects.

Neural Sites of Altered Responsiveness to Painful Stimuli

The brain and spinal cord mediate cannabinoid analgesia. A number of brain areas participate in cannabinoid analgesia and support the role of descending pathways (neural pathways that project from the brain to the spinal cord).[103,105] Although more work is needed to produce a comprehensive map of the sites of cannabinoid analgesia, it is clear that the effects are limited to particular areas, most of which have an established role in pain.

Specific sites where cannabinoids act to affect pain processing include the periaqueductal gray,[104] rostral ventral medulla,[105,110] thalamic nucleus submedius,[102] thalamic ventroposterolateral nucleus,[102] dorsal horn of the spinal cord,[64,65] and peripheral sensory nerves.[64-66,131] Those nuclei also participate in opiate analgesia. Although similar to opiate analgesia, cannabinoid analgesia is not mediated by opioid receptors; morphine and cannabinoids sometimes act synergistically, and opioid antagonists generally have no effect on cannabinoid-induced analgesia.[171] However, a *kappa*-receptor antagonist has been shown to attenuate spinal, but not supraspinal, cannabinoid analgesia.[153,170,171] (*Kappa* opioid receptors constitute one of the three major types of opioid receptors; the other two types are *mu* and *delta* receptors.)

Neurophysiology and Neurochemistry of Cannabinoid Analgesia

Because of the marked effects of cannabinoids on motor function, behavioral studies in animals alone cannot provide sufficient grounds for the conclusion that cannabinoids depress pain perception. Motor behavior is typically used to measure responses to pain, but this behavior is itself affected by cannabinoids. Thus, experimental results include an unmeasured combination of cannabinoid effects on motor and pain systems. The effects on specific neural systems, however, can be measured at the neurophysiological and neurochemical levels. Cannabinoids decrease the response of immediate-early genes (genes that are activated in the early or immediate stage of response to a broad range of cellular stimuli) to noxious stimuli in the spinal cord, decrease response of pain neurons in the spinal cord, and decrease the responsiveness of pain neurons in the ventral posterolateral nucleus of the thalamus.[67,102] Those changes are mediated by cannabinoid receptors, are selective for pain neurons, and are unrelated to changes in skin temperature or depth of anesthesia, and they follow the time course of the changes in behavioral responses to painful stimuli but not the time course of motor changes.[67] On-cells and off-cells in the rostral ventral medulla control pain transmission at the level of the spinal cord, and cannabinoids also modulate their responses in a manner that is very similar to that of morphine.[110]

Endogenous Cannabinoids Modulate Pain

Endogenous cannabinoids can modulate pain sensitivity through both central and peripheral mechanisms. For example, animal studies have shown that pain sensitivity can be increased when endogenous cannabinoids are blocked from acting at CB_1 receptors.[22,62,110,130,158] Administration of cannabinoid antagonists in either the spinal cord[130] or paw[22] increase the sensitivity of animals to pain. In addition, there is evidence that cannabinoids act at the site of injury to reduce peripheral inflammation.[131]

Current data suggest that the endogenous cannabinoid analgesic system might offer protection against the long-lasting central hyperalgesia and allodynia that sometimes follow skin or nerve injuries.[130,158] These results raise the possibility that therapeutic interventions that alter the levels of endogenous cannabinoids might be useful for managing pain in humans.

CHRONIC EFFECTS OF THC

Most substances of abuse produce tolerance, physical dependence, and withdrawal symptoms. *Tolerance* is the most common response to repetitive use of a drug and is the condition in which, after repeated exposure to a drug, increasing doses are needed to achieve the same effect. *Physical dependence* develops as a result of a resetting of homeostatic mechanisms in response to repeated drug use. Tolerance, dependence, and withdrawal are not peculiar to drugs of abuse. Many medicines that are not addicting can produce these types of effects; examples of such medications include clonidine, propranolol, and tricyclic antidepressants. The following sections discuss what is known about the biological mechanisms that underlie tolerance, reward, and dependence; clinical studies about those topics are discussed in chapter 3.

Tolerance

Chronic administration of cannabinoids to animals results in tolerance to many of the acute effects of THC, including memory disruption,[34] decreased locomotion,[2,119] hypothermia,[42,125] neuroendocrine effects,[134] and analgesia.[4] Tolerance also develops to the cardiovascular and psychological effects of THC and marijuana in humans (see also discussion in chapter 3).[55,56,76]

Tolerance to cannabinoids appears to result from both *pharmacokinetic* changes (how the drug is absorbed, distributed, metabolized, and excreted) and *pharmacodynamic* changes (how the drug interacts with target cells). Chronic treatment with the cannabinoid agonist, CP 55,940, increases the activity of the microsomal cytochrome P450 oxidative system,[31] the system through which drugs are metabolized in the liver; this suggests pharmacokinetic tolerance. Chronic cannabinoid treatment also produces changes in brain cannabinoid receptors and cannabinoid receptor mRNA concentrations—an indication that pharmacodynamic effects are important as well.

Most studies have found that brain cannabinoid receptor concentrations usually decrease after prolonged exposure to agonists,[42,119,136,138] although some studies have reported increases[137] or no changes[2] in receptor binding in brain. Differences among studies could be due to the particular agonist tested, the assay used, the brain region examined, or the treatment time. For example, the THC analogue, levonantradol, produces a greater desensitization of adenylyl cyclase inhibition than does THC in cultured neuroblastoma cells.[40] This might be explained by differences in efficacy between these two agonists.[18,147] A time course study revealed differences among brain regins in the rates and magnitudes of receptor down regulation.[16] Those findings suggest that tolerance to different effects of cannabinoids develops at different rates.

Chronic treatment with THC also produces variable effects on cannabinoid-mediated signal transduction systems. It produces substantial desensitization of cannabinoid-activated G proteins in a number of rat brain regions.[147] The time course of this desensitization varies across brain regions.[16]

It is difficult to extend the findings of short-term animal studies to human marijuana use. To simulate long-term use, higher doses are used in animal studies than are normally achieved by smoking marijuana. For example, the average human will feel "high" after injection of THC at a level of 0.06 mg/kg,[118] compared with the 10–20 mg/kg per day used in many chronic rat studies. At the same time, doses of marijuana needed to observe behavioral changes in rats (usually changes in locomotor behavior) are substantially higher than doses at which people feel "high." The pharmacokinetics of THC distribution in the body are also dramatically different between rats and humans and depend heavily on whether it is inhaled, injected, or swallowed. It is likely that some of the same biochemical adaptations to chronic cannabinoid administration occur in laboratory animals and humans, but the magnitude of the effects in humans might be less than that in animals in proportion to the doses used.

Reward and Dependence

Experimental animals that are given the opportunity to self-administer cannabinoids generally do not choose to do so, which has led to the conclusion that they are not reinforcing and rewarding.[38] However, behavioral[95] and brain stimulation[94] studies have shown that THC can be rewarding to animals. The behavioral study used a "place preference" test, in which an animal is given repeated doses of a drug in one place, and is then given a choice between a place where it received the drug and a place where it did not. The animals chose the place where they received the THC. These rewarding effects are highly dose dependent. In all models studied, cannabinoids are only rewarding at midrange; doses that are too low are not rewarding; doses that are too high can be aversive. Mice will self-administer the cannabinoid agonist WIN 55,212-2 but only at low doses.[106] This effect is specifically mediated by CB_1 receptors and indicates that stimulation of those receptors is rewarding to the mice. Antagonism of cannabinoid receptors is also rewarding in rats; in conditioned place preference tests, animals show a preference for the place they receive the cannabinoid antagonist SR 141716A at both low and high doses.[140] Cannabinoids increase dopamine concentrations in the mesolimbic dopamine system of rats, a pathway associated with reinforcement.[25,39,161] However, the mechanism by which THC increases dopamine concentrations appears to be different from that of other abused drugs[51] (see chapter 3 for further discussion of reinforcement). THC-induced increases in dopamine are due to increases in the firing rate of dopamine cells in the ventral tegmental area by Δ^9-THC.[47] However, these increases in firing rate in the ventral tegmental area could not be explained by increases in the firing of the A10 dopamine cell group, where other abused drugs have been shown to act.[51]

Physical dependence on cannabinoids has been observed only under experimental conditions of "precipitated withdrawal" in which animals are first treated chronically with cannabinoids and then given the CB_1 antagonist SR 141716A.[3,166] The addition of the antagonist accentuates any withdrawal effect by competing with the agonist at receptor sites; that is, the antagonist helps to clear agonists off and keep them off receptor sites. This suggests that, under normal cannabis use, the long half-life and slow elimination from the body of THC and the residual bioactivity of its metabolite, 11-OH-THC, can prevent substantial abstinence symptoms. The precipitated withdrawal produced by SR 141716A has some of the characteristics of opiate withdrawal, but it is not affected by opioid antagonists, and it affects motor systems differently. An earlier study with monkeys also suggested that abrupt cessation of chronic THC is associated with withdrawal symptoms.[8] Monkeys in that study were trained to work for food after which they were given THC on a daily basis; when the investigators stopped administering THC, the animals stopped working for food.

A study in rats indicated that the behavioral cannabinoid withdrawal syndrome is consistent with the consequences of withdrawal from other drugs of abuse in that it correlates with the effects of stimulation of central amygdaloid corticotropin-releasing hormone release.[135] However, the withdrawal syndrome for cannabinoids and the corresponding increase in corticotropin-releasing hormone are observed only after administration of the CB_1 antagonist SR 141716A to cannabinoid-tolerant animals.[3,166] The implications of data based on precipitated withdrawal in animals for human cannabinoid abuse have not been established.[166] Furthermore, acute administration of THC also produces increases in corticotropin-releasing hormone and adrenocorticotropin release; both are stress-related hormones.[71] This set of withdrawal studies may explain the generally aversive effects of cannabinoids in animals and could indicate that the increase in corticotropin-releasing hormone is merely a rebound effect. Thus, cannabinoids appear to be conforming to some of the neurobiological effects of other drugs abused by humans, but the underlying mechanisms of these actions and their value for determining the reinforcement and dependence liability of cannabinoids in humans remain undetermined.

CANNABINOIDS AND THE IMMUNE SYSTEM

The human body protects itself from invaders, such as bacteria and viruses through the elaborate and dynamic network of organs and cells referred to as the immune system. Cannabinoids, especially THC, can modulate the function of immune cells in various ways—in some cases enhancing and in others diminishing the immune response[85] (summarized in Table 2.7). However, the natural function of cannabinoids in the immune system is not known. Immune cells respond to cannabinoids in a variety of ways, depending on such factors as drug concentration, timing of drug delivery to leukocytes in relation to antigen stimulation, and type of cell function. Although the chronic effects of cannabinoids on the immune system have not been studied, based on acute exposure studies in experimental animals it appears that THC concentrations that modulate immunological responses are higher than those required for psychoactivity.

The CB_2 receptor gene, which is not expressed in the brain, is particularly abundant in immune tissues, with an expression level 10–100 times higher than that of CB_1. In spleen and tonsils the CB_2 mRNA* content is equivalent to that of CB_1 mRNA in the brain.[48] The rank order, from high to low, of CB_2 mRNA levels in immune cells is B-cells > natural killer cells >> monocytes > polymorphonuclear neutrophil cells > T8 cells > T4 cells. In tonsils the CB_2 receptors appear to be restricted to B-lymphocyte-enriched areas. In contrast, CB_1 receptors are mainly expressed in the central nervous system and, to a lesser extent, in several peripheral tissues such as adrenal gland, heart, lung, prostate, uterus, ovary, testis, bone marrow, thymus, and tonsils.

---

*After a gene is transcribed, it is often spliced and modified into mRNA, or message RNA. The CB-2 mRNA is the gene "message" that moves from the cell nucleus into the cytoplasm where it will be translated into the receptor protein.

TABLE 2.7   Effects of Cannabinoids on the Immune System

Drug Tested	Cell Types Tested or Type of Animal Experiment	Drug Concentration*
THC, 2-AG, 11-OH-THC, CBN	Lymphocytes and splenocytes *in vitro*	0.1–30 µM
THC, 2-AG	Lymphocytes and splenocytes	0.1–25 µM
Anandamide	Splenocytes *in vitro*	1–25 µM
THC, 11-OH-THC, 2-AG	Splenocytes *in vitro*	3–30 µM
THC, CP 55,940, WIN 55,212-2	Lymphocytes *in vitro*	0.1–100 nM (0.0001–0.1 µM)
THC	Drug injected into mice	>5 mg/kg
HU-210	Drug injected into mice	>0.05 mg/kg
THC, 11-OH-THC, CBD, CP 55,940, CBN	Splenocytes *in vitro*	1–30 µM
THC	Drug injected into rodents	3 mg/kg per day for 25 days, 40 mg/kg per day for 2 days
THC, 11-OH-THC	Natural killer cells *in vitro*	0.1–32 µM
THC	Peritoneal macrophages and monocytes	3–30 µM
THC, CBD	Drug injected into mice; in one case, *in vitro* tests done on spleens	>5 mg/kg per day for 4 days or 50 mg/kg every 5 days for up to 8 weeks
THC, CBD	Peripheral blood mononuclear cells *in vitro*	<0.1 µM 30 µM
THC, CBD	Splenocytes and T cells *in vitro*	10 µM
THC	Phorbol myristate acetate-differentiated macrophage *in vitro*	10–20 µM
THC	Endotoxin-activated macrophages *in vitro*	10–30 µM
THC	Peritoneal macrophages *in vitro*	10–30 µM

Result	Reference
Higher doses suppressed T cell proliferation	Luo, 1992; Pross, 1992;[b] Klein, 1985;[c] Specter, 1990;[d] Lee, 1995;[a] Herring, 1998
Lower doses increased T cell proliferation *in vitro*	Luo, 1992; Lee, 1995;[a] Pross, 1992[b]
Little or no effect on T cell proliferation	Lee, 1995;[a] Devane, 1992
Decreased B cell proliferation	Klein, 1985;[c] Lee, 1995[a]
Increased B cell proliferation	Derocq, 1995
Antibody production suppressed	Baczynsky, 1983; Schatz, 1993
Antibody production suppressed	Titishov, 1989
Antibody production suppressed	Klein, 1990; Baczynsky, 1983; Kaminski, 1992, 1994; Herring, 1998
Repeated low doses or a high dose of THC suppressed the activity of natural killer cells	Patel, 1985; Klein, 1987
Doses of ≥10 µM suppressed natural killer cell cytolytic activity; doses <10 µM produced no effect	Klein, 1987; Luo, 1989
Variable doses of THC suppressed macophage functions in vitro	Lopez-Cepero, 1986; Specter, 1991; Tang, 1992
THC suppressed normal immune response; interferons failed to increase when exposed to cytokine inducer; CBD had no suppressive effect	Cabral, 1986; Blanchard, 1986
Increased interferon production Decreased interferon production	Watzl, 1991
Both THC and CBD suppressed interleukin-2 secretion and number of interleukin-2 transcripts	Condie, 1996
Increased tumor necrosis factor production and interleukin-1 supernatant bioactivity	Shivers, 1994
Increased processing and release of interleukin-1 rather than cellular production of interleukin-1	Zhu, 1994
Increased interleukin-1 bioactivity	Klein, 1990

Continued

TABLE 2.7 *Continued*

Drug Tested	Cell Types Tested or Type of Animal Experiment	Drug Concentration*
THC	Drug and sublethal or lethal dose of *Legionella pneumophilia* injected in mice	8 mg/kg before and after bacterial infection <5 mg/kg doses or one 8 mg/kg or 4 mg/kg dose before bacteria infection
THC	Drug and herpes simplex virus injected in immunodeficient mice	100 mg/kg before and after viral infection 100 mg/kg before viral infection

[a]Cell density dependent.
[b]Mitogen dependent.
[c]Dependent on serum concentration in cell culture medium.
[d]Dependent on timing of drug exposure relative to mitogen exposure.
*Drug concentrations are given in the standard format of molarity (M). A 1-M solution is the molecular weight of the compound (in grams) in 1 liter (L) of solution. The molecular

---

Box 2.1 Cells of the Immune System

The various organs of the immune system are positioned throughout the body and include bone marrow, thymus, lymph nodes, and spleen. The cells of the immune system consist of white blood cells, or leukocytes, which are formed in the bone marrow from stem cells—so-called because a great variety of cells descend from them (see below). There are two kinds of leukocytes: lymphocytes and phagocytes. *Lymphocytes* consist of B cells, T cells (B and T refer to where the cells mature, either in the bone marrow [B] or thymus [T]), and natural killer (NK) cells; the major phagocytes are monocytes, macrophages, and neutrophils. *Phagocytes* have many important roles in the immune response; most important is that they initiate the response by engulfing and digesting foreign substances, or antigens (such as bacteria, viruses, and foreign proteins), that enter the body. Once digested, the antigens are exposed to specialized lymphocytes, some of which produce antibodies and effector T cells, which help destroy any antigens remaining in the body. *Antibodies* are proteins produced by B cells that bind to antigens and promote antigen destruction. Effector T cells include killer T cells, which attack and kill antigen laden cells, and helper T cells, which secrete special proteins called cytokines that promote antigen elimination. NK cells are specialized lymphocytes that are also activated by antigen to either kill infected targets or secrete immunoregulatory cytokines.

Result	Reference
Cytokine-mediated septic shock and death occurred with exposure to sublethal dose of bacteria	Klein, 1993, 1994; Newton, 1994
Survival occurred, but with greater susceptiblity to infection when challenged with bacteria and death when challenged with a lethal dose of bacteria	
Two high doses of THC potentiated the effects of herpes simplex and enhanced the progression of death	Specter, 1991
Single dose did not promote death	

weight of THC is 314, so a 1-M solution would be 314 g of THC in 1 L of solution, and a 10-μM solution would be 3.14 mg THC/L.

A 1- to 10-μM concentration will generally elicit a physiologically relevant response in immune cell cultures. Higher doses are often suspected of not being biologically meaningful because they are much larger than would ever be achieved in the body. The doses listed in this table are, for the most part, very high. See text for further discussion.

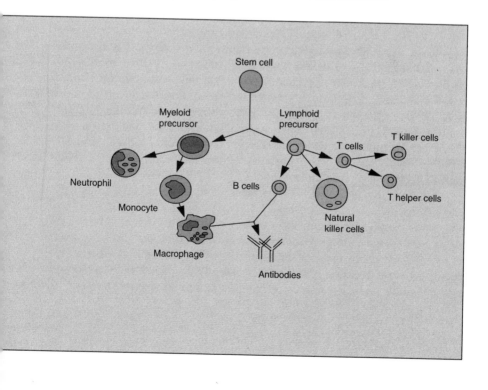

Cannabinoid Receptors and Intracellular Action in Immune Cells

CB_2 appears to be the predominant gene expressed in resting leukocytes.[78,112] The level of CB_1 gene activity is normally low in resting cells but increases with cell activation.[32] Thus the CB_1 receptor might be important only when immune responses are stimulated, but the physiological relevance of this observation remains to be determined. Some of the cannabinoid effects observed in immune systems, especially at high drug concentrations, are likely mediated through nonreceptor mechanisms, but these have not yet been identified.[4]

Ligand binding to either CB_1 or CB_2 inhibits adenylate cyclase, an enzyme that is responsible for cAMP production and is, thus, an integral aspect of intracellular signal transduction (see Figure 2.3).[53,79,91,122,139,151,167] Increases in intracellular cAMP concentrations lead to immune enhancement, and decreases lead to an inhibition of the immune response.[77] Cannabinoids inhibit the rise in intracellular cAMP that normally results from leukocyte activation, and this might be the pathway through which cannabinoids suppress immune cell functions.[28,74,167] In addition, cannabinoids activate other molecular pathways such as the nuclear factor-kB pathway, and therefore these signals might be modified in drug-treated immune cells.[33,74]

T and B Cells

When stimulated by antigen, lymphocytes (see Box 2.1) first proliferate and then mature or differentiate to become potent effector cells, such as B cells that release antibodies or T cells that release cytokines. The normal T-cell proliferation that is seen when human lymphocytes and mouse splenocytes (spleen cells) are exposed to antigens and mitogens* can be inhibited by THC, 11-OH-THC, cannabinol, and 2-AG, as well as synthetic cannabinoid agonists such as CP 55,940; WIN 55,212-2; and HU-210.[61,89,93,99,127,155] In contrast, one study testing anandamide revealed little or no effect on T cell proliferation.[93]

However, these drug effects are variable and depend on experimental conditions, such as the experimental drug dose used, the mitogen used, the percentage of serum in the culture, and the timing of cannabinoid drug exposure. In general, lower doses of cannabinoids increase proliferation and higher doses suppress proliferation. Doses that are effective in suppressing immune function are typically greater than 10 µM in cell culture studies and greater than 5 mg/kg in whole-animal studies.[85] By

---

*Mitogens are substances that stimulate cell division (mitosis) and cell transformation.

comparison, at 0.05 mg/kg, people will experience the full psychoactive effects of THC; however, because of their high metabolic rates, small rodents frequently require drug doses that are 100-fold higher than doses needed for humans to achieve comparable drug effects. Thus, the immune effects of doses of cannabinoids higher than those ever experienced by humans should be interpreted with caution.[93]

As with T cells, B cell proliferation can be suppressed by various cannabinoids, such as THC, 11-OH-THC, and 2-AG, but B cell proliferation is more inhibited at lower drug concentrations than T cell proliferation.[89,93] Conversely, low doses of THC, CP 55,940 and WIN 55,212-2 *increase* B cell proliferation in cultured human cells exposed to mitogen.[35] This effect possibly involves the CB_2 receptor, because the effect appears to be the same when the CB_1 receptor was blocked by the antagonist SR 141716A (which does not block the CB_2 receptor). The reason for the differences in B cell responsiveness to cannabinoids is probably due to differences in cell type and source; for example, B cells collected from mouse spleen might respond to cannabinoids somewhat differently than B cells from human tonsils.

Natural Killer Cells

Repeated injections of relatively low doses of THC (3 mg/kg/day[121*]) or two injections of a high dose (40 mg/kg[86]) suppress the ability of NK cells to destroy foreign cells in rats and mice. THC can also suppress cytolytic activity of the NK cells in cell cultures; 11-OH-THC is even more potent.[86] In contrast, THC concentrations below 10 µM had no effect on NK cell activity in mouse cell cultures.[98]

Macrophages

Macrophages perform various functions, including phagocytosis (ingestion and destruction of foreign substances), cytolysis, antigen presentation to lymphocytes, and production of active proteins involved in destroying microorganisms, tissue repair, and modulation of immune cells. Those functions can be suppressed by THC doses similar to those capable of modulating lymphocyte functions (see above).[88,109]

---

*While 3 mg/kg would be a high dose for humans (see Table 3.1), in rodents, it is a low dose for immunological effects and a moderate dose for behavioral effects.

Cytokines

Cytokines are proteins produced by immune cells. When released from the producing cell, they can alter the function of other cells they come in contact with. In a sense they are like hormones. Thus, cannabinoids can either increase or decrease cytokine production depending upon experimental conditions.

Some cytokines, such as interferon-γ and interleukin-2 (IL-2), are produced by T helper-1 (Th1) cells. These cytokines help to activate cell-mediated immunity and the killer cells that eliminate microorganisms from the body (see Box 2.1). When injected into mice, THC suppresses the production of those cytokines that modulate the host response to infection (see below).[115] Cannabinoids also modulate interferons induced by viral infection,[21] as well as other interferon inducers.[85] Furthermore, in human cell cultures, interferon production can be increased by low concentrations but decreased by high concentrations of either THC or CBD.[168] In addition to Th1 cytokines, cannabinoids modulate the production of cytokines such as interleukin-1 (IL-1), tumor necrosis factor (TNF), and interleukin-6 (IL-6).[145,176] At 8 mg/kg, THC can increase the *in vivo* mobilization of serum acute-phase cytokines, including IL-1, TNF, and IL-6.[90] Finally, although these studies suggest that cannabinoids can induce an increase in cytokines, other studies suggest that they can also suppress cytokine production.[85] The different results might be due to different cell culture conditions or because different cell lines were studied.

Antibody Production

Antibody production is an important measure of humoral immune function as contrasted with cellular (cell-mediated) immunity. Antibody production can be suppressed in mice injected with relatively low doses of THC (>5 mg/kg) or HU-210 (>0.05 mg/kg) and in mouse spleen cell cultures exposed to a variety of cannabinoids, including THC, 11-OH-THC, cannabinol, cannabidiol, CP 55,940, or HU-210.[5,6,61,78,79,84,85,142,164] However, the inhibition of antibody response by cannabinoids was only observed when antibody-forming cells were exposed to T-cell-dependent antigens (the responses require functional T cells and macrophages as accessory cells). Conversely, antibody responses to several T-cell-independent antigens were not inhibited by THC; this suggests that B cells are relatively insensitive to inhibition by cannabinoids.[142]

Resistance to Infection in Animals Exposed to Cannabinoids

Evaluation of bacterial infections in mice that received injections of

THC can suppress resistance to infection, although the effect depends on the dose and timing of drug administration. Mice pretreated with THC (8 mg/kg) one day before infection with a sublethal dose of the pneumonia-causing bacteria *Legionella pneumophilia* and then treated again one day after the infection with THC developed symptoms of cytokine-mediated septic shock and died; control mice that were not pretreated with THC became immune to repeated infection and survived the bacterial challenge.[90] If only one injection of THC was given or doses less than 5 mg/kg were used, all the mice survived the initial infection but failed to survive later challenge with a lethal dose of the bacteria; hence, these mice failed to develop immune memory in response to the initial sublethal infection.[87] Note that these are very high doses and are considerably higher than doses experienced by marijuana users (see Figure 3.1).[115] In rats, doses of 4.0 mg/kg THC are aversive.[95]

Few studies have been done to evaluate the effect of THC on viral infections, and this subject needs further study.[20] Compared to healthy animals, THC might have greater immunosuppressive effects in animals whose immune systems are severely weakened. For example, a very high dose of THC (100 mg/kg) given two days before and after herpes simplex virus infection was shown to be a cofactor with the virus in advancing the progression to death in an immunodeficient mouse model infected with a leukemia virus.[85] However, THC given as a single dose (100 mg/kg) two days before herpes simplex virus infection did not promote the progression to death. Hence, whether THC is immunosuppressive probably depends on the timing of THC exposure relative to an infection.

Antiinflammatory Effects

As discussed above, cannabinoid drugs can modulate the production of cytokines, which are central to inflammatory processes in the body. In addition, several studies have shown directly that cannabinoids can be antiinflammatory. For example, in rats with autoimmune encephalomyelitis (an experimental model used to study multiple sclerosis), cannabinoids were shown to attenuate the signs and the symptoms of central nervous system damage.[100,172] (Some believe that nerve damage associated with multiple sclerosis is caused by an inflammatory reaction.) Likewise, the cannabinoid, HU-211, was shown to suppress brain inflammation that resulted from closed-head injury[146] or infectious meningitis[7] in studies on rats. HU-211 is a synthetic cannabinoid that does not bind to cannabinoid receptors and is not psychoactive;[7] thus, without direct evidence, the effects of marijuana cannot be assumed to include those of HU-211. CT-3, another atypical cannabinoid, suppresses acute and chronic joint inflammation in animals.[178] It is a nonpsychoactive synthetic derivative of 11-THC-oic acid (a breakdown product of THC) and does not appear to bind to cannabinoid receptors.[129] Cannabichromene, a cannabinoid found in marijuana, has also been reported to have antiinflammatory properties.[173] No mechanism of action for possible antiinflammatory effects of cannabinoids has been identified, and the effects of these atypical cannabinoids and effects of marijuana are not yet established.

It is interesting to note that two reports of cannabinoid-induced analgesia are based on the ability of the endogenous cannabinoids, anandamide and PEA, to reduce pain associated with local inflammation that was experimentally induced by subcutaneous injections of dilute formalin.[22,73] Both THC and anandamide can increase serum levels of ACTH and corticosterone in animals.[169] Those hormones are involved in regulating many responses in the body, including those to inflammation. The possible link between experimental cannabinoid-induced analgesia and reported antiinflammatory effects of cannabinoids is important for potential therapeutic uses of cannabinoid drugs but has not yet been established.

Conclusions Regarding Effects on the Immune System

Cell culture and animal studies have established cannabinoids as immunomodulators—that is, they increase some immune responses and decrease others. The variable responses depend on such experimental factors as drug dose, timing of delivery, and type of immune cell examined. Cannabinoids affect multiple cellular targets in the immune system and a variety of effector functions. Many of the effects noted above appear to occur at concentrations over 5 μM *in vitro* and over 5 μg/kg *in vivo*.* By comparison, a 5-mg injection of THC into a person (about 0.06 mg/kg) is enough to produce strong psychoactive effects. It should be emphasized, however, that little is known about the immune effects of chronic low-dose exposure to cannabinoids.

Another issue in need of further clarification involves the potential usefulness of cannabinoids as therapeutic agents in inflammatory diseases. Glucocorticoids have historically been used for these diseases, but nonpsychotropic cannabinoids potentially have fewer side effects and might thus offer an improvement over glucocorticoids in treating inflammatory diseases.

In vitro studies are those in which animal cells or tissue are removed and studied outside the animal; *in vivo* studies are those in which experiments are conducted in the whole animal.

TABLE 2.8 Historical Comparisons Between Cannabinoids and Opiates

Pharmacological Discoveries	Cannabinoids		Opiates	
Discovery of receptor existence	**1988**	(Devane et al. and Dill and Howlett)[36,40]	**1973**	(Pert and Snyder, Simon, and Terenius)[123,149,162]
Identification of receptor antagonist	**1994**	SR 141716A (Rinaldi-Carmona et al.)[132]	Before 1973: naloxone	
Discovery of first endogenous ligand	**1992**	anandamide (Devane et al.)[37]	**1975**	met- and leu-enkephalin (Hughes et al.)[70]
First receptor cloned	**1990** (Matsuda et al.)[107]		**1992**	(Evans et al. and Kieffer et al.)[41,82]
Natural functions	Unknown		Pain, reproduction, mood, movement, and others	

CONCLUSIONS AND RECOMMENDATIONS

Given the progress of the past 15 years in understanding the effects of cannabinoids, research in the next decade is likely to reveal even more. It is interesting to compare how little we know about cannabinoids with how much we know about opiates. Table 2.8 suggests good reason for optimism about the future of cannabinoid drug development. Now that many of the basic tools of cannabinoid pharmacology and biology have been developed, one can expect to see rapid advances that can begin to match what is known of opiate systems in the brain.

Despite the tremendous progress in understanding the pharmacology and neurobiology of brain cannabinoid systems, this field is still in its early developmental stages. A key focus for future study is the neurobiology of endogenous cannabinoids; establishing the precise brain localization (in which cells and where) of cannabinoids, cellular storage and release mechanisms, and uptake mechanisms will be crucial in determining the biological role of this system. Technology needed to establish the biological significance of these systems will be broad based and include such research tools as the transgenic or gene knockout mice, as has already been accomplished for various opioid-receptor types.[26] In 1997, both CB_1 and CB_2 knockout mice were generated by a team of scientists at the National Institutes of Health, and a group in France has developed another strain of CB_1 knockout mice.[92]

Several research tools will greatly aid such investigations, in particular a greater selection of agonists and antagonists that permit discrimination in activation between CB_1 and CB_2 and hydrophilic agonists that can be delivered to animals or cells more effectively than hydrophobic compounds. In the area of drug development, future progress should continue to provide more specific agonists and antagonists for CB_1 and CB_2 receptors, with varying potential for therapeutic uses.

There are certain areas that will provide keys to a better understanding of the potential therapeutic value of cannabinoids. For example, basic biology indicates a role for cannabinoids in pain and control of movement, which is consistent with a possible therapeutic role in these areas. The evidence is relatively strong for the treatment of pain and, intriguing although less well established, for movement disorders. The neuroprotective properties of cannabinoids might prove therapeutically useful, although it should be noted that this is a new area and other, better studied, neuroprotective drugs have not yet been shown to be therapeutically useful. Cannabinoid research is clearly relevant not only to drug abuse but also to understanding basic human biology. Further, it offers the potential for the discovery and development of new therapeutically useful drugs.

CONCLUSION: At this point, our knowledge about the biology of marijuana and cannabinoids allows us to make some general conclusions:

- Cannabinoids likely have a natural role in pain modulation, control of movement, and memory.
- The natural role of cannabinoids in immune systems is likely multi-faceted and remains unclear.
- The brain develops tolerance to cannabinoids.
- Animal research has demonstrated the potential for dependence, but this potential is observed under a narrower range of conditions than with benzodiazepines, opiates, cocaine, or nicotine.
- Withdrawal symptoms can be observed in animals but appear mild compared with those of withdrawal from opiates or benzodiazepines, such as diazepam (Valium).

CONCLUSION: The different cannabinoid receptor types found in the body appear to play different roles in normal physiology. In addition, some effects of cannabinoids appear to be independent of those receptors. The variety of mechanisms through which cannabinoids can influence human physiology underlies the variety of potential therapeutic uses for drugs that might act selectively on different cannabinoid systems.

RECOMMENDATION: **Research should continue into the physiological effects of synthetic and plant-derived cannabinoids and the natural function of cannabinoids found in the body. Because different cannabinoids appear to have different effects, cannabinoid research should include, but not be restricted to, effects attributable to THC alone.**

This chapter has summarized recent progress in understanding the basic biology of cannabinoids and provides a foundation for the next two chapters which review studies on the potential health risks (chapter 3) and benefits of marijuana use (chapter 4).

REFERENCES

1. Abood ME, Martin BR. 1996. Molecular neurobiology of the cannabinoid receptor. *International Review of Neurobiology* 39:197–221.
2. Abood ME, Sauss C, Fan F, Tilton CL, Martin BR. 1993. Development of behavioral tolerance to delta 9-THC without alteration of cannabinoid receptor binding or mRNA levels in whole brain. *Pharmacology, Biochemistry and Behavior* 46:575–579.
3. Aceto MD, Scates SM, Lowe JA, Martin BR. 1995. Cannabinoid precipitated withdrawal by the selective cannabinoid receptor antagonist, SR 141716A. *European Journal of Pharmacology* 282:R1–R2.
4. Adams IB, Martin BR. 1996. Cannabis: Pharmacology and toxicology in animals and humans. *Addiction* 91:1585–1614.
5. Baczynsky WO, Zimmerman AM. 1983a. Effects of delta-9-tetrahydrocannabinol, cannabinol, and cannabidiol on the immune system in mice: I. In vivo investigation of the primary and secondary immune response. *Pharmacology* 26:1–11.
6. Baczynsky WO, Zimmerman AM. 1983b. Effects of delta 9-tetrahydrocannabinol, cannabinol and cannabidiol on the immune system in mice. II. In vitro investigation using cultured mouse splenocytes. *Pharmacology* 26:12–19.
7. Bass R, Engelhard D, Trembovler V, Shohami E. 1996. A novel nonpsychotropic cannabinoid, HU-211, in the treatment of experimental pneumococcal meningitis. *Journal of Infectious Diseases* 173:735–738.
8. Beardsley PM, Balster RL, Harris LS. 1986. Dependence on tetrahydrocannabinol in rhesus monkeys. *Journal of Pharmacology and Experimental Therapeutics* 239:311–319.
9. Ben-Shabat S, Fride E, Sheskin T, Tamiri T, Rhee MH, Vogel Z, Bisogno T, De Petrocellis L, Di Marzo V, Mechoulam R. 1998. An entourage effect: Inactive endogenous fatty acid glycerol esters enhance 2-arachidonoyl-glycerol cannabinoid activity. *European Journal of Pharmacology* 353:23–31.
10. Bennett GJ. 1994. Neuropathic pain. In: Wall PD, Melzack R, Editors, *Textbook of Pain*. Edinburgh: Churchill Livingstone.
11. Bird KD, Boleyn T, Chesher GB, Jackson DM, Starmer GA, Teo RKC. 1980. Inter-cannabinoid and cannabinoid-ethanol interactions and their effects on human performance. *Psychopharmacology* 71:181–188.

12. Bloom AS, Dewey WL, Harris LS, Brosius KK. 1977. 9-nor-9b-hydroxyhexa-hydrocannabinol, a cannabinoid with potent antinociceptive activity: Comparisons with morphine. *Journal of Pharmacology and Experimental Therapeutics* 200:263–270.

13. Bornheim LM, Everhart ET, Li J, Correia MA. 1994. Induction and genetic regulation of mouse hepatic cytochrome P450 by cannabidiol. *Biochemical Pharmacology (England)* 48:161–171.

14. Bornheim LM, Kim KY, Chen B, Correia MA. 1993. The effect of cannabidiol on mouse hepatic microsomal cytochrome P450-dependent anandamide metabolism. *Biochemical and Biophysical Research Communications (United States)* 197:740–746.

15. Bornheim LM, Kim KY, Li J, Perotti BY, Benet LZ. 1995. Effect of cannabidiol pretreatment on the kinetics of tetrahydrocannabinol metabolites in mouse brain. *Drug Metabolism and Disposition (United States)* 23:825–831.

16. Breivogel CS, Sim LJ, Childers SR. 1997. Regional differences in cannabinoid receptor/G-protein coupling in rat brain. *Journal of Pharmacology and Experimental Therapeutics* 282:1632–1642.

17. British Medical Association. 1997. *Therapeutic Uses of Cannabis.* Amsterdam, The Netherlands: Harwood Academic Publishers.

18. Burkey TH, Quock RM, Consroe P, Roeske WR, Yamamura HI. 1997. Delta-9-tetrahydrocannabinol is a partial agonist of cannabinoid receptors in mouse brain. *European Journal of Pharmacology* 323:R3–R4.

19. Buxbaum DM. 1972. Analgesic activity of Δ^9-tetrahydrocannabinol in the rat and mouse. *Psychopharmacology* 25:275–280.

20. Cabral GA , Dove Pettit DA. 1998. Drugs and immunity: Cannabinoids and their role in decreased resistance to infectious disease. *Journal of Neuroimmunology* 83:116–123.

21. Cabral GA, Lockmuller JC, Mishkin EM. 1986. Delta-9-tetrahydrocannabinol decreases alpha/beta interferon response to herpes simplex virus type 2 in the B6C3F1 mouse. *Proceedings of the Society for Experimental Biology and Medicine* 181:305–311.

22. Calignano A, La Rana G, Giuffrida A, Piomelli D. 1998. Control of pain initiation by endogenous cannabinoids. *Nature* 394:277–281.

23. Campbell KA, Foster TC, Hampson RE, Deadwyler SA. 1986a. Delta-9-tetrahydrocannabinol differentially affects sensory-evoked potentials in the rat dentate gyrus. *Journal of Pharmacology and Experimental Therapeutics* 239:936–940.

24. Campbell KA, Foster TC, Hapson RE, Deadwyler SA. 1986b. Effects of delta-9-tetrahydrocannabinol on sensory-evoked discharges of granule cells in the dentate gyrus of behaving rats. *Journal of Pharmacology and Experimental Therapeutics* 239:941–945.

25. Chen J, Marmur R, Pulles A, Paredes W, Gardner EL. 1993. Ventral tegmental microinjection of delta-9-tetrahydrocannabinol enhances ventral tegmental somatodendritic dopamine levels but not forebrain dopamine levels: Evidence for local neural action by marijuana's psychoactive ingredient. *Brain Research* 621:65–70.

26. Childers SR. 1997. Opioid receptors: Pinning down the opiate targets. *Current Biology* 7:R695–R697.

27. Childers SR, Breivogel CS. 1998. Cannabis and endogenous cannabinoid systems. *Drug and Alcohol Dependence* 51:173–187.

28. Coffey RG, Yamamoto Y, Shella E, Pross S. 1996. Tetrahydrocannabinol inhibition of macrophage nitric oxide production. *Biochemical Pharmacology* 52:743–751.

29. Collins DR, Pertwee RG, Davies SN. 1994. The action of synthetic cannabinoids on the induction of long-term potentiation in the rat hippocampal slice. *European Journal of Pharmacology* 259:R7–R8.

30. Collins DR, Pertwee RG, Davies SN. 1995. Prevention by the cannabinoid antagonist, SR141716A, of cannabinoid-mediated blockade of long-term potentiation in the rat hippocampal slice. *British Journal of Pharmacology* 115:869–870.
31. Costa B, Parolaro D, Colleoni M. 1996. Chronic cannabinoid, CP-55,940, administration alters biotransformation in the rat. *European Journal of Pharmacology* 313:17–24.
32. Daaka Y, Friedman H, Klein T. 1996. Cannabinoid receptor proteins are increased in Jurkat, human T-cell line after mitogen activation. *Journal of Pharmacology and Experimental Therapeutics* 276:776–783.
33. Daaka Y, Zhu W, Friedman H, Klein T. 1997. Induction of interleukin-2 receptor α gene by Δ9-tetrahydrocannabinol is mediated by nuclear factor κB and CB_1 cannabinoid receptor. *DNA and Cell Biology* 16:301–309.
34. Deadwyler SA, Heyser CJ, Hampson RE. 1995. Complete adaptation to the memory disruptive effects of delta-9-THC following 35 days of exposure. *Neuroscience Research Communications* 17:9–18.
35. Derocq JM, Segui M, Marchand J, Le Fur G, Casellas P. 1995. Cannabinoids enhance human B-cell growth at low nanomolar concentrations. *FEBS Letters* 369:177–182.
36. Devane WA, Dysarc FA, Johnson MR, Melvin LS, Howlett AC. 1988. Determination and characterization of a cannabinoid receptor in rat brain. *Molecular Pharmacology* 34:605–613.
37. Devane WA, Hanus L, Breuer A, Pertwee RG, Stevenson LA, Griffing F, Gibson D, Mandelbaum A, Etinger A, Mechoulam R. 1992. Isolation and structure of a brain constituent that binds to the cannabinoid receptor. *Science* 258:1946–1949.
38. Dewey WL. 1986. Cannabinoid pharamacology. *Pharmacology Review* 38:151–178.
39. Di Chiara G, Imperato A. 1988. Drugs abused by humans preferentially increase synaptic dopamine concentrations in the mesolimbic system of freely moving rats. *Proceedings of the National Academy of Sciences, USA* 85:5274–5278.
40. Dill JA, Howlett AC. 1988. Regulation of adenylate cyclase by chronic exposure to cannabimimetic drugs. *Journal of Pharmacology and Experimental Therapeutics* 244:1157–1163.
41. Evans DJ, Keith DEJ, Morrison H, Magendzo K, Edwards RH. 1992. Cloning of a delta opioid receptor by functional expression. *Science* 258:1952–1955.
42. Fan F, Tao Q, Abood ME, Martin BR. 1996. Cannabinoid receptor down-regulation without alteration of the inhibitory effect of CP 55,940 on adenylyl cyclase in the cerebellum of CP 55,940-tolerant mice. *Brain Research* 706:13–20.
43. Felder CC, Glass M. 1998. Cannabinoid receptors and their endogenous agonists. *Annual Reviews of Pharmacology and Toxicology* 38:179–200.
44. Felder CC, Nielsen A, Briley EM, Palkovits M, Priller J, Axelrod J, Nguyen DN, Richardson JM, Riggin RM, Koppel GA, Paul SM, Becker GW. 1996. Isolation and measurement of the endogenous cannabinoid receptor agonist, anandamide, in brain and peripheral tissues of human and rat. *FEBS Letters* 393:231–235.
45. Fields HL. 1987. *Pain*. New York: McGraw-Hill.
46. Formukong EA, Evans AT, Evans FJ. 1988. Analgesic and antiinflammatory activity of constituents of Cannabis sativa L. *Inflammation* 12:361–371.
47. French ED. 1997. Delta-9-tetrahydrocannabinol excites rat VTA dopamine neurons through activation of cannabinoid CB_1 but not opioid receptors. *Neuroscience Letters* 226:159–162.
48. Galiegue S, Mary S, Marchand J, Dussossoy D, Carriere D, Carayon P, Bouaboula M, Shire D, Le Fur G, Casellas P. 1995. Expression of central and peripheral cannabinoid receptors in human immune tissues and leukocyte subpopulations. *European Journal of Biochemistry* 232:54–61.

49. Gessa GL, Mascia MS, Casu MA, Carta G. 1997. Inhibition of hippocampal acetylcholine release by cannabinoids: Reversal by SR 141716A. *European Journal of Pharmacology* 327:R1–R2.
50. Gifford AN, Ashby Jr CR. 1996. Electrically evoked acetylcholine release from hippocampal slices is inhibited by the cannabinoid receptor agonist, WIN 55212-2, and is potentiated by the cannabinoid antagonist, SR 141716A. *Journal of Pharmacology and Experimental Therapeutics* 277:1431–1436.
51. Gifford AN, Gardner EL, Ashby CRJ. 1997. The effect of intravenous administration of delta-9-tetrahydrocannabinol on the activity of A10 dopamine neurons recorded *in vivo* in anesthetized rats. *Neuropsychobiology* 36:96–99.
52. Glass M, Dragunow M, Faull RLM. 1997. Cannabinoid receptors in the human brain: A detailed anatomical and quantitative autoradiographic study in the fetal, neonatal and adult human brain. *Neuroscience* 77:299–318.
53. Hadden JW, Hadden EM, Haddox MK, Goldberg ND. 1972. Guanosine 3':5'-cyclic monophosphates: A possible intracellular mediator of mitogenic influences in lymphocytes. *Proceedings of the National Academy of Sciences, USA* 69:3024–3027.
54. Hampson AJ, Grimaldi M, Axelrod J, Wink D. 1998. Cannabidiol and (-)delta-9-tetrahydrocannabinol are neuroprotective antioxidants. *Proceedings of the National Academy of Sciences, USA* 95:8268–8273.
55. Haney M, Ward AS, Comer SD, Foltin RW, Fischman MW. 1999. Abstinence symptoms following oral THC administration to humans. *Psychopharmacology* 141:385–394.
56. Haney M, Ward AS, Comer SD, Foltin RW, Fischman MW. 1999. Abstinence symptoms following smoked marijuana in humans. *Psychopharmacology* 141:395–404.
57. Herkenham M. 1995. Localization of cannabinoid receptors in brain and periphery. In: Pertwee RG, Editor, *Cannabinoid Receptors*. New York: Academic Press. Pp. 145–166.
58. Herkenham M, Lynn AB, de Costa BR, Richfield EK. 1991a. Neuronal localization of cannabinoid receptors in the basal ganglia of the rat. *Brain Research* 547:267–274.
59. Herkenham M, Lynn AB, Johnson MR, Melvin LS, de Costa BR, Rice KC. 1991b. Characterization and localization of cannabinoid receptors in rat brain: A quantative *in vitro* autoradiographic study. *Journal of Neuroscience* 11:563–583.
60. Herkenham M, Lynn AB, Little MD, Johnson MR, Melvin LS, de Costa BR, Rice KC. 1990. Cannabinoid receptor localization in the brain. *Proceedings of the National Academy of Sciences, USA* 87:1932–1936.
61. Herring AC, Koh WS, Kaminski NE. 1998. Inhibition of the cyclic AMP signaling cascade and nuclear factor binding to CRE and kappa B elements by cannabinol, a minimally CNS-active cannabinoid. *Biochemical Pharmacology* 55:1013–1023.
62. Herzberg U, Eliav E, Bennett GJ, Kopin IJ. 1997. The analgesic effects of R(+)-WIN 55,212-2 mesylate, a high affinity cannabinoid agonist, in a rat model of neuropathic pain. *Neuroscience Letters* 221:157–160.
63. Heyser CJ, Hampson RE, Deadwyler SA. 1993. Effects of delta-9-tetrahydrocannabinol on delayed match to sample performance in rats: Alterations in short-term memory associated with changes in task-specific firing of hippocampal cells. *Journal of Pharmacology and Experimental Therapeutics* 264:294–307.
64. Hohmann AG, Briley EM, Herkenham M. 1999. Pre- and postsynaptic distribution of cannabinoid and mu opioid receptors in rat spinal cord. *Brain Research* 822:17–25.
65. Hohmann AG, Herkenham M. 1998. Regulation of cannabinoid and mu opioid receptor binding sites following neonatal capsaicin treatment. *Neuroscience Letters* 252:13–16.

66. Hohmann AG, Herkenham M. 1999. Localization of central cannabinoid CB1 receptor mRNA in neuronal subpopulations of rat dorsal root ganglia: A double-label *in situ* hybridization study. *Neuroscience* 90:923–931.
67. Hohmann AG, Martin WJ, Tsou K, Walker JM. 1995. Inhibition of noxious stimulus-evoked activity of spinal cord dorsal horn neurons by the cannabinoid WIN 55,212-2. *Life Sciences* 56:2111–2119.
68. Hollister LE. 1986. Health aspects of cannabis. *Pharmacological Reviews* 38:1–20.
69. Hollister LE, Gillespie BA. 1975. Interactions in man of delta-9-THC. II. Cannabinol and cannabidiol. *Clinical Pharmacology and Therapeutics* 18:80–83.
70. Hughes J, Smith TW, Kosterlitz HW, Fothergill LA, Morgan BA, Morris HR. 1975. Identification of two related pentapeptides from the brain with potent opiate agonists activity. *Nature* 258:577–580.
71. Jackson AL, Murphy LL. 1997. Role of the hypothalamic-pituitary-adrenal axis in the suppression of luteinizing hormone release by delta-9-tetrahydrocannabinol. *Neuroendocrinology* 65:446–452.
72. Jacob J, Ramabadran K, Campos-Medeiros M. 1981. A pharmacological analysis of levonantradol antinociception in mice. *Journal of Clinical Pharmacology* 21:327S–333S.
73. Jaggar SI, Hasnie FS, Sellaturay S, Rice AS. 1998. The anti-hyperalgesic actions of the cannabinoid anandamide and the putative CB_2 receptor agonist palmitoylethanolamide in visceral and somatic inflammatory pain. *Pain* 76:189–199.
74. Jeon YJ, Yang K-H, Pulaski JT, Kaminski NE. 1996. Attenuation of inducible nitric oxide synthase gene expression by delta-9-tetrahydrocannabinol is mediated through the inhibition of nuclear factor-kB/Rel activation. *Molecular Pharmacology* 50:334–341.
75. Johnson MR, Melvin LS. 1986. The discovery of non-classical cannabinoid analgesics. In: Mechoulam R, Editor, *Cannabinoids as Therapeutic Agents*. Boca Raton, FL: CRC Press, Inc. Pp. 121–145.
76. Jones RT, Benowitz NL, Herning RI. 1981. Clinical relevance of cannabis tolerance and dependence. *Journal of Clinical Pharmacology* 21:143S–152S.
77. Kaminski NE. 1996. Immune regulation by cannabinoid compounds through the inhibition of the cyclic AMP signaling cascade and altered gene expression. *Biochemical Pharmacology* 52:1133–1140.
78. Kaminski NE, Abood ME, Kessler FK, Martin BR, Schatz AR. 1992. Identification of a functionally relevant cannabinoid receptor on mouse spleen cells that is involved in cannabinoid-mediated immune modulation. *Molecular Pharmacology* 42:736–742.
79. Kaminski NE, Koh WS, Yang KH, Lee M, Kessler FK. 1994. Suppression of the humoral immune response by cannabinoids is partially mediated through inhibition of adenylate cyclase by a pertussis toxin-sensitive G-protein coupled mechanism. *Biochemical Pharmacology* 48:1899–1908.
80. Kaminski NE. 1998. Regulation of cAMP cascade, gene expression and immune function by cannabinoid receptors. *Journal of Neuroimmunology* 83:124–132.
81. Karniol IG, Shirakawa I, Kasinski N, Pfeferman A, Carlini EA. 1975. Cannabidiol interferes with the effects of delta-9-tetrahydrocannbinol in man. *European Journal of Pharmacology* 28:172–177.
82. Kieffer BL, Befort K, Gaveriaux-Ruff C, Hirth CG. 1992. The delta-opioid receptor: Isolation of a cDNA by expression cloning and pharmacological characterization. *Proceedings of the National Academy of Sciences, USA* 89:12048–12052.
83. Kirby MT, Hampson RE, Deadwyler SA. 1995. Cannabinoids selectively decrease paired-pulse perforant path synaptic potentials in the dentate gyrus in vitro. *Brain Research* 688:114–120.

84. Klein TW, Friedman H. 1990. Modulation of murine immune cell function by marijuana components. In: Watson R, Editor, *Drugs of Abuse and Immune Function*. Boca
Raton, FL: CRC Press.
85. Klein TW, Friedman H, Specter SC. 1998. Marijuana, immunity and infection. *Journal
of Neuroimmunology* 83:102–115.
86. Klein TW, Newton C, Friedman H. 1987. Inhibition of natural killer cell function by
marijuana components. *Journal of Toxicology and Environmental Health* 20:321–332.
87. Klein TW, Newton C, Friedman H. 1994. Resistance to *Legionella pneumophila* suppressed by the marijuana component, tetrahydrocannabinol. *Journal of Infectious Diseases* 169:1177–1179.
88. Klein TW, Newton C, Friedman H. 1998. Cannabinoid receptors and immunity. *Immunology Today* 19:373–381.
89. Klein TW, Newton C, Widen R, Friedman H. 1985. The effect of delta-9-tetrahydro-
cannabinol and 11-hydroxy-delta-9-tetrahydrocannabinol on T-lymphocyte and B-
lymphocyte mitogen responses. *Journal of Immunopharmacology* 7:451–466.
90. Klein TW, Newton C, Widen R, Friedman H. 1993. Delta-9-tetrahydrocannabinol injection induces cytokine-mediated mortality of mice infected with *Legionella
pneumophila*. *Journal of Pharmacology and Experimental Therapeutics* 267:635–640.
91. Koh WS, Yang KH, Kaminski NE. 1995. Cyclic AMP is an essential factor in immune
responses. *Biochemical and Biophysical Research Communications* 206:703–709.
92. Ledent C , Valverde O, Cossu G, Petitet F, Aubert JF, Beslot F, Bohme GA, Imperato
A, Pedrazzini T, Roques BP, Vassart G, Fratta W, Parmentier M. 1999. Unresponsive-
ness to cannabinoids and reduced addictive effects of opiates in CB1 receptor knockout mice. *Science* 283:401–404.
93. Lee M, Yang KH, Kaminski NE. 1995. Effects of putative cannabinoid receptor ligands,
anandamide and 2-arachidonyl-glycerol, on immune function in B6C3F1 mouse
splenocytes. *Journal of Pharmacology and Experimental Therapeutics* 275:529–536.
94. Lepore M, Liu X, Savage V, Matalon D, Gardner EL. 1996. Genetic differences in delta
9-tetrahydrocannabinol-induced facilitation of brain stimulation reward as measured
by a rate-frequency curve-shift electrical brain stimulation paradigm in three different rat strains. *Life Sciences* 58:365–372.
95. Lepore M, Vorel SR, Lowinson J, Gardner EL. 1995. Conditioned place preference
induced by delta 9-tetrahydrocannabinol: Comparison with cocaine, morphine, and
food reward. *Life Sciences* 56:2073–2080.
96. Lichtman AH, Martin BR. 1991a. Spinal and supraspinal components of cannabinoid-
induced antinociception. *Journal of Pharmacology and Experimental Therapeutics* 258:517–
523.
97. Little PJ, Compton DR, Mechoulam R, Martin BR. 1989. Stereochemical effects of 11-
OH-delta-8-THC-dimethylheptyl in mice and dogs. *Pharmacology, Biochemistry Behavior* 32:661–666.
98. Lu F, Ou DW. 1989. Cocaine or delta-9-tetrahydrocannabinol does not affect cellular
cytotoxicity *in vitro*. *International Journal of Pharmacology* 11:849–852.
99. Luo YD, Patel MK, Wiederhold MD, Ou DW. 1992. Effects of cannabinoids and cocaine on the mitogen-induced transformations of lymphocytes of human and mouse
origins. *International Journal of Immunopharmacology* 14:49–56.
100. Lyman WD, Sonett JR, Brosnan CFER, Bornstein MB. 1989. Delta 9-tetrahydrocan-
nabinol: A novel treatment for experimental autoimmune encephalomyelitis. *Journal
of Neuroimmunology* 23:73–81.
101. Mailleux P, Vanderhaeghen JJ. 1992. Distribution of neuronal cannabinoid receptor in
the adult rat brain: A comparative receptor binding radioautography and *in situ* hybridization histochemistry. *Neuroscience* 48:655–668.

102. Martin WJ, Hohmann AG, Walker JM. 1996. Suppression of noxious stimulus-evoked activity in the ventral posterolateral nucleus of the thalamus by a cannabinoid agonist: Correlation between electrophysiological and antinociceptive effects. *The Journal of Neuroscience* 16:6601–6611.

103. Martin WJ, Patrick SL, Coffin PO, Tsou K, Walker JM. 1995. An examination of the central sites of action of cannabinoid-induced antinociception in the rat. *Life Sciences* 56:2103–2109.

104. Martin WJ , Patrick SL, Coffin PO, Tsou K, Walker JM. 1995. An examination of the central sites of action of cannabinoid-induced antinociception in the rat. *Life Sciences* 56:2103–2109.

105. Martin WJ, Tsou K, Walker JM. 1998. Cannabinoid receptor-mediated inhibition of the rat tail-flick reflex after microinjections into the rostral ventromedial medulla. *Neuroscience Letters* 242:33–36.

106. Martoletta MC, Cossu G, Fattore L, Gessa GL, Fratta W. 1998. Self-administration of the cannabinoid receptor agonist WIN 55,212-2 in drug-naive mice. *Neuroscience* 85:327–330.

107. Matsuda L, Lolait SJ, Brownstein MJ, Young AC, Bonner TI. 1990. Structure of a cannabinoid receptor and functional expression of the cloned cDNA. *Nature* 346:561–564.

108. Mechoulam R, Ben-Shabat S, Hanus L, Ligumsky M, Kaminski NSA, Gopher A, Almog S, Martin BR, Compton D, Pertwee RG, Griffin G, Bayewitch M, Barg J, Vogel Z. 1995. Identification of an endogenous 2-monoglyceride, present in canine gut, that binds to cannabinoid receptors. *Biochemical Pharmacology* 50:83–90.

109. Mechoulam R, Hanus L, Fride E. 1998. Towards cannabinoid drugs—revisited. In: Ellis GP, Luscombe DK, Oxford AW, Editors, *Progress in Medicinal Chemistry.* v. 35. Amsterdam: Elsevier Science. Pp. 199–243.

110. Meng ID, Manning BH, Martin WJ, Fields HL. 1998. An analgesia circuit activated by cannabinoids. *Nature* 395:381–383.

111. Miller AS, Walker JM. 1996. Electrophysiological effects of a cannabinoid on neural activity in the globus pallidus. *European Journal of Pharmacology* 304:29–35.

112. Munro S, Thomas KL, Abu-Shaar M. 1993. Molecular characterization of a peripheral receptor for cannabinoids. *Nature* 365:61–65.

113. Murphy LL, Steger RW, Smith MS, Bartke A. 1990. Effects of delta-9-tetrahydrocannabinol, cannabinol and cannabidiol, alone and in combinations, on luteinizing hormone and prolactin release and on hypothalamic neurotransmitters in the male rat. *Neuroendocrinology* 52:316–321.

114. Narimatsu S, Watanabe K, Matsunaga T, Yamamoto I, Imaoka S, Funae Y, Yoshimura H. 1993. Suppression of liver microsomal drug-metabolizing enzyme activities in adult female rats pretreated with cannabidiol. *Biological and Pharmaceutical Bulletin (Japan)* 16:428–430.

115. Newton CA, Klein T, Friedman H. 1994. Secondary immunity to Legionella pneumophila and Th1 activity are suppressed by delta-9-tetrahydrocannabinol injection. *Infection and Immunity* 62:4015–4020.

116. Norwicky AV, Teyler TJ, Vardaris RM. 1987. The modulation of long-term potentiation by delta-9-tetrahydrocannabinol in the rat hippocampus, in vitro. *Brain Research Bulletin* 19:663.

117. O'Leary D, Block RI, Flaum M, Boles Ponto LL, Watkins GL, Hichwa RD. 1998. Acute marijuana effects on rCBF and cognition: A PET study. *Abstracts—Society for Neuroscience: 28th Annual Meeting.* Los Angeles, November 7–12, 1998. Washington, DC: Society for Neuroscience.

118. Ohlsson A, Lindgren J-E, Wahlen A, Agurell S, Hollister LE, Gillespie HK. 1980. Plasma delta-9-tetrahydrocannabinol concentrations and clinical effects after oral and intravenous administration and smoking. *Clinical Pharmacology and Therapeutics* 28:409–416.

119. Oviedo A, Glowa J, Herkenham M. 1993. Chronic cannabinoid administration alters cannabinoid receptor binding in rat brain: A quantitative autoradiographic study. *Brain Research* 616:293–302.

120. Pacheco MA, Ward SJ, Childers SR. 1993. Identification of cannabinoid receptors in cultures of rat cerebellar granule cells. *Brain Research* 603:102–110.

121. Patel V, Borysenko M, Kumar MSA, Millard WJ. 1985. Effects of acute and subchronic delta-9-tetrahydrocannabinol administration on the plasma catecholamine, beta-endorphin, and corticosterone levels and splenic natural killer cell activity in rats. *Proceedings of the Society for Experimental Biology and Medicine* 180:400–404.

122. Pepe S, Ruggiero A, Tortora G, Ciaardiello F, Garbi C, Yokozaki H, Cho-Chung YS, Clair T, Skalhegg BS, Bianco AR. 1994. Flow cytometric detection of the RI alpha subunit of type-I cAMP-dependent protein kinase in human cells. *Cytometry* 15:73–79.

123. Pert CB, Snyder SH. 1973. Opiate receptor: Demonstration in nervous tissue. *Science* 179:1011–1014.

124. Pertwee RG. 1997b. Pharmacology of cannabinoid CB_1 and CB_2 receptors. *Pharmacology and Therapeutics* 74:129–180.

125. Pertwee RG, Stevenson LA, Griffin G. 1993. Cross-tolerance between delta-9-tetrahydrocannabinol and the cannabimimetic agents, CP 55,940, WIN 55,212-2 and anandamide [published erratum appears in *British Journal of Pharmacology*, 1994, 111(3):968]. *British Journal of Pharmacology* 110:1483–1490.

126. Pertwee RG, Wickens AP. 1991. Enhancement by chlordiazepoxide of catalepsy induced in rats by intravenous or intrapallidal injections of enantiomeric cannabinoids. *Neuropharmacology* 30:237–244.

127. Pross SH, Nakano Y, Widen R, McHugh S, Newton C, Klein TW, Friedman H. 1992. Differing effects of delta-9-tetrahydrocannabinol (THC) on murine spleen cell populations dependent upon stimulators. *International Journal of Immunopharmacology* 14:1019–1027.

128. Razdan RK. 1986. Structure-activity relationships in cannabinoids. *Pharmacology Review* 38:75–149.

129. Rhee MH, Vogel Z, Barg J, Bayewitch M, Levy R, Hanus L, Breuer A, Mechoulam R. 1997. Cannabinol derivatives: Binding to cannabinoid receptors and inhibition of adenyl-cyclase. *Journal of Medicinal Chemistry* 40:3228–3233.

130. Richardson JD, Aanonsen L, Hargreaves KM. 1998. Hypoactivity of the spinal cannabinoid system results in NMDA-dependent hyperalgesia. *Journal of Neuroscience* 18:451–457.

131. Richardson JD, Kilo S, Hargreaves KM. 1998. Cannabinoids reduce hyperalgesia and inflammation via interaction with peripheral CB1 receptors. *Pain* 75:111–119.

132. Rinaldi-Carmona M, Barth F, Heaulme M, Shire D, Calandra B, Congy C, Martinez S, Maruani J, Neliat G, Caput D, Ferrara P, Soubrie P, Breliere JC, Le Fur G. 1994. SR141716A, a potent and selective antagonist of the brain cannabinoid receptor. *FEBS Letters* 350:240–244.

133. Rinaldi-Carmona M, Barth F, Millan J, Defrocq J, Casellas P, Congy C, Oustric D, Sarran M, Bouaboula M, Calandra B, Portier M, Shire D, Breliere J, Le Fur G. 1998. SR144528, the first potent and selective antagonist of the CB_2 cannabinoid receptor. *Journal of Pharmacology and Experimental Therapeutics* 284:644–650.

134. Rodríguez de Fonseca F, Fernández-Ruiz JJ, Murphy LL, Eldridge JC, Steger RW, Bartke A. 1991. Effects of delta-9-tetrahydrocannabinol exposure on adrenal medullary function: Evidence of an acute effect and development of tolerance in chronic treatments. *Pharmacology, Biochemistry and Behavior* 40:593–598.

135. Rodriguez de Fonseca F, Carrera MRA, Navarro M, Koob G, Weiss F. 1997. Activation of corticotropin-releasing factor in the limbic system during cannabinoid withdrawal [see comments *Science* 1997, 276:1967–1968]. *Science* 276:2050–2054.

136. Rodriguez de Fonseca F, Gorriti MA, Fernandez-Ruiz JJ, Palomo T, Ramos JA. 1994. Down-regulation of rat brain cannabinoid binding sites after chronic delta-9-tetrahydrocannabinol treatment. *Pharmacology, Biochemistry and Behavior* 47:33–40.

137. Romero J, Garciá L, Fernández-Ruiz JJ, Cebeira M, Ramos JA. 1995. Changes in rat brain cannabinoid binding sites after acute or chronic exposure to their endogenous agonist, anandamide, or to delta-9-tetrahydrocannabinol. *Pharmacology, Biochemistry and Behavior* 51:731–737.

138. Romero J, Garcia-Palomero E, Castro JG, Garcia-Gil L, Ramos JA, Fernandez-Ruiz JJ. 1997. Effects of chronic exposure to delta-9-tetrahydrocannabinol on cannabinoid receptor binding and mRNA levels in several rat brain regions. *Molecular Brain Research* 46:100–108.

139. Russell DH. 1978. Type I cyclic AMP-dependent protein kinase as a positive effector of growth. *Advances in Cyclic Nucleotide Research* 9:493–506.

140. Sanudo-Pena MC, Tsou K, Delay ER, Hohmann AG, Force M, Walker JM. 1997. Endogenous cannabinoids as an aversive or counter-rewarding system in the rat. *Neuroscience Letters* 223:125–128.

141. Sanudo-Pena MC, Walker JM. 1997. Role of the subthalamic nucleus in cannabinoid actions in the substantia nigra of the rat. *Journal of Neurophysiology* 77:1635–1638.

142. Schatz AR, Koh WS, Kaminski NE. 1993. Delta-9-tetrahydrocannabinol selectively inhibits T-cell dependent humoral immune responses through direct inhibition of accessory T-cell function. *Immunopharmacology* 26:129–137.

143. Schlicker E, Timm J, Zenter J, Goethert M. 1997. Cannabinoid CB_1 receptor-mediated inhibition of noradrenaline release in the human and guinea-pig hippocampus. *Naunyn-Schmiedeberg's Archives of Pharmacology* 356:583–589.

144. Shen M, Piser TM, Seybold VS, Thayer SA. 1996. Cannabinoid receptor agonists inhibit glutamatergic synaptic transmission in rat hippocampal cultures. *Journal of Neuroscience* 16:4322–4334.

145. Shivers SC, Newton C, Friedman H, Klein TW. 1994. Delta 9-tetrahydrocannabinol (THC) modulates IL-1 bioactivity in human monocyte/macrophage cell lines. *Life Sciences* 54:1281–1289.

146. Shohami E, Gallily R, Mechoulam R, Bass R, Ben-Hur T. 1997. Cytokine production in the brain following closed head injury: Dexanabinol (HU-211) is a novel TNF-alpha inhibitor and an effective neuroprotectant. *Journal of Neuroimmunology* 72:169–177.

147. Sim LJ, Hampson RE, Deadwyler SA, Childers SR. 1996. Effects of chronic treatment with delta-9-tetrahydrocannabinol on cannabinoid-stimulated [^{35}S]GTPyS autoradiography in rat brain. *Journal of Neuroscience* 16:8057–8066.

148. Sim LJ, Xiao R, Selley DE, Childers SR. 1996. Differences in G-protein activation by mu- and delta-opioid, and cannabinoid, receptors in rat striatum. *European Journal of Pharmacology* 307:97–105.

149. Simon EJ. 1973. In search of the opiate receptor. *American Journal of Medical Sciences* 266:160–168.

150. Skaper SD, Buriani A, Dal Toso R, Petrelli L, Romanello S, Facci L, Leon A. 1996. The ALIAmide palmitoylethanolamide and cannabinoids, but not anandamide, are protective in a delayed postglutamate paradigm of excitotoxic death in cerebellar granule neurons. *Proceedings of the National Academy of Sciences, USA* 93:3984–3989.

151. Smith JW, Steiner AL, Newberry WM, Parker CW. 1971. Cyclic adenosine 3',5'-monophosphate in human lymphocytes: Alteration after phytohemagglutinin. *Journal of Clinical Investigation* 50:432–441.

152. Smith PB, Compton DR, Welch SP, Razdan RK, Mechoulam R, Martin BR. 1994. The pharmacological activity of anandamide, a putative endogenous cannabinoid, in mice. *Journal of Pharmacology and Experimental Therapeutics* 270:219–227.

153. Smith PB, Welch SP, Martin BR. 1994. Interactions between delta 9-tetrahydrocannabinol and kappa opioids in mice. *Journal of Pharmacology and Experimental Therapeutics* 268: 1381–1387.

154. Sofia RD, Nalepa SD, Harakal JJ, Vassar HB. 1973. Anti-edema and analgesic properties of delta-9-tetrahydrocannabinol (THC). *Journal of Pharmacology and Experimental Therapeutics* 186:646–655.

155. Specter S, Lancz G, Hazelden J. 1990. Marijuana and immunity: Tetrahydrocannabinol mediated inhibition of lymphocyte blastogenesis. *International Journal of Immunophar-macology* 12:261–267.

156. Stefano G, Salzet B, Salzet M. 1997. Identification and characterization of the leech CNS cannabinoid receptor: Coupling to nitric oxide release. *Brain Research* 753:219–224.

157. Stella N, Schweitzer P, Piomelli D. 1997. A second endogenous cannabinoid that modulates long term potentiation. *Nature* 388:773–778.

158. Strangman NM, Patrick SL, Hohmann AG, Tsou K, Walker JM. 1998. Evidence for a role of endogenous cannabinoids in the modulation of acute and tonic pain sensitivity. *Brain Research* 813:323–328.

159. Sulcova E, Mechoulam R, Fride E. 1998. Biphasic effects of anandamide. *Pharmacology, Biochemistry and Behavior* 59:347–352.

160. Szabo B, Dorner L, Pfreundtner C, Norenberg W, Starke K. 1998. Inhibition of GABAergic inhibitory postsynaptic currents by cannabinoids in rat corpus striatum. *Neuroscience* 85:395–403.

161. Tanda G, Pontieri FE, Di Chiara G. 1997. Cannabinoid and heroin activation of mesolimbic dopamine transmission by a common μ1 opioid receptor mechanism. *Science* 276:2048–2049.

162. Terenius L. 1973. Characteristics of the "receptor" for narcotic analgesics in synaptic plasma membrane fraction from rat brain. *Acta Pharmacologica Et Toxicologica* 33:377–384.

163. Terranova JP, Michaud JC, Le Fur G, Soubrié P. 1995. Inhibition of long-term potentiation in rat hippocampal slice by anandamide and WIN55212-2: Reversal by SR141716 A, a selective antagonist of CB_1 cannabinoid receptors. *Naunyn-Schmiedeberg's Archives of Pharmacology* 352:576–579.

164. Titishov N, Mechoulam R, Zimmerman AM. 1989. Stereospecific effects of (−) and (+)-7-hydroxy-delta-6-tetrahydrocannabinol-dimethylheptyl on the immune system of mice. *Pharmacology* 39:337–349.

165. Tsou K, Brown S, Sanudo-Pena MC, Mackie K, Walker JM. 1998. Immunohistochemical distribution of cannabinoid CB_1 receptors in the rat central nervous system. *Neuroscience* 83:393–411.

166. Tsou K, Patrick SL, Walker JM. 1995. Physical withdrawal in rats tolerant to delta-9-tetrahydrocannabinol precipitated by a cannabinoid receptor antagonist. *European Journal of Pharmacology* 280:R13–R15.

167. Watson PF, Krupinski J, Kempinski A, Frankenfield C. 1994. Molecular cloning and characterization of the type VII isoform of mammalian adenylyl cyclase expressed widely in mouse tissues and in S49 mouse lymphoma cells. *Journal of Biological Chemistry* 269:28893–28898.
168. Watzl B, Scuder P, Watson RR. 1991. Marijuana components stimulate human peripheral blood mononuclear cell secretion of interferon-gamma and suppress interleukin-1 alpha in vitro. *International Journal of Immunopharmology* 13:1091–1097.
169. Weidenfeld J, Feldman S, Mechoulam R. 1994. Effect of the brain constituent anandamide, a cannabinoid receptor agonist, on the hypothalamo-pituitary-adrenal axis in the rat. *Neuroendocrinology* 59:110–112.
170. Welch SP. 1993. Blockade of cannabinoid-induced antinociception by norbinaltorphimine, but not N,N-diallyl-tyrosine-Aib-phenylalanine-leucine, ICI 174,864 or naloxone in mice. *Journal of Pharmacology and Experimental Therapeutics* 265:633–640.
171. Welch SP, Thomas C, Patrick GS. 1995. Modulation of cannabinoid-induced antinociception after intracerebroventricular versus intrathecal administration to mice: Possible mechanisms for interaction with morphine. *Journal of Clinical and Experimental Therapeutics* 272:310–321.
172. Wirguin I, Mechoulam R, Breuer A, Schezen E, Weidenfeld J, Brenner T. 1994. Suppression of experimental autoimmune encephalomyelitis by cannabinoids. *Immunopharma-cology* 28:209–214.
173. Wirth PW, Watson ES, ElSohly M, Turner CE, Murphy JC. 1980. Anti-inflammatory properties of cannabichromene. *Life Sciences* 26:1991–1995.
174. Yaksh TL. 1981. The antinociceptive effects of intrathecally administered levonantradol and desacetyl-levonantradol in the rat. *Journal of Clinical Pharmacology* 21:334S–340S.
175. Yoshida H, Usami N, Ohishi Y, Watanabe K, Yamamoto I, Yoshimura H. 1995. Synthesis and pharmacological effects in mice of halogenated cannabinol derivatives. *Chemical and Pharmaceutical Bulletin* 42:335–337.
176. Zhu W, Newton C, Daaka Y, Friedman H, Klein TW. 1994. Delta 9-tetrahydrocannabinol enhances the secretion of interleukin 1 from endotoxin-stimulated macrophages. *Journal of Pharmacology and Experimental Therapeutics* 270:1334–1339.
177. Zuardi AW, Shirakawa I, Finkelfarb E, Karniol IG. 1982. Action of cannabidiol on the anxiety and other effects produced by delta 9-THC in normal subjects. *Psychopharmacology (Berl)* 76:245–250.
178. Zurier RB, Rossetti RG, Lane JH, Goldberg JM, Hunter SA, Burstein SH. 1998. Dimethylheptyl-THC-11 oic acid: A non-psychoactive antiinflammatory agent with a cannabinoid template structure. *Arthritis and Rheumatism* 41:163–170.

3
First, Do No Harm: Consequences of Marijuana Use and Abuse

 Primum non nocere. This is the physician's first rule: whatever treatment a physician prescribes to a patient—first, that treatment must not harm the patient.

The most contentious aspect of the medical marijuana debate is not whether marijuana can alleviate particular symptoms but rather the degree of harm associated with its use. This chapter explores the negative health consequences of marijuana use, first with respect to drug abuse, then from a psychological perspective, and finally from a physiological perspective.

THE MARIJUANA "HIGH"

The most commonly reported effects of smoked marijuana are a sense of well-being or euphoria and increased talkativeness and laughter alternating with periods of introspective dreaminess followed by lethargy and sleepiness (see reviews by Adams and Martin, 1996,[1] Hall and Solowij,[59] and Hall et al. [60]). A characteristic feature of a marijuana "high" is a distortion in the sense of time associated with deficits in short-term memory and learning. A marijuana smoker typically has a sense of enhanced physical and emotional sensitivity, including a feeling of greater interpersonal closeness. The most obvious behavioral abnormality displayed by someone under the influence of marijuana is difficulty in carrying on an intelligible conversation, perhaps because of an inability to remember what was just said even a few words earlier.

The high associated with marijuana is not generally claimed to be integral to its therapeutic value. But mood enhancement, anxiety reduction, and mild sedation can be desirable qualities in medications—particularly for patients suffering pain and anxiety. Thus, although the psychological effects of marijuana are merely side effects in the treatment of some symptoms, they might contribute directly to relief of other symptoms. They also must be monitored in controlled clinical trials to discern which effect of cannabinoids is beneficial. These possibilities are discussed later under the discussions of specific symptoms in chapter 4.

The effects of various doses and routes of delivery of THC are shown in Table 3.1.

Adverse Mood Reactions

Although euphoria is the more common reaction to smoking marijuana, adverse mood reactions can occur. Such reactions occur most frequently in inexperienced users after large doses of smoked or oral marijuana. They usually disappear within hours and respond well to reassurance and a supportive environment. Anxiety and paranoia are the most common acute adverse reactions;[59] others include panic, depression, dysphoria, depersonalization, delusions, illusions, and hallucinations.[1,40,66,69] Of regular marijuana smokers, 17% report that they have experienced at least one of the symptoms, usually early in their use of marijuana.[145] Those observations are particularly relevant for the use of medical marijuana in people who have not previously used marijuana.

DRUG DYNAMICS

There are many misunderstandings about drug abuse and dependence (see reviews by O'Brien[114] and Goldstein[54]). The terms and concepts used in this report are as defined in the most recent *Diagnostic and Statistical Manual of Mental Disorders (DSM-IV)*,[3] the most influential system in the United States for diagnoses of mental disorders, including substance abuse (see Box 3.1). Tolerance, dependence, and withdrawal are often presumed to imply abuse or addiction, but this is not the case. Tolerance and dependence are *normal* physiological adaptations to repeated use of any drug. The correct use of prescribed medications for pain, anxiety, and even hypertension commonly produces tolerance and some measure of physiological dependence.

Even a patient who takes a medicine for appropriate medical indications and at the correct dosage can develop tolerance, physical depen-

TABLE 3.1 Psychoactive Doses of THC in Humans

Investigators	THC Delivery System	THC Dose Administered	Resulting Plasma Concentrations of THC	Subjects' Reactions
Heishman and co-workers (1990)[62a]	One 2.75% THC cigarette smoked	0.32 mg/kg[a]	50–100 ng/ml	At higher level, subjects felt 100% "high" and psychomotor performance was decreased; at 50 ng/ml, subjects felt about 50% "high"
Kelly and co-workers (1993)[85]	1-g marijuana cigarette smoked (2% or 3.5% THC)	0.25–0.50 mg/kg[a]	Not measured	Enough to feel psychological effects of THC
Ohlsson and co-workers (1980)[118]	19-mg THC cigarette smoked (about 1.9% THC)	About 0.22 mg/kg[b]	100 ng/ml	Subjects felt "high"
	5 mg of THC injected intravenously	About 0.06 mg/kg[b]	100 ng/ml	Subjects felt "high"
	Chocolate chip cookie containing 20 mg of THC	About 0.24 mg/kg	8 ng/ml	Subjects rated "high" as only about 40%
Lindgren and co-workers (1981)[95]	19-mg THC cigarette smoked to "desired high"	12 mg smoked (7 mg remained in cigarette butt)	85 ng/ml after 3 min., 35 ng/ml after 15 min.	Subjects felt "high" after 3 min., and maximally high after 10–20 min. (average self-ratings of 5.5 on 10-point scale)
	5 mg of THC injected intravenously	0.06 mg/kg[c]	300 ng/ml after 3 min., 65 ng/ml after 15 min.	Subjects felt maximally "high" after 10 min. (average self ratings of 7.5 on a 10-point scale)

[a]Subjects' weights and cigarette weights were not given. Calculation based on 85-kg body weight and 1-g cigarette weight. Note that some THC would have remained in the cigarette butt and some would have been lost in sidestream smoke, so these represent maximal possible doses. Actual doses would have been slightly less.

[b]Based on estimated average 85-kg weight of 11 men 18–35 years old.

[c]Based on approximate 80-kg weight of subjects (including men and women).

Box 3.1
Definitions

Addiction. Substance dependence.

Craving refers to the intense desire for a drug and is the most difficult aspect of addiction to overcome.

Physiological dependence is diagnosed when there is evidence of either tolerance or withdrawal; it is sometimes, but not always, manifested in substance dependence.

Reinforcement. A drug—or any other stimulus—is referred to as a reinforcer if exposure to it is followed by an increase in frequency of drug-seeking behavior. The taste of chocolate is a reinforcer for biting into a chocolate bar. Likewise, for many people the sensation experienced after drinking alcohol or smoking marijuana is a reinforcer.

Substance dependence is a cluster of cognitive, behavioral, and physiological symptoms indicating that a person continues use of the substance despite significant substance-related problems.

Tolerance is the most common response to repetitive use of a drug and can be defined as the reduction in responses to the drug after repeated administrations.

Withdrawal. The collective symptoms that occur when a drug is abruptly withdrawn are known as withdrawal syndrome and are often the only evidence of physical dependence.

---

dence, and withdrawal symptoms if the drug is stopped abruptly rather than gradually. For example, a hypertensive patient receiving a beta-adrenergic receptor blocker, such as propranolol, might have a good therapeutic response; but if the drug is stopped abruptly, there can be a withdrawal syndrome that consists of tachycardia and a rebound increase in blood pressure to a point that is temporarily higher than before administration of the medication began.

Because it is an illegal substance, some people consider any use of marijuana as substance abuse. However, this report uses the medical definition; that is, substance abuse is a maladaptive pattern of repeated substance use manifested by recurrent and significant adverse consequences.[3] Substance abuse and dependence are both diagnoses of pathological substance use. Dependence is the more serious diagnosis and implies compulsive drug use that is difficult to stop despite significant substance-related problems (see Box 3.2).

Box 3.2
DSM-IV Criteria for Substance Dependence

A maladaptive pattern of substance use, leading to clinically significant impairment or distress, as manifested by three (or more) of the following, occurring at any time in the same 12-month period:

(1) Tolerance, as defined by either of the following:
    (a) A need for markedly increased amount of the substance to achieve intoxication or desired effect.
    (b) Markedly diminished effect with continued use of the same amount of the substance.
(2) Withdrawal, as defined by either of the following:
    (a) The characteristic withdrawal syndrome for the substance.
    (b) The same (or a closely related) substance is taken to relieve or avoid withdrawal symptoms.
(3) The substance is often taken in larger amounts or over a longer period than was intended.
(4) There is a persistent desire or unsuccessful efforts to cut down or control substance use.
(5) A great deal of time is spent in activities necessary to obtain the substance (e.g., visiting multiple doctors or driving long distances), to use the substance (e.g., chain-smoking), or to recover from its effects.
(6) Important social, occupational, or recreational activities are given up or reduced because of substance use.
(7) The substance use is continued despite knowledge of having a persistent or recurrent physical or psychological problem that is likely to have been caused or exacerbated by the substance (e.g., current cocaine use despite recognition of cocaine-induced depression or continued drinking despite recognition that an ulcer was made worse by alcohol consumption).

Substance abuse with physiological dependence is diagnosed if there is evidence of tolerance or withdrawal.
Substance abuse without physiological dependence is diagnosed if there is no evidence of tolerance or withdrawal.

Reinforcement

Drugs vary in their ability to produce good feelings in users, and the more strongly reinforcing a drug is, the more likely it will be abused (G. Koob, Institute of Medicine (IOM) workshop). Marijuana is indisputably reinforcing for many people. The reinforcing properties of even so mild a stimulant as caffeine are typical of reinforcement by addicting drugs (reviewed by Goldstein[54] in 1994). Caffeine is reinforcing for many people at low doses (100–200 mg, the average amount of caffeine in one to two cups of coffee) and is aversive at high doses (600 mg, the average amount of caffeine in six cups of coffee). The reinforcing effects of many drugs are different for different people. For example, caffeine was most reinforcing for test subjects who scored lowest on tests of anxiety but tended not to be reinforcing for the most anxious subjects.

As an argument to dispute the abuse potential of marijuana, some have cited the observation that animals do not willingly self-administer THC, as they will cocaine. Even if that were true, it would not be relevant to human use of marijuana. The value in animal models of drug self-administration is not that they are necessary to show that a drug is reinforcing but rather that they provide a model in which the effects of a drug can be studied. Furthermore, THC is indeed rewarding to animals at some doses but, like many reinforcing drugs, is aversive at high doses (4.0 mg/kg).[93] Similar effects have been found in experiments conducted in animals outfitted with intravenous catheters that allow them to self-administer WIN 55,212, a drug that mimics the effects of THC.[100]

A specific set of neural pathways has been proposed to be a "reward system" that underlies the reinforcement of drugs of abuse and other pleasurable stimuli.[51] Reinforcing properties of drugs are associated with their ability to increase concentrations of particular neurotransmitters in areas that are part of the proposed brain reward system. The median forebrain bundle and the nucleus accumbens are associated with brain reward pathways.[88] Cocaine, amphetamine, alcohol, opioids, nicotine, and THC[144] all increase extracellular fluid dopamine in the nucleus accumbens region (reviewed by Koob and Le Moal[88] and Nestler and Aghajanian[110] in 1997). However, it is important to note that brain reward systems are not strictly "drug reinforcement centers." Rather, their biological role is to respond to a range of positive stimuli, including sweet foods and sexual attraction.

Tolerance

The rate at which tolerance to the various effects of any drug develops is an important consideration for its safety and efficacy. For medical use, tolerance to some effects of cannabinoids might be desirable. Differences in the rates at which tolerance to the multiple effects of a drug develops can be dangerous. For example, tolerance to the euphoric effects of heroin develops faster than tolerance to its respiratory depressant effects, so heroin users tend to increase their daily doses to reach their desired level of euphoria, thereby putting themselves at risk for respiratory arrest. Because tolerance to the various effects of cannabinoids might develop at different rates, it is important to evaluate independently their effects on mood, motor performance, memory, and attention, as well as any therapeutic use under investigation.

Tolerance to most of the effects of marijuana can develop rapidly after only a few doses, and it also disappears rapidly. Tolerance to large doses has been found to persist in experimental animals for long periods after cessation of drug use. Performance impairment is less among people who use marijuana heavily than it is among those who use marijuana only occasionally,[29,104,124] possibly because of tolerance. Heavy users tend to reach higher plasma concentrations of THC than light users after similar doses of THC, arguing against the possibility that heavy users show less performance impairment because they somehow absorb less THC (perhaps due to differences in smoking behavior).[95]

There appear to be variations in the development of tolerance to the different effects of marijuana and oral THC. For example, daily marijuana smokers participated in a residential laboratory study to compare the development of tolerance to THC pills and to smoked marijuana.[61,62] One group was given marijuana cigarettes to smoke four times per day for four consecutive days; another group was given THC pills on the same schedule. During the four-day period, both groups became tolerant to feeling "high" and what they reported as a "good drug effect." In contrast, neither group became tolerant to the stimulatory effects of marijuana or THC on appetite. "Tolerance" does not mean that the drug no longer produced the effects but simply that the effects were less at the end than at the beginning of the four-day period. The marijuana smoking group reported feeling "mellow" after smoking and did not show tolerance to this effect; the group that took THC pills did not report feeling "mellow." The difference was also reported by many people who described their experiences to the IOM study team.

The oral and smoked doses were designed to deliver roughly equivalent amounts of THC to a subject. Each smoked marijuana dose consisted of five 10-second puffs of a marijuana cigarette containing 3.1% THC; the pills contained 30 mg of THC. Both groups also received placebo drugs during other four-day periods. Although the dosing of the two groups was comparable, different routes of administration resulted in different patterns of drug effect. The peak effect of smoked marijuana is usually felt within minutes and declines sharply after 30 minutes[68,95]; the peak effect of oral THC is usually not felt until about an hour and lasts for several hours.[118]

Withdrawal

A distinctive marijuana and THC withdrawal syndrome has been identified, but it is mild and subtle compared with the profound physical syndrome of alcohol or heroin withdrawal.[31,74] The symptoms of marijuana withdrawal include restlessness, irritability, mild agitation, insomnia, sleep EEG disturbance, nausea, and cramping (Table 3.2). In addition to those symptoms, two recent studies noted several more. A group of adolescents under treatment for conduct disorders also reported fatigue and illusions or hallucinations after marijuana abstinence (this study is discussed further in the section on "Prevalence and Predictors of Dependence on Marijuana and Other Drugs").[31] In a residential study of daily

TABLE 3.2   Drug Withdrawal Symptoms

Nicotine	Alcohol	Marijuana	Cocaine	Opioids (e.g., heroin or morphine)
Restlessness		Restlessness		Restlessness
Irritability	Irritability	Irritability		Irritability
Impatience, hostility		Mild agitation		
Dysphoria			Dysphoria	Dysphoria
Depression			Depression	
Anxiety				Anxiety
Difficulty concentrating				
	Sleep disturbance	Insomnia	Sleepiness, fatigue	Insomnia
		Sleep EEG disturbance		
	Nausea	Nausea		Nausea
		Cramping		Cramping
Decreased heart rate	Tachycardia, hypertension		Bradycardia	
	Sweating			Muscle aches
	Seizures			Increased sensitivity to pain
	Alcohol craving		Cocaine craving	Opioid craving
Increased appetite or weight gain	Delirium tremens[a]			
	Tremor			
	Perceptual distortion			

[a]Severe agitation, confusion, visual hallucinations, fever, profuse sweating, nausea, diarrhea, dilated pupils.
SOURCE: O'Brien (1996).[113]

marijuana users, withdrawal symptoms included sweating and runny nose, in addition to those listed above.[62] A marijuana withdrawal syndrome, however, has been reported only in a group of adolescents in treatment for substance abuse problems[31] and in a research setting where subjects were given marijuana or THC daily.[62,74]

Withdrawal symptoms have been observed in carefully controlled laboratory studies of people after use of both oral THC and smoked marijuana.[61,62] In one study, subjects were given very high doses of oral THC: 180–210 mg per day for 10–20 days, roughly equivalent to smoking 9–10 2% THC cigarettes per day.[74] During the abstinence period at the end of the study, the study subjects were irritable and showed insomnia, runny nose, sweating, and decreased appetite. The withdrawal symptoms, however, were short lived. In four days they had abated. The time course contrasts with that in another study in which lower doses of oral THC were used (80–120 mg/day for four days) and withdrawal symptoms were still near maximal after four days.[61,62]

In animals, simply discontinuing chronic heavy dosing of THC does not reveal withdrawal symptoms, but the "removal" of THC from the brain can be made abrupt by another drug that blocks THC at its receptor if administered when the chronic THC is withdrawn. The withdrawal syndrome is pronounced, and the behavior of the animals becomes hyperactive and disorganized.[153] The half-life of THC in brain is about an hour.[16,24] Although traces of THC can remain in the brain for much longer periods, the amounts are not physiologically significant. Thus, the lack of a withdrawal syndrome when THC is abruptly withdrawn without administration of a receptor-blocking drug is probably not due to a prolonged decline in brain concentrations.

Craving

Craving, the intense desire for a drug, is the most difficult aspect of addiction to overcome. Research on craving has focused on nicotine, alcohol, cocaine, and opiates but has not specifically addressed marijuana.[115] Thus, while this section briefly reviews what is known about drug craving, its relevance to marijuana use has not been established.

Most people who suffer from addiction relapse within a year of abstinence, and they often attribute their relapse to craving.[58] As addiction develops, craving increases even as maladaptive consequences accumulate. Animal studies indicate that the tendency to relapse is based on changes in brain function that continue for months or years after the last use of the drug.[115] Whether neurobiological conditions change during the manifestation of an abstinence syndrome remains an unanswered question in drug abuse research.[88] The "liking" of sweet foods, for example, is mediated by opioid forebrain systems and by brain stem systems, whereas "wanting" seems to be mediated by ascending dopamine neurons that project to the nucleus accumbens.[109]

Anticraving medications have been developed for nicotine and alcohol. The antidepressant, bupropion, blocks nicotine craving, while naltrexone blocks alcohol craving.[115] Another category of addiction medication includes drugs that block other drugs' effects. Some of those drugs also block craving. For example, methadone blocks the euphoric effects of heroin and also reduces craving.

MARIJUANA USE AND DEPENDENCE

Prevalence of Use

Millions of Americans have tried marijuana, but most are not regular users. In 1996, 68.6 million people—32% of the U.S. population over 12 years old—had tried marijuana or hashish at least once in their lifetime, but only 5% were current users.[132] Marijuana use is most prevalent among 18- to 25-year-olds and declines sharply after the age of 34 (Figure 3.1).[77,132] Whites are more likely than blacks to use marijuana in adolescence, although the difference decreases by adulthood.[132]

Most people who have used marijuana did so first during adolescence. Social influences, such as peer pressure and prevalence of use by peers, are highly predictive of initiation into marijuana use.[9] Initiation is not, of course, synonymous with continued or regular use. A cohort of 456 students who experimented with marijuana during their high school years were surveyed about their reasons for initiating, continuing, and stopping their marijuana use.[9] Students who began as heavy users were excluded from the analysis. Those who did not become regular marijuana users cited two types of reasons for discontinuing. The first was related to health and well-being; that is, they felt that marijuana was bad for their health or for their family and work relationships. The second type was based on age-related changes in circumstances, including increased responsibility and decreased regular contact with other marijuana users. Among high school students who quit, parental disapproval was a stronger influence than peer disapproval in discontinuing marijuana use. In the initiation of marijuana use, the reverse was true. The reasons cited by those who continued to use marijuana were to "get in a better mood or feel better." Social factors were not a significant predictor of continued use. Data on young adults show similar trends. Those who use drugs in response to social influences are more likely to stop using them than those who also use them for psychological reasons.[80]

The age distribution of marijuana users among the general popula-

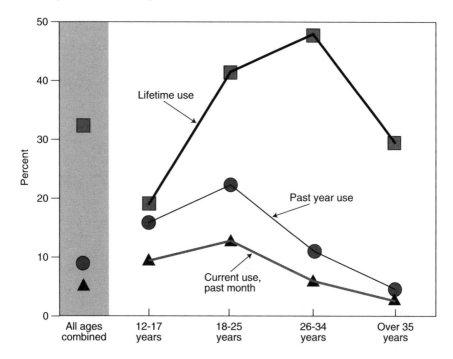

FIGURE 3.1 Age distribution of marijuana users among the general population.

tion contrasts with that of medical marijuana users. Marijuana use generally declines sharply after the age of 34 years, whereas medical marijuana users tend to be over 35. That raises the question of what, if any, relationship exists between abuse and medical use of marijuana; however, no studies reported in the scientific literature have addressed this question.

Prevalence and Predictors of Dependence on Marijuana and Other Drugs

Many factors influence the likelihood that a particular person will become a drug abuser or an addict; the user, the environment, and the drug are all important factors (Table 3.3).[114] The first two categories apply to potential abuse of any substance; that is, people who are vulnerable to drug abuse for individual reasons and who find themselves in an environment that encourages drug abuse are initially likely to abuse the most readily available drug—regardless of its unique set of effects on the brain. The third category includes drug-specific effects that influence the abuse

TABLE 3.3   Factors That Are Correlated with Drug Dependence

Individual Factors
  • Pharmacological effects of the drug
  • Gender
  • Age
  • Genetic factors
  • Individual risk-taking propensities
  • Prior drug use

Environmental Factors
  • Availability of the drug
  • Acceptance of use of that drug in society
  • Balance of social reinforcements and of punishments for use
  • Balance of social reinforcements and of punishments for abstinence

---

SOURCE: Crowley and Rhine (1985).[32]

liability of a particular drug. As discussed earlier in this chapter, the more strongly reinforcing a drug is, the more likely that it will be abused. The abuse liability of a drug is enhanced by how quickly its effects are felt, and this is determined by how the drug is delivered. In general, the effects of drugs that are inhaled or injected are felt within minutes, and the effects of drugs that are ingested take a half hour or more.

The proportion of people who become addicted varies among drugs. Table 3.4 shows estimates for the proportion of people among the general population who used or became dependent on different types of drugs. The proportion of users that ever became dependent includes anyone who was *ever* dependent—whether it was for a period of weeks or years—and thus includes more than those who are currently dependent. Compared to most other drugs listed in this table, dependence among marijuana users is relatively rare. This might be due to differences in specific drug effects, the availability of or penalties associated with the use of the different drugs, or some combination.

Daily use of most illicit drugs is extremely rare in the general population. In 1989, daily use of marijuana among high school seniors was less than that of alcohol (2.9% and 4.2%, respectively).[76]

Drug dependence is more prevalent in some sectors of the population than in others. Age, gender, and race or ethnic group are all important.[8] Excluding tobacco and alcohol, the following trends of drug dependence are statistically significant:[8] Men are 1.6 times as likely than women to become drug dependent, non-Hispanic whites are about twice as likely as blacks to become drug dependent (the difference between non-Hispanic

TABLE 3.4 Prevalence of Drug Use and Dependence[a] in the General Population

Drug Category	Proportion That Have Ever Used (%)	Proportion of Users That Ever Became Dependent (%)
Tobacco	76	32
Alcohol	92	15
Marijuana (including hashish)	46[b]	9
Anxiolytics (including sedatives and hypnotic drugs)	13	9
Cocaine	16	17
Heroin	2	23

[a]Diagnosis of drug dependence used in this study based on DSM-III-R criteria.[2]
[b]The percentage of people who ever used marijuana is higher than that reported by the National Household Survey on Drug Abuse (32%), probably due to different survey methods (for discussion, see Kandel, 1992[76]).
SOURCE: Adapted from Table 2 in Anthony and co-workers (1994).[8]

and Hispanic whites was not significant), and people 25–44 years old are more than three times as likely as those over 45 years old to become drug dependent.

More often than not, drug dependence co-occurs with other psychiatric disorders. Most people with a diagnosis of drug dependence disorder also have a diagnosis of a another psychiatric disorder (76% of men and 65% of women).[76] The most frequent co-occurring disorder is alcohol abuse; 60% of men and 30% of women with a diagnosis of drug dependence also abuse alcohol. In women who are drug dependent, phobic disorders and major depression are almost equally common (29% and 28%, respectively). Note that this study distinguished only between alcohol, nicotine and "other drugs"; marijuana was grouped among "other drugs." The frequency with which drug dependence and other psychiatric disorders co-occur might not be the same for marijuana and other drugs that were included in that category.

A strong association between drug dependence and antisocial personality or its precursor, conduct disorder, is also widely reported in children and adults (reviewed in 1998 by Robins[126]). Although the causes of the association are uncertain, Robins recently concluded that it is more likely that conduct disorders generally lead to substance abuse than the reverse.[126] Such a trend might, however, depend on the age at which the conduct disorder is manifested.

A longitudinal study by Brooks and co-workers noted a significant relationship between adolescent drug use and disruptive disorders in young adulthood; except for earlier psychopathology, such as childhood conduct disorder, the drug use preceded the psychiatric disorders.[18] In contrast with use of other illicit drugs and tobacco, moderate (less than once a week and more than once a month) to heavy marijuana use did not predict anxiety or depressive disorders; but it was similar to those other drugs in predicting antisocial personality disorder. The rates of disruptive disorders increased with increased drug use. Thus, heavy drug use among adolescents can be a warning sign for later psychiatric disorders; whether it is an early manifestation of or a cause of those disorders remains to be determined.

Psychiatric disorders are more prevalent among adolescents who use drugs—including alcohol and nicotine—than among those who do not.[79] Table 3.5 indicates that adolescent boys who smoke cigarettes daily are about 10 times as likely to have a psychiatric disorder diagnosis as those who do not smoke. However, the table does not compare intensity of use among the different drug classes. Thus, although *daily* cigarette smoking among adolescent boys is more strongly associated with psychiatric disorders than is any use of illicit substances, it does not follow that this comparison is true for every amount of cigarette smoking.[79]

Few marijuana users become dependent on it (Table 3.4), but those who do encounter problems similar to those associated with dependence on other drugs.[19,143] Dependence appears to be less severe among people

TABLE 3.5   Relative Prevalence of Diagnoses of Psychiatric Disorders Associated with Drug Use Among Children[a]

Drug Use	Relative Prevalence Estimates[b]	
	Boys	Girls
Weekly alcohol use	6.1	1.6 (n.s.)
Daily cigarette smoking	9.8	2.1 (n.s.)
Any illicit substance use	3.2	5.3

[a]Subjects were from 9 to 18 years old (average, 13 years old).

[b]An estimate of 1 means that the relative prevalence of the disorder is equal in those who do and those who do not use the particular type of drug; that is, there is no measurable association. An estimate greater than 1 indicates that the factor is associated. Substance abuse was excluded because the subjects were already grouped by high drug use. Except where noted (n.s.), all values are statistically significant.

SOURCE: Data from Table 4 in Kandel and co-workers (1997).[79]

who use only marijuana than among those who abuse cocaine or those who abuse marijuana with other drugs (including alcohol).[19,143]

Data gathered in 1990–1992 from the National Comorbidity Study of over 8,000 persons 15–54 years old indicate that 4.2% of the general population were dependent on marijuana at some time.[8] Similar results for the frequency of substance abuse among the general population were obtained from the Epidemiological Catchment Area Program, a survey of over 19,000 people. According to data collected in the early 1980s for that study, 4.4% of adults have, at one time, met the criteria for marijuana dependence. In comparison, 13.8% of adults met the criteria for alcohol dependence and 36.0% for tobacco dependence. After alcohol and nicotine, marijuana was the substance most frequently associated with a diagnosis of substance dependence.

In a 15-year study begun in 1979, 7.3% of 1,201 adolescents and young adults in suburban New Jersey at some time met the criteria for marijuana dependence; this indicates that the rate of marijuana dependence might be even higher in some groups of adolescents and young adults than in the general population.[71] Adolescents meet the criteria for drug dependence at lower rates of marijuana use than do adults, and this suggests that they are more vulnerable to dependence than adults[25] (see Box 3.2).

Youths who are already dependent on other substances are particularly vulnerable to marijuana dependence. For example, Crowley and co-workers[31] interviewed a group of 229 adolescent patients in a residential treatment program for delinquent, substance-involved youth and found that those patients were dependent on an average of 3.2 substances. The adolescents had previously been diagnosed as dependent on at least one substance (including nicotine and alcohol) and had three or more conduct disorder symptoms during their life. About 83% of those who had used marijuana at least six times went on to develop marijuana dependence. About equal numbers of youths in the study had a diagnosis of marijuana dependence and a diagnosis of alcohol dependence; fewer were nicotine dependent. Comparisons of dependence potential between different drugs should be made cautiously. The probability that a particular drug will be abused is influenced by many factors, including the specific drug effects and availability of the drug.

Although parents often state that marijuana caused their children to be rebellious, the troubled adolescents in the study by Crowley and co-workers developed conduct disorders *before* marijuana abuse. That is consistent with reports that the more symptoms of conduct disorders children have, the younger they begin drug abuse,[127] and that the earlier they begin drug use, the more likely it is to be followed by abuse or dependence.[125]

Genetic factors are known to play a role in the likelihood of abuse for drugs other than marijuana,[7,129] and it is not unexpected that genetic factors play a role in the marijuana experience, including the likelihood of abuse. A study of over 8,000 male twins listed in the Vietnam Era Twin Registry indicated that genes have a statistically significant influence on whether a person finds the effects of marijuana pleasant.[97] Not surprisingly, people who found marijuana to be pleasurable used it more often than those who found it unpleasant. The study suggested that, although social influences play an important role in the initiation of use, individual differences—perhaps associated with the brain's reward system—influence whether a person will continue using marijuana. Similar results were found in a study of female twins.[86] Family and social environment strongly influenced the likelihood of ever using marijuana but had little effect on the likelihood of heavy use or abuse. The latter were more influenced by genetic factors. Those results are consistent with the finding that the degree to which rats find THC rewarding is genetically based.[92]

In summary, although few marijuana users develop dependence, some do. But they appear to be less likely to do so than users of other drugs (including alcohol and nicotine), and marijuana dependence appears to be less severe than dependence on other drugs. Drug dependence is more prevalent in some sectors of the population than others, but no group has been identified as particularly vulnerable to the drug-specific effects of marijuana. Adolescents, especially troubled ones, and people with psychiatric disorders (including substance abuse) appear to be more likely than the general population to become dependent on marijuana.

If marijuana or cannabinoid drugs were approved for therapeutic uses, it would be important to consider the possibility of dependence, particularly for patients at high risk for substance dependence. Some controlled substances that are approved medications produce dependence after long-term use; this, however, is a normal part of patient management and does not generally present undue risk to the patient.

Progression from Marijuana to Other Drugs

The fear that marijuana use might cause, as opposed to merely precede, the use of drugs that are more harmful is of great concern. To judge from comments submitted to the IOM study team, it appears to be of greater concern than the harms directly related to marijuana itself. The discussion that marijuana is a "gateway" drug implicitly recognizes that other illicit drugs might inflict greater damage to health or social relations than marijuana. Although the scientific literature generally discusses drug use progression between a variety of drug classes, including alcohol and tobacco, the public discussion has focused on marijuana as a "gateway" drug that leads to abuse of more harmful illicit drugs, such as cocaine and heroin.

There are strikingly regular patterns in the progression of drug use from adolescence to adulthood. Because it is the most widely used illicit drug, marijuana is predictably the first illicit drug that most people encounter. Not surprisingly, most users of other illicit drugs used marijuana first.[81,82] In fact, most drug users do not begin their drug use with marijuana—they begin with alcohol and nicotine, usually when they are too young to do so legally.[82,90]

The gateway analogy evokes two ideas that are often confused. The first, more often referred to as the "stepping stone" hypothesis, is the idea that progression from marijuana to other drugs arises from pharmacological properties of marijuana itself.[82] The second is that marijuana serves as a gateway to the world of illegal drugs in which youths have greater opportunity and are under greater social pressure to try other illegal drugs. The latter interpretation is most often used in the scientific literature, and it is supported, although not proven, by the available data.

The stepping stone hypothesis applies to marijuana only in the broadest sense. People who enjoy the effects of marijuana are, logically, more likely to be willing to try other mood-altering drugs than are people who are not willing to try marijuana or who dislike its effects. In other words, many of the factors associated with a willingness to use marijuana are, presumably, the same as those associated with a willingness to use other illicit drugs. Those factors include physiological reactions to the drug effect, which are consistent with the stepping stone hypothesis, but also psychosocial factors, which are independent of drug-specific effects. There is no evidence that marijuana serves as a stepping stone on the basis of its particular physiological effect. One might argue that marijuana is generally used before other illicit mood-altering drugs, in part, because its effects are milder; in that case, marijuana is a stepping stone only in the same sense as taking a small dose of a particular drug and then increasing that dose over time is a stepping stone to increased drug use.

Whereas the stepping stone hypothesis presumes a predominantly physiological component of drug progression, the gateway theory is a social theory. The latter does not suggest that the pharmacological qualities of marijuana make it a risk factor for progression to other drug use. Instead, the legal status of marijuana makes it a gateway drug.[82]

Psychiatric disorders are associated with substance dependence and are probably risk factors for progression in drug use. For example, the troubled adolescents studied by Crowley and co-workers[31] were dependent on an average of 3.2 substances, and this suggests that their conduct disorders were associated with increased risk of progressing from one drug to another. Abuse of a single substance is probably also a risk factor for later multiple drug use. For example, in a longitudinal study that examined drug use and dependence, about 26% of problem drinkers reported that they first used marijuana after the onset of alcohol-related problems (R. Pandina, IOM workshop). The study also found that 11% of marijuana users developed chronic marijuana problems; most also had alcohol problems.

Intensity of drug use is an important risk factor in progression. Daily marijuana users are more likely than their peers to be extensive users of other substances (for review, see Kandel and Davies[78]). Of 34- to 35-year-old men who had used marijuana 10–99 times by the age 24–25, 75% never used any other illicit drug; 53% of those who had used it more than 100 times did progress to using other illicit drugs 10 or more times. [78] Comparable proportions for women are 64% and 50%.

The factors that best predict use of illicit drugs other than marijuana are probably the following: age of first alcohol or nicotine use, heavy marijuana use, and psychiatric disorders. However, progression to illicit drug use is not synonymous with heavy or persistent drug use. Indeed, although the age of onset of use of licit drugs (alcohol and nicotine) predicts later illicit drug use, it does *not* appear to predict persistent or heavy use of illicit drugs.[90]

Data on the gateway phenomenon are often overinterpreted. For example, one study reports that "marijuana's role as a gateway drug appears to have increased."[55] It was a retrospective study based on interviews of drug abusers who reported smoking crack or injecting heroin daily. The data from the study provide no indication of what proportion of marijuana users become serious drug abusers; rather, they indicate that serious drug abusers usually use marijuana before they smoke crack or inject heroin. Only a small percentage of the adult population uses crack or heroin daily; during the five-year period from 1993 to 1997, an average of three people per 1,000 used crack and about two per 1,000 used heroin in the preceding month.[132]

Many of the data on which the gateway theory is based do not measure dependence; instead, they measure use—even once-only use. Thus, they show only that marijuana users are more likely to use other illicit drugs (even if only once) than are people who never use marijuana, not that they become dependent or even frequent users. The authors of these studies are careful to point out that their data should not be used as evidence of an inexorable *causal* progression; rather they note that identifying stage-based user groups makes it possible to identify the specific risk factors that predict movement from one stage of drug use to the next—the real issue in the gateway discussion.[25]

In the sense that marijuana use typically precedes rather than follows initiation into the use of other illicit drugs, it is indeed a gateway drug.

However, it does not appear to be a gateway drug to the extent that it is the *cause* or even that it is the most significant predictor of serious drug abuse; that is, care must be taken not to attribute cause to association. The most consistent predictors of serious drug use appear to be the intensity of marijuana use and co-occurring psychiatric disorders or a family history of psychopathology (including alcoholism).[78,83]

An important caution is that data on drug use progression pertain to *nonmedical* drug use. It does not follow from those data that if marijuana were available by prescription for *medical* use, the pattern of drug use would be the same. Kandel and co-workers also included nonmedical use of prescription psychoactive drugs in their study of drug use progression.[82] In contrast with the use of alcohol, nicotine, and illicit drugs, there was not a clear and consistent sequence of drug use involving the abuse of prescription psychoactive drugs. The current data on drug use progression neither support nor refute the suggestion that medical availability would increase drug abuse among medical marijuana users. Whether the medical use of marijuana might encourage drug abuse among the general community—not among medical marijuana users themselves but among others simply because of the fact that marijuana would be used for medical purposes—is another question.

LINK BETWEEN MEDICAL USE AND DRUG ABUSE

Almost everyone who spoke or wrote to the IOM study team about the potential harms posed by the medical use of marijuana felt that it would send the wrong message to children and teenagers. They stated that information about the harms caused by marijuana is undermined by claims that marijuana might have medical value. Yet many of our powerful medicines are also dangerous medicines. These two facets of medicine—effectiveness and risk—are inextricably linked.

The question here is not whether marijuana can be both harmful and helpful but whether the perception of its benefits will increase its abuse. For now any answer to the question remains conjecture. Because marijuana is not an approved medicine, there is little information about the consequences of its medical use in modern society. Reasonable inferences might be drawn from some examples. Opiates, such as morphine and codeine, are an example of a class of drugs that is both abused to great harm and used to great medical benefit, and it would be useful to examine the relationship between their medical use and their abuse. In a "natural experiment" during 1973–1978 some states decriminalized marijuana, and others did not. Finally, one can examine the short-term consequences of the publicity surrounding the 1996 medical marijuana campaign in California and ask whether it had any measurable impact on marijuana consumption among youth in California; the consequences of "message" that marijuana might have medical use are examined below.

Medical Use and Abuse of Opiates

Two highly influential papers published in the 1920s and 1950s led to widespread concern among physicians and medical licensing boards that liberal use of opiates would result in many addicts (reviewed by Moulin and co-workers[106] in 1996). Such fears have proven unfounded; it is now recognized that fear of producing addicts through medical treatment resulted in needless suffering among patients with pain as physicians needlessly limited appropriate doses of medications.[27,44] Few people begin their drug addiction problems with misuse of drugs that have been prescribed for medical use.[114] Opiates are carefully regulated in the medical setting, and diversion of medically prescribed opiates to the black market is not generally considered to be a major problem.

No evidence suggests that the use of opiates or cocaine for medical purposes has increased the perception that their illicit use is safe or acceptable. Clearly, there are risks that patients will abuse marijuana for its psychoactive effects and some likelihood of diversion of marijuana from legitimate medical channels into the illicit market. But those risks do not differentiate marijuana from many accepted medications that are abused by some patients or diverted from medical channels for non-medical use. Medications with abuse potential are placed in Schedule II of the Controlled Substances Act, which brings them under stricter control, including quotas on the amount that can be legally manufactured (see chapter 5 for discussion of the Controlled Substances Act). That scheduling also signals to physicians that a drug has abuse potential and that they should monitor its use by patients who could be at risk for drug abuse.

Marijuana Decriminalization

Monitoring the Future, the annual survey of values and lifestyles of high school seniors, revealed that high school seniors in decriminalized states reported using no more marijuana than did their counterparts in states where marijuana was not decriminalized.[72] Another study reported somewhat conflicting evidence indicating that decriminalization had increased marijuana use.[105] That study used data from the Drug Awareness Warning Network (DAWN), which has collected data on drug-related emergency room (ER) cases since 1975. There was a greater increase from 1975 to 1978 in the proportion of ER patients who had used marijuana in states that had decriminalized marijuana in 1975–1976 than in states that had not decriminalized it (Table 3.6). Despite the greater

TABLE 3.6   Effect of Decriminalization on Marijuana Use in Emergency Room (ER) Cases

	Period[b]	Total Reports of Drug Use per ER[a]	
		States That Decriminalized Marijuana	States That Did Not Decriminalize Marijuana
Marijuana use	1975	0.8	1.5
	1978	2.7	2.5
Other drug use	1975	47	55
	1978	55	70

[a]Data are based on patient self-reports.
[b]States that decriminalized marijuana did so after 1975 and before 1978. The 1975 values reflect ER marijuana reports before or in the first months of decriminalization, whereas 1978 values reflect ER reports when decriminalization laws had been in effect at least a year. The 1978 levels are median values for quarters in 1978 and are derived from Figures 1 and 2 in Model (1993).[105]
SOURCE: Adapted from Figures 1 and 2 in Model (1993).[105]

increase among decriminalized states, the proportion of marijuana users among ER patients by 1978 was about equal in states that had and states that had not decriminalized marijuana. That is because the non-decriminalized states had higher rates of marijuana use *before* decriminalization. In contrast with marijuana use, rates of other illicit drug use among ER patients were substantially higher in states that did not decriminalize marijuana use. Thus, there are different possible reasons for the greater increase in marijuana use in the decriminalized states. On the one hand, decriminalization might have led to an increased use of marijuana (at least among people who sought health care in hospital ERs). On the other hand, the lack of decriminalization might have encouraged greater use of drugs that are even more dangerous than marijuana.

The differences between the results for high school seniors from the Monitoring the Future study and the DAWN data are unclear, although the author of the latter study suggests that the reasons might lie in limitations inherent in how the DAWN data are collected.[105]

In 1976, the Netherlands adopted a policy of toleration for possession of up to 30 g of marijuana. There was little change in marijuana use during the seven years after the policy change, which suggests that the change itself had little effect; however, in 1984, when Dutch "coffee shops" that sold marijuana commercially spread throughout Amsterdam, marijuana use began to increase.[98] During the 1990s, marijuana use has continued to increase in the Netherlands at the same rate as in the United States and Norway—two countries that strictly forbid marijuana sale and possession. Furthermore, during this period, approximately equal percentages of American and Dutch 18 year olds used marijuana; Norwegian 18 year olds were about half as likely to have used marijuana. The authors of this study conclude that there is little evidence that the Dutch marijuana depenalization policy led to increased marijuana use, although they note that commercialization of marijuana might have contributed to its increased use. Thus, there is little evidence that decriminalization of marijuana use necessarily leads to a substantial increase in marijuana use.

The Medical Marijuana Debate

The most recent National Household Survey on Drug Abuse showed that among people 12–17 years old the perceived risk associated with smoking marijuana once or twice a week had decreased significantly between 1996 and 1997.[132] (Perceived risk is measured as the percentage of survey respondents who report that they "perceive great risk of harm" in using a drug at a specified frequency.) At first glance, that might seem to validate the fear that the medical marijuana debate of 1996—before passage of the California medical marijuana referendum in November 1997—had sent a message that marijuana use is safe. But a closer analysis of the data shows that Californian youth were an exception to the national trend. In contrast to the national trend, the perceived risk of marijuana use did not change among California youth between 1996 and 1997.[132]* In summary, there is no evidence that the medical marijuana debate has altered adolescents' perceptions of the risks associated with marijuana use.[132]

PSYCHOLOGICAL HARMS

In assessing the relative risks and benefits related to the medical use of marijuana, the psychological effects of marijuana can be viewed both as unwanted side effects and as potentially desirable end points in medical treatment. However, the vast majority of research on the psychological effects of marijuana has been in the context of assessing the drug's intoxicating effects when it is used for nonmedical purposes. Thus, the litera-

---

*Although Arizona also passed a medical marijuana referendum, it was embedded in a broader referendum concerning prison sentencing. Hence, the debate in Arizona did not focus on medical marijuana the way it did in California, and changes in Arizona youths' attitudes likely reflect factors peripheral to medical marijuana.

ture does not directly address the effects of marijuana taken for medical purposes.

There are some important caveats to consider in attempting to extrapolate from the research mentioned above to the medical use of marijuana. The circumstances under which psychoactive drugs are taken are an important influence on their psychological effects. Furthermore, research protocols to study marijuana's psychological effects in most instances were required to use participants who already had experience with marijuana. People who might have had adverse reactions to marijuana either would choose not to participate in this type of study or would be screened out by the investigator. Therefore, the incidence of adverse reactions to marijuana that might occur in people with no marijuana experience cannot be estimated from such studies. A further complicating factor concerns the dose regimen used for laboratory studies. In most instances, laboratory research studies have looked at the effects of single doses of marijuana, which might be different from those observed when the drug is taken repeatedly for a chronic medical condition.

Nonetheless, laboratory studies are useful in suggesting what psychological functions might be studied when marijuana is evaluated for medical purposes. Results of laboratory studies indicate that acute and chronic marijuana use has pronounced effects on mood, psychomotor, and cognitive functions. These psychological domains should therefore be considered in assessing the relative risks and therapeutic benefits related to marijuana or cannabinoids for any medical condition.

Psychiatric Disorders

A major question remains as to whether marijuana can produce lasting mood disorders or psychotic disorders, such as schizophrenia. Georgotas and Zeidenberg[52] reported that smoking 10–22 marijuana cigarettes per day was associated with a gradual waning of the positive mood and social facilitating effects of marijuana and an increase in irritability, social isolation, and paranoid thinking. Inasmuch as smoking *one* cigarette is enough to make a person feel "high" for about 1–3 hours,[68,95,118] the subjects in that study were taking very high doses of marijuana. Reports have described the development of apathy, lowered motivation, and impaired educational performance in heavy marijuana users who do not appear to be behaviorally impaired in other ways.[121,122] There are clinical reports of marijuana-induced psychosis-like states (schizophrenia-like, depression, and/or mania) lasting for a week or more.[112] Hollister suggests that, because of the varied nature of the psychotic states induced by marijuana, there is no specific "marijuana psychosis." Rather, the marijuana experience might trigger latent psychopathology of many types.[66]

More recently, Hall and colleagues[60] concluded that "there is reasonable evidence that heavy cannabis use, and perhaps acute use in sensitive individuals, can produce an acute psychosis in which confusion, amnesia, delusions, hallucinations, anxiety, agitation and hypomanic symptoms predominate." Regardless of which of those interpretations is correct, the two reports agree that there is little evidence that marijuana alone produces a psychosis that persists after the period of intoxication.

Schizophrenia

The association between marijuana and schizophrenia is not well understood. The scientific literature indicates general agreement that heavy marijuana use can precipitate schizophrenic episodes but not that marijuana use can cause the underlying psychotic disorder.[59,96,151] As noted earlier, drug abuse is common among people with psychiatric disorders. Estimates of the prevalence of marijuana use among schizophrenics vary considerably but are in general agreement that it is at least as great as that among the general population.[134] Schizophrenics prefer the effects of marijuana to those of alcohol and cocaine,[35] which they seem to use less often than does the general population.[134] The reasons for this are unknown, but it raises the possibility that schizophrenics might obtain some symptomatic relief from moderate marijuana use. But overall, compared with the general population, people with schizophrenia or with a family history of schizophrenia are likely to be at greater risk for adverse psychiatric effects from the use of cannabinoids.

Cognition

As discussed earlier, acutely administered marijuana impairs cognition.[60,66,112] Positron emission tomography (PET) imaging allows investigators to measure the acute effects of marijuana smoking on active brain function. Human volunteers who perform auditory attention tasks before and after smoking a marijuana cigarette show impaired performance while under the influence of marijuana; this is associated with substantial reduction in blood flow to the temporal lobe of the brain, an area that is sensitive to such tasks.[116,117] Marijuana smoking increases blood flow in other brain regions, such as the frontal lobes and lateral cerebellum.[101,155] Earlier studies purporting to show structural changes in the brains of heavy marijuana users[22] have not been replicated with more sophisticated techniques.[28,89]

Nevertheless, recent studies[14,122] have found subtle defects in cognitive tasks in heavy marijuana users after a brief period (19–24 hours) of marijuana abstinence. Longer term cognitive deficits in heavy marijuana users have also been reported.[140] Although these studies have attempted to match heavy marijuana users with subjects of similar cognitive abilities before exposure to marijuana use, the adequacy of this matching has been questioned.[133] The complex methodological issues facing research in this area are well reviewed in an article by Pope and colleagues.[121] Care must be exercised so that studies are designed to differentiate between changes in brain function caused the effects of marijuana and by the illness for which marijuana is being given. AIDS dementia is an obvious example of this possible confusion. It is also important to determine whether repeated use of marijuana at therapeutic dosages produces any irreversible cognitive effects.

Psychomotor Performance

Marijuana administration has been reported to affect psychomotor performance on a number of tasks. The review by Chait and Pierri[23] not only details the studies that have been done but also points out the inconsistencies among studies, the methodological shortcomings of many studies, and the large individual differences among the studies attributable to subject, situational, and methodological factors. Those factors must be considered in studies of psychomotor performance when participants are involved in a clinical trial of the efficacy of marijuana. The types of psychomotor functions that have been shown to be disrupted by the acute administration of marijuana include body sway, hand steadiness, rotary pursuit, driving and flying simulation, divided attention, sustained attention, and the digit-symbol substitution test. A study of experienced airplane pilots showed that even 24 hours after a single marijuana cigarette their performance on flight simulator tests was impaired.[163] Before the tests, however, they told the study investigators that they were sure their performance would be unaffected.

Cognitive impairments associated with acutely administered marijuana limit the activities that people would be able to do safely or productively. For example, no one under the influence of marijuana or THC should drive a vehicle or operate potentially dangerous equipment.

Amotivational Syndrome

One of the more controversial effects claimed for marijuana is the production of an "amotivational syndrome." This syndrome is not a medical diagnosis, but it has been used to describe young people who drop out of social activities and show little interest in school, work, or other goal-directed activity. When heavy marijuana use accompanies these symptoms, the drug is often cited as the cause, but no convincing data demonstrate a causal relationship between marijuana smoking and these behavioral characteristics.[23] It is not enough to observe that a chronic marijuana user lacks motivation. Instead, relevant personality traits and behavior of subjects must be assessed before and after the subject becomes a heavy marijuana user. Because such research can only be done on subjects who become heavy marijuana users on their own, a large population study—such as the Epidemiological Catchment Area study described earlier in this chapter—would be needed to shed light on the relationship between motivation and marijuana use. Even then, although a causal relationship between the two could, in theory, be dismissed by an epidemiological study, causality could not be proven.

Summary

Measures of mood, cognition, and psychomotor performance should be incorporated into clinical trials evaluating the efficacy of marijuana or cannabinoid drugs for a given medical condition. Ideally, participants would complete mood assessment questionnaires at various intervals throughout the day for a period before; every week during; and, where appropriate, after marijuana therapy. A full psychological screening of research participants should be conducted to determine whether there is an interaction between the mood-altering effects of chronic marijuana use and the psychological characteristics of the subjects. Similarly, the cognitive and psychomotor functioning should be assessed before and regularly during the course of a chronic regimen of marijuana or cannabinoid treatment to determine the extent to which tolerance to the impairing effects of marijuana develops and to monitor whether new problems develop.

When compared with changes produced by either placebo or an active control medication, the magnitude of desirable therapeutic effects and the frequency and magnitude of adverse psychological side effects of marijuana could be determined. That would allow a more thorough assessment of the risk:benefit ratio associated with the use of marijuana for a given indication.

CONCLUSION: The psychological effects of cannabinoids, such as anxiety reduction, sedation, and euphoria, can influence their potential therapeutic value. Those effects are potentially undesirable in some patients and situations and beneficial in others. In addition, psychological effects can complicate the interpretation of other aspects of the drug's effect.

RECOMMENDATION: **Psychological effects of cannabinoids, such as anxiety reduction and sedation, which can influence medical benefits, should be evaluated in clinical trials.**

PHYSIOLOGICAL HARMS: TISSUE AND ORGAN DAMAGE

Many people who spoke to the IOM study team in favor of the medical use of marijuana cited the absence of marijuana overdoses as evidence that it is safe. Indeed, epidemiological data indicate that in the general population marijuana use is not associated with increased mortality.[138] However, other serious health outcomes should be considered, and they are discussed below.

It is important to keep in mind that most of the studies that report physiological harm resulting from marijuana use are based on the effects of marijuana smoking. Thus, we emphasize that the effects reported cannot be presumed to be caused by THC alone or even in combination with other cannabinoids found in marijuana. It is likely that smoke is a major cause of the reported effects. In most studies the methods used make it impossible to weigh the relative contributions of smoke versus cannabinoids.

Immune System

The relationship between marijuana and the immune system presents many facets, including potential benefits and suspected harms. This section reviews the evidence on suspected harms to the immune system caused by marijuana use.

Despite the many claims that marijuana suppresses the human immune system, the health effects of marijuana-induced immunomodulation are still unclear. Few studies have been done with animals or humans to assess the effects of marijuana exposure on host resistance to bacteria, viruses, or tumors.

Human Studies

Several approaches have been used to determine the effects of marijuana on the human immune system. Each has serious limitations, which are discussed below.

Assays of Leukocytes from Marijuana Smokers. One of the more common approaches has been to isolate peripheral blood leukocytes from people who have smoked marijuana in order to evaluate the immune response of those cells in vitro—most often by measuring mitogen-induced cell proliferation, a normal immune response. Almost without exception, this approach has failed to demonstrate any reduction in leukocyte function. The major problem with the approach is that after blood samples are drawn from the study subjects the leukocytes must be isolated from whole blood before they are tested. That is done by high-speed centrifugation followed by extensive washing of the cells, which removes the cannabinoid; perhaps for this reason no adverse effects have been demonstrated in peripheral blood leukocytes from marijuana smokers.[75,91,123,160]

Leukocyte Responses to THC. Another approach is to isolate peripheral blood leukocytes from healthy control subjects who do not smoke marijuana and then to measure the effect of THC on the ability of these cells to proliferate in response to mitogenic stimulation *in vitro*. One important difference between leukocytes isolated from a marijuana smoker, as described above, and leukocyte cell cultures to which THC has been added directly is in the cannabinoid composition. Marijuana smoke contains many distinct cannabinoid compounds of which THC is just one. Moreover, the immunomodulatory activity of many of the other cannabinoid compounds has never been tested, and it is now known that at least one of those—cannabinol (CBN)—has greater activity on the immune system than on the central nervous system,[64] so it is unclear whether the profile of activity observed with THC accurately represents the effects of marijuana smoke on immune competence. Likewise, the extent to which different cannabinoids in combination exhibit additive, synergistic, or antagonistic effects with respect to immunomodulatory activity is unclear. The issue is complicated by the fact that leukocytes express both types of cannabinoid receptors: CB_1 and CB_2.

An additional factor that might affect the immunomodulatory activity of cannabinoids in leukocytes is metabolism. Leukocytes have very low levels of the cytochrome P-450 drug-metabolizing enzymes,[20] so the metabolism of cannabinoids is probably different between *in vivo* and *in vitro* exposure. That last point is pertinent primarily to investigations of chronic, not acute, cannabinoid exposure.

Human-Derived Cell Lines. A third approach for investigating the effects of cannabinoids on human leukocytes has been to study human-derived cell lines.* As described above, the cell lines are treated *in vitro* with cannabinoids to test their responses to different stimuli. Although cell lines

---

*Cell lines are created by removing cells from an organism and then treating them so they are "immortalized," meaning they will continue to divide and multiply indefinitely in culture. Cellular processes can then be studied in isolation from their original source.

are a convenient source of human cells, the problems described above apply here as well. In addition, the cell lines might not be the same as the original cells. For example, cell lines do not necessarily have the same number of cannabinoid receptors as the original human cells.

Rodent Studies

The most widely used approach is to evaluate the effects of cannabinoids in rodents, using rodent-derived cells *in vitro*. The rationale is that the human and rodent immune systems are remarkably similar, and it is assumed that the effects produced by cannabinoids on the rodent immune system will be similar to those produced in humans. Although no substantial species differences in immune system sensitivity to cannabinoids have been reported, the possibility should be considered.

Summary

The complete effect of marijuana smoking on immune function remains unknown. More important, it is not known whether smoking leads to increased rates of infections, tumors, allergies, or autoimmune responses. The problem is how to duplicate the "normal" marijuana smoking pattern while removing other potential immunomodulating lifestyle factors, such as alcohol and tobacco use. Epidemiological studies are needed to determine whether marijuana users have a higher incidence of such diseases, as infections, tumors, allergies, and autoimmune diseases. Studies on resistance to bacterial and viral infection are clearly needed and should involve the collaboration of immunologists, infectious disease specialists, oncologists, and pharmacologists.

Marijuana Smoke

Tobacco is the predominant cause of such lung diseases as cancer and emphysema, and marijuana smoke contains many of the components of tobacco smoke.[69] Thus, it is important to consider the relationship between habitual marijuana smoking and some lung diseases.

Given a cigarette of comparable weight, as much as four times the amount of tar can be deposited in the lungs of marijuana smokers as in the lungs of tobacco smokers.[162] The difference is due primarily to the differences in filtration and smoking technique between tobacco and marijuana smokers. Marijuana cigarettes usually do not have filters, and marijuana smokers typically develop a larger puff volume, inhale more deeply, and hold their breath several times longer than tobacco smokers.[119] However, a marijuana cigarette smoked recreationally typically is not packed as tightly as a tobacco cigarette, and the smokable substance is about half that in a tobacco cigarette. In addition, tobacco smokers generally smoke considerably more cigarettes per day than do marijuana smokers.

Cellular Damage

Lymphocytes: T and B Cells. Human studies of the effect of marijuana smoking on immune cell function are not all consistent with cannabinoid cell culture and animal studies. For example, antibody production was decreased in a group of hospitalized patients who smoked marijuana for four days (12 cigarettes/day), but the decrease was seen in only one subtype of humoral antibody (IgG), whereas two other subtypes (IgA and IgM) remained normal and one (IgE) was increased.[108] In addition, T cell proliferation was normal in the blood of a group of marijuana smokers, although closer evaluation showed an increase in one subset of T cells[161] and a decrease in a different subset (CD8).[157] It appears that marijuana use is associated with intermittent disturbances in T and B cell function, but the magnitude is small and other measures are often normal.[87]

Macrophages. Alveolar macrophages are the principal immune-effector cells in the lung and are primarily responsible for protecting the lung against infectious microorganisms, inhaled foreign substances, and tumor cells. They are increased during tissue inflammation. In a large sample of volunteers, habitual marijuana smokers had twice as many alveolar macrophages as nonsmokers, and smokers of both marijuana and tobacco had twice as many again.[11] Marijuana smoking also reduced the ability of alveolar macrophages to kill fungi, such as *Candida albicans*;* pathogenic bacteria, such as *Staphylococcus aureus*; and tumor target cells. The reduction in ability to destroy fungal organisms was similar to that seen in tobacco smokers. The inability to kill pathogenic bacteria was not seen in tobacco smokers.[10] Furthermore, marijuana smoking depressed production of proinflammatory cytokines, such as TNF-I and IL-6, but not of immunosuppressive cytokines.[10] Cytokines are important regulators of macrophage function, so this marijuana-related decrease in inflammatory cytokine production might be a mechanism whereby marijuana smokers are less able to destroy fungal and bacterial organisms, as well as tumor cells.

The inability of alveolar macrophages from habitual marijuana smokers without apparent disease to destroy fungi, bacteria, and tumor cells

---

Candida albicans is a yeast infection that is particularly prevalent among people whose immune systems are suppressed, such as in AIDS patients.

and to release proinflammatory cytokines, suggests that marijuana might be an immunosuppressant with clinically significant effects on host defense. Therefore, the risks of smoking marijuana should be seriously weighed before recommending its use in any patient with preexisting immune deficits—including AIDS patients, cancer patients, and those receiving immunosuppressive therapies (for example, transplant or cancer patients).

Bronchial and Pulmonary Damage

Animal Studies. A number of animal studies have revealed respiratory tract changes and diseases associated with marijuana smoking, but others have not. Extensive damage to the smaller airways, which are the major site of chronic obstructive pulmonary disease (COPD),* and acute and chronic pneumonia have been observed in various species exposed to different doses of marijuana smoke.[41,42,128] In contrast, rats exposed to increasing doses of marijuana smoke for one year did not show any signs of COPD, whereas rats exposed to tobacco smoke did.[67]

Chronic Bronchitis and Respiratory Illness. Results of human studies suggest that there is a greater chance of respiratory illness in people who smoke marijuana. In a survey of outpatient medical visits at a large health maintenance organization (HMO), marijuana users were more likely to seek help for respiratory illnesses than people who smoked neither marijuana or tobacco.[120] However, the incidence of seeking help for respiratory illnesses was not higher in those who smoked marijuana for 10 years or more than in those who smoked for less than 10 years. One explanation for this is that people who experience respiratory symptoms are more likely to quit smoking and that people who continue to smoke constitute a set of survivors who do not develop or are indifferent to such symptoms. One limitation of this study is that no data were available on the use of cocaine, which when used with marijuana could contribute to the observed differences. Another limitation is that the survey relied on self-reporting; tobacco, alcohol, and marijuana use might have been underreported (S. Sidney, IOM workshop).

When marijuana smokers were compared with nonsmokers and tobacco smokers in a group of 446 volunteers, 15–20% of the marijuana smokers reported symptoms of chronic bronchitis, including chronic

---

*COPD is a slow progressive obstruction of the airways, loss of their elasticity, and loss of lung volume, characterized by chronic shortness of breath, chronic bronchitis, and reduced oxygenation of blood.

cough and phlegm production,[146] and 20–25% of the tobacco smokers reported symptoms of chronic bronchitis. Despite a marked disparity in the amount of each substance smoked per day (three or four joints of marijuana versus more than 20 cigarettes of tobacco), the difference in the percentages of tobacco smokers and marijuana smokers experiencing symptoms of chronic bronchitis was statistically insignificant.[146] Similar findings were reported by Bloom and co-workers,[15] who noted an additive effect of smoking both marijuana and tobacco.

Bronchial Tissue Changes. Habitual marijuana smoking is associated with changes in the lining of the human respiratory tract. Many marijuana or tobacco smokers have increased redness (erythema) and swelling (edema) of the airway tissues and increased mucous secretions.[43,56] In marijuana smokers the number and size of small blood vessels in the bronchial wall are increased, tissue edema is present, and the normal ciliated cells* lining the inner surface of the bronchial wall are largely replaced by mucous-secreting goblet cells. The damage is greater in people who smoke both marijuana and tobacco.[130] Overproduction of mucus by the increased numbers of mucous-secreting cells in the presence of decreased numbers of ciliated cells tends to leave coughing as the only major mechanism to remove mucus from the airways; this might explain the relatively high proportion of marijuana smokers who complain of chronic cough and phlegm production.[148]

A 1998 study has shown that both marijuana and tobacco smokers have significantly more cellular and molecular abnormalities in bronchial epithelium cells than nonsmokers; these changes are associated with increased risk of cancer.[12] The tobacco-only smokers in that study smoked an average of 25 cigarettes per day, whereas the marijuana-only smokers smoked an average of 21 marijuana cigarettes per week. Although the marijuana smokers smoked far fewer cigarettes, their cellular abnormalities were equivalent to or greater than those seen in tobacco smokers. This and earlier studies have shown that such abnormalities are greatest in people who smoke both marijuana and tobacco; hence, marijuana and tobacco smoke might have additive effects on airway tissue.[12,43,56] Tenant[150] found similar results in U.S. servicemen who suffered from respiratory symptoms and were heavy hashish smokers. (Hashish is the resin from the marijuana plant.)

Chronic Obstructive Pulmonary Disease. In the absence of epidemiological data, indirect evidence, such as nonspecific airway hyperrespon-

---

*Ciliated cells have hair-like projections that function to transport mucus toward the mouth by rapid wave-like motion.

siveness and measures of lung function, offers an indicator of the vulnerability of marijuana smokers to COPD.[154] For example, the methacholine provocative challenge test, used to evaluate airway hyperresponsiveness, showed that tobacco smokers develop more airway hyperresponsiveness. But no such correlation has been shown between marijuana smoking and airway hyperresponsiveness.

There is conflicting evidence on whether regular marijuana use harms the small airways of the lungs. Bloom and co-workers found that an average of one joint smoked per day significantly impaired the function of small airways.[15] But Tashkin and co-workers[146] did not observe such damage among heavier marijuana users (three to four joints per day for at least 10 years), although they noted a narrowing of large central airways. Tashkin and co-workers' long-term study, which adjusted for age-related decline in lung function (associated with an increased risk for developing COPD), showed an accelerated rate of decline in tobacco smokers but not in marijuana smokers.[147] Thus, the question of whether usual marijuana smoking habits are enough to cause COPD remains open.

Conclusion. Chronic marijuana smoking might lead to acute and chronic bronchitis and extensive microscopic abnormalities in the cells lining the bronchial passageways, some of which may be premalignant. These respiratory symptoms are similar to those of tobacco smokers, and the combination of marijuana and tobacco smoking augments these effects. At the time of this writing, it had not been established whether chronic smoking marijuana causes COPD, but there is probably an association.

HIV/AIDS Patients

The relationship between marijuana smoking and the natural course of AIDS is of particular concern because HIV patients are the largest group who report using marijuana for medical purposes. Marijuana use has been linked both to increased risk of progression to AIDS in HIV-seropositive patients and to increased mortality in AIDS patients.

For unknown reasons, marijuana use is associated with increased mortality among men with AIDS but not among the general population.[138] (The relative risk of AIDS mortality for current marijuana users in this 12-year study was 1.90, indicating that almost twice as many marijuana users died of AIDS as did noncurrent marijuana users.) Never-married men used twice as much marijuana as married men and accounted for 83% of the AIDS deaths in the study. The authors of the study note that, while marital status is insufficient to adjust for lifestyle factors—particularly, homosexual behavior—a substantial proportion of the never-married men with AIDS were probably homosexuals or bisexuals. That raises the possibility that the association of marijuana use with AIDS deaths might be related to indirect factors, such as use of other drugs or high-risk sexual behavior, both of which increase risks of infection to which AIDS patients are more susceptible. The higher mortality of AIDS patients who were current marijuana users also raises the question of whether this was because patients increased their use of marijuana at the endstages of the disease to treat their symptoms. However, the association between marijuana use and AIDS deaths was similar even when the subjects who died earliest in the first five years of this 12-year study, and who were presumably the most sick, were excluded from the analysis. In summary, it is premature to conclude what the underlying causes of this association might be.

For the general population, the mortality associated with marijuana use was lower than that associated with cigarette smoking, and tobacco smoking was not an independent risk factor in AIDS mortality. The authors of the study described above concluded that therapeutic use of marijuana did not contribute to the increased mortality among men with AIDS.

Marijuana use has been associated with a higher prevalence of HIV seropositivity in cross-sectional studies,[84] but the relationship of marijuana to the progression to AIDS in HIV-seropositive patients is a reasonable question. It remains unclear whether marijuana smoking is an independent risk factor in the progression of AIDS in HIV-seropositive men. Marijuana use did not increase the risk of AIDS in HIV-seropositive men in the Multicenter AIDS Cohort Study, in which 1,795 HIV-seropositive men were studied for 18 months,[84] or in the San Francisco Men's Health Study, in which 451 HIV-seropositive men were studied for six years.[34] In contrast, the Sydney AIDS Project in Australia, in which 386 HIV-seropositive men were studied for 12 months,[152] reported that marijuana use was associated with increased risk of progression to AIDS. The results of the Sydney study are less reliable than those of the other two studies noted; it was the shortest of the studies and, according to the 1993 definition of AIDS, many of the subjects probably already had AIDS at the beginning of the study.*

The most compelling concerns regarding marijuana smoking in HIV/AIDS patients are the possible effects of marijuana on immunity.[111] Reports of opportunistic fungal and bacterial pneumonia in AIDS patients who used marijuana suggest that marijuana smoking either suppresses the immune system[33] or exposes patients to an added burden of patho-

---

*In 1993 the diagnosis of AIDS was expanded to include anyone with a CD4 count of less than 200. Prior to 1993 this alone would have been insufficient for a diagnosis of AIDS.

gens.[21] In summary, patients with preexisting immune deficits due to AIDS should be expected to be vulnerable to serious harm caused by smoking marijuana. The relative contribution of marijuana smoke versus THC or other cannabinoids is not known.

Carcinogenicity

The gas and tar phases of marijuana and tobacco smoke contain many of the same compounds. Furthermore, the tar phase of marijuana smoke contains higher concentrations of polycyclic aromatic hydrocarbons (PAHs), such as the carcinogen benzopyrene. The higher content of carcinogenic PAHs in marijuana tar and the greater deposition of this tar in the lung might act in conjunction to amplify the exposure of a marijuana smoker to carcinogens. For those reasons the carcinogenicity of marijuana smoke is an important concern.

It is more difficult to collect the epidemiological data necessary to establish or refute the link between marijuana smoke and cancer than that between tobacco smoke and cancer. Far fewer people smoke only marijuana than only tobacco, and marijuana smokers are more likely to underreport their smoking.

Case Studies. Results of several case series suggest that marijuana might play a role in the development of human respiratory cancer. Reports indicate an unexpectedly large proportion of marijuana users among people with lung cancer[141,149] and cancers of the upper aerodigestive tract—that is, the oral cavity, pharynx, larynx, and esophagus—that occur before the age of 45.[36,39,149] Respiratory tract cancers associated with heavy tobacco and alcohol consumption are not usually seen before the age of 60,[154] and the occurrence of such cancers in marijuana users younger than 60 suggests that long-term marijuana smoking potentiates the effects of other risk factors, such as tobacco smoking, and is a more potent risk factor than tobacco and alcohol use in the early development of respiratory cancers. Most studies lack the necessary comparison groups to calculate the isolated effect of marijuana use on cancer risk. Many marijuana smokers also smoke tobacco, so when studies lack information regarding cigarette smoking status, there is no way to separate the effects of marijuana smoke and tobacco smoke.

Epidemiological Evidence. As of this writing, Sidney and co-workers[139] had conducted the only epidemiological study to evaluate the association between marijuana use and cancer. The study included a cohort of about 65,000 men and women 15–49 years old. Marijuana users were defined as those who had used marijuana on six or more occasions. Among the 1,421 cases of cancer in this cohort, marijuana use was associated only with an increased risk of prostate cancer in men who did not smoke tobacco. In these relatively young HMO clients, no association was found between marijuana use and other cancers, including all tobacco-related cancers, colorectal cancer, and melanoma. The major limitation associated with interpreting this study is that the development of lung cancer requires a long exposure to smoking, and most marijuana users quit before this level of exposure is achieved. In addition, marijuana use has been widespread in the United States only since the late 1960s; therefore, despite the large cohort size there might not have been a sufficient number of heavy or long-term marijuana smokers to reveal an effect.

Cellular and Molecular Studies. In contrast with clinical studies, cellular and molecular studies have provided strong evidence that marijuana smoke is carcinogenic. Cell culture studies implicate marijuana smoke in the development of cancer. Prolonged exposure of hamster lung cell cultures to marijuana smoke led to malignant transformations,[94] and exposure of human lung explants to marijuana smoke resulted in chromosomal and DNA alterations.[154] The tar from marijuana smoke also induced mutations similar to those produced by tar from the same quantity of tobacco in a common bacterial assay for mutagenicity.[158]

Molecular studies also implicate marijuana smoke as a carcinogen. Proto-oncogenes and tumor suppressor genes are a group of genes that affect cell growth and differentiation. Normally, they code for proteins that control cellular proliferation. Once mutated or activated, they produce proteins that cause cells to multiply rapidly and out of control, and this results in tumors or cancer.* When the production of these proteins was evaluated in tissue biopsies taken from marijuana, tobacco, and marijuana plus tobacco smokers, and nonsmokers, two of them (EGFR and Ki-67) were markedly higher in the marijuana smokers than in the nonsmokers and the tobacco smokers. Moreover, the effects of marijuana and tobacco were additive.[131] Thus, in relatively young smokers of marijuana, particularly those who smoke both marijuana and tobacco, marijuana is implicated as a risk factor for lung cancer.

DNA alterations are known to be early events in the development of cancer, and have been observed in the lymphocytes of pregnant marijuana smokers and in those of their newborns.[4] This is an important study

---

*Some of the genes involved in the development of lung cancer include those that encode for Ki-67 (a nuclear proliferation protein responsible for cell division), the p53 tumor suppressor (a protein that normally suppresses cell growth), and epidermal growth factor receptor (EGFR) (a receptor found on a variety of cell types, especially epithelial cells, that promotes cellular growth and proliferation when bound to epidermal growth factor).

because the investigators were careful to exclude tobacco smokers—a problem in previous studies that cited mutagenic effects of marijuana smoke.[26,53,63,142] The same investigators found similar effects in previous studies among tobacco smokers,[5,6] so the effects cannot be attributed solely to THC or other cannabinoids. Although it can be determined only by experiment, it is likely that the smoke contents—other than cannabinoids—are responsible for a large part of the mutagenic effect.

Preliminary findings suggest that marijuana smoke activates cytochrome P4501A1 (CYP1A1), the enzyme that converts PAHs, such as benz[α]pyrene, into active carcinogens.[99] Bronchial epithelial cells in tissue biopsies taken from marijuana smokers show more binding to CYP1A1 antibodies than do comparable cells in biopsies from nonsmokers (D. Tashkin, IOM workshop). That suggests that there is more of CYP1A1 itself in the bronchial cells of marijuana smokers, but different experimental methods will be needed to establish that possibility.

Conclusions

There is no conclusive evidence that marijuana causes cancer in humans, including cancers usually related to tobacco use. However, cellular, genetic, and human studies all suggest that marijuana smoke is an important risk factor for the development of respiratory cancer. More definitive evidence that habitual marijuana smoking leads or does not lead to respiratory cancer awaits the results of well-designed case control epidemiological studies. It has been 30 years since the initiation of widespread marijuana use among young people in our society, and such studies should now be feasible.

The following studies or activities would be useful in providing data that could more precisely define the health risks of smoking marijuana.

1. **Case control studies to determine whether marijuana use is associated with an increased risk of respiratory cancer.** Despite the lack of compelling epidemiological evidence, findings from the biochemical, cellular, immunological, genetic, tissue, and animal studies cited above strongly suggest that marijuana is a risk factor for human cancer. What is required to address that hypothesis more convincingly is a population-based case control study of sufficiently large numbers of people with lung cancer and upper aerodigestive tumors (cancers of the oral cavity and pharynx, larynx, and esophagus), as well as noncancer controls, to demonstrate a statistically significant association, if one exists. Because of the long period required for induction of human carcinomas and the infrequent use of marijuana in the general U.S. population before 1966, no epidemiological studies so far have been extensive enough to measure the

association between marijuana and cancer adequately. However, epidemiological investigation of this association is probably possible now in that some 30 years have elapsed since the start of widespread marijuana use in the United States among teenagers and young adults.

2. **Molecular markers of respiratory cancer progression in marijuana smokers.** If an epidemiological association between marijuana use and risk of respiratory cancer is demonstrated, studies would be warranted to explore the presence of molecular markers—such as TP53, p16, NATZ, and GSTML—that could be predictive of genetically increased risk of carcinogenesis in marijuana users.

3. **Prospective epidemiological studies of populations with HIV seropositivity or at high risk for HIV infection.** Because HIV/AIDS patients constitute the largest group that reports smoking marijuana for medical purposes and they are particularly vulnerable to immunosuppressive effects, there is a pressing need for a better understanding of the relative risk posed by and the rewards of smoking marijuana. Such studies should include history of marijuana use in the analysis of potential risk factors for seroconversion and acquisition of opportunistic infections or progression to AIDS. The studies could be carried out in the context of any federally approved clinical trials of medical marijuana in immunocompromised patients and should provide a follow-up period long enough to capture potential adverse events.

4. **Regularized recording of marijuana use by patients.** Although marijuana is the most commonly used illicit drug, medical providers often do not question patients about marijuana use and rarely document its use.[102] Among 452 Kaiser Permanente patients who reported daily or almost daily marijuana use, physicians recorded marijuana use in only 3% of their medical records (S. Sidney, IOM workshop).

5. **Additional cellular, animal, and human studies to investigate the effects of THC and marijuana on immune function.** The effects studied should include effects on proinflammatory versus immunosuppressive cytokines and on the function of leukocytes that present antigen to T cells.

The question that needs to be addressed is whether THC or marijuana is a risk factor for HIV infection, for progression to more severe stages of

---

*A *prospective study* is one in which a group of subjects is identified and then studied over the course of time. Such a study allows an experimenter to balance different factors that may contribute to the study outcome. For example, age, family history, and smoking are risk factors for lung cancer. In a prospective study, these factors can be balanced to measure how much smoking increases the risk of lung cancer. A *retrospective study* is one in which people with a particular disease are identified and their histories are studied. Such studies are easier and less expensive to conduct, but they generally lack the explanatory power of prospective studies.

AIDS, or for opportunistic infection among HIV-positive patients. Studies are needed to determine the effects of marijuana use on the function of alveolar macrophages. It would be important to compare the HIV infectivity and replication of alveolar macrophages harvested from habitual marijuana users with those harvested from nonusers or infrequent marijuana users. Cell culture studies could be used to compare the susceptibility of HIV-infected alveolar macrophages to additional infection with opportunistic pathogens. Similarly, further studies on cell cultures of peripheral blood mononuclear cells could be used to assess the effects of exposure to THC on HIV infectivity and replication.

Cardiovascular System

Marijuana smoke and oral THC can cause tachycardia (rapid heart beat) in humans, 20–100% above baseline.[57,85] The increase in heart rate is greatest in the first 10–20 minutes after smoking and decreases sharply and steadily; depending on whether smoked marijuana or oral THC is used, this can last three or five hours, respectively.[68,95] In some cases, blood pressure increases while a person is in a reclining position but decreases inordinately on standing, resulting in postural hypotension (decreased blood pressure due to changing posture from a lying or sitting position to a standing position, which can cause dizziness and faintness). In contrast with acute administration of THC, chronic oral ingestion of THC reduces heart rate in humans.[13]

In animals, THC decreases heart rate and blood pressure.[57,156] However, most of the animal studies have been conducted in anesthetized animals, and anesthesia causes hypertension. Thus, those studies should be interpreted as reports on the effects of cannabinoids in hypertensive subjects. The results of the animal and human studies are consistent with the conclusion that cannabinoids are hypotensive at high doses in animals, as well as humans.[156]

Tolerance can appear after a few days of frequent daily administration (two or three doses per day) of oral THC or marijuana extract, with heart rate decreasing, reclining blood pressure falling, and postural hypotension disappearing.[73] Thus, the intensity of the effects depends on frequency of use, dose, and even body position.

The cardiovascular changes have not posed a health problem for healthy, young users of marijuana or THC. However, such changes in heart rate and blood pressure could present a serious problem for older patients, especially those with coronary arterial or cerebrovascular disease. Cardiovascular diseases are the leading causes of death in the United States (coronary heart disease is first; stroke is third), so any effect of marijuana use on cardiovascular disease could have a substantial impact on public health (S. Sidney, IOM workshop). The magnitude of the impact remains to be determined as chronic marijuana users from the late 1960s enter the age when coronary arterial and cerebrovascular diseases become common. Smoking marijuana is also known to decrease maximal exercise performance. That, with the increased heart rate, could theoretically induce angina (S. Sidney, IOM workshop), so, this raises the possibility that patients with symptomatic coronary artery disease should be advised not to smoke marijuana, and THC might be contraindicated in patients with restricted cardiovascular function.

Reproductive System

Animal Studies. Marijuana and THC can inhibit many reproductive functions on a short-term basis. In both male and female animals, THC injections suppress reproductive hormones and behavior.[107,159] Studies have consistently shown that injections of THC result in rapid, dose-dependent suppression of serum luteinizing hormone (LH).[70] (LH is the pituitary hormone that stimulates release of the gonadal hormones, testosterone and estrogen.) Embryo implantation also appears to be inhibited by THC. But it does not necessarily follow that marijuana use will interfere with human reproduction. With few exceptions, the animal studies are based on acute treatments (single injections) or short-term treatments (THC injections given over a series of days). The results are generally observed for only several hours or in females sometimes for only one ovulatory cycle.

Acute treatments with cannabinoids—including THC, CBD, cannabinol, and anandamide—can decrease the fertilizing capacity of sea urchin sperm.[135-137] The sea urchin is only a distant relative of humans, but the cellular processes that regulate fertilization are similar enough that one can expect a similar effect in humans. However, the effect of cannabinoids on the capacity of sperm to fertilize eggs is reversible and is observed at concentrations of 6–100 µM,[136,137] which are higher than those likely to be experienced by marijuana smokers. The presence of cannabinoid receptors in sperm suggests the possibility of a natural role for anandamide in modulating sperm function during fertilization. However, it remains to be determined whether smoked marijuana or oral THC taken in prescribed doses has a clinically significant effect on the fertilizing capacity of human sperm.

Exposure to THC *in utero* can result in long-term changes. Many *in utero* effects interfere with embryo implantation (see review by Wenger and co-workers[159]). Exposure to THC shortly before or after birth can result in impaired reproductive behavior in mice when they reach adulthood: females are slower to show sexual receptivity, and males are slower to mount.[107]

Although THC can act directly on endocrine tissues, such as the testes and ovaries, it appears to affect reproductive physiology through its actions on the brain, somewhere other than the pituitary. Some of the effects of THC are exerted through its action on stress hormones, such as cortisol.[70]

Human Studies. The few human studies are consistent with the acute animal studies: THC inhibits reproductive functions. However, studies of men and women who use marijuana regularly have yielded conflicting results and show either depression of reproductive hormones, no effect, or only a short-term effect. Overall, the results of human studies are consistent with the hypothesis that THC inhibits LH on a short-term basis but not in long-term marijuana users. In other words, long-term users develop tolerance to the inhibitory effect of THC on LH. The results in men and women are similar, with the added consideration of the menstrual cycle in women; the acute effects of THC appear to vary with cycle stage. THC appears to have little effect during the follicular phase (the phase after menses and before ovulation) and to inhibit the LH pulse during the luteal phase (the phase after ovulation and before menses).[103] In brief, although there are no data on fertility itself, marijuana or THC would probably decrease human fertility—at least in the short term—for both men and women. And it is reasonable to predict that THC can interfere with early pregnancy, particularly with implantation of the embryo. Like tobacco smoke, marijuana smoke is highly likely to be harmful to fetal development and should be avoided by pregnant women and those who might become pregnant in the near future. Nevertheless, although fertility and fetal development are important concerns for many, they are unlikely to be of much concern to people with seriously debilitating or life-threatening diseases. The well-documented inhibition of reproductive functions by THC is thus not a serious concern for evaluating the short-term medical use of marijuana or specific cannabinoids.

The results of studies of the relationship between prenatal marijuana exposure and birth outcome have been inconsistent (reviewed in 1995 by Cornelius and co-workers[30]). Except for adolescent mothers, there is little evidence that gestation is shorter in mothers who smoke marijuana.[30] Several studies of women who smoked marijuana regularly during pregnancy show that they tend to give birth to lower weight babies.[46,65] Mothers who smoke tobacco also give birth to lower weight babies, and the relative contributions of smoking and THC are not known from these studies.

Babies born to mothers who smoked marijuana during pregnancy weighed an average of 3.4 ounces less than babies born to a control group of mothers who did not smoke marijuana; there was no statistically significant difference in either gestational age or frequency of congenital abnormalities.[164] Those results were based on women whose urine tests indicated recent marijuana exposure. However, when the analysis was based only on self-reports of marijuana use (without verification by urine tests), there was no difference in weight between babies born to women who reported themselves as marijuana smokers and those born to women who reported that they did not smoke marijuana. That raises an important concern about the methods used to measure the effects of marijuana smoking in any study, perhaps even more so in studies on the effects of marijuana during pregnancy, when subjects might be less likely to admit to smoking marijuana. (The study was conducted in the last trimester of pregnancy, and there was no information about the extent of marijuana use earlier in pregnancy.)

For most of these studies, much of the harm associated with marijuana use is consistent with that associated with tobacco use, and smoking is an important factor, so the contribution of cannabinoids cannot be confirmed. However, Jamaican women who use marijuana rarely smoke it; but instead prepare it as tea.[37] In a study of neonates born to Jamaican women who did or did not ingest marijuana during pregnancy, there was no difference in neurobehavioral assessments made at three days after birth and at one month.[38] A limitation of the study is that there was no direct measure of marijuana use. Estimates of marijuana use were based on self-reports, which might be more accurate in Jamaica than in the United States because less social stigma is associated with marijuana use in Jamaica but still are less reliable than direct measures.

Newborns of mothers who smoke either marijuana or tobacco have statistically significantly higher mutation rates than those of non-smokers.[4,5]

Since 1978, the Ottawa Prenatal Prospective Study has measured the cognitive functions of children born to mothers who smoked marijuana during pregnancy.[47] Children of mothers who smoked either moderately (one to six marijuana cigarettes per week) or heavily (more than six marijuana cigarettes per week) have been studied from the age of four days to 9–12 years. It is important to keep in mind that studies like this provide important data about the risks associated with marijuana use during pregnancy, but they do not establish the *causes* of any such association.

The children in the different marijuana exposure groups showed no lasting differences in global measures of intelligence, such as language development, reading scores, and visual or perceptual tests. Moderate cognitive deficits were detectable among these children when they were four days old and again at four years, but the deficits were no longer apparent at five years.

Prenatal marijuana exposure was not, however, without lasting effect. At ages 5–6 years and 9–12 years, children in the same study who were prenatally exposed to tobacco smoke scored lower on tests of language skills and cognitive functioning.[48] In another study,[49,50] 9 to 12 year olds who were exposed to marijuana prenatally scored lower than control subjects on tasks associated with "executive function," a term used by psychologists to describe a person's ability to plan, anticipate, and suppress behaviors that are incompatible with a current goal.[50] It was reflected in how the mothers described their children. Mothers of the marijuana-exposed children were more likely to describe their offspring as hyperactive or impulsive than were mothers of control children. The alteration in executive function was not seen in children born to tobacco smokers. The underlying causes might be the marijuana exposure or might be more closely related to the reasons underlying the mothers' use of marijuana during pregnancy.

Mice born to dams injected with the endogenous cannabinoid, anandamide, during the last trimester of pregnancy also showed delayed effects. No effect of anandamide treatment during pregnancy was detected until the mice were adults (40 days old), at which time they showed behavioral changes that are common to the effects of other psychotropic drugs or prenatal stress.[45] As with the children born to mothers who smoked marijuana, it is not known what aspect of the treatment caused the effect. The dams might have found the dose (20 mg/kg of body weight) of anandamide aversive, in which case the effect could have resulted from generalized stress, as opposed to a cannabinoid-specific effect. Either is possible. Despite the uncertainty as to the underlying causes of the effects of prenatal exposure to cannabinoid drugs, it is prudent to advise against smoking marijuana during pregnancy.

SUMMARY AND CONCLUSIONS

This chapter summarizes the harmful effects of marijuana on individual users and, to a lesser extent, on society. The harmful effects on individuals were considered from the perspective of possible medical use of marijuana and can be divided into acute and chronic effects. The vast majority of evidence on harmful effects of marijuana is based on *smoked* marijuana, and, except for the psychoactive effects that can be reasonably attributed to THC, it is not possible to distinguish the drug effects from the effects of inhaling smoke from burning plant material.

For most people the primary adverse effect of *acute* marijuana use is diminished psychomotor performance; it is inadvisable for anyone under the influence of marijuana to operate any equipment that might put the user or others in danger (such as driving or operating complex equipment). Most people can be expected to show impaired performance of complex tasks, and a minority experience dysphoria. People with or at risk of psychiatric disorders (including substance dependence) are particularly vulnerable to developing marijuana dependence, and marijuana use would be generally contraindicated for them. The short-term immunosuppressive effects are not well established; if they exist at all, they are probably not great enough to preclude a legitimate medical use. The acute side effects of marijuana use are within the risks tolerated for many medications.

The *chronic* effects of marijuana are of greater concern for medical use and fall into two categories: the effects of chronic smoking and the effects of THC. Marijuana smoke is like tobacco smoke in that it is associated with increased risk of cancer, lung damage, and poor pregnancy outcome. Smoked marijuana is unlikely to be a safe medication for any chronic medical condition. The second category is that associated with dependence on the psychoactive effects of THC. Despite past skepticism, it has been established that, although it is not common, a vulnerable subpopulation of marijuana users can develop dependence. Adolescents, particularly those with conduct disorders, and people with psychiatric disorders, or problems with substance abuse appear to be at greater risk for marijuana dependence than the general population.

As a cannabinoid drug delivery system, marijuana cigarettes are not ideal in that they deliver a variable mixture of cannabinoids and a variety of other biologically active substances, not all of which are desirable or even known. Unknown substances include possible contaminants, such as fungi or bacteria.

Finally, there is the broad social concern that sanctioning the medical use of marijuana might lead to an increase in its use among the general population. No convincing data support that concern. The existing data are consistent with the idea that this would not be a problem if the medical use of marijuana were as closely regulated as the use of other medications that have abuse potential, but we acknowledge a lack of data that directly address the question. Even if there were evidence that the medical use of marijuana would decrease the perception that it can be a harmful substance, this is beyond the scope of laws regulating the approval of therapeutic drugs. Those laws concern scientific data related to the safety and efficacy of drugs for individual use; they do not address perceptions or beliefs of the general population.

Marijuana is not a completely benign substance. It is a powerful drug with a variety of effects. However, except for the harm associated with smoking, the adverse effects of marijuana use are within the range tolerated for other medications. Thus, the safety issues associated with marijuana do not preclude some medical uses. But the question remains: Is it effective? That question is covered here in two chapters: chapter 2 summarizes what has been learned about the biological activity of cannabinoids in the past 15 years through research in the basic sciences, and chapter 4 reviews clinical data on the effectiveness of marijuana and cannabinoids for the treatment of various medical conditions.

Three factors influence the safety of marijuana or cannabinoid drugs for medical use: the delivery system, the use of plant material, and the side effects of cannabinoid drugs. (1) Smoking marijuana is clearly harmful, especially in people with chronic conditions, and is not an ideal drug delivery system. (2) Plants are of uncertain composition, which renders their effects equally uncertain, so they constitute an undesirable medication. (3) The side effects of cannabinoid drugs are within the acceptable risks associated with approved medications. Indeed, some of the side effects, such as anxiety reduction and sedation, might be desirable for some patients. As with many medications, there are people for whom they would probably be contraindicated.

CONCLUSION: Present data on drug use progression neither support nor refute the suggestion that medical availability would increase drug abuse. However, this question is beyond the issues normally considered for medical uses of drugs, and it should not be a factor in the evaluation of the therapeutic potential of marijuana or cannabinoids.

CONCLUSION: A distinctive marijuana withdrawal syndrome has been identified, but it is mild and short lived. The syndrome includes restlessness, irritability, mild agitation, insomnia, sleep EEG disturbance, nausea, and cramping.

CONCLUSION: Numerous studies suggest that marijuana smoke is an important risk factor in the development of respiratory disease.

RECOMMENDATION: **Studies to define the individual health risks of smoking marijuana should be conducted, particularly among populations in which marijuana use is prevalent.**

REFERENCES

1. Adams IB, Martin BR. 1996. Cannabis: Pharmacology and toxicology in animals and humans. *Addiction* 91:1585–1614.
2. American Psychiatric Association. 1987. *Diagnostic and Statistical Manual of Mental Disorders (DSM-III-R)*. 3rd ed., revised. Washington, DC: American Psychiatric Association.
3. American Psychiatric Association. 1994. *Diagnostic and Statistical Manual of Mental Disorders (DSM-IV)*. 4th ed. Washington, DC: American Psychiatric Association.
4. Ammenheuser MM, Berenson AB, Babiak AE, Singleton CR, Whorton Jr EB. 1998. Frequencies of *hprt* mutant lymphocytes in marijuana-smoking mothers and their newborns. *Mutation Research* 403:55–64.
5. Ammenheuser MM, Berenson NJ, Stiglich EB, Whorton Jr EB, Ward Jr JB. 1994. Elevated frequencies of *hprt* mutant lymphocytes in cigarette-smoking mothers and their newborns. *Mutation Research* 304:285–294.
6. Ammenheuser MM, Hastings DA, Whorton Jr EB, Ward Jr JB. 1997. Frequencies of *hprt* mutant lymphocytes in smokers, non-smokers, and former smokers. *Environmental and Molecular Mutagenesis* 30:131–138.
7. Anthenelli RM, Schuckit MA. 1992. Genetics. In: Lowinson JH, Ruiz P, Millman RB, Editors, *Substance Abuse: A Comprehensive Textbook*. 2nd ed. Baltimore, MD: Williams & Wilkins. Pp. 39–50.
8. Anthony JC, Warner LA, Kessler RC. 1994. Comparative epidemiology of dependence on tobacco, alcohol, controlled substances, and inhalants: Basic findings from the National Comorbidity Survey. *Experimental and Clinical Psychopharmacology* 2:244–268.
9. Bailey SL, Flewelling RL, Rachal JV. 1992. Predicting continued use of marijuana among adolescents: The relative influence of drug-specific and social context factors. *Journal of Health and Social Behavior* 33:51–66.
10. Baldwin GC, Tashkin DP, Buckely DM, Park AN, Dubinett SM, Roth MD. 1997. Marijuana and cocaine impair alveolar macrophage function and cytokine production. *American Journal of Respiratory and Critical Care Medicine* 156:1606–1613.
11. Barbers RG, Gong HJ, Tashkin DP, Oishi J, Wallace J M. 1987. Differential examination of bronchoalveolar lavage cells in tobacco cigarette and marijuana smokers. *American Review of Respiratory Disease* 135:1271–1275.
12. Barsky SH, Roth MD, Kleerup EC, Simmons M, Tashkin DP. 1998. Histopathologic and molecular alterations in bronchial epithelium in habitual smokers of marijuana, cocaine, and/or tobacco. *Journal of the National Cancer Institute* 90:1198–1205.
13. Benowitz NL, Jones RT. 1975. Cardiovascular effects of prolonged delta-9-tetrahydrocannabinol ingestion. *Clinical Pharmacology and Therapeutics* 18:287–297.
14. Block RI, Ghoneim MM. 1993. Effects of chronic marijuana use on human cognition. *Psychopharmacology* 110:219–228.
15. Bloom JW, Kaltenborn WT, Paoletti P, Camilli A, Lebowitz MS. 1987. Respiratory effects of non-tobacco cigarettes. *British Medical Journal* 295:516–518.
16. Bornheim LM, Kim KY, Li J, Perotti BY, Benet LZ. 1995. Effect of cannabidiol pretreatment on the kinetics of tetrahydrocannabinol metabolites in mouse brain. *Drug Metabolism and Disposition (United States)* 23:825–831.
17. British Medical Association. 1997. *Therapeutic Uses of Cannabis*. Amsterdam, The Netherlands: Harwood Academic Publishers.
18. Brook JS, Cohen P, Brook DW. 1998. Longitudinal study of co-occurring psychiatric disorders and substance use. *Journal of the American Academy of Child and Adolescent Psychiatry* 37:322–330.

19. Budney AJ, Radonovich KJ, Higgins ST, Wong CJ. 1998. Adults seeking treatment for marijuana dependence: A comparison with cocaine-dependent treatment seekers. *Experimental and Clinical Psychopharmacology* 6:419–426.
20. Burns LA, Meade BJ, Munson AE. 1996. Toxic responses of the immune system. In: CD Klaassen, MO Amdur, and J Doul, Editors, *Casarett and Doul, Toxicology: The Basic Science of Poisons.* 5th ed. New York: McGraw-Hill. Pp. 355–402.
21. Caiaffa WT, Vlahov D, Graham N, Astemborski J, Solomon L, Nelson KE, Muñoz. 1994. Drug smoking, *Pneumocystis carinii* pneumonia, and immunosuppression increase risk of bacterial pneumonia in human immunodeficiency virus-seropositive injection drug users. *American Journal of Respiratory and Critical Care Medicine* 150:1493–1498.
22. Campbell AM, Evans M, Thompson JL, Williams MR. 1971. Cerebral atrophy in young cannabis smokers. *Lancet* 2:1219–1224.
23. Chait LD, Pierri J. 1992. Effects of smoked marijuana on human performance: A critical review. In: L Murphy and A Bartke, Editors, *Marijuana/Cannabinoids: Neurobiology and Neurophysiology.* Boca Raton, FL: CRC Press. Pp. 387–424.
24. Charalambous A, Marciniak G, Shiue CY, Dewey SL, Schlyer DJ, Wolf AP, Makriyannis A. 1991. PET studies in the primate brain and biodistribution in mice using (–)-5'-18F-delta 8-THC. *Pharmacology Biochemistry and Behavior* 40:503–507.
25. Chen K, Kandel DB, Davies M. 1997. Relationships between frequency and quantity of marijuana use and last year proxy dependence among adolescents and adults in the United States. *Drug and Alcohol Dependence* 46:53–67.
26. Chiesara E, Rizzi R. 1983. Chromosome damage in heroin-marijuana and marijuana addicts. *Archives of Toxicology Supplement* 6:128–130.
27. Cleeland CS, Gonin R, Hatfield AK, Edmonson JH, Blum RH, Stewart JA, Pandya KJ. 1994. Pain and its treatment in outpatients with metastatic cancer. *New England Journal of Medicine* 330:592–596.
28. Co BT, Goodwin DW, Gado M, Mikhael M, Hill SY. 1977. Absence of cerebral atrophy in chronic cannabis users by computerized transaxial tomography. *Journal of the American Medical Association* 237:1229–1230.
29. Cohen MJ, Rickles Jr WH. 1974. Performance on a verbal learning task by subjects of heavy past marijuana usage. *Psychopharmacologia* 37:323–330.
30. Cornelius MD, Taylor PM, Geva D, Day NL. 1995. Prenatal tobacco and marijuana use among adolescents: Effects on offspring gestational age, growth, and morphology. *Pediatrics* 95(5):738–743.
31. Crowley TJ, Macdonald MJ, Whitmore EA, Mikulich SK. 1998. Cannabis dependence, withdrawal, and reinforcing effects among adolescents with conduct symptoms and substance use disorders. *Drug and Alcohol Dependence* 50:27–37.
32. Crowley TJ, Rhine MW. 1985. The substance use disorders. In: Simons RC, Editor, *Understanding Human Behavior in Health and Illness.* 3rd ed. Baltimore, MD: Williams & Wilkins. Pp. 730–746.
33. Denning DW, Follansbee SE, Scolaro M, et al. 1991. Pulmonary aspergillosis in the acquired immunodeficiency syndrome. *New England Journal of Medicine* 324:654–662.
34. Di Franco MJ, Sheppard HW, Hunter DJ, Tosteson TD, Ascher MS. 1996. The lack of association of marijuana and other recreational drugs with progression to AIDS in the San Francisco Men's Health Study. *Annals of Epidemiology* 6:283–289.
35. Dixon L, Haas G, Weiden PJ, Sweeney J, Frances AJ. 1991. Drug abuse in schizophrenic patients: Clinical correlates and reasons for use. *American Journal of Psychiatry* 148:224–230.
36. Donald PJ. 1991. Advanced malignancy in the young marijuana smoker. *Advances in Experimental Medicine and Biology* 288:33–56.

37. Dreher M. 1987. The evolution of a roots daughter. *Journal of Psychoactive Drugs* 19:165–170.
38. Dreher MC, Nugent K, Hudgins R. 1994. Prenatal marijuana exposure and neonatal outcomes in Jamaica: An ethnographic study. *Pediatrics* 93:254–260.
39. Endicott JN, Skipper P, Hernandez L. 1993. Marijuana and head and neck cancer. In: Friedman et al., Editors, *Drugs of Abuse, Immunity and AIDS*. New York: Plenum Press. Pp. 107–113.
40. Fehr K, Kalant H. 1981. Cannabis and health hazards. *Proceedings of an ARF/WHO Scientific Meeting on Adverse Health and Behavioral Consequences of Cannabis Use.* Fehr K, Kalant H, Editors, Toronto, Canada: Addiction Research Foundation.
41. Fleischman RW, Baker JR, Rosenkrantz H. 1979. Pulmonary pathologic changes in rats exposed to marijuana smoke for one year. *Toxicology and Applied Pharmacology* 47:557–566.
42. Fligiel SE, Beals TF, Tashkin DP, Paule MG, Scallet AC, Ali SF, Bailey JR, Slikker WJ. 1991. Marijuana exposure and pulmonary alterations in primates. *Pharmacology, Biochemistry and Behavior* 40:637–642.
43. Fligiel SEG, Roth MD, Kleerup EC, Barsky SH, Simmons M, Tashkin DP. 1997. Tracheobronchial histopathology in habitual smokers of cocaine, marijuana, and/or tobacco. *Chest* 112:319–326.
44. Foley K. 1997. Competent care for the dying instead of physician-assisted suicide. *New England Journal of Medicine* 336:54–58.
45. Fride E, Mechoulam R. 1996. Ontogenetic development of the response to anandamide and delta 9-tetrahydrocannabinol in mice. *Brain Research, Developmental Brain Research* 95:131–134.
46. Fried PA. 1982. Marihuana use by pregnant women and effects on offspring: An update. *Neurobehavioral Toxicology and Teratology* 4:451–454.
47. Fried PA. 1995. The Ottawa Prenatal Prospective Study (OPPS): Methological issues and findings—it's easy to throw the baby out with the bath water. *Life Sciences* 56:2159–2168.
48. Fried PA, O'Connell CM, Watkinson B. 1992. 60- and 72-Month follow-up of children prenatally exposed to marijuana, cigarettes, and alcohol: Cognitive and language assessment. *Developmental and Behavioral Pediatrics* 13:383–391.
49. Fried PA, Watkinson BSLS. 1997. Reading and language in 9- to 12-year-olds prenatally exposed to cigarettes and marijuana. *Neurotoxicology and Teratology* 19:171–183.
50. Fried PA, Watkinson B, Gray R. 1998. Differential effects on cognitive functioning in 9- to 12-year-olds prenatally exposed to cigarettes and marihuana. *Neurotoxicology and Teratology* 20:293–306.
51. Gardner EL. 1992. Brain reward mechanisms. In: Lowinson JH, Ruiz P, Millman RB, Editors, *Substance Abuse: A Comprehensive Textbook*. 2nd ed. Baltimore, MD: Williams and Wilkins. Pp. 70–99.
52. Georgotas A, Zeidenberg P. 1979. Observations on the effects of four weeks of heavy marijuana smoking on group interaction and individual behavior. *Comprehensive Psychiatry* 20:427–432.
53. Gilmore DG, Blood AD, Lele KP, Robbins ES, Maximillian C. 1971. Chromosomal aberrations in users of psychoactive drugs. *Archives of General Psychiatry* 24:268–272.
54. Goldstein A. 1994. Tolerance and Dependence. In: Goldstein A, Editor, *Addiction: From Biology to Drug Policy*. New York: W.H. Freeman. Pp. 73–84.
55. Golub A, Johnson BD. 1994. The shifting importance of alcohol and marijuana as gateway substances among serious drug abusers. *Journal of Studies on Alcohol* 55:607–614.

56. Gong HJ, Fligiel S, Tashkin DP, Barbers RG. 1987. Tracheobronchial changes in habitual, heavy smokers of marijuana with and without tobacco. *American Review of Respiratory Disease* 136:142–149.

57. Graham JDP. 1986. The cardiovascular action of cannabinoids. In: Mechoulam R, Editor, *Cannabinoids as Therapeutic Agents.* Boca Raton, FL: CRC Press. Pp. 159–166.

58. Grant S, London ED, Newlin DB, Villemagne VL, Liu X, Contoreggi C, Phillips RL, Kimes AS, Margolin A. 1996. Activation of memory circuits during cue-elicited cocaine craving. *Proceedings of the National Academy of Sciences, USA* 93:12040–12045.

59. Hall W, Solowij N. 1998. Adverse effects of cannabis. *The Lancet* 352:1611–1616.

60. Hall W, Solowij N, Lemon J. 1994. *The Health and Psychological Consequences of Cannabis Use.* Department of Human Services and Health, Monograph Series, No. 25. Canberra, Australia: Australian Government Publishing Service.

61. Haney M, Ward AS, Comer SD, Foltin RW, Fischman MW. 1999. Abstinence symptoms following oral THC administration to humans. *Psychopharmacology* 141:385–394.

62. Haney M, Ward AS, Comer SD, Foltin RW, Fischman MW. 1999. Abstinence symptoms following smoked marijuana in humans. *Psychopharmacology* 141:395–404.

62a. Heishman SJ, Huestis MA, Henningfield JE, Cone EJ. 1990. Acute and residual effects of marijuana: Profiles of plasma THC levels, physiological, subjective, and performance measures. *Pharmacology, Biochemistry, and Behavior* 37:561-565.

63. Herha J, Obe G. 1974. Chromosomal damage in chronical users of cannabis: In vivo investigation with two-day lymphocyte cultures. *Pharmakopsychiatric* 7:328–337.

64. Herring AC, Koh WS, Kaminski NE. 1998. Inhibition of the cyclic AMP signaling cascade and nuclear factor binding to CRE and kappa B elements by cannabinol, a minimally CNS-active cannabinoid. *Biochemical Pharmacology* 55:1013–1023.

65. Hingson R, Alpert JJ, Day N, Dooling E, Kayn H, Morelock S, Oppenheimer E, Zuckerman B. 1982. Effects of maternal drinking and marihuana use on fetal growth and development. *Pediatrics* 70:539–546.

66. Hollister LE. 1986. Health aspects of cannabis. *Pharmacological Reviews* 38:1–20.

67. Huber GL, Mahajan VK. 1988. The comparative response of the lung to marihuana or tobacco smoke inhalation. In: Chesher G, Consroe P, Musty R, Editors, *Marijuana: An International Research Report: Proceedings of Melbourne Symposium on Cannabis 2-4 September, 1987.* National Campaign Against Drug Abuse Monograph Series No. 7 Edition. Canberra: Australian Government Publishing Service. Pp. 19–24.

68. Huestis MA, Sampson AH, Holicky BJ, Henningfield JE, Cone EJ. 1992. Characterization of the absorption phase of marijuana smoking. *Clinical Pharmacology and Therapeutics* 52:31–41.

69. IOM (Institute of Medicine). 1982. *Marijuana and Health.* Washington, DC: National Academy Press.

70. Jackson AL, Murphy LL. 1997. Role of the hypothalamic-pituitary-adrenal axis in the suppression of luteinizing hormone release by delta-9-tetrahydrocannabinol. *Neuroendocrinology* 65:446–452.

71. Johnson V. 1995. The relationship between parent and offspring comorbid disorders. *Journal of Substance Abuse* 7:267–280.

72. Johnston LD, O'Malley PM, Bachman JG. 1989. Marijuana decriminalization: The impact on youth, 1975–1980. *Journal of Public Health Policy* 10:456.

73. Jones RT, Benowitz NL, Herning RI. 1981. Clinical relevance of cannabis tolerance and dependence. *Journal of Clinical Pharmacology* 21:143S–152S.

74. Jones RT, Benowitz N, Bachman J. 1976. Clinical studies of tolerance and dependence. *Annals of the New York Academy of Sciences* 282:221–239.

75. Kaklamani E, Trichopoulos D, Koutselinis A, Drouga M, Karalis D. 1978. Hashis smoking and T-lymphocytes. *Archives of Toxicology* 40:97–101.

76. Kandel DB. 1992. Epidemiological trends and implications for understanding the nature of addiction. In: O'Brien CP, Jaffe JH, Editors, *Addictive Studies*. New York: Raven Press, Ltd. Pp. 23–40.

77. Kandel DB, Chen KWLA, Kessler R, Grant B. 1997. Prevalence and demographic correlates of symptoms of last year dependence on alcohol, nicotine, marijuana and cocaine in the U.S. population. *Drug and Alcohol Dependence* 44:11–29.

78. Kandel DB, Davies M. 1992. Progression to regular marijuana involvement: phenomenology and risk factors for near-daily use. In: Glantz M, Pickens R, Editors, *Vulnerability to Drug Abuse*. Washington, DC: American Psychological Association. Pp. 211–253.

79. Kandel DB, Johnson JG, Bird HR, Canino G, Goodman SH, Lahey BB, Regier DA, Schwab-Stone M. 1997. Psychiatric disorders associated with substance use among children and adolescents: Findings from the Methods for the Epidemiology of Child and Adolescent Mental Disorders (MECA) Study. *Journal of Abnormal Child Psychology* 25:121–132.

80. Kandel DB, Raveis VH. 1989. Cessation of illicit drug use in young adulthood. *Archives of General Psychiatry* 46:109–116.

81. Kandel DB, Yamaguchi K. 1993. From beer to crack: developmental patterns of drug involvement. *American Journal of Public Health* 83:851–855.

82. Kandel DB, Yamaguchi K, Chen K. 1992. Stages of progression in drug involvement from adolescence to adulthood: Further evidence for the gateway theory. *Journal of Studies in Alcohol* 53:447–457.

83. Kaplan HB, Martin SS, Johnson RJ, Robbins CA. 1996. Escalation of marijuana use: Application of a general theory of deviant behavior. *Journal of Health and Social Behavior* 27:44–61.

84. Kaslow RA, Blackwelder WC, Ostrow DG, et al. 1989. No evidence for a role of alcohol or other psychoactive drugs in accelerating immunodeficiency in HIV-1 positive individuals: A report for the multicenter AIDS cohort study. *Journal of the American Medical Association* 261:3424–3429.

85. Kelly TH, Foltin RW, Fischman MW. 1993. Effects of smoked marijuana on heart rate, drug ratings and task performance by humans. *Behavioural Pharmacology* 4:167–178.

86. Kendler KS, Prescott CA. 1998. Cannabis use, abuse, and dependence in a population-based sample of female twins. *American Journal of Psychiatry* 155:1016.

87. Klein TW, Friedman H, Specter SC. 1998. Marijuana, immunity and infection. *Journal of Neuroimmunology* 83:102–115.

88. Koob GF, Le Moal M. 1997. Drug abuse: Hedonic homeostatic dysregulation. *Science* 278:52–58.

89. Kuehnle J, Mendelson JH, Davis KR, New PF. 1977. Computed tomographic examination of heavy marihuana smokers. *Journal of the American Medical Association* 237:1231–1232.

90. Labouvie E, Bates ME, Pandina RJ. 1997. Age of first use: Its reliability and predictive utility. *Journal of Studies on Alcohol* 58:638–643.

91. Lau RJ, Tubergen DG, Barr MJ, Domino EF, Benowitz N, Jones RT. 1976. Phytohemagglutinin-induced lymphocyte transformation in humans receiving delta-9-tetrahydrocannabinol. *Science* 192:805–807.

92. Lepore M, Liu X, Savage V, Matalon D, Gardner EL. 1996. Genetic differences in delta 9-tetrahydrocannabinol-induced facilitation of brain stimulation reward as measured by a rate-frequency curve-shift electrical brain stimulation paradigm in three different rat strains. *Life Sciences* 58:365–372.

93. Lepore M, Vorel SR, Lowinson J, Gardner EL. 1995. Conditioned place preference induced by delta 9-tetrahydrocannabinol: Comparison with cocaine, morphine, and food reward. *Life Sciences* 56:2073–2080.

94. Leuchtenberger C, Leuchtenberger R. 1976. Cytological and cytochemical studies of the effects of fresh marijuana cigarette smoke on growth and DNA metabolism of animal and human lung cultures. In: Braude MC, Szara S, Editors, *The Pharmacology of Marijuana*. New York: Raven Press.

95. Lindgren JE, Ohlsson A, Agurell S, Hollister LE, Gillespie H. 1981. Clinical effects and plasma levels of delta 9-tetrahydrocannabinol (delta 9-THC) in heavy and light users of cannabis. *Psychopharmacology (Berlin)* 74:208–212.

96. Linzen DH, Dingemans PM, Lenior ME. 1994. Cannabis abuse and the course of recent-onset schizophrenic disorders. *Archives of General Psychiatry* 51:273–279.

97. Lyons MJ., Toomey R, Meyer JM, Green AI, Eisen SA, Goldberg J, True WR, Tsuang MT. 1997. How do genes influence marijuana use? The role of subjective effects. *Addiction* 92:409–417.

98. MacCoun R, Reuter P. 1997. Interpreting Dutch cannabis policy: Reasoning by analogy in the legalization debate. *Science* 278:47–52.

99. Marques-Magallanes JA, Tashkin DP, Serafian T, Stegeman J, Roth MD. 1997. *In vivo* and *in vitro* activation of cytochrome P4501A1 by marijuana smoke. *Symposium on the Cannabinoids of the International Cannabinoid Research Society Program and Abstracts.* Stone Mountain, GA, June 1997.

100. Martellotta MC, Cossu G, Fattore L, Gessa GL, Fratta W. 1998. Self-administration of the cannabinoid receptor agonist WIN 55,212-2 in drug-naive mice. *Neuroscience* 85:327–330.

101. Mathew RJ, Wilson WH, Humphreys DF, Lowe JV, Wiethe KE. 1992. Regional cerebral blood flow after marijuana smoking. *Journal of Cerebral Blood Flow and Metabolism* 12:750–758.

102. Mathre ML. 1998. A survey on disclosure of marijuana use to health care professionals. *Journal of Psychoactive Drugs* 20:117–120.

103. Mendelson JH, Cristofaro P, Ellingboe J, Benedikt R, Mello NK. 1985. Acute effects of marihuana on luteinizing hormone in menopausal women. *Pharmacology, Biochemistry, and Behavior* 23:765–768.

104. Meyer RE, Pillard RC, Shapiro LM, Mirin SM. 1971. Administration of marijuana to heavy and casual marijuana users. *American Journal of Psychiatry* 128:198–204.

105. Model KE. 1993. The effect of marijuana decriminalization on hospital emergency room drug episodes: 1975–1978. *Journal of the American Statistical Association* 88:737–747.

106. Moulin DE, Iezzi A, Amireh R, Sharpe WKJ, Boyd D, Merskey H. 1996. Randomised trial of oral morphine for chronic non-cancer pain. *Lancet* 347:143–147.

107. Murphy LL, Gher J, Szary A. 1995. Effects of prenatal exposure to delta-9-tetrahydrocannabinol on reproductive, endocrine and immune parameters of male and female rat offspring. *Endocrine* 3:875–879.

108. Nahas GG, Osserman EF. 1991. Altered serum immunoglobulin concentration in chronic marijuana smokers. *Advances in Experimental Medicine and Biology* 288:25–32.

109. Nesse RM, Berridge KC. 1997. Psychoactive drug use in evolutionary perspective. *Science* 278:63–66.

110. Nestler EJ, Aghajanian GK. 1997. Molecular and cellular basis of addiction. *Science* 278:58–63.

111. Newell GR, Mansell PW, Wilson MB, Lynch HK, Spitz MR, Hersh EM. 1985. Risk factor analysis among men referred for possible acquired immune deficiency syndrome. *Preventive Medicine* 14:81–91.

112. NIH (National Institutes of Health). 1997. Workshop on the Medical Utility of Marijuana. Report to the Director, National Institutes of Health by the Ad Hoc Group of Experts. Bethesda, MD, February 19–20, 1997. Bethesda, MD: National Institutes of Health.

113. O'Brien CP. 1996. Drug addiction and drug abuse. In: Harmon JG, Limbird LE, Molinoff PB, Ruddon RW, Gilman AG, Editor, *Goodman and Gilman's The Pharmacological Basis of Therapeutics*. 9th ed. New York: McGraw-Hill. Pp. 557–577.

114. O'Brien CP. 1996. Recent developments in the pharmacotherapy of substance abuse. *Journal of Consulting and Clinical Psychology* 64:677–686.

115. O'Brien CP. 1997. A range of research-based pharmacotherapies for addiction. *Science* 278:66–70.

116. O'Leary DS, Andreasen NC, Hurtig RR, Torres IJ, Flashman LA, Kesler ML, Arndt SV, Cizadlo TJ, Ponto LLB, Watkins GL, Hichwa RD. 1997. Auditory and visual attention assessed with PET. *Human Brain Mapping* 5:422–436.

117. O'Leary D, Block RI, Flaum M, Boles Ponto LL, Watkins GL, Hichwa RD. 1998. Acute marijuana effects on rCBF and cognition: A PET study. *Abstracts—Society for Neuroscience: 28th Annual Meeting*. Los Angeles, November 7-12, 1998. Washington, DC: Society for Neuroscience.

118. Ohlsson A, Lindgren J-E, Wahlen A, Agurell S, Hollister LE, Gillespie HK. 1980. Plasma delta-9-tetrahydrocannabinol concentrations and clinical effects after oral and intravenous administration and smoking. *Clinical Pharmacology and Therapeutics* 28:409–416.

119. Peterson RC. 1979. Importance of inhalation patterns in determining effects of marijuana use. *Lancet* 1:727–728.

120. Polen MR, Sidney S, Tekawa IS, Sadler M, Friedman D. 1993. Health care use by frequent marijuana smokers who do not smoke tobacco. *The Western Journal of Medicine* 158:596–601.

121. Pope HG, Gruber AJ, Yurgelun-Todd D. 1995. The residual neuropsychological effects of cannabis: The current status of research. *Drug and Alcohol Dependence* 38:25–34.

122. Pope HG, Yurgelun-Todd D. 1996. The residual cognitive effects of heavy marijuana use in college students. *Journal of the American Medical Association* 275:521–527.

123. Rachelefsky G, Opelz G, Mickey M, Lessin P, Kiuchi M, Silverstein M, Stiehm E. 1976. Intact humoral and cell-mediated immunity in chronic marijuana smoking. *Journal of Allergy and Clinical Immunology* 58:483–490.

124. Rickles Jr WH, Cohen MJ, Whitaker CA, McIntyre KE. 1973. Marijuana-induced state-dependent verbal learning. *Psychopharmacologia* 30:349–354.

125. Robins LN. 1980. The natural history of drug abuse. *Acta Psychiatrica Scandinavica Supplement* 284:7–20.

126. Robins LN. 1998. The intimate connection between antisocial personality and substance abuse. *Social Psychiatry and Psychiatric Epidemiology* 33:393–399.

127. Robins LN, McEvoy LT. 1990. Conduct problems as predictors of substance abuse. In: Robins L, Rutter M, Editors, *Straight and Devious Pathways from Childhood to Adulthood*. New York: Cambridge University Press. Pp. 182–204.

128. Rosenkrantz H, Fleischman RW. 1979. Effects of cannabis on lung. In: Nahas GG, Payton WDH, Editors, *Marijuana: Biological Effects*. Oxford, England: Pergamon Press. Pp. 279–299.

129. Rosenzweig MR, Leiman AL, Breedlove SM. 1996. *Biological Psychology*. Sunderland, MA: Sinauer Associates.

130. Roth MD, Arora A, Barsky SH, Kleerup EC, Simmons MS, Tashkin DP. 1998. Airway inflammation in young marijuana and tobacco smokers. *American Journal of Respiratory and Critical Care Medicine* 157:1–9.

131. Roth MD, Kleerup EC, Arora A, Barsky SH, Tashkin DP. 1996. Endobronchial injury in young tobacco and marijuana smokers as evaluated by visual, pathologic and molecular criteria. *American Review of Respiratory and Critical Care Medicine* 153 (part 2):100A.

132. SAMHSA (Substance Abuse and Mental Health Services Administration). 1998. *National Household Survey on Drug Abuse: Population Estimates 1997.* DHHS Pub. No. (SMA) 98-3250. Rockville, MD: SAMHSA, Office of Applied Studies.

133. Scheier LM, Bovtin GJ. 1996. Cognitive effects of marijuana. *Journal of the American Medical Association* 275:JAMA Letters.

134. Schneier FR, Siris SG. 1987. A review of psychoactive substance use and abuse in schizophrenia: Patterns of drug choice. *Journal of Nervous and Mental Disease* 175:641–652.

135. Schuel H, Berkery D, Schuel R, Chang MC, Zimmerman AM, Zimmerman S. 1991. Reduction of the fertilizing capacity of sea urchin sperm by cannabinoids derived from marihuana. I. Inhibition of the acrosome reaction induced by egg jelly. *Molecular Reproduction and Development* 29:51–59.

136. Schuel H, Chang MC, Berkery D, Schuel R, Zimmerman AM, Zimmerman S. 1991. Cannabinoids inhibit fertilization in sea urchins by reducing the fertilizing capacity of sperm. *Pharmacology, Biochemistry, and Behavior* 40:609–615.

137. Schuel H, Goldstein E, Mechoulam R, Zimmerman AM, Zimmerman S. 1994. Anandamide (arachidonylethanolamide), a brain cannabinoid receptor, agonist, reduces sperm fertilizing capacity in sea urchins by inhibiting the acrosome reaction. *Proceedings of the National Academy of Sciences* 91:7678–7682.

138. Sidney S, Beck JE, Tekawa IS, Quesenberry CP Jr, Friedman GD. 1997a. Marijuana use and mortality. *American Journal of Public Health* 87:585–590.

139. Sidney S, Quesenberry CP Jr, Friedman GD, Tekawa IS. 1997b. Marijuana use and cancer incidence (California, United States). *Cancer Cause and Control* 8:722–728.

140. Solowij N. 1995. Do cognitive impairments recover following cessation of cannabis use? *Life Sciences* 56:2119–2126.

141. Sridhar JS, Raub WA, Weatherby NL, et al. 1994. Possible role of marijuana smoking as a carcinogen in the development of lung cancer at a young age. *Journal of Psychoactive Drugs* 26:285–288.

142. Stenchever MA, Kunysz TJ, Allen MA. 1974. Chromosome breakage in users of marijuana. *American Journal of Gynecology* 118:106–113.

143. Stephens RS, Roffman RA, Simpson EE. 1993. Adult marijuana users seeking treatment. *Journal of Consulting and Clinical Psychology* 61:1100–1104.

144. Tanda G, Pontieri FE, Di Chiara G. 1997. Cannabinoid and heroin activation of mesolimbic dopamine transmission by a common $\mu 1$ opioid receptor mechanism. *Science* 276:2048–2049.

145. Tart CT. 1971. *On Being Stoned: A Psychological Study of Marijuana Intoxication.* Palo Alto, CA: Science and Behavior Books.

146. Tashkin DP, Coulson AH, Clark VA, Simmons M, Bourque LB, Duann S, Spivey GH, Gong H. 1987. Respiratory symptoms and lung function in habitual, heavy smokers of marijuana alone, smokers of marijuana and tobacco, smokers of tobacco alone, and nonsmokers. *American Review of Respiratory Disease* 135:209–216.

147. Tashkin DP, Simmons MS, Sherrill DL, Coulson AH. 1997. Heavy habitual marijuana smoking does not cause an accelerated decline in FEV_1 with age. *American Journal of Respiratory and Critical Care Medicine* 155:141–148.

148. Tashkin E. 1999. Effects of marijuana on the lung and its defenses against infection and cancer. *School Psychology International* 20:23–37.

149. Taylor FM. 1988. Marijuana as a potential respiratory tract carcinogen: A retrospective analysis. *Southern Medical Journal* 81:1213–1216.

150. Tennant FS. 1980. Histopathologic and clinical abnormalities of the respiratory system in chronic hashish smokers. *Substance and Alcohol Actions/Misuse* 1:93–100.

151. Thornicroft G. 1990. Cannabis and psychosis: Is there epidemiological evidence for an association? *British Journal of Psychiatry* 157:25–33.

152. Tindall B, Cooper D, Donovan B, Barnes T, Philpot C, Gold J, Penny R. 1988. The Sydney AIDS Project: Development of acquired immunodeficiency syndrome in a group of HIV seropositive homosexual men. *Australian and New Zealand Journal of Medicine* 18:8–15.

153. Tsou K, Patrick SL, Walker JM. 1995. Physical withdrawal in rats tolerant to delta-9-tetrahydrocannabinol precipitated by a cannabinoid receptor antagonist. *European Journal of Pharmacology* 280:R13–R15.

154. Van Hoozen BE, Cross CE. 1997. Respiratory tract effects of marijuana. *Clinical Reviews in Allergy and Immunology* 15:243–269.

155. Volkow ND, Gillespie H, Mullani N, Tancredi L, Grant C, Valentine A, Hollister L. 1996. Brain glucose metabolism in chronic marijuana users at baseline and during marijuana intoxication. *Psychiatry Research* 67:29–38.

156. Wagner JA, Varga K, Kunos G. 1998. Cardiovascular actions of cannabinoids and their generation during shock. *Journal of Molecular Medicine* 76:824–836.

157. Wallace JM, Tashkin DP, Oishi JS, Barbers RG. 1988. Peripheral blood lymphocyte subpopulations and mitogen responsiveness in tobacco and marijuana smokers. *Journal of Psychoactive Drugs* 20:9–14.

158. Wehner FC, Van Rensburg SJ, Theil PF. 1980. Mutagenicity of marijuana and transkei tobacco smoke condensates in the salmonella/microsome assay. *Mutation Research* 77:135–142.

159. Wenger T, Croix D, Tramu G, Leonardelli J. 1992. Effects of delta-9-tetrahydrocannabinol on pregnancy, puberty, and the neuroendocrine system. In: Murphy L, Bartke A, Editors, *Marijuana/Cannabinoids: Neurobiology and Neurophysiology*. Boca Raton, FL: CRC Press.

160. White SC, Brin SC, Janicki BW. 1975. Mitogen-induced blastogenic responses of lymphocytes from marijuana smokers. *Science* 188:71–72.

161. Whitfield RM, Bechtel LM, Starich GH. 1997. The impact of ethanol and marinol/marijuana usage on HIV+/AIDS patients undergoing azidothymidine, azidothymidine/dideoxycytidine, ordideoxyinosine therapy. *Alcoholism Clinical and Experimental Research* 21:122–127.

162. Wu TC, Tashkin DP, Djahed B, Rose JE. 1988. Pulmonary hazards of smoking marijuana as compared with tobacco. *New England Journal of Medicine* 318:347–351.

163. Yesavage JA, Leirer VO, Denari M, Hollister LE. 1985. Carry-over effects of marijuana intoxication on aircraft pilot performance: A preliminary report. *American Journal of Psychiatry* 142:1325–1329.

164. Zuckerman B, Frank DA, Hingson R, Amaro H, Levenson S, Kayne J, Parker S, Vinci R, Aboagye K, Fried L, Cabral J, Timperi R, Bauchner H. 1989. Effects of maternal marijuana and cocaine use on fetal growth. *New England Journal of Medicine* 320:762–768.

4

The Medical Value of Marijuana and Related Substances

During the course of drug development, a typical compound is found to have some medical benefit and then extensive tests are undertaken to determine its safety and proper dosage for medical use. In contrast, marijuana has been widely used in the United States for decades.[162] In 1996, 68.6 million people—32% of the U.S. population over 12 years old—had tried marijuana or hashish at least once; 5% were current users.[162]

The data on the adverse effects of marijuana are more extensive than the data on its effectiveness. Clinical studies of marijuana are difficult to conduct: researchers interested in clinical studies of marijuana face a series of barriers, research funds are limited, and there is a daunting thicket of regulations to be negotiated at the federal level (those of the Food and Drug Administration, FDA, and the Drug Enforcement Agency, DEA) and state levels (see chapter 5). Consequently, the rapid growth in basic research on cannabinoids contrasts with the paucity of substantial clinical studies on medical uses.

This chapter is devoted to an analysis of the therapeutic value of marijuana and cannabinoids for specific symptoms associated with various conditions. The risks associated with the medical use of marijuana are discussed in chapter 3. It should be noted that THC, the primary active ingredient in marijuana, is an FDA-approved drug referred to as dronabinol and marketed as Marinol. Marijuana is advocated primarily for relief from the symptoms of disease rather than as a cure.

For the most part, the logical categories for the medical use of marijuana are not based on particular diseases but on symptoms—such as nausea, appetite loss, or chronic pain—each of which can be caused by various diseases or even by treatments for diseases. This chapter is therefore organized by symptoms rather than by diseases. There are eight sections. The first section explains clinical trials, the following five deal with specific symptoms and conditions, and the last two summarize the medical benefits of marijuana and cannabinoids. The five sections on symptoms and conditions are as follows: pain, nausea and vomiting, wasting syndrome and appetite stimulation, neurological symptoms (including muscle spasticity), and glaucoma.

The Institute of Medicine (IOM) study team received reports of more than 30 different medical uses of marijuana, more than could be carefully reviewed in a report of this length; even more uses are reported elsewhere.[62,63] For most of the infrequently mentioned medical uses of marijuana there are only a few anecdotal reports. This report reviews only the most prominent symptoms that are reportedly relieved by marijuana. However, many of those diseases not reviewed here share common symptoms, such as pain, nausea and vomiting, and muscle spasms, which might be relieved by cannabinoid drugs.

STANDARDS FOR EVALUATING CLINICAL TRIALS

Before evaluating individual clinical trials concerning the efficacy and safety of medical uses of marijuana and cannabinoids, it is useful to review the general qualities of clinical trials. Clinical trials involve groups of individuals in which different treatments are compared among different groups. Such trials measure the efficacy of a medication and are required by the FDA for approval of any new drug or new use of a drug (discussed further in chapter 5).

The degree of assurance that the outcome of a clinical trial is due to the treatment being tested depends on how well the trial is designed. Three important factors to consider in evaluating the design of a clinical trial are sample selection, subjective effects, and effects that are independent of the treatment. For *sample selection* it is important to ensure that patients are allocated to different treatment groups in such a way that the groups are not biased toward a particular treatment outcome. For example, the health status, gender, and ages of different treatment groups should be equivalent. *Subjective effects* must be controlled because they influence experimental results in two important ways. First, a patient's expectation that a treatment will be effective can influence the degree of its effect (for example, in the control of nausea). Second, the investigator's expectation can influence his or her interpretation of the treatment effect (for example, when assessing the level of pain experienced by a patient).

For these reasons, double blinding, in which neither the subject nor the person who assesses the drug's effect is aware of the subject's treatment group, is particularly important in cannabinoid drug studies. Another important control for subjective effects includes the use of placebo drugs, which are inert substances, or the use of comparison drugs that have effects similar to the experimental drug. Finally, the quality of the experimental design depends on controlling for factors that are unrelated to the test drug but that might nonetheless influence the treatment outcome. *Sequencing effects* are one example of such factors. For example, patients might react differently to the same medication depending on whether the medication was administered after an effective or an ineffective treatment. Likewise, a patient whose symptoms are initially mild might react differently to a drug than would a patient whose symptoms are initially severe. Because psychological effects are associated with cannabinoid drugs, it is important to consider how such side effects might influence the therapeutic value of the treatment. Conditions such as pain and nausea are especially susceptible to subjective influences. For example, depending on the person, THC can reduce or increase anxiety; it is important to determine to what extent this "side effect" contributes to the therapeutic effect.

While double-blind, randomized, controlled clinical trials offer the highest degree of assurance of drug efficacy, such trials are not always feasible. Vulnerable populations, such as children, older patients, and women of child-bearing age, are often excluded from experimental drug trials for safety reasons. Nonetheless, such patients are part of everyday clinical practice. The challenge of integrating the ideal of standardized and rigorous processes for treatment evaluation with everyday clinical practice has encouraged interest in single-patient trials.[67] Methods for such trials have been established and tested in a variety of clinical settings, usually under everyday conditions.[66,105,159] They are particularly valuable when physicians or patients are uncertain about the efficacy of treatment for symptomatic diseases. Controls can be incorporated even in this kind of trial. Such trials can be double blinded and can involve crossover designs in which the patient is treated with alternating treatments, such as placebo-drug-placebo or one drug followed by another drug. As with any other clinical trial, a single-patient trial should be designed to permit objective comparison between treatments.

ANALGESIA

Pain is the most common symptom for which patients seek medical assistance.[5] Pain associated with structural or psychophysiological disorders can arise from somatic, visceral, or neural structures. *Somatic pain* results from activation of receptors outside the brain and is transmitted to the brain via peripheral nerves. *Visceral pain* results from activation of specific pain receptors in the intestine (visceral nociceptive receptors); it is characterized as a deep aching or cramping sensation, but its source is often experienced at sites remote from the site of receptor activation, a phenomenon known as referred pain. *Neuropathic pain* results from injury to peripheral receptors, nerves, or the central nervous system; it is typically burning, the skin feels abnormally unpleasant when gently touched (dysesthesia), and it often occurs in an area of sensory loss, as in the case of postherpetic neuralgia (shingles).

All of the currently available analgesic (pain-relieving) drugs have limited efficacy for some types of pain. Some are limited by dose-related side effects and some by the development of tolerance or dependence. A cannabinoid, or other analgesic, could potentially be useful under any of the following circumstances:

- There is a medical condition for which it is more effective than any currently available medication.
- It has a broad clinical spectrum of efficacy and a unique side effect profile.
- It has synergistic interactions with other analgesics.
- It exhibits "side effects" that are considered useful in some clinical situations.
- Its efficacy is enhanced in patients who have developed tolerance to opioids.

There have not been extensive clinical studies of the analgesic potency of cannabinoids, but the available data from animal studies indicate that cannabinoids could be useful analgesics. In general, cannabinoids seem to be mild to moderate analgesics. Opiates, such as morphine and codeine, are the most widely used drugs for the treatment of acute pain, but they are not consistently effective in chronic pain; they often induce nausea and sedation, and tolerance occurs in some patients. Recent research has made it clear that CB_1 receptor agonists act on pathways that partially overlap with those activated by opioids but through pharmacologically distinct mechanisms (see chapter 2). Therefore, they would probably have a different side effect profile and perhaps additive or synergistic analgesic efficacy.

In light of the evidence that cannabinoids can reduce pain in animals, it is important to re-evaluate the evidence of analgesic efficacy in humans and to ask what clinical evidence is needed to decide whether cannabinoids have any use in the treatment of pain.

Clinical Studies of Cannabinoids

There have been three kinds of studies of the effects of cannabinoids on pain in human volunteers: studies of experimentally induced acute pain, studies of postsurgical acute pain, and studies of chronic pain. Overall, there have been very few studies—only one since 1981—and they have been inconclusive.

Experimentally Induced Acute Pain

Early studies of cannabinoids on volunteers did not demonstrate consistent analgesia when experimental pain models were used. In fact, three early volunteer studies of THC and experimental pain caused by a variety of pain modalities—electrical stimulation, tourniquet pain, and thermal pain—resulted in an *increase* in pain sensitivity (hyperalgesia).[22,84,108]

Other studies also failed to show an analgesic effect of THC, but they were not well designed. Raft and co-workers found no evidence of THC effect on pain thresholds and pain tolerance following electrical stimulation and noxious pressure.[150] But their study suffers from two major methodological problems. First, they measured only the extremes of pain sensation—*threshold* (the lowest intensity at which a particular stimulus is perceived as painful) and *tolerance* (the maximum intensity of pain that a subject can withstand). However, most pain is experienced in an intermediate range, where effects on pain suppression are most detectable. Modern methods of pain assessment in humans typically use ratings of the intensity of the sensation of pain; those methods are superior to assessing the effects of a drug on the extremes of pain.[192] Second, Raft and co-workers did not include a positive control; that is, they did not demonstrate the adequacy of their method by showing that an established analgesic, such as an opiate or narcotic, was effective under their study conditions.

Clark and co-workers[22] tested the effect of smoked marijuana on thermal pain in volunteers and failed to observe an analgesic effect. However, because of the study design, the results are inconclusive. First, there was no positive control to demonstrate the adequacy of their methods; second, the study subjects were habitual marijuana users. During the study, they were hospitalized and allowed free access to marijuana cigarettes for a period of four weeks, consuming an average of four to 17 marijuana cigarettes per day. Pain was tested "approximately every one to two weeks." Thus, it is quite likely that the subjects were tolerant to THC at the time of testing.

Surgical Acute Pain

Raft and co-workers[150] found no analgesic effect of THC on surgical pain induced by tooth extraction. However, that study suffered from several serious limitations: the tooth extraction included treatment with the local anesthetic lidocaine, the pain during the procedure was assessed 24 hours later, and there was no positive control. Levonantradol (a synthetic THC analogue) was tested in 56 patients who had moderate to severe postoperative or trauma pain.[89] They were given intramuscular injections of levonantrodol or placebo 24 hours after surgery. To control for previous drug exposure, patients with a history of drug abuse or addiction and those who received an analgesic, antiinflammatory, tranquilizer, sedative, or anesthetic agent within 24 hours of the test drug were excluded from the study. On average, pain relief was significantly greater in the levonantradol-treated patients than in the placebo-treated patients. Because the authors did not report the number or percentage of people who responded, it is not clear whether the average represents consistent pain relief in all levonantradol-treated patients or whether some people experienced great relief and a few experienced none.

Chronic Pain

The most encouraging clinical data on the effects of cannabinoids on chronic pain are from three studies of cancer pain. Cancer pain can be due to inflammation, mechanical invasion of bone or other pain-sensitive structure, or nerve injury. It is severe, persistent, and often resistant to treatment with opioids. In one study, Noyes and co-workers found that oral doses of THC in the range of 5–20 mg produced analgesia in patients with cancer pain.[139,140] The first experiment was a double-blind, placebo-controlled study of 10 subjects and measured both pain intensity and pain relief.[140] Each subject received all drug treatments: placebo and 5, 10, 15, and 20 mg of THC in pill form; each pill was identical in appearance and given on successive days. The 15- and 20-mg doses of THC produced significant analgesia. There were no reports of nausea or vomiting. In fact, at least half the patients reported increased appetite. With a 20-mg dose of THC, patients were heavily sedated and exhibited "depersonalization," characterized by a state of dreamy immobility, a sense of unreality, and disconnected thoughts. Five of 36 patients exhibited adverse reactions (extreme anxiety) and were eliminated from the study. Only one patient experienced this effect at the 10-mg dose of THC. The mean age of the patients was 51 years, and they were probably not experienced marijuana smokers. A limitation of this study is that there were no positive controls—that is, other analgesics that could provide a better measure of the degree of analgesia produced by THC.

In a later larger single-dose study, the same investigators reported that the analgesic effect of 10 mg of THC was equivalent to that of 60 mg of codeine; the effect of 20 mg of THC was equivalent to that of 120 mg of codeine.[139] (Note that codeine is a relatively weak analgesic.) The side effect profiles were similar, though THC was more sedating than codeine. In a separate publication the same authors published data indicating that patients had improved mood, a sense of well-being, and less anxiety.[139]

The results of the studies mentioned above on cancer pain are consistent with the results of using a nitrogen analogue of THC. Two trials were reported: one compared this analogue with codeine in 30 patients, and a second compared it with placebo or secobarbital, a short-acting barbiturate.[175] For mild, moderate, and severe pain, the THC analogue was equivalent to 50 mg of codeine and superior to placebo and to 50 mg of secobarbital.

Case Reports and Surveys

The few case reports of clinical analgesia trials of cannabinoids are not convincing.[85,120] There are, however, anecdotal surveys that raise the possibility of a role for cannabinoids in some patients who have chronic pain with prominent spasticity. A recent survey of over 100 patients with multiple sclerosis reported that a large number obtained relief from spasticity and limb pain (discussed further under the section on multiple sclerosis).[28] Several said that it relieved their phantom pain and headache.[41]

Migraine Headaches

There is clearly a need for improved migraine medications. Sumatriptan (Imitrex) is the best available medication for migraine headaches, but it fails to abolish migraine symptoms in about 30% of migraine patients.[118,147] Marijuana has been proposed numerous times as a treatment for migraine headaches, but there are almost no clinical data on the use of marijuana or cannabinoids for migraine. Our search of the literature since 1975 yielded only one scientific publication on the subject. It presents three cases of cessation of daily marijuana smoking followed by migraine attacks—not convincing evidence that marijuana relieves migraine headaches.[43] The same result could have been found if migraine headaches were a consequence of marijuana withdrawal. While there is no evidence that marijuana withdrawal is followed by migraines, when analyzing the strength of reports such as these it is important to consider all logical possibilities. Various people have claimed that marijuana relieves their migraine headaches, but at this stage there are no conclusive clinical data or published surveys about the effect of cannabinoids on migraine.

However, a possible link between cannabinoids and migraine is suggested by the abundance of cannabinoid receptors in the periaqueductal gray (PAG) region of the brain. The PAG region is part of the neural system that suppresses pain and is thought to be involved in the generation of migraine headaches.[52] The link or lack thereof between cannabinoids and migraine might be elucidated by examining the effects of cannabinoids on the PAG region.[110] Recent results indicating that both cannabinoid receptor subtypes are involved in controlling peripheral pain[15] suggest that the link is possible. Further research is warranted.

Conclusions: Analgesia

A key question to address is whether there is any receptor selectivity for the analgesic efficacy of cannabinoids. Are the unwanted side effects (amnesia and sedation) caused by the same receptors in the same brain regions as those producing the analgesia? If the answer is *yes*, enhancing efficacy will not solve the problem of sedation. Similarly, are the pleasant side effects due to an action at the same receptor? Can the feelings of well-being and appetite stimulation be separated by molecular design? Recent results indicating that both cannabinoid receptor subtypes are independently involved in controlling peripheral pain[15] (discussed in chapter 2) strongly suggest that this is possible and that further research is warranted.

Further research into the basic circuitry underlying cannabinoid analgesia should be valuable. The variety of neural pathways that underlie the control of pain suggests that a synergistic analgesia "cocktail" would be effective. For example, Lichtman and Martin have shown the involvement of an $\alpha 2$ adrenoreceptor in cannabinoid analgesia.[111] Perhaps a combination of a CB_1 agonist and an $\alpha 2$ agonist (such as clonidine) would provide enhanced analgesia with less severe side effects.

Clinical studies should be directed at pain patients for whom there is a demonstrated need for improved management and where the particular side effect profile of cannabinoids promises a clear benefit over current approaches. The following patient groups should be targeted for clinical studies of cannabinoids in the treatment of pain:

- Chemotherapy patients, especially those being treated for the mucositis, nausea, and anorexia.

- Postoperative pain patients (using cannabinoids as an opioid adjunct to determine whether nausea and vomiting from opioids are reduced).
- Patients with spinal cord injury, peripheral neuropathic pain, or central poststroke pain.
- Patients with chronic pain and insomnia.
- AIDS patients with cachexia, AIDS neuropathy, or any significant pain problem.

In any patient group an essential question to be addressed is whether the analgesic efficacy of opioids can be augmented. The strategy would be to find the ceiling analgesic effect with an opioid (as determined by pain intensity and tolerability of side effects) and then add a cannabinoid to determine whether additional pain relief can be obtained. That would begin the investigation of potential drug combinations. As with any clinical study on analgesic drugs, it will be important to investigate the development of tolerance and physical dependence; these are not themselves reasons to exclude the use of cannabinoids as analgesics, but such information is essential to the management of many drugs that are associated with tolerance or physical dependence.

A secondary question would be whether THC is the only or the best component of marijuana for analgesia. How does the analgesic effect of the plant extract compare with that of THC alone? If there is a difference, it will be important to identify the combinations of cannabinoids that are the most effective analgesics.

In conclusion, the available evidence from animal and human studies indicates that cannabinoids can have a substantial analgesic effect. One exception is the lack of analgesic effect in studies on experimentally induced acute pain, but because of limitations in the design of those studies they were inconclusive. Further clinical work is warranted to establish the magnitude of the effect in different clinical conditions and to determine whether the effect is sustained. Although the usefulness of cannabinoids appears to be limited by side effects, notably sedation, other effects such as anxiolysis, appetite stimulation, and perhaps antinausea and antispasticity effects should be studied in randomized, controlled clinical trials. These very "special" effects might warrant development of cannabinoid drugs for particular clinical populations.

NAUSEA AND VOMITING

Nausea and vomiting (emesis) occur under a variety of conditions, such as acute viral illness, cancer, radiation exposure, cancer chemotherapy, postoperative recovery, pregnancy, motion, and poisoning. Both are produced by excitation of one or a combination of triggers in the gastrointestinal tract, brain stem, and higher brain centers (Figure 4.1, Emesis-stimulating pathways).[127] There are numerous cannabinoid receptors in the nucleus of the solitary tract, a brain center that is important in the control of emesis.[79,80] Although the same mechanisms appear to be involved in triggering both nausea and vomiting, either can occur without the other. Much more is known about the neural mechanisms that produce vomiting than about those that produce nausea, in large part because vomiting is a complex behavior involving coordinated changes in the gastrointestinal tract, respiratory muscles, and posture, whereas nausea is a sensation involving primarily higher brain centers and lacks a discrete observable action.[104,128] Most reports on the antiemetic effects of marijuana or cannabinoids are based on chemotherapy-induced emesis; they are the subject of the following section.

Chemotherapy-Induced Nausea and Vomiting

The use of effective chemotherapeutic drugs has produced cures in some malignancies and retarded the growth of others, but nausea and

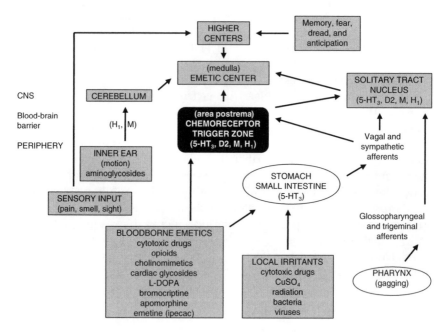

FIGURE 4.1   Emesis-stimulating pathways. SOURCE: Bruton, L.L. 1996. P. 929 in Hardman et al., eds., *The Pharmacological Basis of Therapeutics*, 9th edition. New York: McGraw-Hill. Reprinted with permission.

vomiting are frequent side effects of these drugs. Nausea ranks behind only hair loss as a concern of patients on chemotherapy, and many patients experience it as the worst side effect of chemotherapy. The side effects can be so devastating that patients abandon therapy or suffer diminished quality of life. As a result, the development of effective strategies to control the emesis induced by many chemotherapeutic agents is a major goal in the supportive care of patients with malignancies.

The mechanism by which chemotherapy induces vomiting is not completely understood. Studies suggest that emesis is caused by stimulation of receptors in the central nervous system or the gastrointestinal tract. This stimulation appears to be caused by the drug itself, a metabolite of the drug, or a neurotransmitter.[6,12,35] In contrast with an emetic like apomorphine, there is a delay between the administration of chemotherapy and the onset of emesis. This delay depends on the chemotherapeutic agent; emesis can begin anywhere from a few minutes after the administration of an agent like mustine to an hour for cisplatin.[12]

The most desirable effect of an antiemetic is to control emesis completely, which is currently the primary standard in testing new antiemetic agents (R. Gralla, IOM workshop). Patients recall the number of emetic episodes accurately, even if their antiemetics are sedating or affect memory;[101] thus, the desired end point of complete control is also a highly reliable method of evaluation. The degree of nausea can be estimated through the use of established visual analogue scales.*[21,55,101]

Another consideration in using antiemetic drugs is that the frequency of emesis varies from one chemotherapeutic agent to another. For example, cisplatin causes vomiting in more than 99% of patients who are not taking an antiemetic (with about 10 vomiting episodes per dose), whereas methotrexate causes emesis in less than 10% of patients.[55,82,83] Among chemotherapeutic agents, cisplatin is the most consistent emetic known and has become the benchmark for judging antiemetic efficacy. Antiemetics that are effective with cisplatin are at least as effective with other chemotherapeutic agents. Controlling for the influence of prior chemotherapy and balancing predisposing factors such as, sex, age, and prior heavy alcohol use among study groups are vital for reliability. Reliable randomization of patients and blinding techniques (easier when there are no psychoactive effects) are also necessary to evaluate the control of vomiting and nausea.

---

*The *visual analogue scale* is a continuous line representing all possible levels of a particular sensation. It is an estimation of a patient's subjective evaluation and not a true measurement. Patients select a point anywhere on the line to demonstrate the level of sensation they are experiencing, with one end representing one extreme, such as no sensations, and the other end representing the opposite extreme, such as a maximum level of that sensation.

THC and Marijuana Therapy for Chemotherapy-Induced Nausea and Vomiting

Cannabinoids are mildly effective in preventing emesis in some patients who are receiving cancer chemotherapy. Several cannabinoids have been tested as antiemetics, including THC (both Δ^9-THC and Δ^8-THC) and the synthetic cannabinoids nabilone and levonantradol. Smoked marijuana has also been examined.

Antiemetic Properties of THC

The quality and usefulness of antiemetic studies depend on adherence to the methodological considerations outlined above. Many of the reported clinical experiences with cannabinoids are not based on definitive experimental methods. In studies that compared THC with a placebo, THC was usually found to possess antiemetic properties. However, the chemotherapeutic drug varied in most trials, and some studies included small numbers of patients. In one study THC was found to be superior to a placebo in patients receiving methotrexate, an agent that is not a strong emetic.[18] When the same investigators studied THC in a small number of patients who were receiving a chemotherapeutic drug that is more likely to cause emesis than anthracycline, the antiemetic effect was poor.[19]

Other trials were designed to compare THC with that of Compazine (prochlorperazine).[143,160] In the 1980s, prochlorperazine was one of the more effective antiemetics available, but it was not completely satisfactory, and the search for better agents continued. THC and prochlorperazine given orally showed similar degrees of efficacy, but the studies often used various chemotherapeutic agents. Even when administered in combination, THC and prochlorperazine failed to stop vomiting in two-thirds of patients.[50]

In a carefully controlled double-blind study comparing THC with the antiemetic drug metoclopramide, in which no patient had previously received chemotherapy and in which anticipatory emesis was therefore not a factor, all patients received the same dose of cisplatin and were randomly assigned to the THC group or the metoclopramide group. Complete control of emesis occurred in 47% of those treated with metoclopramide and 13% of those treated with THC.[58] Major control (two or fewer episodes) occurred in 73% of the patients given metoclopramide compared to 27% of those given THC. There were many flaws in experimental methods, but those results suggest that THC has some, but not great, efficacy in reducing chemotherapy-induced emesis.[18,19,50,161] The studies also indicate that the degree of efficacy is not high. In 1985, the

FDA approved THC in the form of dronabinol for this treatment (discussed in chapter 5).

The THC metabolite, 11-OH-THC, is more psychoactive than THC but is a weaker antiemetic.[121] Thus, it might be possible to design antiemetic cannabinoids without the psychological effects associated with marijuana or THC. Δ^8-THC is less psychoactive than THC[151] but was found to completely block both acute and delayed chemotherapy-induced emesis in a study of eight children, ages 3–13 years.* Two hours before the start of each cancer treatment and every six hours thereafter for 24 hours, the children were given Δ^8-THC as oil drops on the tongue or in a bite of bread (18 mg/m² body surface area). The children received a total of 480 treatments. The only side effects reported were slight irritability in two of the youngest children (3.5 and 4 years old). Based on the prediction that the THC-induced anxiety effects would be less in children than in adults, the authors used doses that were higher than those recommended for adults (5–10 mg/m² body surface area).

Antiemetic Properties of Synthetic THC Analogues

Nabilone (Cesamet) and levonantradol were tested in various settings; the results were similar to those with THC. Efficacy was observed in several trials, but no advantage emerged for these agents.[176,185] As in the THC trials, nabilone and levonantradol reduced emesis but not as well as other available agents in moderately to highly emetogenic settings. Neither is commercially available in the United States.

Antiemetic Properties of Marijuana

Among the efforts to study marijuana was a preliminary study conducted in New York state on 56 cancer patients who were unresponsive to conventional antiemetic agents.[188] The patients were asked to rate the effectiveness of marijuana compared with results during prior chemotherapy cycles. In this survey, 34% of patients rated marijuana as moderately or highly effective. The authors concluded that marijuana had antiemetic efficacy, but its relative value was difficult to determine because no control group was used and the patients varied with respect to previous experiences, such as marijuana use and THC therapy.

---

*Note that the authors of this study chose to use Δ^8-THC because it is more stable and easier to produce than Δ^9-THC; it does not follow from this particular study that marijuana, with its mixture of cannabinoids, should be a more powerful antiemetic than Δ^9-THC.

A Canadian oncology group conducted a double-blind, cross-over, placebo-controlled study comparing smoked marijuana with THC in pill form in 20 patients who were receiving various chemotherapeutic drugs.[107] The degree of emetic control was similar: only 25% of patients achieved complete control of emesis; 35% of the patients indicated a slight preference for the THC pills over marijuana, 20% preferred marijuana, and 45% expressed no preference. [107]

Neither study showed a clear advantage for smoked marijuana over oral THC, but neither reported data on the time course of antiemetic control, possible advantages of self-titration with the smoked marijuana, or the degree to which patients were able to swallow the pills. Patients with severe vomiting would have been unlikely to be able to swallow or keep the pills down long enough for them to take effect. The onset of drug effect is much faster with inhaled or injected THC than it is for oral delivery.[87,112,141] Although many marijuana users have claimed that smoked marijuana is a more effective antiemetic than oral THC, no controlled studies have yet been published that analyze this in sufficient detail to estimate the extent to which this is the case.

Side Effects Associated with THC and Marijuana in Antiemetic Therapy

Frequent side effects associated with THC or marijuana are dizziness, dry mouth, hypotension, moderate sedation, and euphoria or dysphoria.[18,19,50,107,143,160,176,185] To patients, dry mouth and sedation are the least troubling side effects. Perhaps the most troubling side effects are orthostatic hypotension and dizziness, which could increase the patient's distress.

There is disagreement as to whether the psychoactive effects of THC correlate with its antiemetic activity. In the prospective double-blind trial comparing THC with metoclopramide, the authors reported no relationship between the occurrence of complete antiemetic control and euphoria or dysphoria.[58] Other investigators believe that the occurrence of euphoria or dysphoria is often associated with improved antiemetic control.[160] Nevertheless, there is a consensus among investigators that dysphoric effects are more common among patients who have had no prior experience with cannabinoids. An important and unexpected problem encountered in the New York state open trial with marijuana was the inability of nearly one-fourth of the patients to tolerate the administration of marijuana by smoking.[188] The intolerance could have been due to inexperience with smoking marijuana and is an important consideration.

Therapy for Chemotherapy-Induced Nausea and Vomiting

Present Therapy

New classes of antiemetics that have emerged over the past 10 years have dramatically reduced the nausea and vomiting associated with cancer chemotherapy and transformed the acceptance of cisplatin by cancer patients. The new antiemetics—including selective serotonin type 3 receptor antagonists, substituted benzamides, corticosteroids, butyrophenones, and phenothiazines—have few side effects when given over a short term and are convenient in various clinical settings.

The most effective commonly used antiemetics are serotonin receptor antagonists (ondansetron and granisetron) with or without corticosteroids.[37,56,88,145,155] In a combination trial of dexamethasone (a corticosteroid) and a serotonin antagonist, complete control of acute cisplatin-induced emesis was observed in about 75% of patients. If the chemotherapy was only moderately emetogenic, up to 90% of the patients who received the combination achieved complete control of emesis. Side effects of those antiemetic agents include headache, constipation, and alterations in liver function, but they are generally well tolerated by most patients.[13]

Other commonly used antiemetics are phenothiazines—prochlorperazine (Compazine) and haloperidol—and metoclopramide. Metoclopramide is somewhat less effective than the serotonin antagonists and has more side effects, including acute dystonic reactions, drowsiness, diarrhea, and depression.[13,37] Side effects associated with phenothiazines are severe or acute dystonic reactions, hypotension, blurred vision, drowsiness, dry mouth, urinary retention, allergic reactions, and occasional jaundice.[13]

The cost of effective antiemetic regimens can vary markedly, depending on the agent, dose, schedule, and route of administration. Overall, oral regimens cost less than intravenous regimens because of lower pharmacy and administration costs, as well as lower acquisition costs in many countries. Regimens with a cost to the pharmacy as low as about $30 to $35 per treatment session have been shown to be effective;[57] these costs are for treatment of acute emesis and delayed emesis with generic agents where available.

Although it is generally not well known by the public, major progress in controlling chemotherapy-induced acute nausea and vomiting has been made since the 1970s. Patients receiving the most difficult to control emetic agents now have no more than about a 20–30% likelihood of experiencing acute emesis,[155] whereas in the 1970s the likelihood was nearly 100% despite antiemetics.[55,86] As has been seen, most antiemetic studies with

BOX 4.1
Attitudes of Oncologists Toward Prescribing Marijuana

In the 1990s, two groups of investigators conducted three surveys on the attitudes of clinical oncologists toward prescribing marijuana as an antiemetic. These studies are arguably out of date in that the antiemetics available now are much more effective than those available when the studies were conducted. Nonetheless, the studies merit attention because they are still often cited as evidence for or against the use of marijuana as an antiemetic.

The two groups' results were contradictory. In 1994, by which time serotonin receptor antagonists (5-HT receptors) had become available, Schwartz and Beveridge[171] concluded that oncologists had little interest in prescribing marijuana to control emesis, whereas Doblin and Kleiman[39] had concluded in 1991 that interest was great. Since 1994, the two groups have debated in the literature as to which study represents the true sentiment among oncologists.[38,172,177] In fact, numerous methodological differences between the two studies might explain the different results.[38,172] Ultimately, these studies are irrelevant. Both deal with perceptions rather than pharmacological realities based on well-designed outcome studies.[177]

cannabinoids had methodological difficulties and are inconclusive. The evidence from the well-conducted trials indicate that cannabinoids reduce emesis in about one-fourth of patients receiving cancer chemotherapy. Cannabinoids are not as effective as several other classes of agents, such as substituted benzamides, serotonin receptor antagonists, and corticosteroids. The side effects associated with cannabinoid use are generally tolerable. Like cannabinoids, smoked marijuana, was apparently effective, but the efficacy was no greater than that of available antiemetic agents now considered to be marginally satisfactory. At present, the most effective antiemetic regimens are combinations of oral serotonin receptor antagonists with dexamethasone in single-dose regimens given before chemotherapy. Neither multiple-dose regimens nor intravenous antiemetics provide better control, and both add unnecessary costs.[59,81]

Future Therapy

Advances in therapy for chemotherapy-induced nausea and vomiting will require discovery of agents that work through mechanisms different from those of existing antiemetics, including the serotonin antagonists. Among the proposed new pathways, neurokinin-1 (NK-1) receptor antagonists appear to be the most promising. Neurokinin receptors are found in brain and intestine and are thought to be involved in motor activity, mood, pain and reinforcement. They might well be involved in mediating intestinal sensations, including nausea. In animal models, agents that block the NK-1 receptor prevent cisplatin-induced emesis. At the time of this writing, clinical trials with NK-1 receptor antagonists were under way (phase II or small phase III comparison studies). Preliminary results indicated that these agents have useful activity in both acute and delayed chemotherapy-induced emesis (that is, beginning or persisting 24 or more hours after chemotherapy) and are safe to administer orally.[102,135]

It is theoretically possible, considering that the mechanism of cannabinoid action appears to differ from that of the serotonin receptor antagonists and of corticosteroids, that THC added to more effective regimens might enhance control of emesis. Such combinations should aim to be as convenient as possible and have few additional side effects. The critical issue is not whether marijuana or cannabinoid drugs might be superior to the new drugs, but whether some group of patients might obtain added or better relief from marijuana or cannabinoid drugs.

Even with the best antiemetic drugs, the control of nausea and vomiting that begins or persists 24 hours after chemotherapy remains imperfect. The pathophysiology of delayed emesis appears different from that of acute emesis, and it is more likely to occur with a strong emetic agent, but it varies from patient to patient. Treatment to prevent this emesis requires dosing both before and after chemotherapy.[103]

Conclusions: Chemotherapy-Induced Nausea

Most chemotherapy patients are unlikely to want to use marijuana or THC as an antiemetic. In 1999, there are more effective antiemetic agents available than were available earlier. By comparison, cannabinoids are only modest antiemetics. However, because modern antiemetics probably act through different mechanisms, cannabinoids might be effective in people who respond poorly to currently used antiemetic drugs, or cannabinoids might be more effective in combination with a new drug than is either alone. For both reasons, studies of the effects of adjunctive cannabinoids on chemotherapy-induced emesis are worth pursuing for patients whose emesis is not optimally controlled with other agents.

While some people who spoke to the IOM study team described the mood-enhancing and anxiety-reducing effects of marijuana as a positive contribution to the antiemetic effects of marijuana, one-fourth of the patients in the New York state study described earlier were unable to tolerate smoked marijuana. Overall, the effects of oral THC and smoked marijuana are similar, but there are differences. For example, in the residential studies of experienced marijuana users by Haney and co-workers, subjects reported that marijuana made them feel "mellow,"[71] whereas comparable doses of oral THC did not.[70] Such differences might be due to the different routes of delivery of THC, as well as the different mixture of cannabinoids found in the marijuana plant. As of this writing, no studies had been published that weighed the relative contributions of those different factors.

The goal of antiemetic medications is to prevent nausea and vomiting. Hence, antiemetics are typically given before chemotherapy, in which case a pill is an effective from of drug delivery. However, in patients already experiencing severe nausea or vomiting, pills are generally ineffective because of the difficulty in swallowing or keeping a pill down and slow onset of the drug effect. Thus, an inhalation (but preferably not smoking) cannabinoid drug delivery system would be advantageous for treating chemotherapy-induced nausea.

Until the development of rapid-onset antiemetic drug delivery systems, there will likely remain a subpopulation of patients for whom standard antiemetic therapy is ineffective and who suffer from debilitating emesis. It is possible that the harmful effects of smoking marijuana for a limited period of time might be outweighed by the antiemetic benefits of marijuana, at least for patients for whom standard antiemetic therapy is ineffective and who suffer from debilitating emesis. Such patients should be evaluated on a case-by-case basis and treated under close medical supervision.

WASTING SYNDROME AND APPETITE STIMULATION

Wasting syndrome in acquired immune deficiency syndrome (AIDS) patients is defined by the Centers for Disease Control and Prevention as the involuntary loss of more than 10% of baseline average body weight in the presence of diarrhea or fever of more than 30 days that is not attributable to other disease processes.[17] Anorexia (loss of appetite) can accelerate wasting by limiting the intake of nutrients. Wasting (cachexia) and anorexia are common end-stage features of some fatal diseases, such as AIDS, and of some types of metastatic cancers. In AIDS, weight loss of as little as 5% is associated with decreased survival, and a body weight about one-third below ideal body weight results in death.[99,158]

There are two forms of malnutrition: starvation and cachexia. Starvation, the deprivation of essential nutrients, results from famine or poverty, malabsorption, eating disorders such as anorexia nervosa, and so on. Starvation leads to metabolic adaptations that deplete body fat before losses of lean tissue. Cachexia results from tissue injury, infection, or tumor and is characterized by a disproportionate loss of lean body mass, such as skeletal muscle. The effects of starvation regardless of the cause can usually be reversed by providing food, whereas the effects of cachexia can be reversed only through control of the underlying disease and—at least for some patients—drugs that stimulate metabolism, such as growth hormone or androgenic-anabolic hormones.

Malnutrition in HIV-Infected Patients

By 1997 more than 30 million people worldwide were infected with human immunodeficiency virus (HIV), and the number is predicted to increase to almost 40 million by the year 2000.[126,186] Malnutrition is common among AIDS patients and plays an independent and important role in their prognosis.[95,100,158] Because treatment for malnutrition depends on whether it is caused by starvation or cachexia, one needs to know the effects of HIV infection on metabolic processes. The answer depends on the clinical situation and can be either or both.[94]

The development of malnutrition in HIV infection has many facets. Malnutrition in HIV-infected patients results in a disproportionate depletion of body cell mass,* total body nitrogen, and skeletal muscle mass; all are consistent with cachexia.[97,194] Body composition studies show that the depletion of body cell mass precedes the progression to AIDS (falling CD4 lymphocyte counts); this suggests that malnutrition is a consequence of the inflammatory response to the underlying viral infection, rather than a general complication of AIDS.[144] In contrast, weight loss is often episodic and related to acute complications, such as febrile opportunistic infections.[113] Mechanisms underlying wasting in HIV-infected patients depend on the stage of HIV infection and on specific associated complications.

The many reasons for decreased food intake among AIDS patients include mouth, throat, or esophageal infections or ulcers (oropharyngeal and esophageal pathology); adverse effects of medications;[196] diarrhea; enteric infection; malabsorption; serious systemic infection; focal or diffuse neurological disease; HIV enteropathy; depression; fatigue; and poverty. Nutrient malabsorption is often the result of microorganism overgrowth or infection in the intestine, especially in the later stages of AIDS.[95,157]

---

*Body cell mass is the fat-free cellular mass. It is composed of the cells of the muscle and organs, plus circulating hematopoietic cells and the aqueous compartment of adipocytes. It is not fat, extracellular water, or extracellular solids (such as tendons).

Marijuana and THC for Malnutrition in HIV-Infected Patients

Despite their frequency of use, little has been published about the effectiveness of marijuana or cannabinoids for the treatment of malnutrition and wasting syndrome in HIV-infected patients. The only cannabinoid evaluated in controlled clinical studies is THC, or dronabinol. Short-term (six-week) and long-term (one-year) therapy with dronabinol was associated with an increase in appetite and stable weight, and in a previous short-term (five-week) clinical trial in five patients, dronabinol was shown to increase body fat by 1%.[8,9,179] In 1992, the FDA approved THC, under the trade name Marinol (dronabinol), as an appetite stimulant for the treatment of AIDS-related weight loss. Megestrol acetate (Megace) is a synthetic derivative of progesterone that can stimulate appetite and cause substantial weight gain when given in high doses (320–640 mg/day) to AIDS patients. Megestrol acetate is more effective than dronabinol in stimulating weight gain, and dronabinol has no additive effect when used in combination with megestrol acetate.[183] HIV/AIDS patients are the largest group of patients who use dronabinol. However, some reject it because of the intensity of neuropsychological effects, an inability to titrate the oral dose easily, and the delayed onset and prolonged duration of its action.[3] There is evidence that cannabinoids modulate the immune system (see chapter 2, "Cannabinoids and the Immune System"), and this could be a problem in immunologically compromised patients. No published studies have formally evaluated use of any of the other cannabinoids for appetite stimulation in wasting.

Anecdotes abound that smoked marijuana is useful for the treatment of HIV-associated anorexia and weight loss.[23,62] Some people report a preference for smoked marijuana over oral THC because it gives them the ability to titrate the effects, which depend on how much they inhale. In controlled laboratory studies of healthy adults, smoked marijuana was shown to increase body weight, appetite, and food intake.[47,119] Unfortunately, there have been no controlled studies of the effect of smoked marijuana on appetite, weight gain, and body composition in AIDS patients. At the time of this writing, Donald Abrams, of the University of California, San Francisco, was conducting the first clinical trial to test the safety of smoked marijuana in AIDS patients, and the results were not yet available.

A major concern with marijuana smoking in HIV-infected patients is that they might be more vulnerable than other marijuana users to immunosuppressive effects of marijuana or to the exposure of infectious organisms associated marijuana plant material (see chapter 3, "Marijuana Smoke").

Therapy for Wasting Syndrome in HIV-Infected Patients

Present Therapy

Generally, therapy for wasting in HIV-infected people focuses on appetite stimulation. Few therapies have proved successful in treatment of the AIDS wasting syndrome. The stimulant studied most is megestrol acetate, which has been shown to increase food intake by about 30% over baseline for reasons that remain unknown. Its effect in producing substantial weight gain is dose dependent, but most of the weight gained is in fat tissue, not lean body mass. Although the findings are still preliminary, anabolic compounds, such as testosterone or growth hormone, might be useful in preventing the loss of or in restoring lean body mass in AIDS patients.[10,44,64,170] Enteral and parenteral nutrition have also been evaluated and shown to increase weight, but again the increase is due more to body fat than to lean body mass.[96,98]

Encouraging advances in the antiviral treatment of HIV infection and developments in the prophylaxis of and therapy for opportunistic infections have recently changed the outlook for the long-term health of HIV-infected people. Death rates have been halved, and the frequency of serious complications, including malnutrition, has fallen markedly.[94,133]

Future Therapy

The primary focus of future therapies for wasting in HIV-infected patients is to increase lean body mass as well as appetite. Active systemic infections are associated with profound anorexia, which is believed to be mediated by cytokines that stimulate inflammation through their actions in and outside the brain.[132] Cytokine inhibitors, such as thalidomide, have been under investigation as potential treatments to increase lean body mass and reduce malnutrition. Even though cannabinoids do not appear to restore lean body mass, they might be useful as adjunctive therapy. For example, cannabinoids could be used as appetite stimulants, in patients with diminished appetite who are undergoing resistance exercises or anabolic therapy to increase lean body mass. They could also be beneficial for a variety of effects, such as increased appetite, while reducing the nausea and vomiting caused by protease inhibitors and the pain and anxiety associated with AIDS.

Considering current knowledge about malnutrition in HIV infection, cannabinoids, by themselves, will probably not constitute primary therapy for this condition but might be useful in combination with other therapies, such as anabolic agents. Specifically, the proposed mechanism of action of increasing food intake would most likely be ineffective in promoting an increase in skeletal muscle mass and functional capacity—the goal in the treatment of cachexia in AIDS patients.

Malnutrition in Cancer Patients

Malnutrition compromises the quality of life of many cancer patients and contributes to the progression of their disease. About 30% of Americans will develop cancer in their lifetimes, and two-thirds of those who get cancer will die as a result of it.[5] Depending on the type of cancer, 50–80% of patients will develop cachexia and up to 50% of them will die, in part, as a result of cachexia.[11,40] The cachexia appears to result from the tumor itself, and cytokines (proteins secreted by the host during an immune response to tumor) are probably important factors in this development. Cachexia does not occur in all cancer patients, but generally occurs in the late stages of advanced cancer of the pancreas, lung, and prostate.

The only cannabinoid evaluated for treating cachexia in cancer patients is dronabinol, which has been shown to improve appetite and promote weight gain.[54] Present treatments for cancer cachexia are similar to that for cachexia in AIDS patients. These treatments are usually indicated in late stages of advanced disease and include megestrol acetate and enteral and parenteral nutrition. Megestrol acetate stimulates appetite and promotes weight gain in cancer patients, although the gain is mostly in fat mass (reviewed by Bruera 1998[14]). Both megestrol acetate and dronabinol have dose-related side effects that can be troublesome for patients: megestrol acetate can cause hyperglycemia and hypertension, and dronabinol can cause dizziness and lethargy. Cannabinoids have also been shown to modulate the immune system (see chapter 2, "Cannabinoids and the Immune System"), and this could be contraindicated in some cancer patients (both the chemotherapy and the cancer can be immunosuppressive).

Future treatments will probably depend on the development of methods that block cytokine actions and the use of selective β2-adrenergic receptor agonists to increase muscle mass.[14,73] Treatments for cancer cachexia will also most likely need to identify individual patients' needs. Some patients might need only a cytokine inhibitor, whereas others could benefit from combined approaches, such as an appetite stimulant and β2-adrenergic receptor agonists. In this respect, such cannabinoids as THC might prove useful as part of a combination therapy as an appetite stimulant, antiemetic, analgesic, and anxiolytic, especially for patients in late stages of the disease.

Anorexia Nervosa

Anorexia nervosa, a psychiatric disorder characterized by distorted body image and self-starvation, affects an estimated 0.6% of the U.S. population, with a greater prevalence in females than males.[5] Its mortality is high, and response to standard treatments is poor.

THC appears to be ineffective in treating this disease. In one study it caused severe dysphoric reactions in three of 11 patients.[65] One possible explanation of the dysphoria is that THC increases appetite and thus intensifies the mental conflict between hunger and food refusal.[13] Furthermore, such patients might have underlying psychiatric disorders, such as schizophrenia and depression, in which cannabinoids might be hazardous (see chapter 3, "Psychological Harms").

Current treatments include psychological techniques to overcome emotional or behavioral problems and dietary intervention to reverse the malnutrition.[195] Pharmacological treatments, such as antidepressants, have been used in addition to psychotherapy but tend to lack the desired level of efficacy.[33] Recently, alterations in a gene for one of the serotonin receptors have been identified in some patients with anorexia nervosa.[45] The possibility of a genetic component suggests a pathway for the development of new drugs to treat this disease.

Conclusions: Wasting Syndrome and Appetite Stimulation

The profile of cannabinoid drug effects suggests that they are promising for treating wasting syndrome in AIDS patients. Nausea, appetite loss, pain, and anxiety are all afflictions of wasting, and all can be mitigated by marijuana. Although some medications are more effective than marijuana for these problems, they are not equally effective in all patients. A rapid-onset (that is, acting within minutes) delivery system should be developed and tested in such patients. Smoking marijuana is not recommended. The long-term harm caused by smoking marijuana makes it a poor drug delivery system, particularly for patients with chronic illnesses.

Terminal cancer patients pose different issues. For those patients the medical harm associated with smoking is of little consequence. For terminal patients suffering debilitating pain or nausea and for whom all indicated medications have failed to provide relief, the medical benefits of smoked marijuana might outweigh the harm.

NEUROLOGICAL DISORDERS

Neurological disorders affect the brain, spinal cord, or peripheral nerves and muscles in the body. Marijuana has been proposed most often as a source of relief for three general types of neurological disorders: muscle spasticity, particularly in multiple sclerosis patients and spinal cord injury victims; movement disorders, such as Parkinson's disease, Huntington's disease, and Tourette's syndrome; and epilepsy. Marijuana is not proposed as a cure for such disorders, but it might relieve some associated symptoms.

Muscle Spasticity

Spasticity is the increased resistance to passive stretch of muscles and increased deep tendon reflexes. Muscles may also contract involuntarily (flexor and extensor spasms). In some cases these contractions are debilitating and painful and require therapy to relieve the spasms and associated pain.

There are numerous anecdotal reports that marijuana can relieve the spasticity associated with multiple sclerosis or spinal cord injury, and animal studies have shown that cannabinoids affect motor areas in the brain—areas that might influence spasticity.[51,78,130,168]

Multiple Sclerosis

Multiple sclerosis (MS) is a condition in which multiple areas of the central nervous system (CNS) are affected. Many nerve fibers become demyelinated, some are destroyed, and scars (sclerosis) form, resulting in plaques scattered throughout the white matter of the CNS. (Myelin is the lipid covering that surrounds nerve cell fibers and facilitates the conduction of signals along nerve cells and ultimately between the brain, the spinal cord, and the rest of the body.) MS exacerbations appear to be caused by abnormal immune activity that causes inflammation and myelin destruction in the brain (primarily in the periventricular area), brain stem, or spinal cord. Demyelination slows or blocks transmission of nerve impulses and results in an array of symptoms such as fatigue, depression, spasticity, ataxia (inability to control voluntary muscular movements), vertigo, blindness, and incontinence. About 90% of MS patients eventually develop spasticity. There are an estimated 2.5 million MS patients worldwide, and spasticity is a major concern of many patients and physicians.[134] Spasticity is variably experienced as muscle stiffness, muscle spasms, flexor spasms or cramps, muscle pain or ache. The tendency for the legs to spasm at night (flexor spasms) can interfere with sleep.

Marijuana is often reported to reduce the muscle spasticity associated with MS.[62,123] In a mail survey of 112 MS patients who regularly use marijuana, patients reported that spasticity was improved and the associated pain and clonus decreased.[287] However, a double-blind placebo-controlled study of postural responses in 10 MS patients and 10 healthy volunteers indicated that marijuana smoking impaired posture and balance in both MS patients and the volunteers.[61] Nevertheless, the 10 MS patients felt that they were clinically improved. The subjective improvement, while intriguing, does not constitute unequivocal evidence that marijuana relieves spasticity. Survey data do not measure the degree of placebo effect, estimated to be as great as 30 percent in pain treatments.[122,131] Furthermore, surveys do not separate the effects of marijuana or cannabinoids on mood and anxiety from the effects on spasticity.

The effects of THC on spasticity were evaluated in a series of three clinical trials testing a total of 30 patients.[24,148,187] They were "open trials," meaning that the patients were informed before treatment that they would be receiving THC. Based on patient report or clinical exam by the investigator, spasticity was less severe after the THC treatment. However, THC was not effective in all patients and frequently caused unpleasant side effects. Spasticity was also reported to be less severe in a single case study after nabilone treatment (Figure 4.2).[117]

In general, the abundant anecdotal reports are not well supported by the clinical data summarized in Table 4.1. But this is due more to the limitation of the studies than to negative results. There are no supporting animal data to encourage clinical research in this area, but there also are no good animal models of the spasticity of MS. Without an appropriate model, studies to determine the physiological basis for how marijuana or THC might relieve spasticity cannot be conducted. Nonetheless, the survey results suggest that it would be useful to investigate the potential therapeutic value of cannabinoids in relieving symptoms associated with MS. Such research would require the use of objective measures of spasticity, such as the pendulum test.* Since THC is mildly sedating, it is also important to distinguish this effect from antispasticity effects in any such investigations. Mild sedatives, such as Benadryl or benzodiazepines, would be useful controls for studies on the ability of cannabinoids to relieve muscle spasticity. The regular use of smoked marijuana, however, would be contraindicated in a chronic condition like MS.

Spinal Cord Injury

In 1990, there were about 15 million patients worldwide with spinal cord injury, and an estimated 10,000 new cases are reported each year in

---

*The *pendulum test* is an objective and accurate measure of MS-induced spasticity. It is done by videotaping a patient who lies supine on a table with his or her leg extending off the edge. The leg is dropped and the resulting motion is mathematically analyzed by computer to provide a quantitative measure of spasticity.

FIGURE 4.2   Effect of nabilone on multiple sclerosis symptoms. This figure shows the results of a trial in which a 45-year-old man with MS was given four-week treatments alternately with placebo and nabilone. The patient served as both experimental subject and control; his treatment sequence was nabilone-placebo-nabilone-placebo. That pattern of alternating treatments reduces the possibility that the observed changes are unrelated to the drug and are not simply due to other factors that changed with time. The results of the trial are consistent with the possibility that THC might relieve spasticity, but although more rigorous than many self-report studies of psychoactive substances, it has problems. First, the patient could not distinguish the treatments at the time of taking them, but after the nabilone treatment he felt sedated. Thus, it is not possible to know how much the expectation of relief contributed to his perception of relief. Second, the study measured his perception of pain, in which spasticity is an important factor but not the only factor. It is not possible to know the extent to which the perception of pain was affected by nabilone and how much by the stimulus that generated the pain—in this case, involuntary muscle contractions. Because it is unaffected by conscious control, the frequency of nocturia is clearer evidence of the effect of THC, although it might also represent how well the patient slept. This trial with a single person is intriguing but not definitive proof that THC can reliably relieve spasticity. SOURCE: Martyn et al. (1995).[117] Reprinted with permission.

TABLE 4.1   Studies on the Effects of Marijuana and Cannabinoids in Multiple Sclerosis

Drug and Dose	Study Design	Results	Reference
Marijuana	Mail survey 112/233 MS patients	Survey was mailed to 233 MS patients, of whom 112 (48%) responded; 97% of respondents reported improved spasticity and reduced pain.	Consroe and co-workers (1997)[28]
Marijuana	Clinical trial 1 MS patient	Reduction in spasticity and improved ataxia.	Meinck and co-workers (1989)[123]
Marijuana	Double-blind, placebo-controlled 10 MS patients; 10 normal individuals	MS patients felt they were improved, but posture and balance were impaired.	Greenberg and co-workers (1994)[61]
Oral THC 5–15 mg every 6 hrs, up to 18 hrs	Open trial 8 MS patients	5 patients experienced subjective but not objective improvement in motor coordination; objective improvement in tremor demonstrated in 2 of the 8 patients.	Clifford (1983)[24]
Oral THC 5 and 10 mg, single doses	Double-blind, placebo controlled 9 MS patients	Spasticity was improved based on examiner ratings.	Petro and Ellenberger (1981)[148]
Oral THC 2.5–15 mg, once or twice daily for 5 days	Double-blind, placebo controlled, crossover 13 MS patients	Patients reported subjective decreases in spasticity at doses of 7.5 mg or greater, but no changes in objective measures of spasticity or weakness were observed.	Ungerleider and co-workers (1987)[187]
Nabilone (THC analogue)	Placebo-controlled 1 MS patient	The patient reported increased well-being, less frequent nocturia, and reduced severity of muscle spasticity during nabilone treatment (Figure 4.2).	Martyn and co-workers (1995)[117]

the United States alone.[134,138] About 60% of spinal cord injuries occur in people younger than 35 years old. Most will need long-term care and some lifelong care.[116]

Many spinal cord injury patients report that marijuana reduces their muscle spasms.[114] Twenty-two of 43 respondents to a 1982 survey of people with spinal cord injuries reported that marijuana reduced their spasticity.[114] One double-blind study of a paraplegic patient with painful spasms in both legs suggested that oral THC was superior to codeine in reducing muscle spasms.[72,120] Victims of spinal cord injury reporting at IOM workshops noted that smoking marijuana reduces their muscle spasms, their nausea, and the frequency of their sleepless nights. The caveats described for surveys of spasticity relief in MS patients also apply here.

Therapy for Muscle Spasticity

Present Therapy. Present therapy for spasticity includes the various medications listed in Table 4.2. Baclofen and tizanidine, the most commonly prescribed antispasticity drugs, relieve spasticity and spasms with various degrees of success. The benefit of these agents is generally only partial. Their use is complicated by the side effects of drowsiness, dry mouth, and increased weakness.

Future Therapy. The discovery of agents that work through mechanisms different from those of existing antispasticity drugs will be an important advance in the treatment of spasticity. The aim of new treatments will be to relieve muscle spasticity and pain without substantially increasing muscle weakness in conditions that result in spasticity. The treatment for MS itself will likely be directed at immunomodulation. Various immunomodulating agents, such as beta-interferon and glatiramer acetate, have been shown to reduce the frequency of symptomatic attacks, the progression of disability, and the rate of appearance of demyelinated lesions as detected by magnetic resonance imaging.[5]

Conclusion: Muscle Spasticity

Basic animal studies described in chapter 2 have shown that cannabinoid receptors are particularly abundant in areas of the brain that control

TABLE 4.2   Classes of Antispasticity Drugs

Drug Class	Drug
GABA$_B$-receptor agonists	Baclofen
α-Receptor agonists	Tizanidine
Noncompetitive GABA$_A$-receptor agonists	Benzodiazepines, including diazepam
Calcium blockers in skeletal muscle	Dantrolene

movement and that cannabinoids affect movement and posture in animals as well as humans. The observations are consistent with the possibility that cannabinoids have antispastic effects, but they do not offer any direct evidence that cannabinoids affect spasticity, even in animals. The available clinical data are too meager to either accept or dismiss the suggestion that marijuana or cannabinoids relieve muscle spasticity. But the few positive reports of the ability of THC and related compounds to reduce spasticity, together with the prevalence of anecdotal reports of the relief provided by marijuana, suggest that carefully designed clinical trials testing the effects of cannabinoids on muscle spasticity should be considered (see chapter 1).[25,62] Such trials should be designed to assess the degree to which the anxiolytic effects of cannabinoids contribute to any observed antispastic effects.

Spasticity occurring at night can be very disruptive to sleep. Thus, a long-lasting medication would be especially useful for MS patients at bedtime—when drowsiness would be a beneficial rather than an unwanted side effect and mood-altering effects would be less of a problem. One caution is related to the effects of THC on the stages of sleep, which should be evaluated in MS patients who have sleep disturbances. If THC is proven to relieve spasticity, a pill might be the preferred route of delivery for nighttime use because of its long duration of action. Compared to the currently available therapies, the long half-life of THC might allow for a smoother drug effect throughout the day. The intensity of the symptoms resulting from spasticity, particularly in MS, can rapidly increase in an unpredictable fashion such that the patient develops an "attack" of intense muscle spasms lasting minutes to hours. An inhaled form of THC (if it were shown to be efficacious) might be appropriate for those patients.

Movement Disorders

Movement disorders are a group of neurological conditions caused by abnormalities in the basal ganglia and their subcortical connections through the thalamus with cortical motor areas. The brain dysfunctions ultimately result in abnormal skeletal muscle movements in the face, limbs, and trunk. The movement disorders most often considered for marijuana or cannabinoid therapy are dystonia, Huntington's disease, Parkinson's disease, and Tourette's syndrome. Movement disorders are often transiently exacerbated by stress and activity and improved by factors that reduce stress. This is of particular interest because for many people marijuana reduces anxiety.

Dystonia

Dystonia can be a sign of other basal ganglion disorders, such as Huntington's disease and tardive dyskinesia (irreversible development of involuntary dyskinetic movements) and can be a primary basal ganglion disorder. Primary dystonias are a heterogeneous group of chronic slowly progressive neurological disorders characterized by dystonic movements—slow sustained involuntary muscle contractions that often result in abnormal postures of limbs, trunk, and neck. Dystonias can be confined to one part of the body, such as spasmodic torticollis (neck) or Meige's syndrome (facial muscles), or can affect many parts of the body, such as dystonia musculorum deformans.[5] Dystonia can cause mild to severe disability and sometimes pain secondary to muscle aching or arthritis. Some dystonias are genetic; others are caused by drugs. The specific neuropathological changes in these diseases have not been determined.

No controlled study of marijuana in dystonic patients has been published, and the only study of cannabinoids was a preliminary open trial of cannabidiol (CBD) that suggested modest dose-related improvements in the five dystonic patients studied.[30] In mutant dystonic hamsters, however, the cannabinoid receptor agonist, WIN 55,212-2, can produce antidystonic effects.[153]

Huntington's Disease

Huntington's disease is an inherited degenerative disease that usually appears in middle age and results in atrophy or loss of neurons in the caudate nucleus, putamen, and cerebral cortex. It is characterized by arrhythmic, rapid muscular contractions (chorea), emotional disturbance, and dementia (impairment in intellectual and social ability). Animal studies suggest that cannabinoids have antichoreic activity, presumably because of stimulation of CB_1 receptors in the basal ganglia.[129,168]

On the basis of positive results in one of four Huntington's disease patients, CBD and a placebo were tested in a double-blind crossover study of 15 Huntington's disease patients who were not taking any antipsychotic drugs. Their symptoms neither improved nor worsened with CBD treatment.[27,164]

The effects of other cannabinoids on patients with Huntington's disease are largely unknown. THC and other CB_1 agonists are more likely candidates than CBD, which does not bind to the CB_1 receptor. Those receptors are densely distributed on the very neurons that perish in Huntington's disease.[152] Thus far there is little evidence to encourage clinical studies of cannabinoids in Huntington's disease.

Parkinson's Disease

Parkinson's disease, a degenerative disease, affects about 1 million Americans over the age of 50.[53] It is characterized by bradykinesia (slowness in movement), akinesia (abrupt stoppage of movement), resting tremor, muscular rigidity, and postural instability.

Theoretically, cannabinoids could be useful for treating Parkinson's disease patients because cannabinoid agonists specifically inhibit the pathways between the subthalamic nucleus and substantia nigra and probably also the pathways between the subthalamic nucleus and globus pallidus (these structures shown in Figure 2.6).[165,169] The latter effect was not directly tested but is consistent with what is known about these neural pathways. Hyperactivity of the subthalamic neurons, observed in both Parkinson's patients and animal models of Parkinson's disease, is hypothesized to be a major factor in the debilitating bradykinesia associated with the disease.[36] Furthermore, although cannabinoids oppose the actions of dopamine in intact rats, they augment dopamine activation of movement in an animal model of Parkinson's disease. This suggests the potential for adjunctive therapy with cannabinoid agonists.[165–167,169]

At the time of this writing, we could find only one published clinical trial of marijuana involving five cases of idiopathic Parkinson's disease.[48] That trial was prompted by a patient's report that smoking marijuana reduced tremor, but the investigators found no improvement in tremor after the five patients smoked marijuana—whereas all subjects benefited from the administration of standard medications for Parkinson's disease (levodopa and apomorphine).[48] Although new animal data might someday indicate a use for cannabinoids in treating Parkinson's disease, current data do not recommend clinical trials of cannabinoids in patients with Parkinson's disease.

Tourette's Syndrome

Tourette's syndrome usually begins in childhood and is characterized by motor and vocal tics (involuntary rapid repetitive movements or vocalizations). It has been suggested that the symptoms might be mediated by a reduction in the activity of limbic-basal ganglia-thalamocortical circuits (shown in Figure 2.4).[42] These circuits, while not well understood, appear to be responsible for translating a person's intentions to move into actual movements. Damage to these structures leads to either involuntary increases in movement (as in Huntington's disease) or the inability to make voluntary movements (as in Parkinson's disease). The nature of the deficit in Tourette's syndrome is unknown.

No clear link has been established between symptoms of Tourette's syndrome and cannabinoid sites or mechanism of action. Pimozide and haloperidol, two widely used treatments for Tourette's syndrome, inhibit effects mediated by the neurotransmitter dopamine, whereas cannabinoids can increase dopamine release.[154,181] The physiological relevance, if any, of these two observations has not been established.

Clinical reports consist of four case histories indicating that marijuana use can reduce tics in Tourette's patients.[75,163] In three of the four cases the investigators suggest that beneficial effects of marijuana might have been due to anxiety-reducing properties of marijuana rather than to a specific antitic effect.[163]

Therapy for Movement Disorders

Various drugs are available (Table 4.3) to treat the different movement disorders. Common side effects of many of these drugs are sedation, lethargy, school and work avoidance, social phobia, and increased risk of parkinsonism and tardive dyskinesia. With some of the medications, like those used for dystonia, efficacy is lacking in up to 50% of the patients. In addition to medications, surgical interventions, such as pallidotomy and neurosurgical transplantation of embryonic substantia nigra tissue into the patient's striatum, have been tried in Parkinson's disease patients. Surgery is generally palliative and is still considered to be in the developmental phase.

TABLE 4.3   Drugs Used to Treat Movement Disorders

Dystonia	Parkinson's disease
Benzodiazepines	Levodopa
Tetrabenazine	Carbidopa+levodopa combination
Intramuscular botulinum toxin	Amantadine
Anticholinergics	Bromocriptine
Baclofen	Pergolide
	Pramipexole
Huntington's disease	Ropinirole
Reserpine	Selegiline
Tetrabenazine	Trihexyphenidyl
Haloperidol	Benztropine
Tourette's syndrome tics	
Pimozide	
Clonidine	
Haloperidol	

Conclusion: Movement Disorders

The abundance of CB_1 receptors in basal ganglia and reports of animal studies showing the involvement of cannabinoids in the control of movement suggest that cannabinoids would be useful in treating movement disorders in humans. Marijuana or CB_1 receptor agonists might provide symptomatic relief of chorea, dystonia, some aspects of parkinsonism, and tics. However, clinical evidence is largely anecdotal; there have been no well-controlled studies of adequate numbers of patients. Furthermore, nonspecific effects might confound interpretation of results of studies. For example, the anxiolytic effects of cannabinoids might make patients feel that their condition is improved, despite the absence of measurable change in their condition.

Compared to the abundance of anecdotal reports concerning the beneficial effects of marijuana on muscle spasticity, there are relatively few claims that marijuana is useful for treating movement disorders. This might reflect a lack of effect or a lack of individuals with movement disorders who have tried marijuana. In any case, while there are a few isolated reports of individuals with movement disorders who report a benefit from marijuana, there are no published surveys indicating that a substantial percentage of patients with movement disorders find relief from marijuana. Existing studies involve too few patients from which to draw conclusions. The most promising reports involve symptomatic treatment of spasticity. If the reported neuroprotective effects of cannabinoids discussed in chapter 2 prove to be therapeutically useful, this could benefit patients with movement disorders, but without further data such a benefit is highly speculative. Since stress often transiently exacerbates movement disorders, it is reasonable to hypothesize that the anxiolytic effects of marijuana or cannabinoids might be beneficial to some patients with movement disorders. However, chronic marijuana smoking is a health risk that could increase the burden of chronic conditions, such as movement disorders. .

Cannabinoids inhibit both major excitatory and inhibitory inputs to the basal ganglia. This suggests that a cannabinoid agonist could produce opposite effects on movement, depending on the type of transmission (excitatory or inhibitory) that is most active at the time of drug administration. This property could be used to design treatments in basal ganglia movement disorders, such as Parkinson's disease where either the excitatory subthalamic input becomes hyperactive or the inhibitory striatal input becomes hypoactive. The dose employed would be a major factor in the therapeutic uses of cannabinoids in movement disorders; low doses should be desirable, while higher doses could be expected to aggravate pathological conditions. Thus, there is a clear reason to recommend pre-

clinical studies; that is, animal studies to test the hypothesis that cannabinoids play an important role in movement disorders.

With the possible exception of multiple sclerosis, the evidence to
recommend clinical trials of cannabinoids in movement disorders is relatively weak. Ideally, clinical studies would follow animal research that
provided stronger evidence than is currently available on the potential
therapeutic value of cannabinoids in the treatment of movement
disorders. Unfortunately, there are no good animal models for these disorders. Thus, double-blind, placebo-controlled clinical trials of isolated
cannabinoids that include controls for relevant side effects should be conducted. Such effects include anxiolytic and sedative effects, which might
either mask or contribute to the potential therapeutic effects of
cannabinoids.

Epilepsy

Epilepsy is a chronic seizure disorder that affects about 2 million
Americans and 30 million people worldwide.[156] It is characterized by recurrent sudden attacks of altered consciousness, convulsions, or other
motor activity. A seizure is the synchronized excitation of large groups of
brain cells. These abnormal electrical events have a wide array of possible
causes, including injury to the brain and chemical changes derived from
metabolic faults of exposure to toxins.[156]

Seizures are classified as partial (focal) or generalized. Partial seizures
are associated with specific sensory, motor, or psychic aberrations that
reflect the function of the part of the cerebral cortex from which the seizures arise. Generalized seizures are usually the result of pathological conditions of brain sites that project to widespread regions of the brain. Such
pathology can produce petit mal seizures or major grand mal convulsions.

Cannabinoids in Epilepsy

There are anecdotal and individual case reports that marijuana controls seizures in epileptics (reviewed in a 1997 British Medical Association
report[13]), but there is no solid evidence. While there are no studies indicating that either marijuana or THC worsen seizures, there is no scientific
basis to justify such studies.

In the only known case-controlled study that was designed to evaluate illicit drug use and the risk of first seizure, Ng and co-workers[137] concluded that marijuana is a protective factor for first-time seizures in men
but not women. Men who used marijuana reportedly had fewer first-time
seizures than men who did not use marijuana. That report was based on a
comparison of 308 patients who had been admitted to a hospital after

their first seizure with a control group of 294 patients. The control group was made up of patients who had not had seizures and were admitted for emergency surgery, such as surgery for appendicitis, intestinal obstruction, or acute cholecystitis. Compared to men who did not use marijuana, the odds ratio of first seizure for men who had used marijuana within 90 days of hospital admission was 0.36 (95% confidence interval = 0.18–0.74). An odds ratio of less than one is consistent with the suggestion that marijuana users are less likely to have seizures. The results for women were not statistically significant. However, this was a weak study. It did not include measures of health status prior to hospital admissions for the patients' serious conditions, and differences in their health status might have influenced their drug use rather than—as suggested by the authors— that differences in their drug use influenced their health.

The potential antiepileptic activity of CBD has been investigated but is not promising. Three controlled trials were conducted in which CBD was given orally to patients who had had generalized grand mal seizures or focal seizures (Table 4.4). Two of these studies were never published, but information about one was published in a letter to the *South African Medical Journal*, and the other was presented at the 1990 Marijuana International Conference on Cannabis and Cannabinoids.[184]

TABLE 4.4   Clinical Trials of Cannabidiol (CBD) in Epileptics

Study Design	Results	Reference
Double-blind placebo-controlled trial 8 epileptic patients were given CBD at 200–300 mg/day in conjunction with standard antiepileptic therapies.	4 of 8 remained almost free of convulsions. Three of the 4 were partially improved for up to 4.5 months.	Cunha and co-workers[34]
Double-blind placebo-controlled study 12 epileptic patients were given CBD at 200–300 mg/day along with standard antiepileptic drugs.	CBD had no effect on seizure frequency.	Ames[4]
Double-blind placebo-controlled, add-on crossover trial 10 epileptic patients were given CBD at 300 mg/day for 6 months.	CBD had no effect on seizures.	Trembly and Sherman, 1990[184] (reviewed in Consroe and Sandyk, 1992[29])
Open trial One patient was given CBD at 900–1,200 mg/day for 10 months.	Seizure frequency was reduced in the patient.	Trembly and Sherman, 1990[184] (reviewed in Consroe and Sandyk, 1992[29])

Even if CBD had antiepileptic properties, these studies were likely too small to demonstrate efficacy. Proving efficacy of anticonvulsants generally requires large numbers of patients followed for months because the frequency of seizures is highly variable and the response to therapy varies depending on seizure type.[4,49]

Therapy for Epilepsy

Present Therapy. Standard pharmacotherapy for partial and generalized seizures, listed in Table 4.5, involves a variety of anticonvulsant drugs. These drugs suppress seizures completely in approximately 60% of patients who have chronic epilepsy and improve seizures in another 15% of patients. All of the anticonvulsants listed in Table 4.5 have side effects, some of the more common of which are drowsiness, mental slowing, ataxia, tremor, hair loss, increased appetite, headache, insomnia, and rash. Nevertheless, recurrent seizures are physically dangerous and emotionally devastating, and preventing them outweighs many undesirable side effects of anticonvulsant drugs.

Future Therapy. The goal of epilepsy treatment is to halt the seizures with minimal or no side effects and then to eradicate the cause. Most of the anticonvulsant research on cannabinoids was conducted before 1986. Since then, many new anticonvulsants have been introduced and cannabinoid receptors have been discovered. At present, the only biological evidence of antiepileptic properties of cannabinoids is that CB_1 receptors are abundant in the hippocampus and amygdala. Both regions are involved in partial seizures but are better known for their role in functions unrelated to seizures.[26] Basic research might reveal stronger links between cannabinoids and seizure activity, but this is not likely to be as fruitful a

TABLE 4.5 Anticonvulsant Drugs for Various Types of Seizures

Generalized grand mal seizures	Partial (focal) seizures
Carbamazepine	Carbamazepine
Valproate	Phenytoin
Phenytoin	Valproate
Phenobarbital	Phenobarbital
	Clonazepam
Generalized petit mal seizures	Gabapentin
Ethosuximide	Lamotrigine
Clonazepam	Tiagabine (as adjunct therapy)
Valproate	

SOURCE: Adapted from Andreoli et al. (1997).[5]

subject of cannabinoid research as others. Given the present state of knowledge, clinical studies of cannabinoids in epileptics are not indicated.

Alzheimer's Disease

Food refusal is a common problem in patients who suffer from Alzheimer's type dementia. The causes of anorexia in demented people are not known but may be a symptom of depression. Antidepressants improve eating in some but not all patients with severe dementia. Eleven Alzheimer's patients were treated for 12 weeks on an alternating schedule of dronabinol and placebo (six weeks of each treatment). The dronabinol treatment resulted in substantial weight gains and declines in disturbed behavior.[190] No serious side effects were observed. One patient had a seizure and was removed from the study, but the seizure was not necessarily caused by dronabinol. Recurrent seizures without any precipitating events occur in 20% of patients who have advanced dementia of Alzheimer's type.[189] Nevertheless, these results are encouraging enough to recommend further clinical research with cannabinoids.

The patients in the study discussed above were in long-term institutional care, and most were severely demented with impaired memory. Although short-term memory loss is a common side effect of THC in healthy patients, it was not a concern in this study. However, the effect of dronabinol on memory in Alzheimer's patients who are not as severely disturbed as those in the above study would be an important consideration.

GLAUCOMA

After cataracts, glaucoma is the second-leading cause of blindness in the world; almost 67 million people are expected to be affected worldwide by the year 2000[149] (for an excellent review, see Alward, 1998[2]). The most common form of glaucoma, primary open-angle glaucoma (POAG), is a slowly progressive disorder that results in loss of retinal ganglion cells and degeneration of the optic nerve, causing deterioration of the visual fields and ultimately blindness. The mechanisms behind the disease are not understood, but three major risk factors are known: age, race, and high intraocular pressure (IOP). POAG is most prevalent among the elderly, with 1% affected in those over 60 years old and more than 9% in those over 80. In African Americans over 80, there is more than a 10% chance of having the disease, and older African Caribbeans (who are less racially mixed than African Americans) have a 20–25% chance of having the disease.[106]

The eye's rigid shape is normally maintained in part by IOP, which is regulated by the circulation of a clear fluid, the aqueous humor,* between the front of the lens and the back of the cornea. Because of impaired outflow of aqueous humor from the anterior chamber of the eye, a high IOP is a risk factor for glaucoma, but the mechanism by which it damages the optic nerve and retinal ganglion cells remains unclear.[174] The two leading possibilities are that high IOP interferes with nutrient blood flow to the region of the optic nerve or that it interferes with transport of nutrients, growth factors, and other compounds within the optic nerve axon (P. Kaufman, IOM workshop). If the interference continues, the retinal ganglion cells and optic nerve will permanently atrophy; the result is blindness.[68] Because high IOP is the only known major risk factor that can be controlled, most treatments have been designed to reduce it. However, reducing it does not always arrest or slow the progression of visual loss.[20,109]

Marijuana and Cannabinoids in Glaucoma

Marijuana and THC have been shown to reduce IOP by an average of 24% in people with normal IOP who have visual-field changes. In a number of studies of healthy adults and glaucoma patients, IOP was reduced by an average of 25% after smoking a marijuana cigarette that contained approximately 2% THC—a reduction as good as that observed with most other medications available today.[1,16,32,76,77,125,193] Similar responses have been observed when marijuana was eaten or THC was given in pill form (10–40 mg) to healthy adults or glaucoma patients.[76,91] But the effect lasts only about three to four hours. Elevated IOP is a chronic condition and must be controlled continuously.

Intravenous administration of Δ^9-THC, Δ^8-THC, or 11-OH-THC to healthy adults substantially decreased IOP, whereas cannabinol, CBD, and β-OH-THC had little effect.[31,146] The cause for the reduction in IOP remains unknown, but the effect appears to be independent of the frequently observed drop in arterial systolic blood pressure (Keith Green, Medical College of Georgia, personal communication).

Three synthetic cannabinoids were investigated; BW29Y, BW146Y, and nabilone. They were given orally to patients who had high IOP. BW146Y and nabilone were as effective as ingesting THC or smoking

---

*The cornea and lens must be optically clear, which means that there cannot be blood circulation in these tissues. The aqueous humor is a clear fluid that functions as alternative circulation across the rear of the cornea and to the lens, providing nutrients and removing waste from these tissues.

marijuana but again with a very short duration of action; BW29Y was ineffective.[136,182]

Topical treatments with cannabinoids have been ineffective in reducing IOP. When Δ^9-THC was applied topically as eye drops, whether once or four times a day, there was no decrease in IOP.[60,90] Suspensions of lipophilic THC tended to be irritating to the eye.

In summary, cannabinoids and marijuana can reduce IOP when administered orally, intravenously, or by inhalation but not when administered topically. Even though a reduction in IOP by standard medications or surgery clearly slows the rate of glaucoma symptom progression, there is no direct evidence of benefits of cannabinoids or marijuana in the natural progression of glaucoma, visual acuity, or optic nerve atrophy.[92,115]

In addition to lowering IOP, marijuana reduces blood pressure and has many psychological effects. Merritt and co-workers reported hypotension, palpitations, and psychotropic effects in glaucoma patients after inhalation of marijuana.[125] Cooler and Gregg[31] also reported increased anxiety and tachycardia after intravenous infusion of THC (1.5–3 mg). All those side effects are problematic, particularly for elderly glaucoma patients who have cardiovascular or cerebrovascular disease. The reduction in blood pressure can be substantial and might adversely affect blood flow to the optic nerve.[124] Many people with systemic hypertension have their blood pressure reduced to manageable and acceptable levels through medication, but this does not seem to affect their IOP. In contrast, there is evidence that reduction in blood pressure to considerably below-normal levels influences IOP and ocular blood flow.[46,74,142] Hence, in the case of an eye with high IOP or an optic nerve in poor condition and susceptibility to high IOP, reduced blood flow to the optic nerve could compromise a functional retina and be a factor in the progression of glaucoma.

Because it is not known how these compounds work, it is also not known how they might interact with other drugs used to treat glaucoma. If the mechanism involves a final common pathway, the effects of cannabinoids might not be additive and might even interfere with effective drugs.

Therapy for Glaucoma

Present Therapy

Six classes of drugs are used to treat glaucoma; all reduce IOP (Table 4.6).[93] In the late 1970s, when early reports of the effects of marijuana on IOP surfaced, only cholinomimetics, epinephrine, and oral carbonic anhydrase inhibitors were available. They are not popular today because of their side effects, such as pupil constriction or dilation, brow ache, tachycardia, and diuresis; all of them have been superseded by the other classes

TABLE 4.6   Classes of Drugs Used to Treat Glaucoma

Cholinergic agonists	α_2-Adrenergic agonists
Pilocarpine	Aproclonidine
	Brimonidine
β_2-Adrenergic agonists	Carbonic anhydrase inhibitors
Epinephrine	Acetazolamide
Dipivefrin	Dorzolamide (Trusopt)
β_2-Adrenergic antagonists	Prostaglandin-F_{2a} analogues
Timolol	Latanoprost
Betaxolol (Betoptic)	Unoprostone

of drugs.[93] Surgical options are also available today to lower IOP, including laser trabeculoplasty, trabeculectomy/sclerostomy, drainage implantation, and cyclodestruction of fluid-forming tissues.[173] Thus, there are now many effective options to slow the progression of glaucoma by reducing IOP.

One important factor in slowing the progression of glaucoma via medications that reduce IOP is patient compliance with dosing regimens. With respect to compliance, the ideal glaucoma drug is one that is applied at most twice a day (P. Kaufman, IOM workshop). If the dose must be repeated every three to four hours, patient compliance becomes a problem; for this reason, marijuana and the cannabinoids studied thus far would not be highly satisfactory treatments for glaucoma. Present therapies, especially combinations of approved topical drugs, can control IOP when administered once or twice a day, at a cost of about $60 per month.

Future Therapy

In all likelihood the next generation of glaucoma therapies will deal with neural protection, neural rescue, neural regeneration, or blood flow, and the optic nerve and neural retina will be treated directly rather than just by lowering IOP (P. Kaufman, IOM workshop). There is some evidence that a synthetic cannabinoid, HU-211, might have neuroprotective effects *in vitro;* this presents a potential approach that has nothing to do with IOP.[197] HU-211 is commonly referred to as a cannabinoid because its chemical structure is similar to THC; however, it does not bind to cannabinoid receptor.

It is known that cannabinoids lower IOP fairly substantially but not how. No one has tested whether the effect is receptor mediated (B. Martin, IOM workshop). To do so, one could test whether a receptor antagonist blocked the effects of THC or other cannabinoids. If the decrease were shown to be receptor mediated, it would be important to know whether it was through CB_1, which mediates central nervous system effects, or CB_2, which is not involved in CNS effects. If it were CB_2, it might be possible to reduce IOP without the CNS side effects. Finally, it is not known whether the endogenous cannabinoid system is a natural regulator of IOP.

Conclusion: Glaucoma

Although glaucoma is one of the most frequently cited medical indications for marijuana, the data do not support this indication. High intraocular pressure (IOP) is a known risk factor for glaucoma and can, indeed, be reduced by cannabinoids and marijuana. However, the effect is too and short lived and requires too high doses, and there are too many side effects to recommend lifelong use in the treatment of glaucoma. The potential harmful effects of chronic marijuana smoking outweigh its modest benefits in the treatment of glaucoma. Clinical studies on the effects of smoked marijuana are unlikely to result in improved treatment for glaucoma.

Future research might reveal a therapeutic effect of isolated cannabinoids. For example, it might be possible to design a cannabinoid drug with longer-lasting effects on IOP and with less psychoactivity than THC.

SUMMARY

Advances in cannabinoid science of the past 16 years have given rise to a wealth of new opportunities for the development of medically useful cannabinoid-based drugs. The accumulated data suggest a variety of indications, particularly for pain relief, antiemesis, and appetite stimulation. For patients such as those with AIDS or who are undergoing chemotherapy, and who suffer simultaneously from severe pain, nausea, and appetite loss, cannabinoid drugs might offer broad-spectrum relief not found in any other single medication. The data are weaker for muscle spasticity but moderately promising. The least promising categories are movement disorders, epilepsy, and glaucoma. Animal data are moderately supportive of a potential for cannabinoids in the treatment of movement disorders and might eventually yield stronger encouragement. The therapeutic effects of cannabinoids are most well established for THC, which is the primary psychoactive ingredient of marijuana. But it does not follow from this that smoking marijuana is good medicine.

Although marijuana smoke delivers THC and other cannabinoids to the body, it also delivers harmful substances, including most of those found in tobacco smoke. In addition, plants contain a variable mixture of biologically active compounds and cannot be expected to provide a precisely defined drug effect. For those reasons there is little future in smoked marijuana as a medically approved medication. If there is any future in cannabinoid drugs, it lies with agents of more certain, not less certain, composition. While clinical trials are the route to developing approved medications, they are also valuable for other reasons. For example, the personal medical use of smoked marijuana—regardless of whether or not it is approved—to treat certain symptoms is reason enough to advocate clinical trials to assess the degree to which the symptoms or course of diseases are affected. Trials testing the safety and efficacy of marijuana use are an important component to understanding the course of a disease, particularly diseases such as AIDS for which marijuana use is prevalent. The argument against the future of smoked marijuana for treating any condition is not that there is no reason to predict efficacy but that there is risk. That risk could be overcome by the development of a nonsmoked rapid-onset delivery system for cannabinoid drugs.

There are two caveats to following the traditional path of drug development for cannabinoids. The first is timing. Patients who are currently suffering from debilitating conditions unrelieved by legally available drugs, and who might find relief with smoked marijuana, will find little comfort in a promise of a better drug 10 years from now. In terms of good medicine, marijuana should rarely be recommended unless all reasonable options have been eliminated. But then what? It is conceivable that the medical and scientific opinion might find itself in conflict with drug regulations. This presents a policy issue that must weigh—at least temporarily—the needs of individual patients against broader social issues. Our assessment of the scientific data on the medical value of marijuana and its constituent cannabinoids is but one component of attaining that balance.

The second caveat is a practical one. Although most scientists who study cannabinoids would agree that the scientific pathways to cannabinoid drug development are clearly marked, there is no guarantee that the fruits of scientific research will be made available to the public. Cannabinoid-based drugs will become available only if there is either enough incentive for private enterprise to develop and market such drugs or sustained public investment in cannabinoid drug research and development. The perils along this pathway are discussed in chapter 5. Although marijuana is an abused drug, the logical focus of research on the therapeutic value of cannabinoid-based drugs is the treatment of specific symptoms or diseases, not substance abuse. Thus, the most logical research sponsors would be the several institutes within the National Institutes of Health or organizations whose primary expertise lies in the relevant symptoms or diseases.

CONCLUSION: Scientific data indicate the potential therapeutic value of cannabinoid drugs, primarily THC, for pain relief, control of nausea and vomiting, and appetite stimulation; smoked marijuana, however, is a crude THC delivery system that also delivers harmful substances.

RECOMMENDATION: **Clinical trials of cannabinoid drugs for symptom management should be conducted with the goal of developing rapid-onset, reliable, and safe delivery systems.**

RECOMMENDATION: **Clinical trials of marijuana use for medical purposes should be conducted under the following limited circumstances: trials should involve only short-term marijuana use (less than six months), should be conducted in patients with conditions for which there is reasonable expectation of efficacy, should be approved by institutional review boards, and should collect data about efficacy.**

RECOMMENDATION: **Short-term use of smoked marijuana (less than six months) for patients with debilitating symptoms (such as intractable pain or vomiting) must meet the following conditions:**

- **failure of all approved medications to provide relief has been documented,**
- **the symptoms can reasonably be expected to be relieved by rapid-onset cannabinoid drugs,**
- **such treatment is administered under medical supervision in a manner that allows for assessment of treatment effectiveness, and**
- **involves an oversight strategy comparable to an institutional review board process that could provide guidance within 24 hours of a submission by a physician to provide marijuana to a patient for a specified use.**

Until a nonsmoked rapid-onset cannabinoid drug delivery system becomes available, we acknowledge that there is no clear alternative for people suffering from *chronic* conditions that might be relieved by smoking marijuana, such as pain or AIDS wasting. One possible approach is to treat patients as *n*-of-1 clinical trials, in which patients are fully informed of their status as experimental subjects using a harmful drug delivery system and in which their condition is closely monitored and documented under medical supervision, thereby increasing the knowledge base of the risks and benefits of marijuana use under such conditions. We recommend these n-of-1 clinical trials using the same oversight mechanism as that proposed in the above recommendations.

OTHER REPORTS ON MARIJUANA AS MEDICINE

Since 1996, five important reports pertaining to the medical uses of marijuana have been published, each prepared by deliberative groups of medical and scientific experts (Appendix E). They were written to address different facets of the medical marijuana debate, and each offers a somewhat different perspective. With the exception of the report by the Health Council of the Netherlands, each concluded that marijuana can be moderately effective in treating a variety of symptoms. They also agree that current scientific understanding is rudimentary; indeed, the sentiment most often stated is that more research is needed. And these reports record the same problem with herbal medications as noted here: the uncertain composition of plant material makes for an uncertain, and hence often undesirable, medicine.

The 1996 report by the Health Council of the Netherlands concluded that there is insufficient evidence to justify the medical use of marijuana *or* THC, despite the fact that the latter is an approved medication in the United States and Britain. However, that committee addressed only whether there was sufficient evidence to warrant the prescription of marijuana or cannabinoids, not whether the data are sufficient to justify clinical trials. Conclusions of the Health Council of the Netherlands contrast with that country's tolerance of marijuana use. The health council's report noted that marijuana use by patients in the terminal stages of illness is tolerated in hospitals. It also said that the council did "not wish to judge patients who consume marihuana (in whatever form) because it makes them feel better. . . ."

In contrast, the American Medical Association House of Delegates, National Institutes of Health (NIH), and the British Medical Association recommend clinical trials of smoked marijuana for a variety of symptoms. The NIH report, however, was alone in recommending clinical studies of marijuana for the treatment of glaucoma—and even then there was disagreement among the panel members (William T. Beaver, chair, NIH Ad Hoc Expert Panel on the Medical Use of Marijuana, personal communication, 1998).

Recent reviews that have received extensive attention from those who follow the medical marijuana debate have been written by strong advocates *for* (Grinspoon and Bakalar, 1993[62]; Zimmer and Morgan, 1997[198]) or *against* (Voth and Schwartz, 1997[191]) the medical use of marijuana. Those reports represent the individual views of their authors, and they are not reviewed here but have been reviewed in major scientific journals.[7,69,178,180]

REFERENCES

1. Alm A, Camras CB, Watson PG. 1997. Phase III latanoprost studies in Scandanavia, the United Kingdom and the United States. *Survey of Ophthalmology* 41:S105–S110.
2. Alward WL. 1998. Medical management of glaucoma. *The New England Journal of Medicine* 339:1298–1307.
3. AMA (American Medical Association Council on Scientific Affairs). 1997. *Report to the AMA House of Delegates.* Chicago: AMA.
4. Ames FR. 1986. Anticonvulsant effect of cannabidiol. *South African Medical Journal* 69:14.
5. Andreoli TE, Carpenter CC, Bennet CJ, Plum F, eds. 1997. *Cecil Essentials of Medicine.* Fourth Edition. Philadelphia: W.B. Saunders Co.
6. Andrews PL, Davis CJ. 1995. The physiology of emesis induced by anti-cancer therapy. In: Reynolds DJ, Andrews PL, Davis CJ, Editors, *Serotonin and the Scientific Basis of Anti-Emetic Therapy.* Oxford: Oxford Clinical Communications. Pp. 25–49.
7. Bayer R, O'Connell TJ, Lapey JD. 1997. Medicinal uses of marijuana (Letter to the Editor). *Annals of Internal Medicine* 127:1134–1135.
8. Beal JE, Olson RLL, Morales JO, Bellman P, Yangco B, Lefkowitz L, Plasse TF, Shepard KV. 1995. Dronabinol as a treatment for anorexia associated with weight loss in patients with AIDS. *Journal of Pain and Symptom Management* 10:89–97.
9. Beal JE, Olson R, Lefkowitz L, Laubenstein L, Bellman P, Yangco B, Morales JO, Murphy R, Powderly W, Plasse TF, Mosdell KW, Shepard KV. 1997. Long-term efficacy and safety of dronabinol for acquired immunodeficiency syndrome-associated anorexia. *Journal of Pain and Symptom Management* 14:7–14.
10. Bhasin S, Storer TW, Asbel-Sethi N, Kilbourne A, Hays R, Sinha-Hikim I, Shen R, Arver S, Beall G. 1998. Effects of testosterone replacement with a nongenital, transdermal system, Androderm, in human immunodeficiency virus-infected men with low testosterone levels. *Journal Clinical of Endocrinology and Metabolism* 83:3155–3162.
11. Billingsley KG, Alexander HR. 1996. The pathophysiology of cachexia in advanced cancer and AIDS. In: Bruera E, Higginson I, Editors, *Cachexia-Anorexia in Cancer Patients.* New York: Oxford Universtiy Press. Pp. 1–22.
12. Borison HL, McCarthy LE. 1983. Neuropharmacology of chemotherapy-induced emesis. *Drugs* 25:8–17.
13. British Medical Association. 1997. *Therapeutic Uses of Cannabis.* Amsterdam, The Netherlands: Harwood Academic Publishers.
14. Bruera E. 1998. Pharmacological treatment of cachexia: Any progress? *Supportive Care of Cancer* 6:109–113.
15. Calignano A, La Rana G, Giuffrida A, Piomelli D. 1998. Control of pain initiation by endogenous cannabinoids. *Nature* 394:277–281.
16. Camras CB, Alm A, Watson P, Stjernschantz J. 1996. Latanoprost, a prostaglandin analog, for glaucoma therapy: Efficacy and safety after 1 year of treatment in 198 patients. Latanoprost Study Groups. *Ophthalmology* 103:1916–1924.
17. (CDC) Centers for Disease Control. 1992. 1993 revised classification system for HIV infection and expanded surveillance case definition for AIDS among adolescents and adults. *MMWR (Morbidity Mortality Weekly Report)* 41(RR-17):1–19.
18. Chang AE, Shiling DJ, Stillman RC, et al. 1979. Delta-9-tetrahydrocannabinol as an antiemetic in patients receiving high-dose methotrexate: A prospective, randomized evaluation. *Annals of Internal Medicine* 91:819–824.
19. Chang AE, Shiling DJ, Stillman RC, Goldberg NH, Seipp CA, Barofsky I, Rosenberg SA. 1981. A prospective evaluation of delta-9-tetrahydrocannabinol as an antiemetic in patients receiving adriamycin and cytoxan chemotherapy. *Cancer* 47:1746–1751.

20. Chauhan BC, Drance SM. 1992. The relationship between intraocular pressure and visual field progression in glaucoma. *Graefe's Archives for Clinical and Experimental Ophthalmology* 230:521–526.
21. Clark RA, Tyson LB, Frisone M. 1985. A correlation of objective and subjective parameters in assessing antiemetic regimens. *Proceedings of the Tenth Anniversary Congress of the Oncology Nursing Society* 2:96.
22. Clark WC, Janal MN, Zeidenberg P, Nahas GG. 1981. Effects of moderate and high doses of marihuana on thermal pain: A sensory decision theory analysis. *Journal of Clinical Pharmacology* 21:299S–310S.
23. Clarke RC. 1995. *Marijuana Botany—An Advanced Study: The Propagation and Breeding of Distinctive Cannabis*. Berkeley, CA: Ronin Publishing.
24. Clifford DB. 1983. Tetrahydrocannabinol for tremor in multiple sclerosis. *Annals of Neurology* 13:669–671.
25. Consroe P. 1998a. Clinical and experimental reports of marijuana and cannabinoids in spastic disorders. In: Nahas GG, Sutin KM, Harvey DJ, Agurell S, Editors, *Marijuana and Medicine*. Totowa, NJ: Humana Press.
26. Consroe P. 1998b. Brain cannabinoid systems as target for the treatment of neurological disorders. *Neurobiology of Disease* 5:534–551.
27. Consroe P, Laguna J, Allender J, Snider S, Stern L, Sandyk R, Kennedy K, Schram K. 1991. Controlled clinical trial of cannabidiol in Huntington's disease. *Pharmacology, Biochemistry and Behavior (New York)* 40:701–708.
28. Consroe P, Musty R, Rein J, Tillery W, Pertwee RG. 1997. The perceived effects of smoked cannabis on patients with multiple sclerosis. *European Neurology* 38:44–48.
29. Consroe P, Sandyk R. 1992. Potential role of cannabinoids for therapy of neurological disorders. In: Bartke A, Murphy LL, Editors, *Marijuana/Cannabinoids: Neurobiology and Neurophysiology*. Boca Raton, FL: CRC Press. Pp. 459–524.
30. Consroe P, Sandyk R, Snider SR. 1986. Open label evaluation of cannabidiol in dystonic movement disorders. *International Journal of Neuroscience* 30:277–282.
31. Cooler P, Gregg JM. 1977. Effect of delta–9–tetrahydrocannabinol on intraocular pressure in humans. *Southern Medical Journal* 70:951–954.
32. Crawford WJ, Merritt JC. 1979. Effects of tetrahydrocannabinol on arterial and intraocular hypertension. *International Journal of Clinical Pharmacology and Biopharmacy* 17:191–196.
33. Crow S. 1997. Investigational drugs for eating disorders. *Expert Opinion on Investigational Drugs* 6:427–436.
34. Cunha JM, Carlini EA, Pereira AE, Ramos OL, Pimentel C, Gagliardi R, Sanvito WL, Lander N, Mechoulam R. 1980. Chronic administration of cannabidiol to healthy volunteers and epileptic patients. *Pharmacology* 21:175–185.
35. Davis CJ. 1995. Emesis research: A concise history of the critical concepts and experiments. In: Reynolds DJ, Andrews PL, Davis CJ, Editors, *Serotonin and the Scientific Basis of Anti-Emetic Therapy*. Oxford : Oxford Clinical Communications. Pp. 9–24.
36. DeLong MR, Georgopoulos AP, Crutcher MD, Mitchell S J, Richardson RT, Alexander GE. 1984. Functional organization of the basal ganglia: Contributions of single-cell recording studies. *CIBA Foundation Symposium* 107:64–82.
37. DeMulder PH, Seynaeve C, Vermorker JB, et al. 1990. Ondansetron compared with high-dose metoclopramide in prophylaxis of acute and delayed cisplatin-induced nausea and vomiting: A multicenter, randomized, double-blind, crossover study. *Annals of Internal Medicine* 113:834–840.
38. Doblin R, Kleiman MA. 1995. The medical use of marijuana: The case for clinical trials [editorial; comment]. *Journal of Addictive Diseases* 14:5–14; Comment in *Journal of Addictive Diseases* 1994, 13(1):53–65.

39. Doblin R, Kleiman M. 1991. Marijuana as antiemetic medicine: A survey of oncologists' experiences and attitudes. *Journal of Clinical Oncology* 9:1314–1319.
40. Dunlop R. 1996. Clinical epidemiology of cancer cachexia. In: Bruera E, Higginson I, Editors, *Cachexia-Anorexia in Cancer Patients*. Vol. 5. Oxford: Oxford University Press. Pp. 76–82.
41. Dunn M, Davis R. 1974. The perceived effects of marijuana on spinal cord injured males. *Paraplegia* 12:175.
42. Eidelberg D, Moeller JR, Antonini A, Kazumata K, Dhawan V, Budman C, Feigin A. 1997. The metabolic anatomy of Tourette's syndrome. *Neurology* 48:927–934.
43. El-Mallakh RS. 1987. Marijuana and migraine. *Headache* 27:442–443.
44. Engelson ES, Rabkin JG, Rabkin R, Kotler DP. 1996. Effects of testosterone upon body composition. *Journal of Acquired Immune Deficiency Syndrome and Human Retrovirology* 11:510–511.
45. Enoch M, Kaye WH, Rotondo A, Greenberg BD, Murphy DL, Goldman D. 1998. 5-HT2A promoter polymorphism-1438G/A, anorexia nervosa, and obsessive-compulsive disorder. *The Lancet* 351:1785–1786.
46. Follmann P, Paltotas C, Suveges I, Petrovits A. 1996–1997. Nocturnal blood pressure and intraocular pressure measurement in glaucoma patients and healthy controls. *International Ophthalmology* 20:83–87.
47. Foltin RW, Fischman MW, Byrne MF. 1988. Effects of smoked marijuana on food intake and body weight of humans living in a residential laboratory. *Appetite* 11:1–14.
48. Frankel JP, Hughes A, Lees AJ, Stern GM. 1990. Marijuana for Parkinsonian tremor. *Journal of Neurology, Neurosurgery and Psychiatry* 53:436.
49. French J. 1998. The art of antiepileptic trial design. *Advances in Neurology* 76:113–123.
50. Frytak S, Moertel CG, O'Fallon J, et al. 1979. Delta-9-tetrahydrocannabinol as an antiemetic in patients treated with cancer chemotherapy: A double comparison with prochloperazine and a placebo. *Annals of Internal Medicine* 91:825–830.
51. Glass M, Dragunow M, Faull RLM. 1997. Cannabinoid receptors in the human brain: A detailed anatomical and quantitative autoradiographic study in the fetal, neonatal and adult human brain. *Neuroscience* 77:299–318.
52. Goadsby PJ, Gundlach AL. 1991. Localization of [3H]-dihydroergotamine binding sites in the cat central nervous system: Relevance to migraine. *Annals of Neurology* 29:91–94.
53. Gonzalez EC, Brownlee HJ. 1998. Movement disorders. In: Taylor RB, Editor, *Family Medicine: Principles and Practice*. 5th Edition. New York: Springer-Verlag. Pp. 565–573.
54. Gorter R. 1991. Management of anorexia-cachexia associated with cancer and HIV infection. *Oncology (Supplement)* 5:13–17.
55. Gralla RJ, Itri LM, Pisko SE, et al. 1981. Antiemetic efficacy of high dose metoclopramide: Randomized trials with placebo and prochlorperazine in patients with chemotherapy-induced nausea and vomiting. *New England Journal of Medicine* 305:905–909.
56. Gralla RJ, Navari RM, Hesketh PJ, et al. 1998. Single-dose oral granisetron has equivalent antiemetic efficacy to intravenous ondansetron for highly emetogenic cisplatin-based chemotherapy. *Journal of Clinical Oncology* 16:1–7.
57. Gralla RJ, Rittenberg CN, Lettow LA, et al. 1995. A unique all-oral, single-dose, combination antiemetic regimen with high efficacy and marked cost saving potential. *Proceedings of the American Society for Clinical Oncology* 14:526.
58. Gralla RJ, Tyson LB, Borden LB, et al. 1984. Antiemetic therapy: A review of recent studies and a report of a random assignment trial comparing metoclopramide with delta-9-tetrahydrocannabinol. *Cancer Treatment Reports* 68:163–172.

59. Grandara DR, Roila F, Warr D, Edelman MJ, Perez EA, Gralla RJ. 1998. Consensus proposal for 5HT3 antagonists in the prevention of acute emesis related to highly emetogenic chemotherapy: Dose, schedule, and route of administration. *Supportive Care in Cancer* 6:237–243.

60. Green K, Roth M. 1982. Ocular effects of topical administration of delta-9-tetrahydrocannabinol in man. *Archives of Ophthalmology* 100:265–267.

61. Greenberg HS, Werness SA, Pugh JE, Andrus RO, Anderson DJ, Domino EF. 1994. Short-term effects of smoking marijuana on balance in patients with multiple sclerosis and normal volunteers. *Clinical Pharmacology and Therapeutics* 55:324–328.

62. Grinspoon L, Bakalar JB. 1993. *Marijuana: The Forbidden Medicine.* New Haven: Yale University Press.

63. Grinspoon L, Bakalar JB, Zimmer L, Morgan JP. 1997. Marijuana addiction [Letter]. *Science* 277:749; discussion, 750–752.

64. Grinspoon S, Corcoran C, Askari H, Schoenfeld D, Wolf L, Burrows B, Walsh M, Hayden D, Parlman K, Anderson E, Basgoz N, Klibanski A. 1998. Effects of androgen administration in men with the AIDS wasting syndrome. *Annals of Internal Medicine* 129:18–26.

65. Gross H, Egbert MH, Faden VB, Godberg SC, Kaye WH, Caine ED, Hawks R, Zinberg NE. 1983. A double-blind trial of delta-9-THC in primary anorexia nervosa. *Journal of Clinical Psychopharmacology* 3:165–171.

66. Guyatt GH, Keller JL, Jaeschke R, Rosenbloom D, Adachi JD, Newhouse MT. 1990. The N-of-1 randomized controlled trial—clinical usefulness: Our three-year experience. *Annals of Internal Medicine* 112:293–299.

67. Guyatt GH, Sackett D, Taylor DW, Chong J, Roberts R, Pugsley S. 1986. Determining optimal therapy: Randomized trials in individual patients. *New England Journal of Medicine* 314:889–892.

68. Guyton AC. 1986. *Textbook of Medical Physiology.* 7th ed. Philadelphia: WB Saunders Company.

69. Hall W. 1997. An ongoing debate. *Science* 278:75.

70. Haney M, Ward AS, Comer SD, Foltin RW, Fischman MW. 1999. Abstinence symptoms following oral THC administration to humans. *Psychopharmacology* 141:385–394.

71. Haney M, Ward AS, Comer SD, Foltin RW, Fischman MW. 1999. Abstinence symptoms following smoked marijuana in humans. *Psychopharmacology* 141:395–404.

72. Hanigan WC, Destree R, Truong XT. 1986. The effect of delta-9-THC on human spasticity. *Clinical Pharmacology and Therapeutics* 39:198.

73. Hardin TC. 1993. Cytokine mediators of malnutrition: Clinical implications. *Nutrition in Clinical Practice* 8:55–59.

74. Hayreh SS, Zimmerman MB, Podhajsky P, Alward W. 1994. Nocturnal arterial hypotension and its role in optic nerve head and ocular ischemic disorders. *American Journal of Ophthalmology* 117:603–624.

75. Hemming M, Yellowlees PM. 1993. Effective treatment of Tourette's syndrome with marijuana. *Journal of Psychopharmacology* 7:389–391.

76. Hepler RS, Frank IM, Petrus R. 1976. Ocular effects of marijuana smoking. In: Braude MC, Szara S, Editors, *The Pharmacology of Marijuana.* New York: Raven Press. Pp. 815–824.

77. Hepler RS, Frank IR. 1971. Marihuana smoking and intraocular pressure. *Journal of the American Medical Association* 217(10):1392.

78. Herkenham M, Lynn AB, de Costa BR, Richfield EK. 1991a. Neuronal localization of cannabinoid receptors in the basal ganglia of the rat. *Brain Research* 547:267–274.

79. Herkenham M, Lynn AB, Johnson MR, Melvin LS, de Costa BR, Rice KC. 1991b. Characterization and localization of cannabinoid receptors in rat brain: A quantitative *in vitro* autoradiographic study. *Journal of Neuroscience* 11:563–583.

80. Herkenham M, Lynn AB, Little MD, Johnson MR, Melvin LS, de Costa BR, Rice KC. 1990. Cannabinoid receptor localization in the brain. *Proceedings of the National Academy of Sciences of the United States of America* 87:1932–1936.

81. Herrstedt J, Aapro MS, Smyth JF, Del Favero A. 1998. Corticosteroids, dopamine antagonists and other drugs. *Supportive Care in Cancer* 6:204–214.

82. Hesketh PJ, Gralla RJ, duBois A, Tonato M. 1998. Methodology of antiemetic trials: Response assessment, evaluation of new agents and definition of chemotherapy emetogenicity. *Supportive Care in Cancer* 6:221–227.

83. Hesketh PJ, Kris MG, Grunberg SM, Beck T, Hainsworth JD, Harker G, Aapro MS, Gandara D, Lindley CM. 1997. Proposal for classifying the acute emetogenicity of cancer chemotherapy. *Journal of Clinical Oncology* 15:103–109.

84. Hill SY, Schwin R, Goodwin DW, Powell BJ. 1974. Marihuana and pain. *Journal of Pharmacology and Experimental Therapeutics* 188:415–418.

85. Holdcroft A, Smith M, Jacklin A, Hodgson H, Smith B, Newton M, Evans F. 1997. Pain relief with oral cannabinoids in familial Mediterranean fever. *Anaesthesia* 5:483–486.

86. Homesley HD, Gainey JM, Jobson VN, et al. 1982. Double-blind placebo-controlled study of metoclopramide in cisplatin-induced emesis. *New England Journal of Medicine* 307:250–251.

87. Huestis MA, Henningfield JE, Cone EJ. 1992. Blood cannabinoids. I. Absorption of THC and formation of 11-OH-THC and THCCOOH during and after smoking marijuana. *Journal of Analytical Toxicology* 16:276–282.

88. Italian Group for Antiemetic Trials. 1995. Dexamethasone, granisetron, or both for the prevention of nausea and vomiting during chemotherapy for cancer. *New England Journal of Medicine* 332:332–337.

89. Jain AK, Ryan JR, McMahon FG, Smith G. 1981. Evaluation of intramuscular levonantradol and placebo in acute postoperative pain. *Journal of Clinical Pharmacology* 21:320S–326S.

90. Jay WM, Green K. 1983. Multiple-drop study of topically applied 1% Δ^9-tetrahydrocannabinol in human eyes. *Archives of Ophthalmology* 101:591–593.

91. Jones RT, Benowitz NL, Herning RI. 1981. Clinical relevance of cannabis tolerance and dependence. *Journal of Clinical Pharmacology* 21:143S–152S.

92. Kass MA, Gordon MO, Hoff MR, Pardinson JM, Kolker AE, Hart WM, Becker B. 1989. Topical timolol administration reduces the incidence of glaucomatous damage in ocular hypertensive individuals: A randomized, double-masked, long-term clinical trial. *Archives of Ophthalmology* 107:1590–1598.

93. Kaufman P, Mittag TW. 1994. Medical therapy of glaucoma. In: Kaufman P, Mittag TW, Editors, *Textbook of Ophthalmology*. Volume 7. London: Mosby-Yearbook.

94. Kotler DP. 1997. Wasting Syndrome Pathogenesis and Clinical Markers. *Institute of Medicine Workshop*. Irvine, CA, December 15, 1997. Pp. 56–66. Washington, DC: Institute of Medicine.

95. Kotler DP, Gaetz HP, Klein EB, Lange M, Holt PR. 1984. Enteropathy associated with the acquired immunodeficiency syndrome. *Annals of Internal Medicine* 101:421–428.

96. Kotler DP, Tierney AR, Culpepper-Morgan JA, Wang J, Peirson RN. 1990. Effect of home total parental nutrition on body composition in patients with acquired immunodeficiency syndrome. *Journal of Parenteral Nutrition* 14:454–458.

97. Kotler DP, Tierney AR, Dilmanian FA, Kamen Y, Wang J, Pierson Jr RN, Weber D. 1991. Correlation between total body potassium and total body nitrogen in patients with acquired immunodeficiency syndrome. *Clinical Research* 39:649A.

98. Kotler DP, Tierney AR, Ferraro R, et al. 1991. Enteral alimentation and repletion of body cell mass in malnourished patients with acquired immunodeficiency syndrome. *American Journal of Clinical Nutrition* 53:149–154.

99. Kotler DP, Tierney AR, Wang J, Pierson RN. 1989. Magnitude of body-cell-mass depletion and the timing of death from wasting in AIDS. *American Journal of Clinical Nutrition* 50:444–447.

100. Kotler DP, Wang J, Pierson RN. 1985. Studies of body composition in patients with the acquired immunodeficiency syndrome. *American Journal of Clinical Nutrition* 42:1255–1265.

101. Kris MG, Gralla RJ, Clark RA, et al. 1987. Antiemetic control and prevention of side effects of anticancer therapy with lorazepam or diphenhydramine when used in combination with metoclopramide plus dexamethasone: A double-blind randomized trial. *Cancer* 60:2816–2822.

102. Kris MG, Radford JE, Pizzo BA, et al. 1997. Use of an NK-1 receptor antagonist to prevent delayed emesis following cisplatin. *Journal of the National Cancer Institute* 89:817–818.

103. Kris MG, Roila F, De Mulder PH, Marty M. 1998. Delayed emesis following anticancer chemotherapy. *Supportive Care in Cancer* 6:228–232.

104. Lang IM, Sarna SK. 1989. Motor and myoelectric activity associated with vomiting, regurgitation, and nausea. In: Wood JD, Editor, *Handbook of Physiology: The Gastrointestinal System.* 1, Motility and Circulation. Bethesda, MD: American Physiological Society. Pp. 1179–1198.

105. Larson EB, Ellsworth AJ, Oas J. 1993. Randomized clinical trials in single patients during a 2-year period. *Journal of the American Medical Association* 270:2708–2712.

106. Leske MC, Connell AM, Schachat AP, Hyman L. 1994. The Barbados Eye Study: Prevalence of open angle glaucoma. *Archives of Ophthalmology* 112:821–829.

107. Levitt M, Faiman C, Hawks R, et al. 1984. Randomized double-blind comparison of delta-9-THC and marijuana as chemotherapy antiemetics. *Proceedings of the American Society for Clinical Oncology* 3:91.

108. Libman E, Stern MH. 1985. The effects of delta-9-tetrahydrocannabinol on cutaneous sensitivity and its relation to personality. *Personality, Individuality and Difference* 6:169–174.

109. Lichter PR. 1988. A wolf in sheep's clothing. *Ophthalmology* 95:149–150.

110. Lichtman AH, Cook SA, Martin BR. 1996. Investigation of brain sites mediating cannabinoid-induced antinociception in rats: Evidence supporting periaqueductal gray involvement. *Journal of Pharmacology and Experimental Therapeutics* 276:585–593.

111. Lichtman AH, Martin BR. 1991. Cannabinoid-induced antinociception is mediated by a spinal alpha-noradrenergic mechanism. *Brain Research* 559:309–314.

112. Lindgren JE, Ohlsson A, Agurell S, Hollister LE, Gillespie H. 1981. Clinical effects and plasma levels of delta 9-tetrahydrocannabinol (delta 9-THC) in heavy and light users of cannabis. *Psychopharmacology (Berlin)* 74:208–212.

113. Macallan DC, Noble C, Baldwin C, Foskett M, McManus T, Griffin GE. 1993. Prospective analysis of patterns of weight change in stage IV human immunodeficiency virus infection. *American Journal of Clinical Nutrition* 58:417–424.

114. Malec J, Harvey RF, Cayner JJ. 1982. Cannabis effect on spasticity in spinal cord injury. *Archives of Physical Medicine and Rehabilitation* 63:116–118.

115. Mao LK, Stewart WC, Shields M. 1991. Correlation between intraocular pressure control and progressive glaucomatous damage in primary open-angle glaucoma. *American Journal of Ophthalmology* 111:51–55.
116. Marotta JT. 1995. Spinal injury. In: Rowland LP, Editor, *Merrit's Textbook of Neurology.* 9th Edition. Philadelphia: Lea and Febiger. Pp. 440–447.
117. Martyn CN, Illis LS, Thom J. 1995. Nabilone in the treatment of multiple sclerosis [Letter]. *Lancet* 345:579.
118. Mathew NT. 1997. Serotonin 1D (5-HT 1D) agonists and other agents in acute migraine. *Neurologic Clinics* 15:61–83.
119. Mattes RD, Engelman K, Shaw LM, Elsohly MA. 1994. Cannabinoids and appetite stimulation. *Pharmacology, Biochemistry and Behavior* 49:187–195.
120. Maurer M, Henn V, Dittrich A, Hoffman A. 1990. Delta-9-tetrahydrocannabinol shows antispastic and analgesic effects in a single case double-blind trial. *European Archives of Psychiatry and Clinical Neuroscience* 240:1–4.
121. McCarthy LE, Flora KP, Vishnuvajjala BR. 1984. Antiemetic properties and plasma concentrations of delta-9-tetrahydrocannabinol against cisplatin vomiting in cats. In: Agurell S, Dewey WL, Willette RE, Editors, *The Cannabinoids: Chemical, Pharmacologic and Therapeutic Aspects.* Orlando, FL: Academic Press. Pp. 859–870.
122. McQuay H, Carroll D, Moore A. 1996. Variation in the placebo effect in randomised controlled trials of analgesics: All is as blind as it seems. *Pain* 64:331–335.
123. Meinck HM, Schonle PW, Conrad B. 1989. Effect of cannabinoids on spasticity and ataxia in multiple sclerosis. *Journal of Neurology* 236:120–122.
124. Merritt JC, Cook CE, Davis KH. 1982. Orthostatic hypotension after delta 9-tetrahydrocannabinol marihuana inhalation. *Ophthalmic Research* 14:124–128.
125. Merritt JC, Crawford WJ, Alexander PC, Anduze AL, Gelbart SS. 1980. Effect of marihuana on intraocular and blood pressure in glaucoma. *Ophthalmology* 87:222–228.
126. Mertens TE, Low-Beer D. 1996. HIV and AIDS: Where is the epidemic going? *Bulletin of the World Health Organization* 74:121–129.
127. Miller AD. 1998. Nausea and vomiting: Underlying mechanisms and upcoming treatments. *Journal of the Japanese Broncho-Esophagological Society* 49:57–64.
128. Miller AD, Nonaka S, Siniaia MS, Jakus J. 1995. Multifunctional ventral respiratory group: Bulospinal expiratory neurons play a role in pudendal discharge during vomiting. *Journal of the Autonomic Nervous System* 54:253–260.
129. Miller AS, Walker JM. 1995. Effects of a cannabinoid on spontaneous and evoked neuronal activity in the substantia nigra pars reticulata. *European Journal of Pharmacology* 279:179–185.
130. Miller AS, Walker JM. 1996. Electrophysiological effects of a cannabinoid on neural activity in the globus pallidus. *European Journal of Pharmacology* 304:29–35.
131. Moertel CG, Taylor WF, Roth A, Tyce FA. 1976. Who responds to sugar pills? *Mayo Clinic Proceedings* 51:96–100.
132. Moldawer LL, Andersson C, Gelin J, Lundholm KG. 1988. Regulation of food intake and hepatic protein synthesis by recombinant-derived cytokines. *American Journal of Physiology* 254:G450–G456.
133. Mulligan K, Tai VW, Schambelan M. 1997. Cross-sectional and longitudinal evaluation of body composition in men with HIV infection. *Journal of Acquired Immunodeficiency Syndrome* 15:43–48.
134. Murray CJL, Lopez AD. 1996. *Global Health Statistics: A Compendium of Incidence, Prevalence, and Mortality Estimates for Over 200 Conditions.* Global Burden of Disease and Injury Series, Volume II. Boston, MA: The Harvard School of Public Health.

135. Navari RM, Reinhardt RR, Gralla RJ, Kris MG, Hesketh PJ, et al. 1999. Reduction of cisplatin-induced emesis by a selective neurokinin-1-receptor antagonist. *The New England Journal of Medicine* 340:190–195.
136. Newell FW, Stark P, Jay WM, Schanzlin DJ. 1979. Nabilone: A pressure-reducing synthetic benzopyran in open-angle glaucoma. *Ophthalmology* 86:156–160.
137. Ng SKC, Brust JCM, Hauser WA, Susser M. 1990. Illicit drug use and the risk of new-onset seizures. *American Journal of Epidemiology* 132:47–57.
138. NIH. 1997. Spinal cord injury: Emerging concepts: An NIH workshop. *Proceedings of an NIH Workshop on Spinal Cord Injury.* Bethesda, MD, September 30–October 1, 1996. Bethesda, MD: National Institute of Neurological Disorders and Stroke.
139. Noyes R, Jr, Brunk SF, Avery DH, Canter A. 1975b. The analgesic properties of delta-9-tetrahydrocannabinol and codeine. *Clinical Pharmacology and Therapeutics* 18:84–89.
140. Noyes Jr R, Brunk SF, Baram DA, Canter A. 1975a. Analgesic effect of delta-9-tetrahydrocannabinol. *Journal of Clinical Pharmacology* 15:139–143.
141. Ohlsson A, Lindgren J-E, Wahlen A, Agurell S, Hollister LE, Gillespie HK. 1980. Plasma delta-9-tetrahydrocannabinol concentrations and clinical effects after oral and intravenous administration and smoking. *Clinical Pharmacology and Therapeutics* 28:409–416.
142. Orgul S, Kaiser HJ, Flammer J, Gasser P. 1995. Systemic blood pressure and capillary blood-cell velocity in glaucoma patients: A preliminary study. *European Journal of Ophthalmology* 5:88–91.
143. Orr LE, McKernan JF, Bloome B. 1980. Antiemetic effect of tetrahydrocannabinol. Compared with placebo and prochlorperazine in chemotherapy-associated nausea and emesis. *Archives of Internal Medicine* 140:1431–1433.
144. Ott M, Lambke B, Fischer H, Jagre R, Polat H, Geier H, Rech M, Staszeswki S, Helm EB, Caspary WF. 1993. Early changes of body composition in human immunodeficiency virus-infected patients: Tetrapolar body impedance analysis indicates significant malnutrition. *American Journal of Clinical Nutrition* 57:15–19.
145. Perez EA, Chawla SP, Kaywin PK, et al. 1997. Efficacy and safety of oral granisetron versus IV ondansetron in prevention of moderately emetogenic chemotherapy-induced nausea and vomiting. *Proceedings of the American Society for Clinical Oncology* 16:43.
146. Perez-Reyes M, Wagner D, Wall ME, Davis KH. 1976. Intravenous administration of cannabinoids and intraocular pressure. In: *The Pharmacology of Marihuana*, New York: Raven Press. Pp. 829–832.
147. Peroutka SJ. 1996. Drugs effective in the therapy of migraine. In: Hardman JG, Limbird LE, Editors, *Goodman and Gilman's The Pharmacological Basis of Therapeutics.* 9th Edition. New York: McGraw-Hill. Pp. 487–502.
148. Petro D, Ellenberger Jr C. 1981. Treatment of human spasticity with delta 9-tetrahydrocannabinol. *Journal of Clinical Pharmacology* 21:413S–416S.
149. Quigley HA. 1996. Number of people with glaucoma worldwide. *British Journal of Ophthalmology* 80:389–393.
150. Raft D, Gregg J, Ghia J, Harris L. 1977. Effects of intravenous tetrahydrocannabinol on experimental and surgical pain: Psychological correlates of the analgesic response. *Clinical Pharmacology and Therapeutics* 21:26–33.
151. Razdan RK. 1986. Structure-activity relationships in cannabinoids. *Pharmacology Review* 38:75–149.
152. Richfield EK, Herkenham M. 1994. Selective vulnerability in Huntington's disease: Preferential loss of cannabinoid receptors in lateral globus pallidus. *Annals of Neurology* 36:577–584.

153. Richter A, Loscher W. 1994. (+)-WIN55,212-2 A novel cannabinoid receptor agonist, exerts antidystonic effects in mutant dystonic hamsters. *European Journal of Pharmacology* 264:371–377.
154. Rodriguez de Fonseca F, Carrera MRA, Navarro M, Koob G, Weiss F. 1997. Activation of corticotropin-releasing factor in the limbic system during cannabinoid withdrawal [see comments *Science* 1997., 276:1967–1968]. *Science* 276:2050–2054.
155. Roila F, Tonato M, Cognetti F, et al. 1991. Prevention of cisplatin-induced emesis: A double-blind multicenter randomized crossover study comparing ondansetron and ondansetron plus dexamethasone. *Journal of Clinical Oncology* 9:674–678.
156. Rosenzweig MR, Leiman AL, Breedlove SM. 1996. *Biological Psychology*. Sunderland, MA: Sinauer Associates, Inc.
157. Roth RI, Owen RL, Keren DF, Volberding PA. 1985. Intestinal infection with Mycobacterium avium in acquired immune deficiency syndrome (AIDS): Histological and clinical comparison with Whipple's disease. *Digestive Disease Science* 30:497–504.
158. Süttmann U, Ockenga J, Selberg O, Hoogestraat L, Deicher H, Müller MJ. 1995. Incidence and prognostic value of malnutrition and wasting in human immunodeficiency virus—infected outpatients. *Journal of Acquired Immune Deficiency Syndrome and Human Retrovirology* 8:239–246.
159. Sackett D, Rosenberg W, Haynes B, Richardson S. 1997. *Evidence-Based Medicine: How to Practice and Teach EBM*. New York: Churchhill Livingston.
160. Sallan SE, Cronin CM, Zelen M, et al. 1980. Antiemetics in patients receiving chemotherapy for cancer: A randomized comparison of delta-9-tetrahydrocannabinol and prochlorperazine. *New England Journal of Medicine* 302:135–138.
161. Sallan SE, Zinberg NE, Frei E. 1975. Antiemetic effect of delta-9-THC in patients receiving cancer chemotherapy. *New England Journal of Medicine* 293:795–797.
162. SAMHSA (Substance Abuse and Mental Health Services Administration). 1998. *National Household Survey on Drug Abuse: Population Estimates 1997*. DHHS Pub. No. (SMA) 98-3250. Rockville, MD: SAMHSA, Office of Applied Studies.
163. Sandyk R, Awerbuch G. 1988. Marijuana and Tourette's syndrome. *Journal of Clinical Psychopharmacology* 8:444–445.
164. Sandyk R, Consroe P, Stern P, Biklen D. 1988. Preliminary trial of cannabidiol in Huntington's disease. Chesher G, Consroe P, Musty R., Editors, *Marijuana: An International Research Report*. Canberra: Australian Government Publishing Service.
165. Sanudo-Pena MC, Patrick SL, Patrick RL, Walker JM. 1996. Effects of intranigral cannabinoids on rotational behavior in rats: Interactions with the dopaminergic system. *Neuroscience Letters* 206:21–24.
166. Sanudo-Pena MC, Tsou K, and Walker JM. Cannabinoid dopamine interactions in the basal ganglia in an animal model of Parkinson disease. (in preparation).
167. Sanudo-Pena MC, Tsou K, and Walker JM. Superior colliculus and turning: Dopamine and cannabinoids. (in preparation).
168. Sanudo-Pena MC, Walker JM. 1997. Role of the subthalamic nucleus in cannabinoid actions in the substantia nigra of the rat. *Journal of Neurophysiology* 77:1635–1638.
169. Sanudo-Pena MC, Walker JM. 1998. Effects of intrastriatal cannabinoids on rotational behavior in rats: Interactions with the dopaminergic system. *Synapse* 30:221–226.
170. Schambelan M, Mulligan K, Grunfeld C, Daar ES, LaMarca A, Kotler DP. 1996. Recombinant human growth hormone in patients with HIV-associated wasting: A randomized, placebo-controlled trial: Serostim Study Group. *Annals of Internal Medicine* 125:873–882.
171. Schwartz RH, Beveridge RA. 1994. Marijuana as an antiemetic drug: How useful is it today? Opinions from clinical oncologists [see Comments]. *Journal of Addictive Diseases* 13:53–65.

172. Schwartz RH, Voth EA. 1995. Marijuana as medicine: Making a silk purse out of a sow's ear. *Journal of Addictive Diseases* 14:15–21.
173. Shields MB. 1998. *Textbook of Glaucoma*. 4th Edition. Baltimore, MD: Williams & Wilkins.
174. Sommer A, Tielsch JM, Katz J, Quigley HA, Gottsch JD, Javitt J, Singh K. 1991. Relationship between intraocular pressure and primary open angle glaucoma among white and black Americans: The Baltimore Eye Survey. *Archives of Ophthalmology* 109:1090–1095.
175. Staquet M, Gantt C, Machin D. 1978. Effect of a nitrogen analog of tetrahydrocannabinol on cancer pain. *Clinical Pharmacology and Therapeutics* 23:397–401.
176. Steele N, Gralla RJ, Braun Jr DW. 1980. Double-blind comparison of the antiemetic effects of nabilone and prochlorperazine on chemotherapy-induced emesis. *Cancer Treatments Report* 64:219–224.
177. Stimmel B. 1995. Medical marijuana: To prescribe or not to prescribe, that is the question [Editorial]. *Journal of Addictive Diseases* 14:1–3.
178. Strassman RJ. 1998. *Marijuana: The Forbidden Medicine* (book review). *Journal of the American Medical Association* 279:963–964.
179. Struwe M, Kaempfer SH, Geiger CJ, Pavia AT, Plasse TF, Shepard KV, Ries K, Evans TG. 1993. Effect of dronabinol on nutritional status in HIV infection. *Annals of Pharmacotherapy* 27:827–831.
180. Swift RM. 1994. *Marijuana: The Forbidden Medicine* (book review). *The New England Journal of Medicine* 331:749–750.
181. Tanda G, Pontieri FE, Di Chiara G. 1997. Cannabinoid and heroin activation of mesolimbic dopamine transmission by a common μ1 opioid receptor mechanism. *Science* 276:2048–2049.
182. Tiedeman JS, Shields MB, Weber PA, Crow JW, Cocchetto DM, Harris WA, Howes JF. 1981. Effect of synthetic cannabinoids on elevated intraocular pressure. *Ophthalmology* 88:270–277.
183. Timpone JG, Wright DJ, Li N, Egorin MJ, Enama ME, Mayers J, Galetto G, DATRI 004 Study Group. 1997. The safety and pharmacokinetics of single-agent and combination therapy with megestrol acetate and dronabinol for the treatment of HIV wasting syndrome: The DATRI 004 study group. *AIDS Research and Human Retroviruses* 13:305–315.
184. Trembly B, Sherman M. 1990. Double-blind clinical study of cannabidiol as a secondary anticonvulsant. Unpublished manuscript presented at the Marijuana '90 International Conference on Cannabis and Cannabinoids. Kolympari, Crete, July 8–11.
185. Tyson LB, Gralla RJ, Clark RA, et al. 1985. Phase I trial of levonantradol in chemotherapy-induced emesis. *American Journal of Clinical Oncology* 8:528–532.
186. UNAIDS, WHO. 1998. *Report on the Global HIV/AIDS Epidemic, June 1998.*
187. Ungerleider JT, Andrysiak TA, Fairbanks L, Ellison GW, Myers LW. 1987. Delta-9-THC in the treatment of spasticity associated with multiple sclerosis. *Advances in Alcohol and Substance Abuse* 7:39–50.
188. Vinciguerra V, Moore T, Brennan E. 1988. Inhalation marijuana as an antiemetic for cancer chemotherapy. *New York State Journal of Medicine* 88:525–527.
189. Volicer L, Smith S, Volicer BJ. 1995. Effect of seizures on progression of dementia of the Alzheimer type. *Dementia* 6:258–263.
190. Volicer L, Stelly M, Morris J, McLaughlin J, Volicer BJ. 1997. Effects of dronabinol on anorexia and disturbed behavior in patients with Alzheimer's disease. *International Journal of Geriatric Psychiatry* 12:913–919.
191. Voth EA, Schwartz RH. 1997. Medicinal applications of delta-9-tetrahydrocannabinol and marijuana. *Annals of Internal Medicine* 126:791–798.

192. Wall PD, Melzack R. 1994. *Textbook of Pain.* Edinburgh: Churchill Livingstone.
193. Walters TR. 1996. Development and use of brimonidine in treating acute and chronic elevations of intraocular pressure: A review of safety, efficacy, dose response, and dosing studies. *Survey of Ophthalmology* 41(Suppl. 1):S19–S26.
194. Wang ZM, Visser M, Ma R, Baumgartner RN, Kotler DP, Gallagher D, Heymsfield SB. 1996. Skeletal muscle mass: Validation of neutron activation and dual energy X-ray absorptiometry methods by computerized tomography. *Journal of Applied Physiology* 80:824–831.
195. Whitney EN, Cataldo CB, Rolfes SR. 1994. *Understanding Normal and Clinical Nutrition.* 4th Edition. Minneapolis, MN: West Publishing Co.
196. Wood. 1998. HIV-protease inhibitors. *Drug Therapy* 338:1281–1292.
197. Yoles E, Belkin M, Schwartz M. 1996. HU-211, a nonpsychotropic cannabinoid, produces short- and long-term neuroprotection after optic nerve axotomy. *Journal of Neurotrauma* 13:49–57.
198. Zimmer L, Morgan JP. 1997. *Marijuana Myths, Marijuana Facts.* New York: The Lindesmith Center.

5

Development of Cannabinoid Drugs

Medicines today are expected to be of known composition and quality. Even in cases where marijuana can provide relief of symptoms, the crude plant mixture does not meet this modern expectation. The future of medical marijuana lies in classical pharmacological drug development, and indeed there has been a resurgence of scientific, as well as public, interest in the therapeutic applications of cannabinoids. After an initial burst of scientific activity in the 1970s, today's renewed interest has been fueled by major scientific discoveries discussed in previous chapters: the identification and cloning of endogenous cannabinoid receptors, the discovery of endogenous substances that bind to these receptors, and the emergence of synthetic cannabinoids that also bind to cannabinoid receptors. These scientific accomplishments have propelled interest in developing new drugs that can treat more effectively or more safely the constellation of symptoms for which cannabinoids might have therapeutic benefit (see chapter 4). Through the process of what is referred to as "rational drug design," scientists manipulate the chemical structures of known cannabinoids to design better therapeutic agents. Several new cannabinoids are being developed for human use, but none has reached the stage of human testing in the United States.

The purpose of this chapter is to describe the process of and analyze the prospects for development of cannabinoid drugs. It first discusses the regulatory hurdles that every new drug encounters en route to market. It then proceeds to describe the regulatory and market experiences of dronabinol (tetrahydrocannabinol, or THC, in sesame oil), the only approved cannabinoid in the United States. These sections serve as a road map to determine whether the therapeutic potential of cannabinoids is likely to be exploited commercially to meet patient needs. Finally, the chapter describes what would be needed to bring marijuana to market as a medicinal plant.

The term *cannabinoids* is used in this chapter to refer to a group of substances that are structurally related to THC—by virtue of a tricyclic chemical structure—or that bind to cannabinoid receptors, such as the natural ligand anandamide. From a chemist's point of view, this definition encompasses a variety of distinct chemical classes. But because the purpose of this chapter is to explore prospects for drug development, both chemical structure and pharmacological activity are important; therefore, the broader definition of cannabinoids is used.

FEDERAL DRUG DEVELOPMENT POLICY

Like controlled substances, cannabinoids developed for medical use encounter a gauntlet of public health regulatory controls administered by two federal agencies: the Food and Drug Administration (FDA) of the U.S. Department of Health and Human Services (DHHS) and the Drug Enforcement Administration (DEA) of the U.S. Department of Justice. The FDA regulates human testing and the introduction of new drugs into the marketplace, whereas the DEA determines the schedule of and establishes production quotas for drugs with potential for abuse to prevent their diversion to illicit channels. The DEA also authorizes registered physicians to prescribe controlled substances. Some drugs, such as marijuana, are labeled Schedule I in the Controlled Substance Act, and this adds considerable complexity and expense to their clinical evaluation. It is important to point out that Schedule I status does not necessarily apply to all cannabinoids.

Food and Drug Administration

Under the Federal Food, Drug, and Cosmetic (FD&C) Act, the FDA approves new drugs for entry into the marketplace after their safety and efficacy are established through controlled clinical trials conducted by the drugs' sponsors.[23] FDA approval of a drug is the culmination of a long, research intensive process of drug development, which often takes well over a decade.[19,44] Drug development is performed largely by pharmaceutical companies, but some targeted drug development programs are sponsored by the National Institutes of Health (NIH) to stimulate further development and marketing by the private sector. The NIH's drug development programs—including those for AIDS, cancer, addiction, and epilepsy—have been instrumental in ushering new drugs to market in collaboration with pharmaceutical companies.[33] In fact, as noted later, most of the preclinical and clinical research on dronabinol was supported by NIH.

Drug development begins with discovery, that is, the synthesis and purification of a new compound with expected biological activity and therapeutic value. The next major step is the testing of the compound in animals to learn more about its safety and efficacy and to predict its utility for humans. Those early activities are collectively referred to as the preclinical phase. When evidence from the preclinical phase suggests a promising role in humans, the manufacturer submits an Investigational New Drug (IND) application to the FDA. The IND submission contains a plan for human clinical trials and includes the results of preclinical testing and other information.[20] Absent FDA objection, the IND becomes effective after 30 days, allowing the manufacturer to conduct clinical testing (testing in humans), which generally involves three phases (see Figure 5.1). The three stages of clinical testing are usually the most time-consuming phases of drug development, lasting five years on average.[22] The actual time depends on the complexity of the drug, availability of patients, duration of use, difficulty of measuring clinical end points, therapeutic class, and indication (the disease or condition for which the drug has purported benefits).[31]

Drug development is a long and financially risky process. For every drug that ultimately reaches clinical testing through an IND, thousands of drugs are synthesized and tested in the laboratory. And only about one in five drugs initially tested in humans successfully secures FDA approval for marketing through a new drug application (NDA).[19]

The manufacturer submits an NDA to the FDA to gain approval for marketing when clinical testing is complete. An NDA is a massive document, the largest portion of which contains the clinical data from Phase I–III testing. The other technical sections of an NDA include chemistry, manufacturing, and controls; nonclinical pharmacology and toxicology; and human pharmacokinetics and bioavailability.[23] In the case of a new cannabinoid, an abuse liability assessment would also probably be part of an NDA submission. In 1996 the median time for FDA review of an NDA, from submission to approval, was 15.1 months, a review period considerably shorter than that in 1990, when the figure was 24.3 months.[22] The shortening of approval time is an outgrowth of the Prescription Drug User Fee Act of 1992, which authorized the FDA to hire additional review staff with so-called user fees paid by industry and imposed clear deadlines for FDA action on an NDA. With respect to the cost of a single drug's development, a number of recent studies have provided a range of estimates of

196

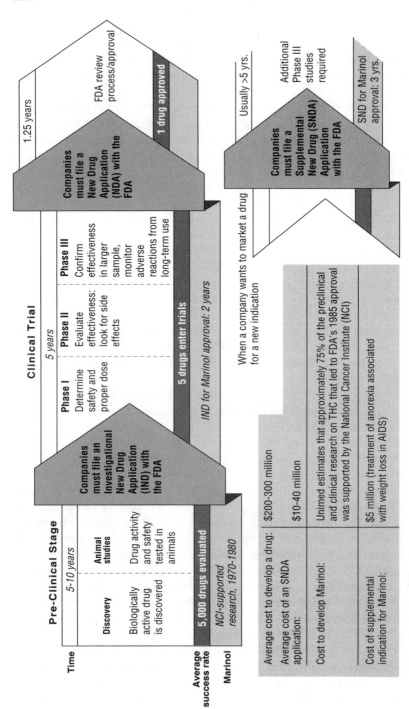

FIGURE 5.1 Stages of clinical testing.

about $200–$300 million, depending on the method and year of calculation.[33,44]

With FDA approval of an NDA, the manufacturer is permitted to market the drug for the *approved indication*. At that point, although any physician is at liberty to prescribe the approved drug for another indication (an "off-label use"), the manufacturer cannot promote it for that indication unless the new indication is granted separate marketing approval by the FDA.* To obtain such approval, the manufacturer is required to compile another application to the FDA for what is known variously as an "efficacy supplement," a "supplemental application," or a "supplemental new drug application." Those terms connote that the application is supplemental to the NDA. In general, collecting new data for FDA approval of an efficacy supplement is not as intensive a process as that for an NDA; it generally requires the firm to conduct two additional Phase III studies, although under some circumstances only one additional study of the drug's efficacy is needed.[24] The preclinical studies, for example, ordinarily need not be replicated. The average cost to the manufacturer for obtaining approval for the new indication is typically about $10–$40 million.[33] The review time to obtain FDA approval for the new indication can be considerable; a recent study of supplemental indications approved by the FDA in 1989–1994 found the approval time to exceed that for the original NDA,[18] a reflection, in part, of the lower priority that the FDA accords to the review of efficacy supplements as opposed to new drugs.[23]

The manufacturer also must apply to the FDA to receive marketing approval for a new formulation of a previously approved drug. A new formulation is a new dosage form, including a new route of administration. An example of such a new formulation is an inhaled version of Marinol, which is currently approved only in capsule form. The manufacturer is required to establish bioequivalence, safety, and efficacy of the new formulation. The amount of evidence required for approval is highly variable, depending on the similarities between the new formulation and the approved formulation. New formulations are evaluated case by case by the FDA. In the case of Marinol, for example, an inhaled version is likely to require not only new studies of efficacy but also new studies of abuse liability. There appear to be no published peer-reviewed studies of the average cost and time for approval of a new formulation.

Two other FDA programs might be relevant to the potential availabil-

---

*FDA policies for off-label use are being transformed as a result of the Food and Drug Administration Modernization Act of 1997. The FDA recently promulgated new rules to give manufacturers greater flexibility to disseminate information about off-label uses (FDA, 1998b[24a]). As of this writing, however, court decisions have left the status of the new rules somewhat unclear.

ity of new cannabinoids. One program is authorized under the Orphan Drug Act of 1983, which provides incentives to manufacturers to develop drugs to treat "orphan diseases." An orphan disease, as defined in an amendment to the act, is one that affects 200,000 or fewer people in the United States.* The act's most important incentive is a period of exclusive marketing protection of seven years, during which time the FDA is prohibited from approving the same drug for the same indication.[5,6] Some of the medical conditions for which cannabinoids have been advocated— Huntington's disease, multiple sclerosis, and spinal cord injury (see chapter 4)—might meet the definition of an orphan disease and thus enable manufacturers to take advantage of the act's financial incentives to bring products to market. If a disease affects more than 200,000 people, the manufacturer sometimes subdivides the patient population into smaller units to qualify. For example, a drug for the treatment of Parkinson's disease is not likely to receive an orphan designation because its prevalence exceeds 200,000, but orphan designation has been accorded to drugs for subsets of Parkinson's patients, such as those suffering from early-morning motor dysfunction in the late stages of the disease.[25]

The other program is the Treatment-IND program, which was established by regulation in 1987 (and codified into law in 1997) to allow patients with serious and life-threatening diseases to obtain experimental medications, such as marijuana, before their general marketing.† Treatment INDs may be issued during Phase III studies to patients who are not enrolled in clinical trials, provided among other requirements that no comparable alternative drug is available.[22,32,33] Thus, the treatment IND program can provide a mechanism for some patients to obtain a promising new cannabinoid before its widespread commercial availability if it reached the late stages of clinical testing for a serious or life-threatening disease.

Drug Enforcement Administration

The DEA is responsible for scheduling controlled substances, that is, drugs and other agents that possess a potential for abuse. *Abuse* is generally defined as nonmedical use that leads to health and safety hazards, diversion from legitimate channels, self-administration, and other untoward results.[15,21] The legislation that gives DEA the authority to regulate

---

*The FDA can grant orphan designation to a drug intended for a condition that affects a larger population if the manufacturer's estimated expenses are unlikely to be recovered by sales in the United States (Public Law 98-551).

†Marijuana cigarettes were available under a special FDA-sponsored Compassionate Investigational New Drug Program for desperately ill patients until March 1992, when the program was closed to new participants.[48]

drugs of abuse is the Controlled Substances Act, which was passed in 1970 and amended several times. The overall purpose of the CSA is to restrict or control the availability of drugs to prevent their abuse.

Under the CSA, the DEA places each drug that has abuse potential into one of five categories. The five categories, referred to as Schedules I–V, carry different degrees of restriction. Schedule I is the most restrictive, covering drugs that have "no accepted medical use" in the United States and that have high abuse potential. The definitions of the categories and examples of drugs in each are listed in Appendix C. Each schedule is associated with a distinct set of controls that affect manufacturers, investigators, pharmacists, practitioners, patients, and recreational users. The controls include registration with the DEA, labeling and packaging, production quotas, security, recordkeeping, and dispensing.[15] For instance, patients with a legitimate medical need for drugs in Schedule II, the most restrictive schedule for drugs "currently with accepted medical use," can neither refill their prescriptions nor have them telephoned to a pharmacy (except in an emergency).

The scheduling of substances under the CSA is handled case by case. It may be initiated by DEA, by DHHS, or by petition from an interested party, including the drug's manufacturer or a public-interest group.[15] The final decision for scheduling rests with the DEA, but for this purpose the secretary of DHHS is mandated to provide a recommendation. The secretary's recommendation* to DEA is based in part on results from abuse liability testing that the FDA requires of the manufacturer seeking approval of a new drug. Abuse liability testing is not a single test; it is a compilation of several *in vitro* human and animal studies, of which some of the best known are drug self-administration and drug discrimination studies.[21,34] The secretary's recommendation for scheduling is formally guided by eight legal criteria, including the drug's actual or relative potential for abuse, scientific evidence of its pharmacological effect, risk to public health, and its psychic or physiological dependence liability (21 U.S.C. § 811 (b), (c)). Once the DEA receives a scheduling recommendation, its scheduling decision, including the requirement for obtaining public comment, usually takes weeks to months.[33] In practice, the DEA usually adheres to the recommendation of the secretary.† Beyond the DEA,

---

*The FDA and the National Institute of Drug Abuse, two agencies of DHHS, work jointly to develop the medical and scientific analysis that is forwarded to the secretary, who makes a recommendation to the administrator of the DEA (DEA, 1998[15]).

†Under the CSA, "the recommendations of the Secretary to the Attorney General shall be binding on the Attorney General as to such scientific and medical matters, and if the Secretary recommends that a drug or other substance not be controlled, the Attorney General shall not control the drug or other substance" (21 U.S.C.§ 811 (b)).

various state scheduling laws also affect the manufacture and distribution of controlled substances.[33,50]

Under the CSA, marijuana and THC* are in Schedule I, the most restrictive schedule. The scheduling of any other cannabinoid under this act first hinges on whether it is found *in the plant*. All cannabinoids in the plant are automatically in Schedule I because they fall under the act's definition of marijuana (21 U.S.C. § 802 (16)). In addition, under DEA's regulations, synthetic equivalents of the substances contained in the plant and "synthetic substances, derivatives, and their isomers" whose "chemical structure and pharmacological activity" are "similar" to THC also are automatically in Schedule I (21 CFR § 1308.11(d)(27). Based on the examples listed in the regulations, the word *similar* probably limits the applicability of the regulation to isomers of THC, but DEA's interpretation of its own regulations would carry significant weight in any specific situation.

Prompted by a 1995 petition from Jon Gettman, a former president of the National Organization for the Reform of Marijuana Laws (NORML), to remove marijuana and THC from Schedule I, DEA gathered information which was then submitted to DHHS for a medical and scientific recommendation and scheduling recommendation, as required by the CSA. For the reasons noted above, any changes in scheduling of marijuana and THC would also affect other plant cannabinoids. For the present, however, any cannabinoid found in the plant is automatically controlled in Schedule I.

Investigators are affected by Schedule I requirements even if their research is being conducted *in vitro* or on animals. For example, researchers studying cannabinoids found in the plant are required under the CSA to submit their research protocol to DEA, which issues a registration that is contingent on FDA's evaluation and approval of the protocol (21 CFR § 1301.18). DEA also inspects the researcher's security arrangements. However, the regulatory implications are quite different for cannabinoids *not found in the plant*. Such cannabinoids appear to be unscheduled unless the FDA or DEA decides that they are sufficiently similar to THC to be placed automatically into Schedule I under the regulatory definition outlined above or the FDA or the manufacturer deems them to have potential for abuse, thereby triggering *de novo* the scheduling process noted above. Thus far, the cannabinoids most commonly used in preclinical research (Table 5.1) appear to be sufficiently distinct from THC that they are not currently considered controlled substances by definition (F. Sapienza, DEA, personal communication, 1998). No new cannabinoids other than

---

*Technically, the CSA and the regulations use the term "tetrahydrocannabinols."

TABLE 5.1 Cannabinoids and Related
Compounds Commonly Used in Research

Agonists
THC
WIN 55,212-2
CP-55940
HU-210
Anandamide (natural ligand)
2-Arachidonylglycerol (natural ligand)

Antagonists
SR 141716A
SR 144528

SOURCES: Felder and Glass (1998)[26] and Mechoulam et al. (1998).[36]

THC have yet been clinically tested in the United States, so scheduling experience is limited. The unscheduled status of some cannabinoids might change as research progresses. Results of early clinical research could lead a manufacturer to proceed with or lead the FDA to require abuse liability testing. Depending on the results of such studies, DHHS might or might not recommend scheduling *de novo* to DEA, which makes the final decision case by case.

Will newly discovered cannabinoids be subject to scheduling? That is a complex question that has no simple answer. The answer depends entirely on each new cannabinoid—whether it is found in the plant, its chemical and pharmacological relationship to THC, and its potential for abuse. Novel cannabinoids with strong similarity to THC are likely to be scheduled at some point before marketing, whereas those with weak similarity might not be. The manufacturer's submission to FDA, which contains its own studies and its request for a particular schedule, can also shape the outcome. Cannabinoids found in the plant are automatically in Schedule I until the manufacturer requests and provides justification for rescheduling. The CSA does permit DEA to reschedule a substance (move it to a different schedule) and to deschedule a substance (remove it from control under the CSA) according to the scheduling criteria (see Appendix F) and the process outlined above.

The possibility of scheduling is a major determinant of whether a manufacturer proceeds with drug development.[33] In general, pharmaceutical firms perceive scheduling to be a deterrent because it limits their ability to achieve market share for the following reasons: restricted access, physician disinclination to prescribe scheduled substances, stigma, the additional expense for abuse liability studies, and expensive delays in reaching the market due to federal and state scheduling processes.[33] Empirical evidence to support that widely held perception is difficult to find, but at least one large survey of physicians found them to have moderate concerns about prescribing opioids because of actual or perceived pressure from regulatory agencies, such as DEA.[57] On the basis of a legal analysis and widespread complaints from researchers and pharmaceutical executives, the Institute of Medicine (IOM, 1995)[33] recommended changes in the CSA to eliminate the act's barriers to undertaking clinical research and development of controlled substances; this position was supported in a later report on marijuana.[40]

DEVELOPMENT AND MARKETING OF MARINOL

The following material is based on the published literature (where cited), workshops sponsored by the IOM, and an interview with Robert Dudley, senior vice president of Unimed Pharmaceuticals, Inc., the manufacturer of Marinol and the holder of the NDA. Unimed markets Marinol jointly with Roxane Laboratories, Inc.

Marinol (dronabinol) is the only cannabinoid with approval for marketing in the United States.* The following description covers its development, regulatory history, pharmacokinetics, adverse effects, abuse liability, and market growth. The experience with Marinol can serve as a possible bellwether for the regulatory and commercial fate of new cannabinoids being considered for development.

Development and Regulatory History

Marinol is manufactured as a capsule containing THC in sesame oil; it is taken orally. It was approved by the FDA in 1985 for the treatment of nausea and vomiting associated with cancer chemotherapy. In 1992, the FDA approved marketing of dronabinol for the treatment of anorexia associated with weight loss in patients with AIDS.[45] The preclinical and clinical research on THC that culminated in the FDA's 1985 approval was supported primarily by the National Cancer Institute (NCI), whose research support goes back to the 1970s. NCI's contribution appears pivotal, considering that Unimed, the pharmaceutical company that holds

---

*The only cannabinoid licensed outside the United States is nabilone (Cesamet), which is an analogue of THC available in the United Kingdom for the management of nausea and vomiting associated with cancer chemotherapy (Pertwee, 1997).[46]

the NDA, estimates its contribution to have been only about 25% of the total research effort. The FDA's review and approval of Marinol took about two years after submission of the NDA, according to Unimed. To obtain approval for Marinol's second indication (through an efficacy supplement), the FDA required two more relatively small Phase III studies. The studies lasted three years and cost $5 million to complete.

Physical Properties, Pharmacokinetics, and Adverse Events

Marinol is synthesized in the laboratory rather than extracted from the plant. Its manufacture is complex and expensive because of the numerous steps needed for purification. The poor solubility of Marinol in aqueous solutions and its high first-pass metabolism in the liver account for its poor bioavailability; only 10–20% of an oral dose reaches the systemic circulation.[45,60] The onset of action is slow; peak plasma concentrations are not attained until two to four hours after dosing.[45,56] In contrast, inhaled marijuana is rapidly absorbed. In a study comparing THC administered orally, by inhalation, and intravenously, plasma concentration peaked almost instantaneously after both inhalation and intravenous administration; most participants' peak plasma concentrations after oral administration occurred at 60 or 90 minutes. Variation in individual responses is highest for oral THC and bioavailability is lowest.[42]

Marinol's most common adverse events are associated with the central nervous system (CNS): anxiety, confusion, depersonalization, dizziness, euphoria, dysphoria, somnolence, and thinking abnormality.[8,9,45,59] In two recent clinical trials, CNS adverse events occurred in about one-third of patients, but only a small percentage discontinued the drug because of adverse effects.[8,9] Lowering the dose of dronabinol can minimize side effects, especially dysphoria (disquiet or malaise).[47]

Abuse Potential and Scheduling

On commercial introduction in 1985, Marinol was placed in Schedule II. This schedule, the second most restrictive, is reserved for medically approved substances that have "high potential for abuse" (21 U.S.C. § 812 (b) (2)). Unimed did not encounter any delays in marketing as a result of the scheduling process because the scheduling decision was made by the DEA before FDA's approval for marketing. Nor did Unimed encounter any marketing delays as a result of state scheduling laws. Unimed was not specifically asked by the FDA to perform abuse liability studies for the first approval, presumably because such studies had been conducted earlier.

Unimed later petitioned the DEA to reschedule Marinol from Schedule II to Schedule III, which is reserved for medically approved substances that have some potential for abuse (21 U.S.C. § 812 (b) (3)). To buttress its request for rescheduling, Unimed supported an analysis of Marinol's abuse liability by researchers at the Haight Ashbury Free Clinic of San Francisco, which treats many cannabis-dependent patients and people who have HIV/AIDS. The analysis found no evidence of abuse or diversion of Marinol after a literature review and surveys and interviews of medical specialists in addiction, oncology, cancer research, and treatment of HIV, and people in law enforcement. The authors attribute Marinol's low abuse potential to its slow onset of action, its dysphoric effects, and other factors.[12] On November 5, 1998, the DEA announced a proposal to reschedule Marinol to Schedule III.[17] As of this writing, no formal action on that proposal had been taken.

The rescheduling of a drug from Schedule II to Schedule III is considered important because it lifts some of the restrictions on availability. For example, Unimed expects a sales increase of about 15–20% as a result of rescheduling. In its judgment and that of many other pharmaceutical companies,[33] scheduling limits market penetration; the more restrictive the schedules, the greater the limitation. The reasons are that physicians and other providers are reluctant to prescribe Schedule II drugs; patients are deterred from seeking prescriptions because of Schedule II prohibition of refills, as opposed to other commercially available scheduled substances; additional restrictions are imposed by several states, such as quantity restrictions (for example, 30-day supply limits) and triplicate prescriptions;[50] and some Schedule II drugs are excluded from hospital formularies because of onerous security and paperwork requirements under federal and state controlled substances laws.

Market Growth and Transformation

Annual sales of Marinol are estimated at $20 million, according to Unimed. Of Marinol's patient population 80% use it for HIV, 10% for cancer chemotherapy, and about 5–10% for other reasons. The latter group is thought to consist of Alzheimer's patients drawn to the drug by a recently published clinical study indicating Marinol's promise for the treatment of their anorexia and disturbed behavior.[58] As noted earlier, Unimed cannot promote Marinol for this unlabeled indication, but physicians are free to prescribe it for such an indication. Unimed is conducting additional research in pursuit of FDA approval of a new indication for Marinol in the treatment of Alzheimer disease.

The 1992 approval of Marinol for the treatment of anorexia in AIDS patients marked a major transformation in the composition of the patient population. Marinol's use had been restricted to oncology patients. The oncology market for Marinol gradually receded as a result of the introduction of newer medications, including such serotonin antagonists as ondansetron, which are more effective (see chapter 4, "Nausea and Vomiting) and are not scheduled. Much of the recent growth of the market for Marinol (which is about 10% per year) is attributed to its increasing use by HIV patients being treated with combination antiretroviral therapy. Marinol appears to have a dual effect, not only stimulating appetite but also combating the nausea and vomiting associated with combination therapy. Unimed is supporting a Phase II study to examine this combined effect and, with promising results, plans to seek FDA approval for this new indication.

Unimed has two forms of market protection for Marinol. In December 1992, the FDA granted Marinol seven years of exclusive marketing under the Orphan Drug Act. The market exclusivity is related to Marinol's use in anorexia associated with AIDS. Because of the designated orphan indication, the active ingredient, THC, cannot be marketed by another manufacturer for the same indication until December 1999. Other pharmaceutical manufacturers are not constrained from manufacturing and marketing THC for its *other* indication, antiemesis for cancer chemotherapy, but none appears to be interested in what is, by pharmaceutical company standards, a small market. In addition to market exclusivity, Unimed secured in June 1998 a "use patent" for dronabinol for the treatment of disturbed patients with dementia; this confers patent protection to Unimed for this use for 20 years from the date of filing of the application,* assuming that this indication eventually gains FDA approval.

The rate-limiting factors in the growth of the market for Marinol, according to Unimed are the lack of physician awareness of the drug's efficacy, its adverse effects, and its restricted availability as a result of placement in Schedule II. Unimed perceives only a small percentage of its market to be lost to "competition" from marijuana itself, but there are, admittedly, no reliable statistics on the number of people who have chosen to treat their symptoms with illegally obtained marijuana, despite their ability to obtain Marinol.

New Routes of Administration

It is well recognized that Marinol's oral route of administration hampers its effectiveness because of slow absorption and patients' desire for

---

*A use patent—also known as a process patent—accords protection for a method of using a composition or compound. A use patent is not considered as strong as a product patent, which prohibits others from manufacturing, using, or selling the product for all uses, rather than for the specific use defined in a use patent.

more control over dosing. A drug delivered orally is first absorbed from the stomach or small intestine and then passed through the liver, where it undergoes some metabolism before being introduced into the circulation. To overcome the deficiencies of oral administration, Unimed activated an IND in 1998 as a step toward developing new formulations for Marinol. Four new formulations—deep lung aerosol, nasal spray, nasal gel, and sublingual preparation—are under study in Phase I clinical studies being conducted in conjunction with Roxane Laboratories. These formulations seek to deliver Marinol to the circulation more rapidly and directly. The first two fall under inhalation as a route of administration. Inhalation is considered the most promising method, owing to the rapidity of onset of its effects and potential for better titration of the dose by the patient, but it might also carry an increased potential for abuse. The abuse of a drug correlates with its rapidity of onset (G. Koob, IOM workshop). Sublingual route (under the tongue) administration also affords rapid absorption into the circulation, in this case from the oral mucosa. Other researchers are pursuing the delivery of THC through rectal suppositories, but this slower route might not be acceptable to many patients. Transdermal (skin patches) administration, which is best suited to hydrophilic drugs, is precluded by the lipophilicity of THC. Thus, the choice of routes of administration depends heavily on the physicochemical characteristics of the drug and on its safety, abuse liability, and tolerability.

Unimed expects the FDA to require it to conduct studies of the bioavailability, efficacy, and possibly abuse liability of any new formulation it seeks to market. Any formulation that expedites Marinol's onset of action, as suggested above, is thought to carry greater possibility of abuse. The cost of developing each new formulation is estimated by Unimed at $7–$10 million.

Unimed and Roxane are developing, or considering development of, five new indications for Marinol: disturbed behavior in Alzheimer's disease, nausea and vomiting in HIV patients who are receiving combination therapy, spasticity in multiple sclerosis, intractable pain, and anorexia in cancer and renal disease.

Costs of Marinol and Marijuana

During the IOM public workshops held during the course of this study, many people commented that an important advantage of using marijuana for medical purposes is that it is much less expensive than Marinol. But this comparison is deceptive. While the direct costs of marijuana are relatively low, the indirect costs can be prohibitive. Individuals who violate federal or state marijuana laws risk a variety of costs associated with engaging in criminal activity, ranging from increased vulnerability to theft and personal injury legal fees to long prison terms. In addition, when purchasing illicit drugs there is no guarantee that the product purchased is what the seller claims it is or that it is not contaminated.

The price of Marinol for its most commonly used indication, anorexia in AIDS, is estimated at $200 per month. The less common indication—nausea and vomiting with cancer chemotherapy—is not as expensive because it is not chronic. Regardless of indication, patients' out-of-pocket expenses tend to be much less—often minimal—because of reimbursement through public or private health insurance. For indigent patients who are uninsured, Roxane sponsors a patient assistance program to defray the cost.

The street value of marijuana, according to the DEA's most recent figures, is about $5–$10 per bag of loose plant.[16*] At the California buyers' clubs, the price is $2–$16 per gram, depending on the grade of marijuana. The cost to a patient using marijuana depends on the number of cigarettes smoked each day, their THC content, and the duration of use. Insurance does not cover the cost of marijuana. In addition, it is possible for a person to cultivate marijuana privately with little financial investment.

Thus, Marinol appears to be less expensive than marijuana for patients with health insurance or with financial assistance from Roxane. But if the full cost of Marinol is borne out of pocket by the patient, the cost comparison is not so unambiguous. In this case the daily cost in relation to marijuana varies according to the number of cigarettes smoked: If the patient smokes two or more marijuana cigarettes per day, Marinol might be less expensive than marijuana; if the patient smokes only one marijuana cigarette per day, Marinol might be more expensive than marijuana, according to an analysis submitted to the DEA by Unimed. The cost comparisons will depend on fluctuations in the retail price and street value of Marinol and marijuana, respectively, and will vary if marijuana becomes commercially available.

In summary, Marinol has been on the U.S. market since 1985. Its commercial development depended heavily on research supported by the NIH. Marinol's market has grown to $20 million in annual sales. Further market growth is expected but is still constrained by lack of awareness, adverse effects, the oral route of administration, and restrictions imposed by drug scheduling. The manufacturer is proceeding with research on new forms of delivery to overcome the problems associated with oral administration. The manufacturer also is proceeding with research on an array of new indications for Marinol.

---

*The DEA did not provide an estimate of the weight of marijuana per bag.

MARKET OUTLOOK FOR CANNABINOIDS

The potential therapeutic value of cannabinoids is extremely broad. It extends well beyond antiemesis for chemotherapy and appetite stimulation for AIDS, the two indications for which the FDA has approved dronabinol (Marinol). Chapter 4 of this report assesses the possible wider therapeutic potential of marijuana and THC in neurological disorders, glaucoma, and analgesia—all conditions for which clinical research has been under way to fulfill unmet patient needs. New therapeutic uses are being explored in preclinical research. For any of these therapeutic indications, will novel cannabinoids reach the market to satisfy the medical needs of patients?

Economic Factors in Development

The outcomes of preclinical and clinical research determine whether a drug is sufficiently safe and effective to warrant FDA approval for marketing. But the decisions to launch preclinical research and to proceed to clinical trials if early results are promising are dictated largely by economic factors. A pharmaceutical company must decide whether to invest in what is universally regarded as a long and risky research path. For any given drug the question is, Will there be an adequate return on investment? The investment in this case is the high cost of developing a drug. The expectation of high financial returns on investment is what drives drug development.[44,53]

Market analyses are undertaken to forecast whether a drug will reap a substantial return on investment. The market analysis for a cannabinoid is likely to be shaped by various factors. The average cost of developing a cannabinoid is likely to be higher than that of developing other drugs if its clinical indication is in the therapeutic categories of neuropharmaceutical or nonsteroidal antiinflammatory drug, the two therapeutic categories associated with the highest research and development costs.[19] One reason for higher costs is the need to satisfy the DEA's regulatory requirements related to drug scheduling.

On the "market return" side are multiple factors. A market analysis examines the expected returns from the possible markets for which a cannabinoid could be clinically pursued. The financial size of each market is calculated mostly on the basis of the current and projected patient prevalence (for a given clinical indication), sales data (if available), and competition from other products. The duration of use is also factored in—a drug needed for long-term use in a condition with an early age of onset is desirable from a marketing perspective. Factors that can augment or diminish market return include patentability and other forms of market protection,

TABLE 5.2 Cannabinoids Under Development for Human Use

Name of Drug	Investigator	Stage of Development	Pharmacology	U.S. FDA Status	Possible Indication(s)
HU-211	Pharmos Corp.	Clinical Phase II in Israel	NMDA receptor antagonist	None	Neuroprotection (neurotrauma, stroke, Parkinson's, Alzheimer's)
CT-3	Atlantic Pharmaceuticals	Preclinical	Nonpsychoactive	None	Antiinflammatory analgesia
THC	Unimed Roxane Labs	Clinical Phase I	Cannabinoid receptor agonist	IND	(See text)
Marijuana plant	HortaPharm GW Pharmaceuticals	Clinical in England[a]	Cannabinoid mixture	None	Multiple sclerosis
	Donald Abrams, M.D.	Clinical Phase I	Cannabinoid mixture	IND	HIV-related appetite stimulation
	Ethan Russo, M.D.		Cannabinoid mixture	IND pending	Migraine

[a]Clinical trials are to proceed in the next few years under a license from the British Home Office.[10]
SOURCES: Glain, 1998[27]; Atlantic Pharmaceuticals, 1997[7]; Striem et al., 1997[55]; Nainggolan, 1997[37]; Zurier et al., 1998[61]; D. Abrams and E. Russo, personal communications, 1998; R. Dudley, personal communication, 1998; Pharmaprojects Database, 1998.

reimbursement climate, restrictions in access due to drug scheduling, social attitudes, adverse effect profile, and drug interactions.[33,53] New cannabinoids generally can receive product patents, giving the patent holder 20 years of protection from others seeking to manufacture or sell the same product. According to U.S. patent law, the product must be novel and "nonobvious" in relation to prior patents.[28]

Cannabinoids under Development

From publicly available sources, the IOM was able to learn of several cannabinoids being developed for human use (Table 5.2). With the exception of Marinol and marijuana, all are in the preclinical phase of testing in the United States. This list might not be comprehensive, inasmuch as other compounds could be under development, but that information is proprietary.* The table does not list the full complement of cannabinoids, both agonists and antagonists, being used in research as tools to understand the pharmacology of cannabinoids (for more comprehensive lists of cannabinoids, see Felder and Glass, 1998[26]; Mechoulam et al., 1998[36]; Howlett, 1995[30]; Pertwee 1997[46]). Nor does it list cannabinoids once considered for development but later discontinued. An 18-year survey of analgesics in development in 1980–1998 found that six of the nine cannabinoids under development for analgesia were discontinued or undeveloped,[49,†] but work on most of these was halted before 1988, when the first endogenous cannabinoid receptor was discovered (chapter 3).

Three points can be made on the basis of Table 5.2. First, virtually all of the listed cannabinoids are being developed by small pharmaceutical companies or by individuals. In general, that implies that their development is considered especially risky from a commercial standpoint in that small companies are often willing to assume greater development risks than larger more established firms (W. Schmidt, personal communication, 1998). Without the benefit of sales revenues, small companies are able to fund their research through financing from venture capital, stock offerings, and relationships with established pharmaceutical companies.[43]

Second, with the exception of THC, no constituents of the marijuana plant appear to be undergoing development by pharmaceutical companies. A number of plant compounds have been tested in experimental models and humans. For example, the antiemetic properties and negligible side effects of Δ^8-THC were demonstrated in a clinical trial in children who were undergoing cancer chemotherapy,[1] but no sponsor was interested in developing Δ^8-THC for commercial purposes (R. Mechoulam, Hebrew University, personal communication, 1998). The absence of plant cannabinoids under development implies that the specter of automatic placement in Schedule I under the CSA is an important deterrent, even though rescheduling would occur before marketing.[††] The point from the earlier discussion is that automatic, as opposed to de novo, scheduling appears to cast a pall over development of a cannabinoid found in the plant. Another impediment is that a cannabinoid extracted

---

*Information about the existence of an IND is proprietary; it can be confirmed only by the manufacturer, not the FDA.

†Discontinued: levonantradol, nabitan, nantradol, and pravadoline. Undeveloped: CP-47497 and CP-55244.

††As a result of the FDA's approval of an NDA, the drug would be, at a minimum, rescheduled in Schedule II. Depending on abuse liability data supplied by the manufacturer and the FDA's recommendation, the drug could be moved to a less restrictive schedule or be descheduled.

from the plant is not likely to fulfill the criteria for a product patent, although other forms of market protection are possible. Marinol, for example, was accorded orphan drug status and its manufacturer obtained a use patent.

Third, cannabinoids are being developed for therapeutic applications beyond those discussed earlier in this chapter and in chapter 4. One of the most prominent new applications of cannabinoids is for "neuroprotection," the rescue of neurons from cell death associated with trauma, ischemia, and neurological diseases.[29,36] Cannabinoids are thought to be neuroprotective—through receptor-dependent[51] as well as receptor-independent pathways; both THC, which binds to CB_1 receptors, and CBD, which does not, are potent antioxidants, effective neuroprotectants because of their ability to reduce the toxic forms of oxygen (free radicals) that are formed during cellular stress.[29] The synthetic cannabinoid HU-211 (dexanabinol) is an antioxidant and an antagonist of the NMDA receptor, rather than an agonist at the cannabinoid receptor.[52] Earlier research demonstrated that HU-211 protects neurons from neurotoxicity induced by excess concentrations of the excitatory neurotransmitter glutamate. Excess release of glutamate, which acts by binding to the NMDA receptor, is associated with trauma and disease.[54] As an NMDA antagonist, HU-211 blocks the damaging action of glutamate and other endogenous neurotoxic agents.[52,55] After having been studied in the United Kingdom in Phase I clinical trials, HU-211 progressed to Phase II clinical trials in Israel for treatment of severe closed-head trauma (Knoller et al., 1998).[35]

Market Prospects

It is difficult to gauge the market prospects for new cannabinoids. There certainly appears to be scientific interest, particularly for the discovery of new cannabinoids, but whether this interest can be sustained commercially through the arduous course of drug development is an open question. Research and development experience is limited; only one cannabinoid, dronabinol, is commercially available, and most of its research and development costs were shouldered by the federal government. Furthermore, the size of dronabinol's market (at about $20 million) is modest by pharmaceutical company standards. None of the other cannabinoids in development has reached clinical testing in the United States. Their scientific, regulatory, and commercial fates are likely to be very important in shaping future investment patterns. Experience with the drug scheduling process also is likely to be watched very carefully. If the early products are heavily regulated in the absence of strong abuse liability, future development might be deterred. For the present, what seems to be clear from the dearth of products in development and the small size of the companies sponsoring them is that cannabinoid development is seen as especially risky.

One scenario is that cannabinoids will be pursued for lucrative markets that reflect large unmet medical needs. Of the therapeutic needs for which cannabinoid receptor agonists have been tested, analgesia is by far the largest. The annual U.S. prescription and over-the-counter analgesic market in 1997 was $4.4 billion.[49] Given the long-standing need for less addictive, safer, easier to use, and more effective drugs for acute and chronic pain, it would not be surprising to see cannabinoids developed to treat some segments of the current analgesic market, if their safety and effectiveness were clearly established in clinical trials.

In addition to cannabinoid receptor agonists, two classes of cannabinoid-related drugs might prove therapeutically useful: cannabinoid antagonists and inverse agonists, compounds that bind to receptors but produce effects opposite those of agonists. Neither would be subject to the same scheduling concerns as cannabinoid agonists because they are not found in marijuana and would be highly unlikely to have any abuse potential. Another set of cannabinoid-related drugs, such as those that affect the synthesis, uptake, or inactivation of endogenous cannabinoids might, however, have abuse potential because they would influence the signal strength of endogenous cannabinoids.

The development of specific cannabinoid antagonists, like SR141716A for CB_1 receptors and SR144528 for CB_2 receptors, has provided a substantial impetus to understand cannabinoid actions. Those compounds block many of the effects of THC in animals, and their testing in humans has just begun. Cannabinoid antagonists have physiological effects on their own, in the absence of THC. They might have important therapeutic potential in a variety of clinical situations. For example, THC reduces short-term memory, so it is possible that a CB_1 antagonist like SR141716A could act as a memory-enhancing agent. Similarly, for conditions in which cannabinoids decrease immune function (presumably by binding to CB_2 receptors in immune cells), a CB_2 antagonist might be useful as an immune stimulant.

Cannabinoid inverse agonists would exert effects opposite those of THC and might thus cause appetite loss, short-term memory enhancement, nausea, or anxiety. Those effects could possibly be separated by molecular design, in which case inverse agonists might have some therapeutic value. One report has been published suggesting that the CB_1 receptor antagonist, SR141617A,[11] is an inverse agonist, and there will likely be others.

REGULATION OF AND MARKET OUTLOOK FOR MARIJUANA

Marijuana is not legally marketed in the United States.* No sponsor has ever sought marketing approval from the FDA for medical use of marijuana. One sponsor has an IND for a clinical safety study on HIV anorexia (D. Abrams, University of California at San Francisco, personal communication, 1998). Another has an IND pending for the treatment of migraine headaches (E. Russo, Western Montana Clinic, personal communication, 1998). Since 1970, marijuana's manufacture and distribution have been tightly restricted under the CSA, which places marijuana in Schedule I, which is reserved for drugs or other substances with "a high potential for abuse," "no currently accepted medical use," and "lack of accepted safety for use . . . under medical supervision" (21 U.S.C. § 812 (b)(1)).

Marijuana has remained in Schedule I despite persistent efforts at rescheduling since the 1970s by advocacy groups, such as NORML. Through petitions to the DEA, advocacy groups contend that marijuana does not fit the legal criteria for a Schedule I substance, owing to its purported medical uses and lack of high abuse liability.[3,4,48] Another rescheduling petition, which was filed in 1995, is being evaluated by the FDA and DEA.

Availability for Research

To use marijuana for research purposes, researchers must register with the DEA, as well as adhere to other relevant requirements of the CSA and other federal statutes, such as the FD&C act. The National Institute on Drug Abuse (NIDA), one of the institutes of NIH, is the only organization in the United States licensed by the DEA to manufacture and distribute marijuana for research purposes. NIDA performs this function under its Drug Supply Program.† Through this program, NIDA arranges for marijuana, to be grown and processed through contracts with two organizations: the University of Mississippi and the Research Triangle Institute. The University of Mississippi grows, harvests, and dries marijuana; and the institute processes it into cigarettes. A researcher can obtain marijuana free of charge from NIDA through an NIH-approved research grant to investigate marijuana, or through a separate protocol review.[39] Research grant approvals are handled through the conventional NIH peer review

---

*Under the CSA, its only legal use is in research under strictly defined conditions.

†This is also the program through which several patients receive marijuana under a compassionate use program monitored by the FDA. For history and information on this effort, see Randall (1993).[48]

process for extramural research, a highly competitive process with a success rate in 1997 of 32% of approved NIDA grants.[41] Through the separate protocol review, in which a researcher funds research independently of an NIH grant, NIDA submits the researcher's protocol to several external reviewers who evaluate the protocol on the basis of scientific merit and relevance to the mission of NIDA and NIH.

Through those two avenues marijuana has been supplied to several research groups—most of those that apply. While there has been much discussion of NIDA's alleged failure to supply marijuana for research purposes, we are unaware of recent cases in which they failed to supply marijuana to an investigator with an NIH-approved grant for research on marijuana. Donald Abrams's difficulty in obtaining research funding and marijuana from NIDA has been much discussed,[2] but the case of a single individual should not be presumed to be representative of the community of marijuana researchers. Failure of investigators who apply to NIH for marijuana research grants to receive funding is hardly exceptional: in 1998 less than 25% of *all* first-time investigator-initiated grant applications (known as RO1s) to the NIH were funded.[38]

To import marijuana under the CSA for research purposes, the procedures are more complex. Under DEA regulations, marijuana can be imported, provided that the researcher is registered with the DEA, has approval for marijuana research (21 CFR § 1301.11, .13, and .18), and has a DEA-approved permit for importation (21 CFR § 1312.11, .12, and .13), and that the exporter in the foreign country has appropriate authorization by the country of exportation. Importation would enable U.S. researchers to conduct research on marijuana grown by HortaPharm, a company that has developed unique strains of marijuana. However, no U.S. researcher has imported HortaPharm's marijuana because Dutch authorities have refused to issue an export permit, despite the issuance of an import permit by the DEA (D. Pate, HortaPharm, personal communication, 1998).*

HortaPharm, which is in the Netherlands, grows marijuana as a raw material for the manufacture of pharmaceuticals. Through selective breeding and controlled production, HortaPharm has developed marijuana strains that feature single cannabinoids, such as THC or cannabidiol. The plants contain a consistently "clean" phytochemical profile and a higher

---

*It might eventually be possible to import HortaPharm's marijuana from England, where HortaPharm is growing its marijuana strains for research use in clinical trials for multiple sclerosis (Boseley, 1998).[10] England, as the country of origin, would have to provide appropriate authorization for export of the strains to the United States. Permission to export for research purposes is part of the basis for HortaPharm's participation in this project with GW Pharmaceuticals through a special set of licenses with the British Home Office (David Pate, HortaPharm, personal communication, 1998).

concentration of THC (16%) or other desired cannabinoids than seized marijuana. Marijuana seized in the United States in 1996 had a THC content averaging about 5%.[16] Consistency of THC content is desirable because it overcomes the natural variability due to latitude, weather, and soil conditions. Product consistency is a basic tenet of pharmacology because it enables standardized dosing for regulatory and treatment purposes.

The difficulties of conducting research on marijuana were noted in the 1997 NIH report[40] that recommended that NIH facilitate clinical research by developing a centralized mechanism to promote design, approval, and conduct of clinical trials.

Regulatory Hurdles to Market

For marijuana to be marketed legally in the United States, a sponsor with sufficient resources would be obliged to satisfy the regulatory requirements of both the FD&C act and the CSA.

Under the FD&C act, a botanical product like marijuana *theoretically* might be marketed in oral form as a dietary supplement;* however, as a practical matter, only a new drug approval is likely to satisfy the provisions of the CSA, which require prescribing and distribution controls on drugs of abuse that also have an "accepted medical use." (The final paragraphs of this section clarify the criteria for "accepted medical use.")

Bringing marijuana to market as a new drug is uncharted terrain. The route is fraught with uncertainty for at least three pharmacological reasons: marijuana is a botanical product, it is smoked, and it is a drug with abuse potential. In general, botanical products are inherently more difficult to bring to market than are single chemical entities because they are complex mixtures of active and inactive ingredients. Concerns arise about product consistency, potency of the active ingredients, contamination, and stability of both active and inactive ingredients over time. These are among the concerns that a sponsor would have to overcome to meet the requirements for an NDA, especially those related to safety and to chemistry, manufacturing, and control.

A handful of botanical preparations are on the market, but none received formal approval as a new drug by today's standards of safety and efficacy (FDA, Center for Drug Evaluation and Research, personal communication, 1998). The three marketed botanical preparations are older drugs that came to market years before safety and efficacy studies were required by legislative amendments in 1938 and 1962, respectively.

---

*Inhaled products may not lawfully be marketed as dietary supplements.

One of the botanical preparations is the prescription product digitalis. Because it came to market before 1938, it is available today, having been "grandfathered" under the law; but it does not necessarily meet contemporary standards for safety and effectiveness.[20] Two other botanical preparations, psyllium and senna, came to market between 1938 and 1962. Drugs entering the market during that period were later required to be evaluated by the FDA in what is known as the over-the-counter drug review process,[20] through which psyllium and senna were found to be generally recognized as safe and effective and so were allowed to remain on the market as over-the-counter drugs.* Although no botanical preparations have been approved as new drugs, it is important to point out that a number of individual plant constituents, either extracted or synthesized *de novo*, have been approved (for example, taxol and morphine). But these drug approvals were for single constituents rather than botanical preparations themselves. The FDA is developing guidance for industry to explain how botanicals are reviewed as new drugs, but the final document might not be available before 1999.

That marijuana is smoked might pose an even greater regulatory challenge. The risks associated with smoking marijuana are described in chapter 2. The FDA would have to weigh those risks with marijuana's therapeutic benefits to arrive at a judgment about whether a sponsor's NDA for marijuana met the requirements for safety and efficacy under the FD&C act. Marijuana delivered in a novel way that avoids smoking would overcome some, but not all, of the regulatory concerns. Vaporization devices that permit inhalation of plant cannabinoids without the carcinogenic combustion products found in smoke are under development by several groups; such devices would also require regulatory review by the FDA.

The regulatory hurdles to market posed by the CSA are formidable but not insurmountable. If marijuana received market approval as a drug by the FDA, it would most likely be rescheduled under the CSA, as was the case for dronabinol. That is because a new drug approval satisfies the "accepted medical use" requirement under the CSA for manufacture and distribution in commerce.[13] But a new drug approval is not the *only* means to reschedule marijuana under the CSA.[14] For years advocates for rescheduling have argued that marijuana does enjoy "accepted medical use," even in the absence of a new drug approval. Although advocates have been unsuccessful in rescheduling efforts, their actions prompted

---

*Over-the-counter monographs for these products have been issued as tentative final monographs (proposed rules) but have not yet been issued in final form as final rules (FDA, Center for Drug Evaluation and Research, personal communication, 1998).

the DEA to specify the criteria by which it would determine whether a substance had "accepted medical use." In the DEA's 1992 denial of a re-scheduling petition, it listed these elements as constituting "accepted medical use": the drug's chemistry must be known and reproducible, there must be adequate safety studies, there must be adequate and well-controlled studies proving efficacy, the drug must be accepted by quali-fied experts, and the scientific evidence must be widely available.[14]

Assuming that all of those criteria were satisfied, marijuana could be rescheduled—but into which schedule? The level of scheduling would be dictated primarily by a medical and scientific recommendation to the DEA made by the secretary of DHHS.* As noted earlier, this recommendation is determined by the five scheduling criteria listed in the CSA. However, scheduling in a category less restrictive than Schedule II might be prohib-ited by international treaty obligations. The Single Convention on Nar-cotic Drugs, a treaty ratified by the United States in 1967, restricts sched-uling of the plant and its resin to at least Schedule II (the more restrictive Schedule I is another option).[13]

Market Outlook

The market outlook for the development of marijuana as a new drug, on the basis of the foregoing analysis, is not favorable, for a host of scien-tific, regulatory, and commercial reasons. From a scientific point of view, research is difficult because of the rigors of obtaining an adequate supply of legal, standardized marijuana for study. Further scientific hurdles are related to satisfying the exacting requirements for FDA approval of a new drug. The hurdles are even more exacting for a botanical product because of the inherent problems with, for example, purity and consistency. Fi-nally, the health risks associated with smoking pose another barrier to FDA approval unless a new smoke-free route of administration is demon-strated to be safe. Depending on the route of administration, an addi-tional overlay of regulatory requirements might have to be satisfied.

From a commercial point of view, uncertainties abound. The often-cited cost of new drug development, about $200–$300 million, might not apply, but there are probably additional costs needed to satisfy the FDA's requirements for a botanical product. As noted above, no botanical prod-ucts have ever been approved as new drugs by the FDA under today's stringent standards for safety and efficacy. Satisfying the legal require-

---

*At present, there is no practical mechanism for generating such a recommendation out-side the new drug approval process, although such a mechanism could, theoretically, be developed.[33]

ments of the CSA also will add substantially to the cost of development. On the positive side, so much research already has been done that some development costs will be lower. The cost of bringing dronabinol to market, for example, was reduced dramatically as a result of clinical trials supported with government funding. Nevertheless, it is impossible to estimate the cost of developing marijuana as a new drug. Estimating return on investment is similarly difficult. A full-fledged market analysis would be required for the indication being sought. Such an analysis would take into account the market limitations resulting from drug scheduling restrictions, stigma, and patentability.

The plant does not constitute patentable subject matter under U.S. patent law because it is unaltered from what is found in nature. So-called products of nature are not generally patentable.[28] New marijuana strains, however, could be patentable in the United States under a product patent or a plant patent because they *are* altered from what is found in nature. (A product patent prohibits others from manufacturing, using, or selling each strain for 20 years; a plant patent carries somewhat less protection.) HortaPharm has not yet sought any type of patent for its marijuana strains in the United States, but it has received approval for a plant registration in Europe (David Watson, HortaPharm, personal communication, 1998).

In short, development of the marijuana plant is beset by substantial scientific, regulatory, and commercial obstacles and uncertainties. The prospects for its development as a new drug are unfavorable unless return on investment is not a driving force. It is noteworthy that no pharmaceutical firm has sought to bring it to market in the United States. The only interest in its development appears to be in England in a small pharmaceutical firm (see Boseley, 1998[10]) and in the United States among physicians without formal ties to pharmaceutical firms (D. Abrams, University of California at San Francisco, and E. Russo, Western Montana Clinic, personal communications, 1998).

CONCLUSIONS

Cannabinoids are an interesting group of compounds with potentially far-reaching therapeutic applications. There is a surge of scientific interest in their development as new drugs, but the road to market for any new drug is expensive, long, risky, and studded with scientific, regulatory, and commercial obstacles. Experience with the only approved cannabinoid, dronabinol, might not illuminate the pathway because of the government's heavy contribution to research and development, dronabinol's scheduling history, and its small market.

There appear to be only two novel cannabinoids actively being developed for human use, but they have yet to be tested in humans in the

United States. Their experience is likely to be more predictive of the marketing prospects for other cannabinoids. It is too early to forecast the prospects for cannabinoids, other than to note that their development at this point is considered to be especially risky, to judge by the paucity of products in development and the small size of the pharmaceutical firms sponsoring them.

The market outlook in the United States is distinctly unfavorable for the marijuana plant and for cannabinoids found in the plant. Commercial interest in bringing them to market appears nonexistent. Cannabinoids in the plant are automatically placed in the most restrictive schedule of the Controlled Substances Act, and this is a substantial deterrent to development. Not only is the plant itself subject to the same scheduling strictures as are individual plant cannabinoids, but development of marijuana also is encumbered by a constellation of scientific, regulatory, and commercial impediments to availability.

REFERENCES

1. Abrahamov A, Abrahamov A, Mechoulam R. 1995. An efficient new cannabinoid antiemetic in pediatric oncology. *Life Sciences* 56:2097–2102.
2. Abrams DI. 1998. Medical marijuana: Tribulations and trials. *Journal of Psychoactive Drugs* 30:163–169.
3. AMA (American Medical Association Council on Scientific Affairs). 1997. *Report to the AMA House of Delegates.* Chicago: AMA.
4. Annas GJ. 1997. Reefer madness—the federal response to California's medical-marijuana law. *The New England Journal of Medicine* 337:435–439.
5. Arno PS, Bonuck K, Davis M. 1995. Rare diseases, drug development, and AIDS: The impact of the Orphan Drug Act. *Milbank Quarterly* 73:231–252.
6. Asbury C. 1991. The Orphan Drug Act: The first seven years. *Journal of the American Medical Association* 265:893–897.
7. Atlantic Pharmaceuticals. 1997. Atlantic Pharmaceuticals' proprietary compound shows promising anti-inflammatory effects in pre-clinical trials [WWW document]. URL http://www.atlan.com/p-11-10-97ct3zurier.htm (accessed September 1998).
8. Beal JE, Olson RLL, Morales JO, Bellman P, Yangco B, Lefkowitz L, Plasse TF, Shepard KV. 1995. Dronabinol as a treatment for anorexia associated with weight loss in patients with AIDS. *Journal of Pain and Symptom Management* 10:89–97.
9. Beal JE, Olson R, Lefkowitz L, Laubenstein L, Bellman P, Yangco B, Morales JO, Murphy R, Powderly W, Plasse TF, Mosdell KW, Shepard KV. 1997. Long-term efficacy and safety of dronabinol for acquired immunodeficiency syndrome-associated anorexia. *Journal of Pain and Symptom Management* 14:7–14.
10. Boseley S. 1998. Multiple sclerosis victims to test medicinal effects of marijuana [WWW document].URL http://www.anomalous-images/news/news/227.HTML (accessed September 8, 1998).

11. Bouaboula M, Perrachon S, Milligan L, Canat X, Rinaldi-Carmona M, Portier MB, Calandra B, Pecceu F, Lupker J, Maffrand JP, Le Fur G, Casellas P. 1997. A selective inverse agonist for central cannabinoid receptor inhibits mitogen-activated protein kinase activation stimulated by insulin or insulin-like growth factor 1. Evidence for a new model of receptor/ligand interactions. *Journal of Biological Chemistry* 272:22330–22339.

12. Calhoun, SR, Galloway GP , Smith DE . 1998. Abuse potential of dronabinol (Marinol). *Journal of Psychoactive Drugs* 30:187–196.

13. Cooper RM. 1980. Therapeutic use of marijuana and heroin: The legal framework. *Food Drug Cosmetic Law Journal* 35:68–82.

14. DEA (Drug Enforcement Administration). 1992. Marijuana scheduling petition; denial of petition; remand. *Federal Register* 57:10499–10508.

15. DEA. 1998. Drugs of abuse [WWW document].URL http://www.usdoj.gov/dea/pubs/abuse/contents.htm (accessed September 1998).

16. DEA. 1996. The National Narcotics Intelligence Consumers Committee (NNICC) report [WWW document].URL www.usdoj.gov/dea/pubs/intel/nnicc97.htm (accessed September 1998).

17. DEA. 1998b. Rescheduling of synthetic dronabinol from Schedule II to Schedule III. *Federal Register* 63:59751–59753.

18. DiMasi JA, Brown JS, Lasagna L. 1996. An analysis of regulatory review times of supplemental indications for already-approved drugs: 1989–1994. *Drug Information Journal* 30:315–337.

19. DiMasi JA, Hanson RW, Grabowski HG, Lasagna L. 1995. Research and development costs for new drugs by therapeutic category: A study of the U.S. pharmaceutical industry. *PharmacoEconomics* 7:152–169.

20. FDA (Food and Drug Administration). 1990. *From Test Tube to Patient: New Drug Development in the United States.* Rockville, MD: U.S. Department of Health and Human Services.

21. FDA. 1997b. *Draft Guidelines for Research Involving the Abuse Liability Assessment of New Drugs.* Rockville, MD: U.S. Department of Health and Human Services. Division of Anesthetic, Critical Care and Addiction Drug Products.

22. FDA. 1997a. Center for Drug Evaluation and Research Fact Book [WWW document]. URL http://www.fda.gov/cder/homepage (accessed September 1998).

23. FDA. 1998a. Center for Drug Evaluation and Research Handbook [WWW document]. URL http://www.fda/cder/handbook.htm (accessed September 1998).

24a. FDA. 1998b. FDA proposes rules for dissemination information on off label uses (press release, June 5). Washington, DC: U.S. Department of Health and Human Services.

24. FDA. 1998c. Guidance for industry: Providing clinical evidence of effectiveness for human drugs and biological products. Center for Drug Evaluation and Research, Center for Biologics Evaluation and Research. May 1998 [WWW document].URL http://www.fda.gov/cder/guidance/1397fnl.pdf (accessed September 1998).

25. FDA. 1998d. Office of Orphan Products Development Program Overview [WWW document].URL http://www.fda.gov/orphan/DESIGNAT/recent.htm (accessed October 14, 1998).

26. Felder CC, Glass M. 1998. Cannabinoid receptors and their endogenous agonists. *Annual Reviews of Pharmacology and Toxicology* 38:179–200.

27. Glain SJ. 1998. I. *Wall Street Journal.*

28. Gollin MA. 1994. Patenting recipes from nature's kitchen: How can a naturally occurring chemical like taxol be patented? *Biotechnology (NY)* 12:406–407.

29. Hampson AJ, Grimaldi M, Axelrod J, Wink D. 1998. Cannabidiol and (–)delta-9-tetrahydrocannabinol are neuroprotective antioxidants. *Proceedings of the National Academy of Sciences USA* 95:8268–8273.
30. Howlett AC. 1995. Pharmacology of cannabinoid receptors. *Annual Review of Pharmacology and Toxicology* 35:607–634.
31. IOM (Institute of Medicine). 1990. *Modern Methods of Clinical Investigation.* Washington, DC: National Academy Press.
32. IOM. 1991. *Expanding Access to Investigational Therapies for HIV Infection and AIDS.* Washington, DC: National Academy Press.
33. IOM. 1995. *The Development of Medications for the Treatment of Opiate and Cocaine Addictions: Issues for the Government and Private Sector.* Washington, DC: National Academy Press.
34. IOM. 1996. *Pathways of Addiction: Opportunities in Drug Abuse Research.* Washington, DC: National Academy Press.
35. Knoller N, Levi L, Israel Z, Razon N, Reichental E, Rappaport Z, Ehrenfreund N, Biegon A. Safety and outcome in a Phase II clinical trail of dexanabinol in severe head trauma. Congress of Neurological Surgeons Annual Meeting. Seattle, WA, Oct. 7, 1998.
36. Mechoulam R, Hanus L, Fride E. 1998. Towards cannabinoid drugs—revisited. In: Ellis GP, Luscombe DK, Oxford AW, Editors, *Progress in Medicinal Chemistry.* vol. 35. Amsterdam: Elsevier Science. Pp. 199–243.
37. Nainggolan L. 1997. Marijuana—a missed market opportunity? *Scrip Magazine.*
38. National Institutes of Health (NIH). 1999. http://www.nih.gov/grants/award/award.htm.
39. NIDA (National Institute on Drug Abuse). 1996. *Research Resources: Drug Supply System, 10th Edition.* Rockville, MD.
40. NIH (National Institutes of Health). 1997. Workshop on the Medical Utility of Marijuana. Report to the Director, National Institutes of Health by the Ad Hoc Group of Experts. Bethesda, MD, February 19–20, 1997. Bethesda, MD: National Institutes of Health.
41. NIH. 1998. FY (1970–1997 NIH (Preliminary) competing research project applications [WWW document].URL http:/silk.nih.gov/public/cbz2rfm.@www.comic.dsncc (accessed October 1998).
42. Ohlsson A, Lindgren JE, Wahlen A, Agurell S, Hollister LE, Gillespie HK. 1980. Plasma delta-9-tetrahydrocannabinol concentrations and clinical effects after oral and intravenous administration and smoking. *Clinical Pharmacology and Therapeutics* 28:409–416.
43. OTA (Office of Technology Assessment). 1991. *Biotechnology in a Global Economy.* OTA-BA-494. Washington, DC: U.S. Government Printing Office.
44. OTA. 1993. *Pharmaceutical R&D: Costs, Risks and Rewards.* OTA-H-522. Washington, DC: U.S. Government Printing Office.
45. PDR (Physicians' Desk Reference). 1996. *Physicians' Desk Reference.* 50th ed. Montvale, NJ: Medical Economics Co.
46. Pertwee RG. 1997. Cannabis and cannabinoids: Pharmacology and rationale for clinical use. *Pharmaceutical Science* 3:539–545.
47. Plasse TF, Gorter RW, Krasnow SH, Lane M, Shepard KV, Wadleigh RG. 1991. Recent clinical experience with dronabinol. *Pharmacology Biochemistry and Behavior* 40:695–700.
48. Randall IV B. 1993. *Medical Use of Marijuana: Policy and Regulatory Issues.* 93-308 SPR. Washington, DC: Congressional Research Service.

49. Schmidt WK. 1998. Overview of current investigational drugs for the treatment of chronic pain. National Managed Health Care Congress, Second Annual Conference on Therapeutic Developments in Chronic Pain. Annapolis, MD, May 18, 1998.

50. Shapiro RS. 1994. Legal bases for the control of analgesic drugs. *Journal of Pain and Symptom Management* 9:153–159.

51. Shen M, Piser TM, Seybold VS, Thayer SA. 1996. Cannabinoid receptor agonists inhibit glutamatergic synaptic transmission in rat hippocampal cultures. *Journal of Neuroscience* 16:4322–4334.

52. Shohami E, Weidenfeld J, Ovadia H, Vogel Z, Hanus L, Fride E, Breuer A, Ben-Shabat S, Sheskin T, Mechoulam R. 1996. Endogenous and synthetic cannabinoids: Recent advances. *CNS Drug Reviews* 2:429–451.

53. Spilker B. 1989. *Multinational Drug Companies: Issues in Drug Discovery and Development.* New York: Raven Press.

54. Standaert DG, Young AB. 1996. Treatment of central nervous system degenerative disorders. In: Hardman JG, Limbird LE, Molinoff PB, Ruddon RR, Gilman AG, Editors, *Goodman & Gilman's: The Pharmacological Basis of Therapeutics.* 9th ed. New York: McGraw-Hill. Pp. 503–519.

55. Striem S, Bar-Joseph A, Berkovitch Y, Biegon A. 1997. Interaction of dexanabinol (HU-211), a novel NMDA receptor antagonist, with the dopaminergic system. *European Journal of Pharmacology* 388:205–213.

56. Timpone JG, Wright DJ, Li N, Egorin MJ, Enama ME, Mayers J, Galetto G, DATRI 004 Study Group. 1997. The safety and pharmacokinetics of single-agent and combination therapy with megestrol acetate and dronabinol for the treatment of HIV wasting syndrome. The DATRI 004 study group. *AIDS Research and Human Retroviruses* 13:305–315.

57. Turk DC, Brody MC, Akiko OE. 1994. Physicians' attitudes and practices regarding the long-term prescribing of opioids for non-cancer pain. *Pain* 59:201–208.

58. Volicer L, Stelly M, Morris J, McLaughlin J, Volicer BJ. 1997. Effects of dronabinol on anorexia and disturbed behavior in patients with Alzheimer's disease. *International Journal of Geriatric Psychiatry* 12:913–919.

59. Voth EA, Schwartz RH. 1997. Medicinal applications of delta-9-tetrahydrocannabinol and marijuana. *Annals of Internal Medicine* 126:791–798.

60. Wall ME, Sadler BM, Brine D, Taylor H, Perez-Reyes M. 1983. Metabolism, disposition, and kinetics of delta-9-tetrahydrocannabinol in men and women. *Clinical Pharmacology and Therapeutics* 34:352–363.

61. Zurier RB, Rossetti RG, Lane JH, Goldberg JM, Hunter SA, Burstein SH. 1998. Dimethylheptyl-THC-11 oic acid: A non-psychoactive antiinflammatory agent with a cannabinoid template structure. *Arthritis and Rheumatism* 41:163–170.

Appendixes

APPENDIX A
Individuals and Organizations That Spoke or Wrote to the Institute of Medicine About Marijuana and Medicine

Donald I. Abrams
University of California at San
    Francisco

Jill Aguilera
Colorado Federation of Parents

William F. Alden
D.A.R.E. America

Roger D. Anderson
Anderson Clinical Research

M. Douglas Anglin
UCLA Drug Abuse Research
    Center

Dave Baleria
Jackson County Sheriff's Office

Joe Barker

Frank Bartosic
Minister of Universal Life
    Church

Dana Beal
Cures Not Wars

J. Bellam
Center for Drug Information

Sandra S. Bennett
Northwest Center for Health and
    Safety

Anna T. Boyce
California Senior Legislature
    (Prop 215)

William Britt

Richard Brookhiser
National Review

Ronald Brooks
California Narcotic Officers
    Association

Bonnie Broussard
L.A. Takes a Stand, Inc.

Al Byrne
Patients Out of Time

Marvin Edward Chavez, Sr.
O.C. Patient-Doctor-Nurse
    Support Group Cannabis
    Co-Op

Steven Childers
Bowman Gray School of
    Medicine
Wake Forest University

Barb Christensen
Prevention Partners

Gale Cincotta
National People's Action

Carol Coburn
Prevention Partners

Chris Conrad
Author of *Hemp for Health*

Paul Consroe
University of Arizona

J. Richard Crout
Private Consultant

Judy Cushing
Oregon Partnership, National
    Family Partnership

John De Miranda
Peninsula Health Concepts

Mahendra Dedhiya
Roxane Laboratories, Inc.

Robert Deitch
Cannabis Freedom Fund

Philip Diaz
Physicians for Prevention

Stephen L. Dilts
American Academy of Addiction
    Psychiatry

Rick Doblin
MAPS and Kennedy School of
    Government

Del Dolton

Barbara Douglass

Drug-Free Youth—USA

Robert Dudley
UNIMED

Victoria Duran
National Parents and Teachers
    Association

David Edwards

Edward Ehman
Certified Prevention Specialist

Mahmoud ElSohly
University of Mississippi

Mouncey Ferguson

Howard L. Fields
University of California at San
    Francisco

Jody Fitt

Richard W. Foltin
Columbia University

Etienne Fontan
Cannabis Alliance of Veterans,
1st CAV

Meg Foster

Phyllis Gardner
ALZA Corporation

Charles V. Giannasio
American Academy of Addiction
Psychiatry

Dale Gieringer
California NORML, Friends of
215

Mark Gold
University of Florida Brain
Institute

Richard Gralla
OCHSNER Cancer Institute

Linda Hall
Pride, Omaha, Inc.

Margaret Haney
Columbia University

Ann Hansen
Michigan Communities in Action
for Drug-Free Youth

Jim Hardin

Terry Hensley
Drug-Free America Foundation

Kimberly Hessel
American Cancer Society and
Muscatine General Hospital

Michele Hodak
National Education Association

Leo Hollister
Harris County Psychiatric Center

Jennifer Hudson
Oregonians Against Dangerous
Drugs

Paul Isford

Becki Jelinek
Family Service/South Omaha
Counseling

Jeffery Jones
Oakland Cannabis Buyers'
Cooperative

Linda R. Wolf Jones
Therapeutic Communities of
America

Norbert E. Kaminski
Michigan State University

Robert Kampia
Marijuana Policy Project

Paul L. Kaufman
University of Wisconsin Medical
School

Andrew Kinnon

Thomas Klein
University of South Florida
College of Medicine

Audra Koerber
Orange County Patient, Doctor,
Nurse Support Group

Ellen Komp
San Luis Obispo Citizens for
    Medical Marijuana

George Koob
Scripps Research Institute

Thomas R. Kosten
American Academy of Addiction
    Psychiatry

Donald Kotler
St. Luke's-Roosevelt Hospital

Michael Krawitz
Disabled American Veterans,
    American Legion

Kiyoshi Kuromiya
Critical Path AIDS Project

Karin Kyles
Connecticut Communities for
    Drug-Free Youth, Inc.

Eric Larson
University of Washington
    Medical Center

Linda B. Ledger
O. J. Federation for Drug-Free
    Communities

Carla Lowe

Ray Lozano
C.A.D.F.Y.

Patrick Magee
Orange County Hemp Council

Robert L. Maginnis
Family Research Council

Billy R. Martin
Virginia Commonwealth
    University

Mary Lynn Mathre
Patients Out of Time

Jeane McCarty
West Coast Neonatology

Todd McCormick

JoAnna McKee
Green Cross Patient Co-Op

Manon McKinnon
Empower America

George McMahon

Peter McWilliams

John Edward Mendelson
University of California at
    San Francisco

Bonnie Metcalf
Yuba County Compassionate Use
    Co-Op

R. Mikin
American Academy of Addiction
    Psychiatry

Alan D. Miller
The Rockefeller University

Jim Montgomery

John P. Morgan
City University of New York
    Medical School

Arlene Munoz
Office of Substance Abuse,
San Joaquin County

Elvy Musikka

Richard E. Musty
University of Vermont

Edgar P. Nace
American Academy of Addiction
Psychiatry

Joyce Nalepka
America Cares

Tammera Nauts
Great Falls Public Schools

Dan Noelle
Multnomah County Sheriff

Stephen O'Brien
East Bay Aids Center

Jerry Olli
Michigan Elks and Michigan
Communities in Action for
Drug-Free Youth

Lynn Osburn
Access Unlimited

Robert Pandina
Rutgers, The State University of
New Jersey

David Pate
HortaPharm B.V.

Maggie Petito
Drug Watch International

Stephen Popolizio
The International Association of
Lions Clubs

Jo Prang
NFP Networker (Oregon
Partnership)
Adolescent Substance Abuse
Prevention, Inc./MEDICAP
Pharmacy

Beny Primm
Addiction Research and
Treatment Corporation

Carol Reeves
Greenville Family Partnership

Irvin Rosenfeld
Stockbroker

Michael Rowbotham
University of California at
San Francisco

A. Kenison Roy
American Society of Addiction

Reid Rubsamen
Aradigm

Sue Rusche
National Families in Action

Clara Sanudo-Pena
Brown University

Peggy Sapp
Informed Families

C. Robert Schuster
Wayne State University School of
Medicine

Greg Scott

Richard Scribner
Louisiana State University
    Medical School

Betty S. Sembler
S.O.S.

Richard W. Sharke
McDowell Drug Task Force/
    CADCA

Lynette Shaw
Marin Alliance for Medical
    Marijuana

John Sheridan
New York City Marijuana
    Buyers' Club

Cathy Shipp
PRIDE-Omaha, Inc.

Stephen Sidney
Kaiser Permanente

Brian Slater

Kenneth Smuland
Women's Alliance for Medical
    Marijuana

Mark Stone
Washington, D.C., Police
    Department

Barb Sweeney
Flower Therapy

Donald Tashkin
University of California at Los
    Angeles School of Medicine

Dana Taub

Chuck Thomas
Marijuana Policy Project
    Foundation

Bill Tiuen
Gainesville Family Partnership

Joyce Tobias
Parents' Association to
    Neutralize Drug and Alcohol
    Abuse, Inc.

Jeanne Trumble
American Academy of Addiction
    Psychiatry

Barbara Urist-Fenton
OCHC

Eric A. Voth
International Drug Strategy
    Institute

Michelle Voth
Kansas Family Partnership

C. Gary Wainwright
American Civil Liberties Union

J. Michael Walker
Brown University

Gene Weeks
Southern California Medical
    Cannabis Consumers' Co-Op

Sandra Welch
Medical College of Virginia

Tracy Wells
Family Service–Healthy
  Alternatives for Little Ones

Sgt. Larry L. Welty
Oregon State Police

Sis Wenger
National Association of Children
  of Alcoholics

Lennice Werth
Virginians Against Drug
  Violence

Casey Wilbanks
Green Cross

Carol Wortman
Drug Watch Pennsylvania

Kevin Zeese
Common Sense for Drug Policy

Appendix B

Workshop Agendas

**Workshop on Perspectives on the Medical Use of Marijuana:
Basic and Clinical Science**

December 14–16, 1997
Beckman Center, Irvine, California

AGENDA

Sunday, December 14, 1997

2:00 p.m.   Introduction
Constance Pechura, *IOM Division Director,*
Neuroscience and Behavioral Health

2:30 p.m.   Public Input Session, *5 minutes per person*
Moderator: Stanley Watson, Jr., *IOM Study Investigator,*
University of Michigan

5:30 p.m.   ADJOURN

Monday, December 15, 1997

CANNABINOID NEUROSCIENCE

8:30 a.m. **Moderator:** Stanley Watson, *IOM Study Investigator,*
University of Michigan

8:45 a.m. **Neuropharmacology of Cannabinoids and Their Receptors**
Steven R. Childers, Wake Forest University School of
Medicine

9:15 a.m. **Precipitated Cannabinoid Withdrawal and Sensory
Processing of Painful Stimuli**
J. Michael Walker, Brown University

9:45 a.m. **Role of Cannabinoids in Movement**
Clara Sanudo, Brown University

10:15 a.m. **Tolerance and Cannabinoid-Opioid Interactions**
Sandra P. Welch, Medical College of Virginia

10:45 a.m. BREAK

MEDICAL USES OF MARIJUANA:
CLINICAL DATA AND BASIC BIOLOGY

11:10 a.m. **Moderator:** John A. Benson, Jr., *IOM Study Investigator,*
Oregon Health Sciences University

11:15 a.m. **Profile of Medical Marijuana Users**
John Mendelson, University of California at San Francisco

11:45 a.m. **Immune Modulation by Cannabinoids**
Norbert Kaminski, Michigan State University

12:15 p.m. **Psychological Effects of Marijuana Use**
Charles R. Schuster, Wayne State University

12:45 p.m. LUNCH

1:45 p.m.   **Marijuana and Glaucoma**
            Paul Kaufman, University of Wisconsin

2:15 p.m.   **Effects of Marijuana and Cannabinoids in Neurological Disorders**
            Paul Consroe, University of Arizona Health Sciences Center

2:45 p.m.   **Neural Mechanisms of Cannabinoid Analgesia**
            Howard Fields, University of California at San Francisco

3:15 p.m.   **Pain Management**
            Michael Rowbotham, University of California at San Francisco

3:45 p.m.   **Wasting Syndrome Pathogenesis and Clinical Markers**
            Donald Kotler, St. Luke's-Roosevelt Hospital

4:15 p.m.   **Clinical Experience with Marijuana**
            Stephen O'Brien, East Bay AIDS Center

4:45 p.m.   ADJOURN

Tuesday, December 16, 1997

MEDICAL USES OF MARIJUANA:
CLINICAL DATA AND BASIC BIOLOGY

8:30 a.m.   **Moderator:** John A. Benson, Jr., *IOM Study Investigator,* Oregon Health Sciences University

8:45 a.m.   **Marijuana in AIDS Wasting: Tribulations and Trials**
            Donald I. Abrams, University of California at San Francisco

9:15 a.m.   **Nausea and Vomiting: Underlying Mechanisms and Upcoming Treatments**
            Alan D. Miller, The Rockefeller University

9:45 a.m.   **Postchemotherapy Nausea and Antiemetics**
            Richard J. Gralla, Ochsner Cancer Center

10:15 a.m.   BREAK

SUMMARY VIEWS

10:30 a.m.   **Marijuana Is Different from THC: A Review of Basic
Research and State Studies of Antiemesis**
Richard E. Musty, University of Vermont

11:00 a.m.   **Medical Uses of Crude Marijuana: Medical and
Social Issues**
Eric A. Voth, The International Drug Strategy Institute

11:30 a.m.   **General Questions**
Moderator: John A. Benson, Jr., *IOM Study Investigator*

12:00 noon   ADJOURN

Workshop on
Acute and Chronic Effects of Marijuana Use

January 22–23, 1998
New Orleans Marriott Hotel
New Orleans, Louisiana

AGENDA

Thursday, January 22, 1998

2:00 p.m.   Introduction
             Constance Pechura, *IOM Division Director,*
             Neuroscience and Behavioral Health

2:30 p.m.   Public Input Session, *5 minutes per person*
             Moderator: Stanley Watson, Jr., *IOM Study Investigator,*
             University of Michigan

4:30 p.m.   ADJOURN

Friday, January 23, 1998

8:30 a.m.   **Moderator:** John A. Benson, Jr., *IOM Study Investigator,*
             Oregon Health Sciences University

HEALTH CONSEQUENCES OF MARIJUANA USE

9:00 a.m.   **Health Consequences of Marijuana Use: Epidemiological
             Studies**
             Stephen Sidney, Kaiser Permanente, Oakland, CA

9:30 a.m.   **Immunity, Infections, and Cannabinoids**
             Thomas Klein, University of South Florida

10:00 a.m.   **Pulmonary Effects of Smoked Marijuana**
             Donald Tashkin, Unversity of California at Los Angeles

10:30 a.m.   BREAK

10:45 a.m.   **Is Marijuana Carcinogenic?:   Epidemiological and Biological Evidence**

               Panel Discussion
                Stephen Sidney
                Donald Tashkin

12:00 noon   LUNCH

EFFECTS OF MARIJUANA ON BEHAVIOR

1:30 p.m.   **Marijuana: Addictive and Amotivational States, the Scientific Evidence**
John Morgan, City University of New York Medical School

2:00 p.m.   **Marijuana's Acute Behavioral Effects in Humans**
Richard Foltin, Columbia University

2:30 p.m.   **Tolerance and Dependence Following Chronic Administration of Oral THC or Smoked Marijuana to Humans**
Margaret Haney, Columbia University

3:00 p.m.   **Patterns of Continuity and Discontinuity of Marijuana Use in Relationship to Other Drugs**
Robert Pandina, Rutgers University

3:30 p.m.   ADJOURN

Workshop on Prospects for Cannabinoid Drug Development

February 23–24, 1998
National Academy of Sciences Building
Washington, D.C.

AGENDA

Monday, February 23, 1998

1:30 p.m.   Introduction
                Constance Pechura, *IOM Division Director,*
                Neuroscience and Behavioral Health

2:00 p.m.   Public Input Session, *5 minutes per person*
                Moderator: John A. Benson, Jr., *IOM Study Investigator,*
                Oregon Health Sciences University

5:30 p.m.   ADJOURN

Tuesday, February 24, 1998

8:30 a.m.   Introduction
                Constance Pechura, *IOM Division Director*
                Neuroscience and Behavioral Health

                Moderator: Stanley J. Watson, Jr., *IOM Study Investigator,*
                University of Michigan

OVERVIEWS OF PRECEDING WORKSHOPS

8:45 a.m.   **Acute and Chronic Effects of Marijuana**
                Billy R. Martin, Medical College of Virginia

9:25 a.m.   **Perspectives on the Medical Use of Marijuana**
                Eric B. Larson, University of Washington Medical School

9:55 a.m.   **The Neurobiology of Cannabinoid Dependence**
                George F. Koob, Scripps Research Institute

10:25 a.m.   BREAK

DRUG DEVELOPMENT

10:45 a.m. **Regulatory Requirements Affecting Marijuana**
J. Richard Crout, Crout Consulting

11:15 a.m. **Marinol and the Market**
Robert E. Dudley, Unimed Pharmaceuticals, Inc.

11:45 a.m. **Development of Cannabis-based Therapeutics**
Dave Pate, HortaPharm, B.V.

12:15 p.m. LUNCH

DRUG DELIVERY

1:30 p.m. **Alternative Drug Delivery Technologies for the Therapeutic Use of Marijuana**
Phyllis I. Gardner, ALZA Corporation, Stanford University

2:00 p.m. **Delivery of Analgesics via the Respiratory Track**
Reid M. Rubsamen, Aradigm Corporation

2:30 p.m. **Current Concepts for Delivery of THC**
Mahendra G. Dedhiya, Roxanne Laboratories, Inc.

3:00 p.m. **Δ^9-THC-Hemisuccinate in Suppository Formulation: An Alternative to Oral and Smoked THC**
Mahmoud A. ElSohly, University of Mississippi, ElSohly Laboratories, Inc.

3:30 p.m. **Concluding Remarks**
John A. Benson, Jr., *IOM Study Investigator*, Oregon Health Sciences University

3:45 p.m. ADJOURN

Appendix C

Scheduling Definitions

SCHEDULING DEFINITIONS ESTABLISHED BY THE CONTROLLED SUBSTANCES ACT OF 1970

Schedule I (includes heroin, LSD, and marijuana)

(A) The drug or other substance has a high potential for abuse.

(B) The drug or other substance has no currently accepted medical use in treatment in the United States.

(C) There is a lack of accepted safety for the use of the drug or other substance under medical supervision.

Schedule II (includes Marinol, methadone, morphine, methamphetamine, and cocaine)

(A) The drug or other substance has a high potential for abuse.

(B) The drug or other substance has a currently accepted medical use in treatment in the United States or a currently accepted medical use with severe restrictions.

(C) Abuse of the drug or other substances may lead to severe psychological or physical dependence.

Schedule III (includes anabolic steroids)

(A) The drug or other substance has a potential of abuse less than the drugs or other substances in Schedules I and II.

(B) The drug or other substance has a currently accepted medical use in treatment in the United States.

(C) Abuse of the drug or other substance may lead to moderate or low physical dependence or high psychological dependence.

Schedule IV (includes Valium and other tranquilizers)

(A) The drug or other substance has a low potential for abuse relative to the drugs or other substances in Schedule III.

(B) The drug or other substance has a currently accepted medical use in treatment in the United States.

(C) Abuse of the drug or other substance may lead to limited physical dependence or psychological dependence relative to the drugs or other substances in Schedule III.

Schedule V (includes codeine-containing analgesics)

(A) The drug or other substance has a low potential for abuse relative to the drugs or other substances in Schedule IV.

(B) The drug or other substance has a currently accepted medical use in treatment in the United States.

(C) Abuse of the drug or other substance may lead to limited physical dependence or psychological dependence relative to the drugs or other substances in Schedule IV.

SOURCES: LeCraw (1996) and 21 U.S.C. 812.

APPENDIX D

Statement of Task

The study will assess what is currently known and not known about the medical use of marijuana. It will include a review of the science base regarding the mechanism of action of marijuana, an examination of the peer-reviewed scientific literature on the efficacy of therapeutic uses of marijuana, and the costs of using various forms of marijuana versus approved drugs for specific medical conditions (e.g., glaucoma, multiple sclerosis, wasting diseases, nausea, and pain).

The study will also include an evaluation of the acute and chronic effects of marijuana on health and behavior; a consideration of the adverse effects of marijuana use compared with approved drugs; an evaluation of the efficacy of different delivery systems for marijuana (e.g., inhalation vs. oral); an analysis of the data concerning marijuana as a gateway drug; and an examination of the possible differences in the effects of marijuana due to age and type of medical condition.

SPECIFIC ISSUES

Specific issues to be addressed fall under three broad categories: the science base, therapeutic use, and economics.

Science Base

- Review of neuroscience related to marijuana, particularly the relevance of new studies on addiction and craving.
- Review of behavioral and social science base of marijuana use, par-

ticularly assessment of the relative risk of progression to other drugs following marijuana use.

• Review of the literature determining which chemical components of crude marijuana are responsible for possible therapeutic effects and for side effects.

Therapeutic Use

• Evaluation of any conclusions on the medical use of marijuana drawn by other groups.

• Efficacy and side effects of various delivery systems for marijuana compared to existing medications for glaucoma, wasting syndrome, pain, nausea, or other symptoms.

• Differential effects of various forms of marijuana that relate to age or type of disease.

Economics

• Costs of various forms of marijuana compared with costs of existing medications for glaucoma, wasting syndrome, pain, nausea, or other symptoms.

• Assessment of the differences between marijuana and existing medications in terms of access and availability.

These specific areas along with the assessments described above will be integrated into a broad description and assessment of the available literature relevant to the medical use of marijuana.

Recommendations Made in Recent Reports on the Medical Use of Marijuana

Recommendations from five recent key reports pertaining to the medical use of marijuana are listed below by subject. Recommendations made on issues outside the scope of this report, such as drug law and scheduling decisions, are not included here. The following reports were reviewed:

- Health Council of the Netherlands, Standing Committee on Medicine. 1996. *Marihuana as Medicine.* Rijswikj, the Netherlands: Health Council of the Netherlands.
- *Report of the Council on Scientific Affairs.* 1997. Report to the American Medical Association House of Delegates. Subject: Medical Marijuana. Chicago: AMA.
- British Medical Association. 1997. *Therapeutic Uses of Cannabis.* United Kingdom: Harwood Academic Publishers.
- National Institutes of Health. 1997. *Workshop on the Medical Utility of Marijuana.* Bethesda, MD: National Institutes of Health.
- World Health Organization. 1997. *Cannabis: A Health Perspective and Research Agenda.* Geneva: WHO.

In November 1998, the British House of Lords Science and Technology Committee published *Medical Use of Cannabis,* in which the committee reported its conviction that "cannabis almost certainly does have genuine medical applications." The House of Lords report was released too late in the preparation of the present Institute of Medicine report to permit careful analysis and is not summarized here. It is available on the Internet at: *www.parliament.uk.*

GENERAL RECOMMENDATIONS

Health Council of the Netherlands

In order to assess the efficacy of marijuana and cannabinoids, the committee studied literature published during the past 25 years. Based on those findings, the committee concluded that there was insufficient evidence to justify the medical use of marijuana.

AMA House of Delegates

Adequate and well-controlled studies of smoked marijuana should be conducted in patients who have serious conditions for which preclinical, anecdotal, or controlled evidence suggests possible efficacy, including AIDS wasting syndrome, severe acute or delayed emesis induced by chemotherapy, multiple sclerosis, spinal cord injury, dystonia, and neuropathic pain.

British Medical Association

Research on the clinical indications for medical prescription of cannabinoids should be undertaken. For all indications listed below (antiemetics, pain, epilepsy, glaucoma, asthma, immunological effects, multiple sclerosis, spinal cord injury, and other spastic disorders) further research is required to establish suitable methods of administration, optimal dosage regimens, and routes of administration. A central registry should be kept of patients prescribed cannabinoids so that the effects can be followed up over the long term.

National Institutes of Health

For at least some potential indications, marijuana looks promising enough to recommend that new controlled studies be done. The indications in which varying levels of interest were expressed are the following: appetite stimulation and wasting, chemotherapy-induced nausea and vomiting, neurological and movement disorders, analgesia, [and] glaucoma. Until studies are done using scientifically acceptable clinical trial design and subjected to appropriate statistical analysis, the question concerning the therapeutic utility of marijuana will likely remain largely unanswered. To the extent that the NIH can facilitate the development of a scientifically rigorous and relevant database, the NIH should do so.

World Health Organization

Therapeutic uses of cannabinoids warrant further basic pharmacological and experimental investigation and clinical research into their effectiveness. More research is needed on the basic neuropharmacology of THC and other cannabinoids so that better therapeutic agents can be found.

ANALGESIA

Health Council of the Netherlands

No recommendations made.

AMA House of Delegates

Controlled evidence does not support the view that THC or smoked marijuana offers clinically effective analgesia without causing significant adverse events when used alone. Preclinical evidence suggests that cannabinoids can potentiate opioid analgesia and that cannabinoids may be effective in animal models of neuropathic pain. Further research into the use of cannabinoids in neuropathic pain is warranted.

British Medical Association

The prescription of nabilone, THC, and other cannabinoids should be permitted for patients with intractable pain. Further research is needed into the potential of cannabidiol as an analgesic in chronic, terminal, and postoperative pain.

National Institutes of Health

Evaluation of cannabinoids in the management of neuropathic pain, including HIV-associated neuropathy, should be undertaken.

World Health Organization

No recommendations made, although the report notes that some newly synthesized cannabinoids are extremely potent analgesics; however, separation of the analgesia and side effects remains to be demonstrated.

NAUSEA AND VOMITING

Health Council of the Netherlands

No recommendations made.

AMA House of Delegates

THC and smoked marijuana are considerably less effective than currently available therapies to treat acute nausea and vomiting caused by chemotherapy, although certain patients still do not respond adequately to conventional therapy. Research involving THC and smoked marijuana should focus on their possible use in treating delayed nausea and vomiting and their adjunctive use in patients who respond inadequately to 5-HT_3 antagonists. The use of an inhaled substance has the potential to benefit ambulatory patients who are experiencing the onset of nausea and are thus unable to take oral medications.

British Medical Association

Further research is needed on the use of Δ^8-THC as an antiemetic, the use of cannabidiol in combination with THC, and the relative effectiveness of cannabinoids compared with 5-HT_3 antagonists. Further research is needed in other cases, such as postoperative nausea and vomiting.

National Institutes of Health

Inhaled marijuana merits testing in controlled, double-blind, randomized trials for nausea and vomiting.

World Health Organization

More basic research on the central and peripheral mechanisms of the effects of cannabinoids on gastrointestinal function may improve the ability to alleviate nausea and emesis.

WASTING SYNDROME AND APPETITE STIMULATION

Health Council of the Netherlands

No recommendations made.

AMA House of Delegates

THC is moderately effective in the treatment of AIDS wasting, but its long duration of action and intensity of side effects preclude routine use. The ability of patients who smoke marijuana to titrate their dosage according to need and the lack of highly effective, inexpensive options to treat this debilitating disease create the conditions warranting formal clinical trials of smoked marijuana as an appetite stimulant in patients with AIDS wasting syndrome.

British Medical Association

Allowing the prescription of nabilone and THC for cancer chemotherapy and HIV/AIDS seems justified for preventing weight loss and treating anorexia in HIV/AIDS irrespective of whether the patient is experiencing nausea and/or vomiting.

National Institutes of Health

Areas of study for the potential appetite-stimulating properties of marijuana include the cachexia of cancer, HIV/AIDS symptomatology, and other wasting syndromes. Investigations should be designed to assess long-term effects on immunology status, the rate of viral replication, and clinical outcomes in participants as well as weight gain. In therapeutic trials of cachexia, research should attempt to separate out the effect of marijuana on mood versus appetite. Some questions need to be answered in the studies: (1) Does smoking marijuana increase total energy intake in patients with catabolic illness? (2) Does marijuana use alter energy expenditure? (3) Does marijuana use alter body weight and to what extent? (4) Does marijuana use alter body composition and to what extent?

World Health Organization

No specific recommendations are made, although the report notes that dronabinol is an effective appetite stimulant for patients with AIDS wasting syndrome.

MUSCLE SPASTICITY

Health Council of the Netherlands

No recommendations made.

AMA House of Delegates

Considerably more research is required to identify patients who may benefit from THC or smoked marijuana and to establish whether responses are primarily subjective in nature. A therapeutic trial of smoked marijuana or THC may be warranted in patients with spasticity who do not derive adequate benefit from available oral medications, prior to their considering intrathecal baclofen therapy or neuroablative procedures.

British Medical Association

A high priority should be given to carefully controlled trials of cannabinoids in patients with chronic spastic disorders that have not responded to other drugs are indicated. In the meantime, there is a case for the extension of the indications for nabilone and THC for use in chronic spastic disorders unresponsive to standard drugs.

National Institutes of Health

No recommendations are made, although the report notes that marijuana or the use of other cannabinoids as human therapies might be considered for treating spasticity and nocturnal spasms complicating multiple sclerosis and spinal cord injury.

World Health Organization

The report notes that cannabinoids have not yet been proven useful in treating multiple sclerosis, but therapeutic uses of cannabinoids are being demonstrated by controlled studies as an antispasmodic. Research in this area should continue.

MOVEMENT DISORDERS

Health Council of the Netherlands

No recommendations made.

AMA House of Delegates

Considerably more research is required to identify dystonic patients who may benefit from THC or smoked marijuana and to establish whether responses are primarily subjective in nature.

British Medical Association

The potential of (+)-HU-210 for neruodegenerative disorders should be explored through further research.

National Institutes of Health

No recommendations made, although the report notes that marijuana or the use of other cannabinoids as human therapies might be considered for treating for some forms of dystonia.

World Health Organization

No recommendations made, although the report notes that cannabinoids have not yet been proven useful in the treatment of movement disorders.

EPILEPSY

Health Council of the Netherlands

No recommendations made.

AMA House of Delegates

No recommendations made.

British Medical Association

Trials with cannabidiol (which is nonpsychoactive), used to enhance the activity of other drugs in cases not well controlled by other anticonvulants, are needed.

National Institutes of Health

No recommendations made, although the report notes that marijuana or the use of other cannabinoids as human therapies might be considered for treating various active epilepsy states.

World Health Organization

No recommendations made, although the report notes that cannabinoids have not yet been proven useful in the treatment of convulsant disorders, but therapeutic uses of cannabinoids are being demonstrated by controlled studies as an anticonvulsant.

GLAUCOMA

Health Council of the Netherlands

No recommendations made.

AMA House of Delegates

Neither smoked marijuana nor THC is a viable approach in the treatment of glaucoma, but research on their mechanism of action may be important in developing new agents that act in an additive or synergistic manner with currently available therapies.

British Medical Association

Cannabinoids do not at present look promising for this indication, but much further basic and clinical research is needed to develop and investigate cannabinoids that lower intraocular pressure, preferably by topical application (e.g., eye drops, inhalant aerosols), without producing unacceptable systemic and central nervous system effects.

National Institutes of Health

Further studies to define the mechanism of action and to determine the efficacy of Δ^9-tetrahydrocannabinol and marijuana in the treatment of glaucoma are justified. There does not appear to be any obvious reason to use smoked marijuana as a primary "stand-alone" investigational therapy, as there are many available agents for treatment, and these topical preparations seem to be potentially ideal. An approach that may be useful is to study smoked marijuana in incomplete responders to standard therapies. The suggested design for clinical studies is to add marijuana, oral THC, or placebo to standard therapy under double-blind conditions: (1) Establish dose-response and dose-duration relationships for intraocular pressure

(IOP) and central nervous system effects. (2) Relate IOP and blood pressure measurements longitudinally to evaluate potential tolerance development to cardiovascular effects. (3) Evaluate central nervous system effects longitudinally for tolerance development.

World Health Organization

No recommendations made, although the report notes that, while THC has long been known to reduce the increased intraocular pressure of glaucoma, it has not been fully studied therapeutically. The report also notes that therapeutic uses of cannabinoids are being demonstrated by controlled studies in the treatment of glaucoma.

PHYSIOLOGICAL HARMS

Health Council of the Netherlands

No recommendations made.

AMA House of Delegates

No recommendations made.

British Medical Association

Further research is needed to establish the suitability of cannabinoids for immunocompromised patients, such as those undergoing cancer chemotherapy or those with HIV/AIDS.

National Institutes of Health

Risks associated with smoked marijuana must be considered not only in terms of immediate adverse effects but also long-term effects in patients with chronic diseases. The possibility that frequent and prolonged marijuana use might lead to clinically significant impairments of immune system function is great enough that relevant studies should be part of any marijuana medication development research.

Additional studies of long-term marijuana use are needed to determine if there are or are not important adverse pulmonary, central nervous system, or immune system problems.

World Health Organization

Further studies are needed on the fertility effects in cannabis users in view of the high rate of use during the early reproductive years. Further clinical and experimental research is required on the effects of cannabis on respiratory function and respiratory diseases. More studies are needed to show whether cannabis affects the risk of lung malignancies and at what level of use that may occur. In addition, more studies are needed to clarify the rather different results of pulmonary histopathological studies in animals and man.

More clinical and experimental research is needed on the effects of cannabis on immunological function. More clarity should be sought concerning the molecular mechanisms responsible for immune effects, including both cannabinoid receptor and nonreceptor events.

The possibility that chronic cannabis use has adverse effects on the cardiovascular system should have a priority in epidemiological research.

Research on chronic and residual cannabis effects is also needed. The pharmacokinetics of chronic cannabis use in humans are poorly described, and this lack of knowledge restricts the ability of researchers to relate drug concentrations in blood or other fluids and observed effects.

PSYCHOLOGICAL HARMS

Health Council of the Netherlands

No recommendations made.

AMA House of Delegates

No recommendations made.

British Medical Association

No recommendations made.

National Institutes of Health

No recommendations made.

World Health Organization

There is a need for controlled studies investigating the relationships between cannabis use, schizophrenia, and other serious mental disorders.

There is also a need for case-controlled studies comparing those experiencing cannabis problems with people who have, and do not have, alcohol and other psychoactive substance use problems.

There is a need for better delineation of the clinical features of cannabis dependence and for studies of its responsiveness to interventions aimed at assisting users to stop.

Insufficient research has been undertaken on the "amotivational" syndrome which may or may not result from heavy cannabis use. It is not clear that the syndrome exists, even though heavy cannabis use is sometimes associated with reduced motivation to succeed in school and work. New research is needed to show whether the reduced motivation seen in some cannabis users is due to other psychoactive substance use and whether it precedes cannabis use.

Further development of cognitive and psychomotor tests for controlled studies that are sensitive to the performance effects of cannabis use and that reflect the complexity of specific daily functions (e.g., driving, learning, reasoning) also need additional research.

More research is needed to examine the relationship between THC concentrations in blood and other fluids and the degree of behavioral impairment produced.

SMOKED MARIJUANA AND USE OF PLANTS AS MEDICINE

Health Council of the Netherlands

The committee believes that physicians cannot accept responsibility for a product of unknown composition that has not been subjected to quality control.

AMA House of Delegates

No specific recommendations made, but related issues are discussed in the general recommendation and drug development sections.

British Medical Association

Prescription formulations of cannabinoids or substances acting on the cannabinoid receptors should not include either cigarettes or herbal preparations with unknown concentrations of cannabinoids or other chemicals.

National Institutes of Health

Smoked marijuana should be held to standards equivalent to other medications for efficacy and safety considerations. There might be some patient populations for whom the inhalation route might offer advantages over the currently available capsule formulation. Smoking plant material poses difficulties in standardizing testing paradigms, and components of the smoke are hazardous, especially in the immunocompromised patient. Therefore, the experts generally favored the development of alternative dosage forms, including an inhaler dosage form into which a controlled unit dose of THC could be placed and volatilized.

World Health Organization

Not discussed in the context of medical use, although many health hazards associated with chronic marijuana smoking are noted.

DRUG DEVELOPMENT

Health Council of the Netherlands

Not discussed.

AMA House of Delegates

The National Institutes of Health should use its resources to support the development of a smoke-free inhaled delivery system for marijuana or THC to reduce the health hazards associated with the combustion and inhalation of marijuana.

British Medical Association

Pharmaceutical companies should undertake basic laboratory investigations and develop novel cannabinoid analogs that may lead to new clinical uses.

National Institutes of Health

NIH should use its resources and influence to rapidly develop a smoke-free inhaled delivery system for marijuana or THC. A recommendation was made for the development of insufflation/inhalation devices or dosage forms capable of delivering purer THC or cannabinoids to the lungs free of dangerous combustion byproducts.

World Health Organization

Not discussed.

Appendix F

Rescheduling Criteria

DRUG ENFORCEMENT AGENCY'S
FIVE-FACTOR TEST FOR RESCHEDULING*

1. The drug's chemistry must be known and reproducible.

The substance's chemistry must be scientifically established to permit it to be reproduced in dosages which can be standardized. The listing of the substance in a current edition of one of the official compendia, as defined by section 201(j) of the Food, Drug, and Cosmetic Act, 21 USC 321(f), is sufficient generally to meet this requirement.

2. There must be adequate safety studies.

There must be adequate pharmacological and toxicological studies done by all methods reasonably applicable on the basis of which it could be fairly and responsibly concluded, by experts qualified by scientific training and experience to evaluate the safety and effectiveness of drugs, that the substance is safe for treating a specific, recognized disorder.

3. There must be adequate and well-controlled studies proving efficacy.

There must be adequate, well-controlled, well-designed, well-conducted, and well-documented studies, including clinical investigations, by experts qualified by scientific training and experience to evaluate

---

*Formulated in 1992 in response to a court challenge to scheduling.

the safety and effectiveness of drugs on the basis of which it could fairly and responsibly be concluded by such experts that the substance will have its intended effect in treating a specific, recognized disorder.

4. The drug must be accepted by qualified experts.

The drug must have a New Drug Application (NDA) approved by the Food and Drug Administration . . . or, a consensus of the national community of experts, qualified by scientific training and experience to evaluate the safety and effectiveness of drugs, accepts the safety and effectiveness of the substance for use in treating a specific, recognized disorder. A material conflict of opinion among experts precludes a finding of consensus.

5. The scientific evidence must be widely available.

In the absence of NDA approval, information concerning the chemistry, pharmacology, toxicology, and effectiveness of the substance must be reported, published, or otherwise widely available in sufficient detail to permit experts, qualified by scientific training and experience to evaluate the safety and effectiveness of drugs, to fairly and responsibly conclude the substance is safe and effective for use in treating a specific, recognized disorder.

SOURCES: LeCraw (1996) and 57 *Federal Register* 10499 (1992).

Index

A

Addiction, *see* Craving; Dependence; Tolerance; Withdrawal symptoms
Adjunctive therapy, general, 4, 10, 145, 153, 157, 167, 172, 247
    see also Pain, treatment of
Administration of drugs, *see* Drug delivery
Adolescents, 6, 15, 16, 90, 91, 96, 97, 98, 99, 101, 102, 104, 123, 126
Affinity, receptors, 42, 44, 46, 51
    defined, 42(footnote)
African Americans, 173
Age factors, 9, 16, 22, 92-93, 94, 95, 100, 117
    adolescents, 6, 15, 16, 90, 91, 96, 97, 98, 99, 101, 102, 104, 123, 126
    children, 96, 97, 101, 124-125, 139, 149, 167, 210
    clinical trials, 139, 142
    prenatal exposure, effects of, 124-125
    see also Elderly persons
Agonists, receptor, 34, 37, 38, 39, 43-47, 54, 56-57, 58, 64, 70
    glaucoma, 176-177
    listed, 44
    market considerations, 209, 210, 212
    neurological disorders, 166, 167, 168
    see also SR 141716A; SR 144528
AIDS, *viii*, 16, 18, 21, 22, 23, 107, 115-117, 120-121, 145, 178, 252

AIDS wasting, 4, 8, 23, 154-158, 159, 177, 204-205, 207, 209, 234, 246, 248
    clinical trials, 8, 156, 213, 245
    defined, 154
    individual patient account, 27-28
    smoking of marijuana, 27-28, 156
Alaska, *vii*, 17
Alcohol use and abuse, 6, 88, 90, 92, 95, 96, 97, 100, 101, 117, 254
    nausea and vomiting, 147
Alternative medicine, general, 19, 20, 180, 215, 216, 217-218, 254-255
Alzheimer's disease, 173, 204, 205, 209
American Medical Association, 180, 244-255 (passim)
Amotivational syndrome, *see* Motivation
Amphetamines, 21, 88, 240
Analgesia, *see* Pain, treatment of
Anandamide, 34, 41, 43-47, 48, 54, 194
Animal studies, 3, 35, 36-81, 88, 89, 91, 111, 120, 122-123, 125, 140, 145, 195, 199, 212, 246
    movement disorders, 164-165, 167, 170
    relevance of, general, 36
Anorexia, *see* Appetite; Wasting syndrome
Anorexia nervosa, 159
Antagonist, receptor, 34, 37, 39, 44, 55, 58, 70
    market considerations, 205, 210, 211
    nausea and vomiting, 151, 152-153
Antiemesis, *see* Vomiting

259

Antigens, 59, 64, 66, 120
Anxiety, 4, 10, 36, 84, 90, 109, 127, 142, 153, 165, 168, 203
    see also Dysphoria; Euphoria; Sedation
Appetite, *viii*, 3, 4, 10, 21, 23, 142, 144, 156-159 (passim), 173, 205, 209, 245, 248
    see also Nausea; Vomiting; Wasting syndrome
Arachidonic acid, 46, 47, 57
Arachidonyl glycerol (2-AG), 43, 45, 46, 47, 64, 65
Arizona, *vii*, 1, 17, 18, 104(footnote)
Arthritis, 28-29
Attitudes
    patients, 27-29, 153, 205-206
    physicians, prescribing marijuana, 152, 202
    risk perception, 104

B

Barbiturates, 143, 172
Basal ganglia, 48-52, 164-166, 168
B cells, 62, 64, 65, 66, 112
    see also Lymphocytes, general
Benzodiazepines, 3, 70, 161, 164, 168
Blood pressure
    hypertension, 48, 84, 86, 90, 121, 158, 175
    hypotension, 121, 150, 151, 175
Brain, general, 3, 35, 36-37, 48-49, 69, 70, 92, 170
    basal ganglia, 48-52, 164-166, 168
    cannabinoid receptors, 37-65, 69-70
    cerebellum, 46, 49, 50, 51, 53, 121, 122
    endogenous cannabinoid system, 43-51, 70
    globus pallidus, 49, 52, 53, 167
    hippocampus, 45-46, 49, 53
    putamen, 49, 52, 53, 166
    striatum, 46, 51, 53
    substantia nigra, 49, 51, 52, 53, 167, 168
    thalamus, 46, 49, 51, 52, 53, 55, 165, 167, 169
    see Neurons, general
British Medical Association, 180, 244-255 (passim)
Bronchi, 113-114, 115, 119
Buyers' clubs, see Cannibis buyers' clubs

C

Cachexia, 145, 154, 155, 158
    see also AIDS wasting; Appetite; Wasting syndrome

Caffeine, 88
California, *vii*, 1, 16, 17, 18, 101-102, 104, 204, 207
Canada, 150
Cancer
    smoking of marijuana as cause, 5, 114, 115, 117-121, 237
    treatment of, 22, 23, 142, 145, 154, 158, 159, 204-205; see also Chemotherapy
Cannabidiol (CBD), 3, 36-37, 47, 60-61, 66, 122, 166, 171-172, 214
Cannabinoids, general, *vii*, *viii-ix*, 2-4
    defined, 2, 25-26, 194
    defined substances, 4
    standards, general, 19, 213, 216, 217
    see also THC
Cannabinol, 25, 37, 64, 66, 110
    see also THC
Cannibis buyers' clubs, *viii*, 16, 20, 21, 22, 207
    defined, 20
Cardiovascular system, 121-122, 251
    see also Blood pressure
Case studies, 15, 27-29, 117, 119-120, 254
    individual patient accounts, 27-29
    single-patient clinical trials, 139, 162
CBD, see Cannabidiol
Cellular biology, 5, 25, 35-59, 69-70, 118-119, 120-121
    see also Genetics; Immune system; Receptors; Signal transduction
Cerebellum, 46, 49, 50, 51, 53, 121, 122
Cesamet, see Nabilone
Chemotherapy, *viii*, 4, 16, 23, 144, 146-153 (passim), 177, 205, 207, 234, 245, 247, 248
Children, 96, 97, 101, 124-125, 139, 149, 167, 210
    see also Adolescents
Chronic obstructive pulmonary disease, 114-115
Clinical studies, 15, 30, 34-35, 137, 206, 233-234
    glaucoma, 177, 251
    movement disorders, 166, 169-170
    smoking of marijuana, 9-10
Clinical trials, 7-8, 9-10, 34, 137, 141, 142-143, 203, 209, 211, 218
    age factors, 139, 142
    AIDS wasting, 8, 156, 213, 245
    animal studies *vs*, 36
    epilepsy, 170-172, 173
    Investigational New Drugs, 195, 196

movement disorders, 167, 168
nausea and vomiting, 7-8, 142, 145-154,
   179, 245, 247
pain, 7-8, 141-145, 179
psychological effects, 5, 10, 109, 149
recommendations, 4, 5, 7-8, 9-10, 178,
   179-180, 215, 245-255 (passim)
regulatory requirements, 195, 196, 200,
   202, 208, 211, 213, 218, 256-257
single-patient trials, 139, 162
spasticity, 160-164, 165, 249
standards for, 7-8, 10, 138-139, 179-180
Cocaine, 3, 20, 70, 88, 90, 95, 102, 240
Colorado, *vii*, 1
Codeine, 143, 241
Cognitive effects, 49, 83-84, 89, 105, 106-
   107, 108, 124-125
   disorientation, 4, 142, 203
   memory, 35, 49, 53, 56, 84, 89, 106, 144,
      173, 212
   see also Psychological effects
Connecticut, 17
Controlled Substance Act, 16-17, 102, 198-
   204 (passim), 210, 213-219 (passim)
   scheduling, 17, 102, 194, 198-213
      (passim), 216-217, 218, 240-241, 256-
      257
Convulsions, *see* Seizures
Cost factors, 9, 16, 206-207, 243
   antiemetics, 151, 152
   drug development, 195, 196, 203, 206,
      217-218
CP 47,497, 210
CP 55,244, 210
CP 55,940, 44, 46, 56, 201
Craving, 9, 90, 91-92
CT-3, 67, 209
Cytokines, 62, 66, 67, 112, 120, 157

D

DEA, *see* Drug Enforcement
   Administration
Delivery modes, *see* Drug delivery
Department of Health and Human
   Services, 199, 200, 201, 217
   see also National Institutes of Health
Dependence, 6, 9, 57-59, 70, 84, 86, 237
   animal research, 35
   criteria, 87
   legal issues, 16

marijuana as a gateway drug, 6-7, 9, 20-
   21, 98-101
   predictors of, 93-98, 99, 100, 101, 126
   see also Craving; Tolerance; Withdrawal
      symptoms
Depression, 22, 23, 29, 84, 95, 105, 155, 159
   fluoxetine, 48
   see also Dysphoria
*Diagnostic and Statistical Manual of Mental
   Disorders*, 84, 87
Diarrhea, 24, 155
District of Columbia, 17
Dizziness, 27, 121, 150, 158, 203
Dopamine, 58, 88, 92, 167, 168
Dosage factors, 137, 245, 248, 256
   affinity, 42(footnote)
   AIDS wasting, 156, 157, 158
   caffeine, 88
   cardiovascular effects, 121
   CBD, 36, 60-61
   cognitive effects, 107
   glaucoma treatment, 176, 177, 251
   immune system effects, 60-63, 64-67, 68
   morphine, 37
   multiple sclerosis treatment, 163
   neurological disorder treatment, 166, 169
   overdosing, 37, 109, 206
   pain treatment, 102, 142, 143, 149
   psychological effects, 84, 85, 105
   psychomotor effects, 51, 53, 85
   reproductive effects, 122, 125
   respiratory effects, 113
   THC, 88, 89, 91, 122, 142, 176, 203, 206,
      215, 255
      anxiety, 36, 142, 149
      glaucoma treatment, 176, 177, 251
      pain treatment, 102, 142, 143, 149
      psychoactive doses, 85
      vomiting, 147, 154
   vomiting, 147, 151, 152, 154
   see also Dependence; Tolerance
Dronabinol, *see* Marinol
Drug Awareness Warning System, 102-103
Drug delivery, 7, 9, 151, 197, 199, 217, 239,
   242, 245
   inhalation, 7, 9, 57, 94, 150, 154, 165, 175,
      197, 203, 206, 215(footnote), 216,
      242, 247, 251, 255; *see* Smoking,
      marijuana
   injection, 39, 54, 57, 66, 67, 68, 85, 88, 94,
      100, 122, 150, 151, 152, 159, 174, 175,
      203

oral, 4, 9, 16, 57, 84, 89, 91, 121, 122, 142,
      148-156 (passim), 163, 164, 165, 171,
      174, 175, 202, 203, 205, 206, 207, 215,
      242, 247, 249, 251
   suppositories, 206
   topical, 175, 176, 251
Drug Enforcement Administration (DEA),
      137, 198-202, 203-204, 208, 213, 214,
      217
Dysphoria, 5, 84, 126, 150, 159, 203
   see also Anxiety; Depression
Dystonia, 166, 168, 245, 250

                        E

Economic factors
   access and availability, general, 9, 194-
      198, 206-208, 213-214
   health insurance, 207
   malnutrition, 154, 155
   private investment, 178, 195-219
   public investment, 4, 137, 178, 211, 214, 218
   see also Cost factors
Efficacy, 9, 11, 14, 19, 20, 30, 54, 57, 88, 107,
      108, 126, 144, 179, 217, 243, 256
   defined, 4-5
   regulatory requirements, 197, 212, 215
   see also Clinical studies; Clinical trials
Elderly persons, 21
   clinical trials, 139
   psychological effects, 4, 175
Emesis, see Vomiting
Emotional factors, see Psychological effects
Endorphins (endogenous opioids), 35, 43
Epidemiological Catchment Area Program,
      97
Epilepsy, 29, 170-173, 177, 245, 250-251
Euphoria, 5, 16, 83-84, 85, 87, 88, 89, 92, 108,
      144, 150, 203
Eye diseases, see Glaucoma

                        F

Federal government, 194-202
   see also Department of Health and
      Human Services; Drug Enforcement
      Administration; Food and Drug
      Administration; Legal issues and
      legislation; Public investment
Fluoxetine, 48

Food and Drug Administration, 17, 20, 137,
      138, 149, 156, 194-198, 199, 200, 202-
      203, 204, 205, 208, 209, 213, 215, 216,
      217, 257
Food and Drug Administration
      Modernization Act, 197(footnote)
Food, Drug, and Cosmetic Act, 194, 213,
      215, 256
Foreign countries, see International
      perspectives; specific countries
France, 69
Funding, see Public investment

                        G

Gamma-aminobutyric acid (GABA), 50
Gateway theory, 6-7, 9, 20-21, 98-101
Gender factors, 20, 22, 94, 95, 115, 170-171
Genetics, 5, 38, 42, 69, 118-119, 120
   dependence, 94, 97-98
   drug development, 19-20
   gene regulation, 37, 38
   reproductive system effects, 122-125
   transduction, 37, 38, 40-41, 43, 57; see also
      Agonists, receptor
   see also Cellular biology; Receptor
      binding; Receptors
Glaucoma, 9, 22, 24, 173-177, 234, 251-252
   agonists, receptor, 176-177
   dose effects, 176, 177, 251
   intraocular pressure, 175, 176, 251-252
   smoking of marijuana, 174, 175, 177, 251
Globus pallidus, 49, 52, 53, 167

                        H

Hallucinations, 84, 90, 106
Headaches, 151
   see also Migraine headaches
Health insurance, 207
Heart, see Cardiovascular system
Herbal medicine, general, see Alternative
      medicine, general
Heroin, 88, 90, 92, 95, 99, 100, 240
Hippocampus, 45-46, 49, 53
Hispanics, 94-95
Historical perspectives, 118
   antiemetics, 151
   legal issues, 16-18
   medicinal uses of marijuana, 16-19

research on marijuana, 33-34, 244-255
HIV, *see* AIDS
Hormones, 37, 48, 58-59, 66, 122, 123, 155, 157
HortaPharm, 214-215, 218
HU-210/HU-211, 44, 60, 64, 66, 67, 176, 201, 209, 211, 250
Huntington's disease, 49, 166, 198
Hyperalgesia, 54, 56, 141
Hypertension, 48, 84, 86, 90, 121, 158, 175
Hypotension, 121, 150, 151, 175

I

Immune system, 5, 37, 42, 51, 59-68, 70, 109-111, 112-113, 116-117, 120, 156, 158, 212, 233, 236, 245, 248, 252
    antigens, 59, 64, 66, 120
    cytokines, 62, 66, 67, 112, 120, 157
    dose effects, 60-63, 64-67, 68
    infections, 66-67, 112-113, 155, 236
    inflammatory/antiinflammatory effects, 67-68, 112-113, 142, 155, 209
    leukocytes, 59, 62, 64, 109-111, 120
    lymphocytes, general, 59, 62, 64, 112, 118, 155
        B cells, 62, 64, 65, 66, 112
        T cells, 59, 62, 64-65, 66, 112
    macrophages, 66, 112-113, 121
    multiple sclerosis, 160
    see also AIDS
Inactivation, 36, 46, 47, 48, 212
Infections, 66-67, 112-113, 155, 236
    see also AIDS; Receptors
Inflammatory/antiinflammatory effects, 67-68, 112-113, 142, 155, 209
Information dissemination, *see* Public information
Insurance, *see* Health insurance
International perspectives, 180, 244-255
    exporter of marijuana for research, 214-215, 218
    marijuana laws, 103-104
    seizure treatment, 171
    Single Convention on Narcotic Drugs, 217
    see also specific countries
Internet, *viii*, 16, 245
Intraocular pressure, *see* Glaucoma
Investigational New Drug applications (FDA), 195, 196, 198, 206, 213
Israel, 209

L

Legal issues and legislation, 14, 16-18, 86, 126, 206-207, 215-216
    Controlled Substance Act, 16-17, 102, 198-204 (passim), 210, 213-219 (passim)
    scheduling, 17, 102, 194, 198-213 (passim), 216-217, 218, 240-241, 256-257
    Food and Drug Administration Modernization Act, 197(footnote)
    Food, Drug, and Cosmetic Act, 194, 213, 215, 256
    foreign/international, 103-104, 217
    Marijuana Tax Act, 16
    National Organization for the Reform of Marijuana Legislation, 17, 18, 200, 213
    Orphan Drug Act, 198, 205, 211
    patent law, 208-210
    Prescription Drug User Fee Act, 195
    referenda, *vii*, 1, 17, 18
    Single Convention on Narcotic Drugs, 217
    state legislation, 17, 18, 102-103, 200, 206-207
    see also Regulatory issues
Lethargy, *see* Motivation
Leukocytes, 59, 62, 64, 109-111, 120
Levonantradol, 44, 57, 142, 148, 149, 210
Ligands, 37, 39, 40-41, 42, 45, 53, 64, 194
    see also Agonists, receptor; Antagonist, receptor; Receptor binding
Lipophilic substances, 25, 39, 175, 206
Louisiana, 17
LSD, 240
Lungs, 5, 111-115, 117, 118, 119, 126, 236, 253
Lymphocytes, general, 59, 64, 112, 118, 155
    B cells, 64, 65, 66, 112
    T cells, 59, 64-65, 66, 112

M

Macrophages, 66, 112-113, 121
Malnutrition, *see* Appetite; Nutrition
Marijuana, general
    active constituents, 36-37
    defined, 2, 24-25
    prevalence of use, 92-93, 137

Marijuana and Health, 2, 33
Marijuana Tax Act, 16
Marinol (dronabinol), 16, 44, 137, 149, 156,
        158, 173, 194, 195, 240, 248
    development of, 193-194, 195, 197, 202-
        208, 210, 211, 216, 218
Medical Use of Cannabis, 244-245
Memory, 35, 49, 53, 56, 84, 89, 106, 144, 212
    Alzheimer's disease, 173
Men, *see* Gender factors
Metabolic processes, 36-37, 65, 110, 203
    starvation, 154-155
Methadone, 92, 240
Methodology
    drug development, 19-20, 137, 193-219,
        238-239, 255; *see also* Drug
        Enforcement Administration; Food
        and Drug Administration
    costs of, 195, 196, 203, 206, 217-218
    other research, 20-22, 24, 119-121, 162,
        163, 213-214
    recommendations by non-committee
        organizations, 244-257
    psychological research, 104-105
    study at hand, 15-16, 225-243
    see also Case studies; Clinical studies;
        Clinical trials
Migraine headaches, 22, 23, 143-144, 209, 213
Minority groups, *see* Racial/ethnic factors
Mood effects, 21, 69, 84, 89, 92, 99, 105, 108,
        143, 144, 153, 154, 161, 165, 248
    see also Anxiety; Depression; Dysphoria;
        Euphoria; Sedation
Morphine, 37, 41, 55, 240
Motivation, 58, 105, 107-108, 158, 168, 237, 254
Motor effects, *see* Movement disorders;
        Psychomotor effects
Movement disorders, 4, 160, 165-170, 177,
        233, 245, 249-250
    animal studies, 164-165, 167, 170
    Parkinson's disease, 49, 167, 168, 198, 209
    seizures, 22, 29, 90, 170-173, 177, 245,
        250-251
    Tourette's syndrome, 167-168
    see also Basal ganglia; Psychomotor
        performance; Spasticity
Mucositis, 144
Multiple sclerosis, 9, 22, 23, 143, 160-161,
        162, 163, 170, 198, 209, 245
    individual patient account, 28
Muscle spasticity, *see* Spasticity

N

Nabilone, 44, 148, 149, 161, 162, 163, 174,
        202, 246, 248, 249
Naloxone, 37, 92
National Cancer Institute, 202
National Household Survey on Drug
        Abuse, 104
National Institute of Drug Abuse, 213-214
National Institutes of Health, 178, 180, 194-
        195, 202, 213-214, 215, 244-255
        (passim)
National Organization for the Reform of
        Marijuana Legislation, 17, 18, 200, 213
Nausea
    antagonist, receptors 151, 152-153
    clinical trials, 7-8, 142, 145-154, 245, 247
    opioids, 140
    palliation, 3, 4, 7-8, 9, 10, 16, 21, 23, 27,
        29, 142, 144, 145-154, 159, 164, 202,
        205, 207, 234, 245, 247, 248
    withdrawal symptoms, 6, 90, 127
    see also Appetite; Vomiting
Netherlands, 103-104, 180, 214, 244, 245,
        246, 249-255 (passim)
Neurology and neurological disorders, 233,
        234, 242, 245, 246, 251
    Alzheimer's disease, 173, 204
    dizziness, 27, 121, 150, 158, 203
    glaucoma, 173-176 (passim)
    seizures, 22, 29, 90, 170-173, 177, 245,
        250-251
    see Brain; Movement disorders; Multiple
        sclerosis; Spasticity; Spinal cord
Neurons, general, 2, 37, 38, 46, 47, 48, 49-50,
        53, 55, 167, 211
Neuroprotection, 47, 67, 70, 176, 209, 211
Neurotransmitters, 37, 38, 43, 48, 50, 53, 54,
        88, 147, 168, 211
    dopamine, 58, 88, 92, 167, 168
    see also Endorphins; Gamma-
        aminobutyric acid; Serotonin
Nevada, *vii*, 1, 17
New drug applications (FDA), 195-197, 203,
        215, 257
New Hampshire, 17
Nicotine, 3, 70, 88, 90, 92, 96, 97, 100
    see also Tobacco
Norway, 104
Nutrition, 154-156, 158
    anorexia nervosa, 159
    see also Appetite; Wasting syndrome

O

Office of National Drug Control Policy, *vii*, 1
Ohio, 17
Older persons, *see* Elderly persons
Opioids, 3, 35, 37, 43, 53, 54, 55, 58, 69, 70, 88, 92, 102, 233, 246
  heroin, 88, 90, 92, 95, 99, 100, 240
  morphine, 37, 41, 55, 240
  pain treatment, 140, 142
Oregon, *vii*, 1, 17
Orphan Drug Act, 198, 205, 211

P

Pain, treatment of, *viii*, 3, 4, 7, 9, 10, 11, 20-22, 23, 24, 28-29, 84, 159, 164, 210, 233, 234, 241, 245-247
  clinical trials, 7-8, 141-145, 179
  dose effects, 102, 142, 143, 149
  hyperalgesia, 54, 56, 141
  market for, 210, 212
  neurophysiology of, 35, 53-56, 70
  sedation, 5, 10, 109, 127, 140, 144, 145, 150, 161, 164, 168, 241
  standards of analgesic usefulness, general, 140-141
  usefulness of analgesics, general, 140-141
Pain, types of, 141-145, 166
  acute, 54, 67-68, 141-142
  chronic, 8, 21, 22, 23, 30, 53, 54, 67-68, 138, 142-143
  definitional issues, 139-140, 141
  depression, 22, 23, 29, 48, 84, 95, 105, 155, 159
  dysphoria, 5, 84, 126, 150, 159, 203
  inflammatory/antiinflammatory effects, 67-68, 112-113, 142, 155, 209
  surgical, 142, 145, 247
  withdrawal, 3, 6, 35, 58-59, 70, 84, 86, 87, 89-91, 127, 143-144
Paranoia, 84, 105
Parkinson's disease, 49, 167, 168, 198, 209
  see also Substantia nigra
Peer review, 9, 15
Performance, *see* Psychomotor performance
Pharmaceutical companies, *see* Private sector
Political and social factors, *vii*, 1, 2, 6-7, 13-15, 17-19, 92, 93, 94, 98, 99, 202, 234

National Organization for the Reform of Marijuana Legislation, 17, 18, 200, 213
  see also Legal issues and legislation; Referenda
Polycyclic aromatic hydrocarbons, 117, 119
Potency, 41, 46, 214-215
Pregnancy, 122-125, 126, 139, 145
Prescription Drug User Fee Act, 195
Private sector, 178, 195-219
Prostaglandins, 44, 46, 176
Prozac, *see* Fluoxetine
Psychiatric disorders, *see* Schizophrenia
Psychological effects, 3, 4-5, 44, 54, 65, 83-92, 101, 104-109, 126, 233, 237, 253-254
  anorexia nervosa, 159
  anxiety, 4, 10, 36, 84, 90, 109, 127, 142, 153, 165, 168, 203
  clinical trials, 5, 10, 109, 149
  dependence predictors, 95-96, 99, 100, 101, 126
  depression, 22, 23, 29, 48, 84, 95, 105, 155, 159
  dose effects, 84, 85, 105
  DSM-IV, 84, 87
  dysphoria, 5, 84, 126, 150, 159, 203
  elderly patients, 4, 175
  euphoria, 5, 16, 83-84, 88, 92, 108, 150, 203
  hallucinations, 84, 90, 106
  mood disorders, general, 23, 24
  motivation, 58, 105, 107-108, 158, 168, 237, 254
  paranoia, 84, 105
  receptor physiology, 35
  schizophrenia, 105, 106, 159, 253
  seizures, impacts of, 172
  smoking of marijuana, 5-6, 10-11, 104-109
  withdrawal, 3, 6, 35, 58-59, 70, 84, 86, 87, 89-91, 127, 143-144
  see also Cognitive effects
Psychomotor performance, 5, 85, 89, 107, 108, 125-126, 254
  dizziness, 27, 121, 150, 158, 203
  dose effects, 51, 53, 85
  movement disorders
  physiology of, 35, 49, 51-53, 55
  see also Spasticity
Public information, *viii*, 101
  Internet, *viii*, 16, 245
Public investment, 4, 137, 178, 211, 214, 218
Putamen, 49, 52, 53, 166

R

Racial/ethnic factors, 94-95, 173
Receptor binding, 37, 39-45, 64, 194, 211
  affinity, 42, 44, 46, 51
  ligands, 37, 39, 40-41, 42, 45, 53, 64, 194
  potency, 41, 46
  see also Agonists, receptor; Antagonist,
    receptor
Receptors, 2, 3, 33, 34, 35, 37-65, 69-71, 86,
    110, 144, 159, 169, 172, 176-177
  anandamide, 34, 41, 43-47, 48, 54, 194
  brain, 41, 49, 51-59
  immune system, 59-64
  nausea and vomiting, 146, 147, 152, 153
  serotonin, 48, 151, 152-153, 159, 205
Referenda, vii, 1, 17, 18
Regulatory issues, 14, 211, 213-218
  clinical trials, 195, 196, 200, 202, 208, 211,
    213, 218, 256-257
  THC, 200-208, 214-215
  see also Drug Enforcement
    Administration; Food and Drug
    Administration; Legal issues and
    legislation; Standards
Reproductive system effects, 122-125, 126,
    139, 145, 253
Research methodology, see Methodology
Respiratory system, 5-6, 10, 88, 113-115,
    119-120, 127, 146, 236, 253
  see also Lungs

S

Scheduling, 17, 102, 194, 198-213 (passim),
    216-217, 218, 240-241, 256-257
Schizophrenia, 105, 106, 159, 253
Sedation, 5, 10, 109, 127, 140, 144, 145, 150,
    161, 164, 168, 241
Seizures, 22, 29, 90, 170-173, 177, 245, 250-251
  types of, 170
Serotonin, 48, 151, 152-153, 159, 205
Side effects, general, 9, 27, 28, 127, 138, 140,
    151, 203, 243, 246
  marijuana use, 34, 145, 150, 152, 158, 161,
    170, 172, 173, 177
  see also Anxiety; Chemotherapy;
    Memory; Nausea; Sedation;
    Vomiting
Signal transduction, 37, 38, 40-41, 43, 57
  see also Agonists, receptor; Cellular
    biology

Single Convention on Narcotic Drugs, 217
Sleep, 6, 27, 37, 49, 83, 90, 127, 160, 164, 165
Smoking, marijuana, 2, 4, 5, 7-8, 47, 83, 85,
    91, 104, 111-127, 177-178, 216, 254-
    255
  AIDS wasting, 27-28, 156
  carcinogenic effects, 5, 114, 115, 117-121,
    237
  defined, 2
  glaucoma, 174, 175, 177, 251
  individual patient accounts, 27-29
  movement disorders, 167
  physiological effects, 5-6, 10-11, 104-109
  spasticity, 161, 163
  tolerance, 57, 89
  vomiting, control of, 150, 152, 153, 154,
    179, 247
  wasting syndrome, 27-28, 156, 159
Smoking, tobacco, see Tobacco
Social factors, see Political and social factors
Spasticity, 23, 24, 143, 169, 245, 249
  clinical trials, THC, 160-164, 165, 249
  multiple sclerosis, 9, 22, 23, 28, 143, 160-
    161, 162, 163, 198
  smoking of marijuana, 161, 163
Spinal cord, 49, 54, 55-56,
  injury, 23, 145, 159-160, 161, 163-164, 198,
    245, 249
Spleen, 46, 59, 64, 66
SR 141716A, 34, 44, 57-58, 65, 69
SR 144528, 34, 44
Standards
  analgesic usefulness, general, 140-141
  cannabinoid drugs, 19, 213, 216, 217
  clinical trials, 7-8, 10, 138-139, 179-180
  DSM-IV, 84, 87
State-level action
  legislation, 17, 18, 102-103, 200, 206-207
  referenda, vii, 1, 17, 18
  see also specific states
Striatum, 46, 51, 53
Substantia nigra, 49, 51, 52, 53, 167, 168

T

Tardive dyskinesia, 166, 168
Taxes, 16
T cells, 59, 62, 64-65, 66, 112, 120
  see also Lymphocytes, general
Tetrahydrocannabinol, see Marinol; THC
Thalamus, 46, 49, 51, 52, 53, 55, 165, 167, 169

THC, *viii*, 2, 3, 4, 5, 10, 25, 26, 36-37, 39, 41,
   71, 85, 88, 107, 109, 127, 177, 212,
   234, 246, 247, 255
  analogues, 44
  Alzheimer's disease, 173
  cardiovascular system, 121-122
  dependence, 57-59
  dose effects, 88, 89, 91, 122, 142, 176, 203,
    206, 215, 255
    anxiety, 36, 142, 149
    glaucoma treatment, 176, 177, 251
    pain treatment, 102, 142, 143, 149
    psychoactive doses, 85
    vomiting, 147, 154
  endogenous cannabinoids and, 43-48
  epilepsy, 170
  glaucoma, 174-175, 176-177, 251-252
  immune system, 59-68 (passim), 110, 117
  levonantradol, 44, 57, 142, 148, 149, 210
  Marinol (dronabinol), 16, 44, 137, 149,
    156, 158, 173, 194, 195, 240, 248
    development of, 193-194, 195, 197,
     202-208, 210, 211, 216, 218
  pain treatment, 7-8, 102, 141-145, 149, 179
  regulatory issues, 200-208, 214-215
  reproductive system effects, 122-125
  spasticity, clinical trials, 160-164, 165, 249
  tolerance, 56-57, 89, 121
  vomiting, clinical trials, 148-150, 153
Tobacco, *viii*, 5, 6, 95, 96, 97, 111-112, 113-
   114, 117, 118-119, 123
  see also Nicotine
Tolerance, 3, 56-57, 70, 84, 86, 88-89, 121,
   126-127, 233, 237
  analgesics, usefulness of, 140
  defined, 86, 87
  smoking of marijuana, 57, 89
  THC, 56-57, 89, 121
  see also Dependence
Tourette's syndrome, 167-168
2-AG, *see* Arachidonyl glycerol

U

Unimed Pharmaceuticals, Inc., 202-205
United Kingdom, 180, 209, 211, 218, 244-
   255 (passim)

V

Vermont, 17
Virginia, 17
Vomiting, 3, 4, 10, 21, 23, 27, 29, 202, 205,
   207, 210, 234, 248
  antagonists, receptors, 151, 152-153
  clinical trials, 7-8, 142, 145-154, 179, 245,
    247
  cost of antiemetics, 151, 152
  dose effects, 147, 151, 152, 154
  drug delivery route, 148-154 (passim),
    179, 247
  smoking of marijuana, 150, 152, 153, 154,
    179, 247
  THC, 148-150, 153
  see also Nausea

W

Washington, D.C., *see* District of Columbia
Washington State, *vii*, 1, 17
Wasting syndrome, 9, 23, 24, 28-29, 144,
   154-159, 234, 248
  Alzheimer's disease, 173
  definitions, 153-154
  smoking of marijuana, 27-28, 156, 159
  see also AIDS wasting; Appetite
WIN 55,212, 42, 44, 64, 65, 88
Wisconsin, 17
Withdrawal symptoms, 3, 6, 35, 58-59, 70,
   84, 86, 89-91, 127, 143-144
  defined, 86, 87
Women, *see* Pregnancy; Reproductive
   system effects
World Health Organization, 244-255
   (passim)
World Wide Web, *see* Internet

BLACK & WHITE & NOIR

BLACK & WHITE & NOIR
AMERICA'S PULP MODERNISM

Paula Rabinowitz

COLUMBIA UNIVERSITY PRESS NEW YORK

COLUMBIA UNIVERSITY PRESS
Publishers Since 1893
New York   Chichester, West Sussex

Copyright © 2002 Columbia University Press
All rights reserved

Library of Congress Cataloging-in-Publication Data
Rabinowitz, Paula.
Black & white & noir : America's pulp modernism /
Paula Rabinowitz.
p. cm.
Includes bibliographical references and index.
ISBN 0–231–11480–X (cloth)
ISBN 0–231–11481–8 (paper)
1. Film noir–United States–History and criticism.
2. Popular culture–United States–History–20th century.
I. Title: Black and white and noir. II. Title.

PN1995.9.F54 R33   2002
791.43'655–dc21   2002019270

Columbia University Press books are printed
on permanent and durable acid-free paper.

Printed in the United States of America
Designed by Audrey Smith

c 10 9 8 7 6 5 4 3 2 1
p 10 9 8 7 6 5 4 3 2 1

For Charlotte Nekola
sisters under the screen

CONTENTS

Preface and Acknowledgments ix

Introduction: On Pulp Modernism 1

PART I BLACK: ROOMS AND RAGE

1. Already Framed: Esther Bubley Invents Noir 25
2. Domestic Labor: Film Noir, Proletarian Literature, and Black Women's Fiction 60
3. Double Cross: Wri(gh)ting as *The Outsider* 82

PART 2 WHITE: WORK AND MEMORY

4. Blanc Noir: Rural Pulp and Documentary Modernism 105
5. Melodrama/Male Drama: The Sentimental Contract of American Labor Films 121
6. Not "Just the Facts, Ma'am": Social Workers as Private Eyes 142

PART 3 NOIR: HOUSEHOLD OBJECTS

7. Barbara Stanwyck's Anklet 171
8. Medium Uncool: Avant-Garde Film and Uncanny Feminism 193
9. Mapping Noir 225

Notes 245

Index 295

After her beautiful face has been permanently disfigured, scarred by a pot of hot coffee hurled at her primary asset by Vince Stone (Lee Marvin), her gangster lover in *The Big Heat*, Debby Marsh (Gloria Grahame) takes a trip to visit Bertha Duncan (Jeanette Nolan), the more respectable but still utterly corrupt widow of a police officer. Debby finds Bertha dressed in mink, a coat far more luxurious than one might afford on a policeman's pension, all ready to party. She knows that Bertha too is hooked up with the syndicate that controls the city and their lives, and Debby pleads with her to come clean and expose Mike Lagana's racket. Debby's terse observation thrills: "We're sisters under our minks," she tells Bertha. Fritz Lang's bleak depiction of the widespread sleaze oozing from the rackets to the police department also reveals a central theme of a temporarily submerged feminism—marriage, like prostitution, is just another form of the rackets. A man can offer no real protection for a woman, so she needs to get whatever goods she can by any means. Cloaked in her dark mink, Debby kills Bertha, ultimately sacrificing herself to save Dave Bannion (Glenn Ford), whose loyal but sexy wife was blown up by the mob in retaliation for his investigation into Duncan's suicide, and thus all the women end up sisters six feet under the earth. Their thick furs provide no protection from the coldness of death; yet, as Gilles Deleuze shows in his brilliant gloss on Leopold von Sacher-Masoch's *Venus in Furs*, the texture of mink covering the icy white body of the desired woman resexualizes death itself: "icy—sentimental—cruel," he calls her (51). It's a grim and perverse picture, and, like the many film noirs it mirrors, it fascinates me.

Since 1972, when I was living two blocks away from the Orson Welles Cinema on Massachusetts Avenue in Cambridge and wandered one afternoon into a screening of *Double Indemnity*, returning every day for the entire month-long revival of film noirs, I have spent long hours in cafes or on the telephone with my girlfriends recounting the plots of these movies. Back then, I quit my noir job at a Central Square florist shop, which fronted for a bookie joint, in order to soak up these films that seemed oddly familiar yet chillingly strange. I could not get over Fred McMurray—that sweet, funny, single dad of Chip and his brothers from *My Three Sons*—wisecracking double entendres much less murdering two people. And Barbara Stanwyck—that soft, sloppy, over-the-top mom in *Stella Dallas*—turned out to be, as she says, "a hard, rotten case." I had never seen anything like these films, I thought; yet they seemed utterly recognizable. I knew them all—the characters, settings, plots, dialogue, and lighting—from somewhere, sometime, outside the plush red velvet seats of the movie theater. In fact, I had been watching these B-movies all my life on the afternoon television shows, *Million Dollar Movies* or *Dialing for Dollars* or the midnight reruns crowding late 1950s and early 1960s television sets. So had my friends; they were our education into a bizarre grown-up adulthood far from that of our parents' staid lives, a black-and-white world glimpsed in snapshots from their pasts in the ghettoes of New York: the men dashing, dressed in uniforms returned from war; the women, hair marcelled, posing on the stoops before setting out to jobs in the city.

I came up with the title of this book five years ago, while lying on my couch in my dream apartment overlooking Trastevere. I was on a Fulbright scholarship in Rome, the culmination of a quarter-century fantasy of mine, rereading all the great American novels—*Moby-Dick*, *The Scarlet Letter*, *Daisy Miller*, because these were what was available in the used English-language bookstore down the block— I had loved as an undergraduate, but which I had not looked at in decades. On late-night television, RAI Uno played old black-and-white American movies dubbed into Italian, and the nearby cinema club was named Detour. So I spent many hours trying to figure out why, old and weird as the history of Rome was, it could not be a noir city, despite the murders of Beatrice Cenci, Giordano Bruno, and the martyrs of Fosse Ardeatino. I realized I had been writing around these questions—why America is so perverse in its racism and its Puritanism—for years. It was time to write about my secret obsession. But when I came to finish the book in the foggy, time-frozen noir-like town of Corvallis, Oregon, a place whose downtown still sports a bright orange Rexall Drugstore sign and whose outskirts are ringed by paper mills stinking of pulp, I found I still avoided investigating film noir as such. This book, instead, interrogates noir sensibility, the "effetto noir" as an exhibition mounted in the summer of 2000 in the Italian Alps called it, but it barely talks about the movies I love so much. In part this is because there are already many excellent books on the subject—the bibliography on this style, genre, form, code, whatever you want to call it, is long and rich—but it is also that I find I resist writing about them. Talking is one thing, writing another. So this is a book in which a deep debt to noir is paid through avoidance; it's a typical noir strategy, I'm afraid. Still, I hope I say something new about film noir; I know film noir has much to offer photography, literature, politics, and history. Call it political theory masking as pulp, or, more accurately, pulp masking as political history; at any rate, this book interrogates the essential trashiness of modern American culture, America's pulp modernism.

Many people and institutions have helped me research and write this book, sustaining me financially and intellectually. Support has come from the University of Minnesota: its Graduate School Grants-in-Aid of Research, which funded my terrific graduate assistants, Carol Mason, Rebecca Hill, and Laura Schere; International Travel Grants; Scholar of the College Award, and help with juggling leaves. I thank Shirley Nelson Garner, former chair of the Department of English Language and Literature, who unstintingly endorsed my many requests for time and money. I was lucky to have been named senior fellow at the Oregon State University Center for the Humanities during 2000–2001 so that I could complete the manuscript. In addition to a generous stipend, Peter Copek, Wendy Madar, and Jerry Sabin gave me a lovely corner office, solitude, and expert computer assistance. Tragically, Peter Copek died unexpectedly just weeks after I completed this manuscript. I have had the opportunity to present much of this work before rigorous audiences in the United States and in Europe. I thank Daniele Fiorentino at Rome's Centro Studi Americani for inviting me to participate in the Third and Fourth Seminars on American Studies there; portions of the book were developed for a symposium at the Centro on American women writers and a conference on the American city, both organized by Cristina Giorcelli, my colleague at Roma Tre where I taught as Fulbright Professor of American Studies. I delivered lectures from some of the material at the Universities of Siena and Arezzo. Many thanks to Rick McCormick of the University of Minnesota's German Forum for inviting me to his conference on "Thirty Years After: The Legacy of 1968 in German and American Culture," at which I delivered much of chapter 8. Thanks also to Giuliana Colaizzi, Marta Selva, and the women at Drac Magic in Barcelona for inviting me to deliver an address to the Sixth International Exhibition of Women's Films. Other places where I delivered parts of this book include the Rethinking Marxism conference at University of Massachusetts-Amherst, the Weisman Art Museum at the University of Minnesota, the Center for the Humanities at Oregon State University, and SUNY Albany. In addition, I have been lucky to have taught a number of intensive undergraduate seminars on political pulp and film noir to some of Minnesota's smartest, hippest students; they immediately recognized, in the words of one, that "Melville [both Herman and Jean-Pierre] is way weirder than Anne Rice."

I received enormous help from reference librarians at the Wilson Library at the University of Minnesota, the Library of Congress in Washington, D.C., the New York Public Library, and the Centro Studi Americani in Rome; David Klaassen archivist at the Social Welfare History Archive at the University of Minnesota aided my search for arcane information on Caroline Slade. Jean Bubley, executor of Esther Bubley's estate, along with her archivist, Tracy Schmid, gave me free rein to examine Esther's private papers, contact sheets, and unpublished photographs. I met her through the help of Bonnie Yochelson. Maureen Heher at Yale University's Beinecke Rare Book and Manuscript Library in addition to helping me while I was working there, valiantly retrieved my corrupted files after I'd left. Sharon Frost (NYPL), Nancy Goldman (PFA), Maja Keech and Barbara Oliver (LOC), Mary Corliss (MOMA), David Ferber, Dorothy Wiley, and Gunvor Nelson helped with images. Everyone at London's BFI was helpful, digging up ancient prints of *Yield to the Night* and many other British noirs from their collection for me to watch. I could not have written this book without the existence of repertory theaters willing to recycle old movies for the abject; Bob Cowgill and the Oak Street Cinema run a weekly film noir series for those of us in Minneapolis. I owe him a huge debt for letting me see dozens of black-and-white movies during the past five years. My editors at Columbia University Press, Ann Miller and Jennifer Crewe, and assistant editors, Jennifer Barager and Godwin Chu, saw the book through from idea to print.

Many of the chapters in this book began as essays invited by others for special issues of journals or anthologies. Each of the editors cut me enough slack so that my contribution could serve two purposes—that of their volumes and that of mine. A version of chapter 2 appears in a *Modern Fiction Studies* special issue on working-class literature, edited by Stephen Ross; a condensed version of chapter 3 appeared in *Città Reali ed Immaginaire*, edited by Cristina Giorcelli, Camilla Catarulla, and Anna Scacchi. Chapter 4 began as an essay in *Brave New Words: Strategies of Language and Communication in the United States of the 1930s*, edited by Biancamaria Bosco Tedeschini-Lalli and Maurizio Vaudagna. Versions of chapter 5 have appeared in a special issue on documentary of *Media International Australia* and in Janet Walker and Diane Waldman's superb collection *Feminism and Documentary*, published by University of Minnesota Press. Parts of chapter 6 appeared in *Legacy*'s special issue on class and gender, edited by Jeanne Pfaelzer, and in an issue of *Social Text* that was devoted to welfare. A shorter version of chapter 7 appears in volume four (accessories) of *Abito e Identità*, edited by Cristina Giorcelli. Chapter 8 appears in a slightly different form in a special issue on 1960s cultural politics of *Science and Society*, edited by Alan Wald and Paul Mishler; a section of chapter 9 was collected in Amitava Kumar's *Poetics/Politics*, published by St. Martin's Press. I thank all of these friends and colleagues for encouraging my work to develop in so many directions.

Most of my intellectual debts go to my many friends and relatives who have spent hours listening to me go on and on about movies and everything else. My son Raphael Rabinowitz is always willing to see any film noir; moreover, he remembers every plot twist and each character's name. My other son, Jacob Bernstein, and their father, David Bernstein, however, refuse to join me in my decadent pleasures; nevertheless, they too are willing to talk endlessly about the noirish elements of America's past. Countless conversations and movie dates over the years with Lake of the Isles walking partners Maria J. Fitzgerald and Cecily Marcus were essential to distilling my ideas. Past and present Minnesota colleagues Rita Copeland, Maria Damon, John Wright, Jani Scandura, John Mowitt, Mary Roth, Rita Raley, and Tom Pepper talk to me about history, theory, and politics in astounding ways. Coffee and phone calls with Patty Zimmermann, Ruth Bradley, Kathleen Fraser, Connie Samaras, Sara Antonelli, Alice Echols, Sandro Portelli, Cheryl Johnson, Bruce Robbins, Nelson Lichtenstein, Bradley Butterfield, Alan Wald, Sheri Stein, and my mother, Shirley Rabinowitz, kept me going through long winters and short summers. Finally, this book is dedicated to my sister under the screen, Charlotte Nekola, the blonde always available on the other end of the line.

BLACK & WHITE & NOIR

INTRODUCTION: ON PULP MODERNISM

> The only town for certain where a Philadelphia first-baseman can answer an attractive brunette's invitation to step into her room: "I have a surprise for you"—and meet a shotgun blast under the heart. "The urge kept nagging at me and the tension built up. I thought killing someone would relieve it."
> —*Nelson Algren on Richard Wright's Chicago*

> But is not every square inch of our cities the scene of a crime? Every passer-by a culprit?
> —*Walter Benjamin on Eugene Atget's Paris*

EMPTYING THE STREETS

Driving through Los Angeles with her friend N[athalie Sorokine Moffat] in February 1947, feminist philosopher and tourist par excellence Simone de Beauvoir notes: "We cross one suburb after another—nothing but suburbs. The city slips away like a phantom city. The streets thrown down any which way on the sides of hills, in the hollows of valleys, have been laid out at random as needed."[1] Her view echoes Theodor Adorno's baleful commentary from 1944 on the "shortcoming of the American landscape . . . that it bears no traces of the human hand. This applies not only to the lack of arable land, the uncultivated woods often no higher than scrub, but above all to the roads. These are always inserted directly in the landscape, and the more impressively smooth and broad they are, the more unrelated and violent their gleaming track appears against its wild, overgrown surroundings." The roads through are "uncomforted and comfortless;" glimpsed by "the hurrying eye . . . from the car . . .

the vanishing landscape leaves no more traces behind than it bears upon itself."[2] This nightmare vision, however, thrills de Beauvoir. Highly attuned, as she is, to the cinematic quality of her tour, almost all of America comes to resemble a film noir. "American cities are too big. At night their dimensions proliferate," she comments as she describes how difficult it was to walk to a movie house to see *The Killers*. "We set out on foot. . . . Suddenly, we were on a dark road lined with tracks, unmoving trains, and hangars, crossed now and then by other deserted streets. We were in the heart of town yet in a desert. It began to rain violently, and in the wind and rain, we felt as forlorn as on a treeless plain—no shelter, no cars in sight" (139). Eventually, they find some workmen and a pay phone to call a cab and make it to the theater in time for the movie.

De Beauvoir, who spent only four months in the United States, cannot see the country outside of the movies she constantly uses as reference points—California deserts equal Von Stroheim's *Greed* (157), Las Vegas nightclubs bring out "Edward G. Robinson [a movie actor known for gangster roles]" (159), the Sierra Nevada mountains make her "think of the snow in *The Gold Rush* (145). San Francisco is "the perfect place for Humphrey Bogart to murder his wife and claim it was an accident" (131). For de Beauvoir, America was dreamed through its movies. Particularly through its crime films, America circulated its fantasy of dangerous modernity, of pulpy concerns with sex and violence, that both repelled this sophisticated European and entranced her: "Movies show a conventional, papier-mache America in which only the landscapes and the material details have some reality" (173). Mary McCarthy would skewer de Beauvoir, "Mlle. Gulliver," she called her, for her fatuous conflation of image and reality; but then she was on a moral rampage against this trait she found in all Stalinists.[3] De Beauvoir's prose fuses her actual views of America with its cinematic construction that she had feasted on in the immediate postwar years in Paris, where she and Richard Wright, to whom she dedicated *America Day by Day*, often watched newly arrived American movies together. The United States itself, noir America, was a land of weirdly empty cities, of neon motel signs looming out of its deserts, of movie palaces tucked into lonely corners. It was crisscrossed with highways stopping abruptly to detour through washed-out small towns where a steak and whiskey might be had.

Her travel journal is filled with the names of the black-and-white pictures she has seen: *Gilda*, *The Best Years of Our Lives*, *Lost Weekend*, *Lady in the Lake*. These films provide metaphor and perspective; they offer a landscape. They not only invest the sights she sees with significance, they invent it. Upon arriving in New York, she takes the ferryboat to the Statue of Liberty because "I just want to see a view of Battery as I've so often seen it in the movies." This view and her visit to the hairdresser make her feel "less uprooted." America is fabricated in and through its fabrications. In the immediate postwar moment, those constructions were brilliantly differentiated between deep shadows and key lighting; the precise definition between sun and shadow, the insistent vertical lines of New York seem "fragile. . . . What a field day a bomber would have!" she concludes. The "house of cards" that is postwar America becomes apparent only through the obscure, darkly-lit films flowing from this sun-filled nation. After Pearl Harbor, no bombers would have a field day on this terrain. But de Beauvoir's instincts are correct, the potential for destruction is ever present. She knew this from the movies she saw and the highways she traveled. The explosions to come, however, the fire next time, would erupt from the bedrock below these glittering cities, the dark shadows "where no sun penetrates" that she discerned while walking Broadway (9).[4]

Cities—living cities, according to Jane Jacobs—are places where people walk the streets. Random people, many people, night and day, collide amid the traffic of commerce, industry, leisure, and play. But the cities of postwar North American popular imagination—cities perhaps reflecting the devastation of bombings abroad, or presentiments of urban renewal and planning at home, appeared dead and lifeless: empty streets filled menacingly not with bodies but with deep shadows, silent pools of light and the sound of one lone man's steps on the pavement, where anyone might just find that dame with a surprise, because, as Nelson Algren said of Chicago, "every 3 A.M. corner looks hired" and "every day is D-day under the El."[5] In this noir world, a man walks to the outskirts of town, collar turned up against the rain, and hopes for a ride; a man wanders into the bleak city night alone—the glow of a cigarette dangling from his lips the only light to guide his way; a man curls against the side of a building, his white shirt stained black as a pool of blood leaks from him;

a man runs desperately through the fog, nobody follows, yet still he runs. These scenes from 1940s B-movies—*Detour, Out of the Past, Double Indemnity, Night and the City*—are among the hundreds made, sometimes in two or three weeks for as little as $30,000, between 1942 and 1958. We know them: a lone man, a regular Joe, an average guy, perhaps slightly crooked or a bit too interested in the beautiful blonde whom he happens upon by chance—if there is such thing in this determined world—gets in over his head; the past catches up with him; the frame is too big; and he ends up, where? Dead, if he's lucky; walking those lonely streets, waiting, if he's not. The French called them *films noirs*, and they are emblematic of a cultural process, the pulp modernism of America.[6]

When the War ended, Hollywood turned the documentary techniques of the 1930s and early 1940s on its own backyard, filming the many 1930s hard-boiled detective novels of James M. Cain, Dashiell Hammett, and Raymond Chandler set in California. In the words of a *Life* magazine report, "homicide, always popular, became an obsession with the movies in 1946, and thrillers that racked up less than four or five murders before the final fade-out seemed almost sissified. Movie killers were no longer drawn exclusively from the ranks of gangsters, however. Hollywood's sudden discovery of psychology late in 1945 meant that any character in a film might turn out to be an undiscovered murderer."[7] French movie critics celebrated these dark thrillers, finding art in the chiaroscuro lighting, poetry in the clipped dialogue, philosophy in the doomed insatiable desire, and a smoldering sexuality in the curves of snake women played by such all-American ethnic working girls as Barbara Stanwyck and Rita Hayworth.[8] Un-American, yet thoroughly American. Like the HUAC hearings convening simultaneously, these films tracked urban anxiety, contracting the city into a region of inner terror as they spread its claustrophobia across the vast landscape of the nation.

The heroes of these films are often returning vets, out of place in the newly scrubbed world of home appliances and of women's shoulder-padded assertiveness. After the violence of war, they encounter a new world not of their making and strangely dangerous beyond imagination. The America they left behind, crumbling under the weight of the Depression—a country still located on Main Street—is gone forever. They had no address there anyway, so good riddance, but their place was at least secured—"If you're white, you're all right," croaks Algren in his anti-ode to Chicago. Now, nothing is certain; yet with used car lots full of Chevys and neon spilling from bar and hotel windows, a man can slip into an unknown and invisible life: change his name, head west, walk in some else's shoes. The anonymity of the living, teeming city gives way to another, scarier form: the uniformity of the Garden City; tidy bungalows rimming the Los Angeles hills house an inner violence. These regular guys can't go home. As early as the 1930s, urban planners had been dreaming of the city's disappearance. Rexford G. Tugwell, director of the Farm Security Administration responsible for the New Deal's Green Belt suburbs, put it bluntly: "My idea is to go just outside centers of populations, pick up cheap land, build a whole community and entice people into it. Then go back into the cities and tear down whole slums and make parks of them."[9] These slums, since the great migration of the 1910s and 1920s, had become home to millions of African Americans, as well as impoverished Eastern and Southern European, Mexican and, to some extent, Asian immigrants who had entered the United States before the 1924 Immigration Act restrictions. The face of the city had quite literally darkened; but it took postwar defense subsidies for highways and housing to fulfill Tugwell's dream.

The rise of 1950s car culture was smoothly integrated into home furnishings and women's fashion. The efforts of manufacturers to lure female consumers with car interiors decorated like living rooms culminated in a 1957 Chrysler model, La Femme, whose pink exterior and rose embroidered interior came complete with matching lipstick and nail polish (the exterior paint job) and raincoat and umbrella (the upholstery). The image of 1950s endless effortless mobility—both social, as working-class white ethnics slid into middle-class suburbia (parking the ubiquitous 1956 Chevy in the garage), and geographic, as families headed out on the same road as the Beats ("See the U.S.A. in your Chevrolet," crooned Dinah Shore)—is part of the noir story. The development of Levittown and other cheap suburbs as well as the visions of urban planners, such as New York's Robert Moses, doomed most U.S. cities, crisscrossing neighborhoods with thruways, tearing down tenements for high rises. Film noirs reveal what happened both within those evacuated, blackening cities and behind the doors of the well-kept, bleached suburbs.

PULP MODERNISM

Film noir provides a medium for understanding the peculiar ways in which America expressed its uniquely hokey modernism. The films offer a theory of its pulp modernity. Pulp, the byproduct of the timber industry that helped build the nation, is at once useless waste, clotting the landscape, and recycled goods, making possible the paperback revolution democratizing letters. By activating the world of scandal and trash and relocating it within the domestic melodrama, these films archived changing sexual, gender, and racial mores during the embourgeoisement of white working-class ethnics. Echoing Ann Douglas's assessment of nineteenth-century America, Andreas Huyssen sees modernism as staging a tough-guy fight against a femme-fatale mass culture.[10] However, modernism itself—at least as it was performed within the American frame—could never escape its stake in kitsch.[11] At this millennial moment, it seems we just cannot get enough of modernism—there's New Deal Modernism, there's Hollywood Modernism, there's Modernism Inc., there's vernacular modernism, modernism "we have wanted to forget," "low modernism and modernism of the street," Afro-American modernism, transnational modernism, among many others.[12] These many and proliferating modernisms relocate modernism onto American soil with, in Michael Denning's terms, a "plebian" flavor. Extracted from the ruins of European imperialism found in the gassed and traumized, defeated and fragile, bodies on the Western Front, modernism is reinvigorated through the stirring figure of working-class solidarity. The Depression and fascism form its background, not World War I and the Jazz Age. The twin spectres of unemployment and mass murder, and the burgeoning popular culture of Hollywood movies and other mass media are the sources for America's pulp modernism.

Salvador Dali's 1935 cartoon hanging in the Menil Collection in Houston, Texas, "Gangsterisms; or the Goofy Visions of New York," tracks the interconnections among Hollywood gangster films, proletarian culture, and modern urban settings that were also the basis for Kenneth Fearing's ominous poems from the mid-1930s. Alan Wald calls Fearing a "Marxist Noir" poet who brought a new and nasty aesthetic of the popular to the older literary radicals orbiting the *New*

Masses. Fearing's 1930s poems, especially his collection *Dead Reckon-ing* (1935–1938), like Dali's drawing, map what will become, after World War II, film noir. Film noir, in turn, charts more than post-war traumas of nuclear annihilation; it aids in understanding our current crisis and horror-stained landscape of destruction and war. Fearing wrote his poems with the nightmares of National Socialism's rise in Germany and the defeat of the Loyalists in Spain as backdrop. "C Stands for Civilization" anticipates CNN coverage of the wars in Iraq and Afghanistan: "zooming through the night in Lockheed mono-planes the / witches bring accurate pictures of the latest disaster ex- / actly on time."[13] Relying on the newly created mass-media adver-tising devices—captions, boldface type, repetition, slogans—the poems produce jarring dissonances between the cheery affect of the sales pitch and the grimness of the object being purveyed.

His jazzy, headline-poaching songs—dirges, elegies, requiems—speak the language of noir, sing their lyrics: "smoke the last ciga-rette, drink the last tall drink, go with the / last long whistle of the midnight train" ("Lunch with the Sole Survivor" 102) "Tear up the letters and bury the clothes, throw away the keys, / file the number from the gun, burn the record of birth, / smash the name from the tomb, bathe the fingers in acid, / wrap the bones in lime, / Forget the street, the house, the name, the day" ("Escape" 49). Like a scene from any number of 1940s films (perhaps *The Big Clock* from Fear-ing's roman noir, his lyric, "Memo," asks "is there still any shadow there, on the rainwet window of the / coffee pot, / Between the haberdasher's and the pinball arcade, / . . . // Is there on tonight's damp, heelpocked pavement somewhere the / mark of a certain toe, and especial nail, or the butt of a particular dropped cigarette?" (77). Death is all around "the night of love, and murder, and reckoning, and sleep" ("American Rhapsody (1)" 43). Yet the goofy settings of daily life repeat endlessly—lunch counters, and movie theaters and dime stores: "Whether we found a greater, deeper, more perfect love, by / courtesy of Camels, over NBC; whether the comics / amused us, or the newspapers carried a hunger death / and a White House prayer for mother's day" ("No Credit" 58). These purveyors of the emerging "culture of abundance," as Rita Barnard calls it,[14] serve as the backdrop for the wrecked but profoundly moving lives of men and women passing through a "city for sale, for rent" with "ghost horizons" ("Manhattan" 110) full of "shattered glass"

("Debris" 98). This gloomy image of the city—"No name, any name, nowhere, nothing, no one, none" ("Escape" 50)—returns in visual form in the post-war documents called film noir. What Fearing, with incredible prescience, scripted was the scenario for hundreds of B-movies. Fearing's intimations that fascism was both a threat from afar and from within the ghost horizons of our second-rate cities were reimagined during the cold war as nuclear annihilation and threats of a resurgent native fascism in McCarthyism or fears of communist terror from Asia and eastern Europe and from the son and daughters of their emigrants within—Jews for the most part, the supposed threat to German nationalism now seen as destabilizing America, an America that dropped atomic bombs destroying cities and gassed a mother and father for disclosing its "secrets."

Left-wing iconography from the 1930s attempts to shore up the "Hollow Men" as Mike Gold, glossing T. S. Eliot, called those intellectuals failing to join the CPUSA. The hungry bodies of unemployed men limned a crisis in American manhood as much as an economic crisis. *New Masses* cartoonist Hugo Gellert's lithographs and worker-writer H. H. Lewis's poems were terribly concerned with rebuilding the solid musculature of the working class in order to fight decadent fat cats and emaciated vampires of capitalism. It's homophobic and homoerotic overcompensation with a vengeance that has a frightening commonality with what Klaus Theweleit identified motivating the German Freikorps, the shock troops that formed the core of Hitler's SA—fear of the new woman, of modern female sexuality and mobility felt as aggression.[15] Because gendered metaphors aligning the bourgeoisie with femininity, suffrage, the unconscious, the new woman, women's education, autonomy and emergence as citizens lurk behind much of the call to fraternal arms to solidarity. Even the word "solidarity" suggests anxieties about softness, flaccidity, and so forth.

Film noir fixated on this dangerous scenario—the woman left alone to work the machinery of the homefront while her man was off fighting on the battlefront, often returning a damaged man. Demobilized vets numbed, perhaps maimed, by the horror of war they have experienced, remembering the emptiness of pre-war Depression life, come home to nightclubs glittering with bejeweled women—sisters under our minks, as Gloria Grahame calls them in *The Big Heat*—on the prowl, aggressively seeking money and sex in a new world of pleasure and commodities. A world filled with toasters and refrigerators and radios playing bebop and bulbous black cars, with supermarkets piled high with canned peaches and peas, with women sporting short tight skirts and spiked heels that clatter across the pavement like artillery fire. The terror of this place, home, yet not home—the uncanny home, was first envisioned in the surreal nightmare of Maya Deren's *Meshes of the Afternoon* and the bleak Office of War Information photographs of women in rooming houses and Washington, D.C., bars shot by the misnamed Esther Bubley (both 1943) and spread across popular culture in the iconography of noir spilling out of Hollywood throughout the 1940s and '50s. This time, *Dead Reckoning*, with Humphrey Bogart and Lizabeth Scott (1947), tracks a woman who has rubbed out her first husband and secretly married a gangster only to seduce her dead husband's army buddy as he investigates what happened to his friend. Men can be together in America only by dying together, or through the triangle with the third, the other woman, who dies instead. Bogart's saved when Scott dies in a flaming car crash. Like Barbara Stanwyck in *The File on Thelma Jordan*, like Lana Turner in *The Postman Always Rings Twice*, like Jane Greer in *Out of the Past*—and on and on.

C. L. R. James understood the connection between "the popular arts and modern society" as one in which the "characteristic of modern American life—an enormous tension" is expressed "in well-made gangster films" (126). The tension keeps building up, as it did for Algren's brunette, and pulling the trigger seems to relieve it. These works "are a form of art which must satisfy the mass, the individual seeking individuality in a mechanized, socialized society, where his life is ordered and restricted at every turn. . . . Gangsters get what they want, trying it for a while, they are killed. In the end 'crime does not pay,' but for an hour and a half, highly skilled actors and a huge organization of production and distribution have given to many millions a sense of active living, and in the bloodshed, the violence, the freedom from restraint to allow pent-up feelings free play, they have released the bitterness, hate, fear and sadism which simmer just below the surface" (127). James's insight into the connection between the world of the gangster, one that celebrates the rising, raging individual who functions within a highly organized organization, and the system of Hollywood film stars and film production suggests how film noir can offer a theory of American modernity. The crime film provides a template for its expression and experience. He cites Humphrey Bogart and Ida Lupino in *High Sierra*, but any number of films might do. In their reliance on individuating the masses—through stars, as gangsters—these popular crime films collapse the difference between example and theory, particular and general. According to James, "[O]ne after the other, these films pour out, vying with each other in bloodshed and violence, cruelty, sadism and disregard for all established standards" (132). They offered mass audiences a cogent and fulfilling entry into the workings of power: "They stamp on his face, they crush his jaw, when he is knocked out, they hold him up and beat him, they revel in violence. A succession of evil women has appeared, as cruel and ruthless as cobras" (130). This was the reason audiences lapped them up. The scenarios James outlines and the characters within them— the guy whose face is stamped and the cruel, ruthless women— repeat the classic outlines of masochistic dreams. "Disavowal, suspense, waiting, fetishism and fantasy together make up the specific constellation of masochism," notes Gilles Deleuze.[16] They suggest that while America may have emerged on top of the twentieth century—which Henry Luce had declared to be "The American Century"—in its fantasy life, America resembled a perennial bottom. America's pulp modernism continually restages the "coldness and cruelty," as Deleuze calls it, of masochistic fantasy. James and de Beauvoir commented on postwar American culture as outsiders, left-wing alien observers. They shared much in common with the many expatriate directors creating these parables of modern American life with the aesthetic hammers of Expressionism and the ideological nails of Marxism they brought with them from abroad.

They were not as appalled as some were. Observing Hollywood, Theodor Adorno, aghast at the vision of modern times it afforded, quipped: "The modern has really become unmodern."[17] The danger Adorno saw in film was precisely its ability to concretize the reactionary shift of the modern into a regressive sentimentality through the reification of subjectivity, "a mere function of the production process," in art into saleable goods that administer to the public its own inward emotions (214–15). This sentimentality was precisely what made American desire so perverse. It turned everything into "catchwords for a hit song, designed to boost it." Doubling back on itself as object and sales pitch, America's pulp modernism offers up a sloppy melodrama. "Illuminated in the neon-light switched on by these words," Adorno notes in "English Spoken," "culture displays its character as advertising" (*Minima Moralia*, 47). It is the foundation for the repetitive masochistic fantasy. Whether one agrees with James's more optimistic vision of popular culture providing an analysis of modern America to its subjects or with Adorno's sense that America's modern subjects were hopeless objects of its consumer culture is, to my mind, less important than seeing how both these theorists of American modernity turn to the popular to understand its expression. I should amend my statement—not only do Americans dream modernity through the movies, foreigners dream America in them as well. That is why, despite claims for a British cycle of film noir for instance, it is, as Alain Silver and Elizabeth Ward call it, "an American style," requiring the peculiar geographical history of the nation.[18] Great Britain is an island, too small to allow for escape, too established to enable anarchic invisibility, too accustomed to maintaining a stiff upper lip and bearing up; after all, its highway detours are called "diversions."

Jacques Tourneur's noir psychological horror film *Cat People* (1942) traces the tensions both James and Adorno refer to in the mutable body of Irene, the Serbian artist working as a dress designer whom the smitten Oliver meets while she is sketching a black leopard in the Central Park Zoo. She claims its sleek black coat offers fashion inspirations, but the crumpled paper she discards, tossing it defiantly onto the pavement rather than the trashcan nearby, belies another story. It is a picture of the leopard impaled on a sword, the masochist's vision of "Venus in furs." Oliver's work as an engineer designing ships contrasts with Irene's, although he too draws: he measures precisely and has an office full of assistants. He's an "Americano," he tells Irene, who has never been unhappy in his life until his marriage to her installs him in her dark claustrophobic studio apartment, close to the nighttime growls of the leopard, where she works at her easel alone. His assistant, Alice, ultimately reveals her love for Oliver, declaring herself to be "a new kind of other woman." As Oliver's wholesome workmate, she will not lure him into the clutches of ancient rituals associated with the violent past of another's race as Irene has. Alice may be the blonde girl next door, but she too demonstrates an aggressive mobility and autonomy. Leaving Oliver late one night to walk home alone, she tells him she's a "big girl" who knows how to take care of herself. She wants to have a sexual relationship with Oliver, while Irene, haunted by the legend of her village that demands she kill whomever she kisses, sleeps alone behind a locked door.

This blood legacy from a medieval Eastern Europe connects Irene to the anti-Semitic iconography circulating in and from Nazi Germany. She is the Jew; as such she is also the African presence in America.[19] Alice suggests to Oliver that Irene might be helped out of her shell by seeing a psychiatrist; however, the doctor's dapper urbanity in accent, manner, and dress, and his profession as a mind doctor link him to Irene. No pragmatic engineer who uses measurements to improve a ship's design, Dr. Judd, like the Viennese Dr. Freud driven from his city by fascism, knows about the unconscious and its uncanny desire for death. Forcing Irene to kiss him, Dr. Judd unleashes the deadly feline within her. A few years earlier, Rosita Forbes documenting "women called wild," had tracked women who had turned into beasts through Central America and Africa; a few years later, *Amazing Stories* featured a cover story depicting the "Tiger Woman of Shadow Valley."[20] But the American cobras, as James had called them, roaming New York or San Francisco, expected full access to the sites zoned for men—the streets at night, bars and nightclubs, jobs and apartments.

Made shortly after the United States entered the Second World War, *Cat People* crystallizes central tropes of film noir—human annihilation, female desire, racial history, social mobility, and the production and replication of objects and machinery—that play themselves out as camp in Robert Aldrich's *Kiss Me Deadly* thirteen years later. Like so many film noirs, these two films implicate art and science—both high-end concepts trying to divorce themselves from the tackiness of American life—in the big business of capitalist production. In *Kiss Me Deadly*, Mike Hammer drives through Los Angeles in his full-metal-jacket sports car searching for the anonymous woman he picked up hitchhiking. This woman, barefoot and naked under her trenchcoat, quotes Christina Rossetti and listens to opera and classical music stations on the radio and has literally swallowed the key to human survival. Hammer ultimately discovers the "big whassit" he's been tracking by interpreting the lines of poetry recited to him by his strange passenger. Literary criticism unlocks the secret bomb that annihilates the Malibu beach house where the

FIGURE 1. Isobel Beard, "Women into Beast," from Rosita Forbes, *Women Called Wild* (1937).

crooks are keeping it, and with it, the entire world. For both films, literary analysis—the talking cure of the psychiatrist, the textual study of the poem—becomes part of the violent actions of men bent on piercing the surface, solving the mystery. Strange women— aliens, asylum escapees, poets—possess dark knowledge, secrets locked within their bodies that threaten death and destruction if they are plumbed. These women are irresistible, hiding a darkness, like America itself.

My take on film noir, like James's and Adorno's, is symptomatic. This book is less about film noir as a subject of study than as a leit-motif running thorough mid-twentieth-century American culture. James Naremore's superb study, *More Than Night*, places, as its sub-title asserts, "film noir in its contexts." Instead, I view film noir *as* the context; its plot structure and visual iconography make sense of America's landscape and history. The terrifying size and emptiness of the American continent are tamed by the incessant crossings of tele-phone wires, linked by a never-ending web of female operators rout-ing calls through their switchboards, highways traversed by lone roadsters driving through the night, and road houses where a satin-sheathed chanteuse sits alone on her cigarette break. Film noir shows how communication, transportation, and entertainment shade into pulp. These systems, major industries that dominate the nation and the world, enable crime; in fact, they are criminal enterprises. Noir offers a template for analyzing how cultural formations achieve legi-bility through stable repetitions of instability, predictable renderings of chaos, sinister animations of immobile objects. The hazy smoke clouding the diner counter, hotel lobby, or nightclub suggests that the straight lines—Route 66, the Empire Builder, telephone poles ris-ing with regularity—connecting city to city and city to small town are dotted with hidden dangers. These transgressive sites provide spaces for the illicit expression of sexuality and greed. They house a restless, mobile population, dislocated by hunger, war, and desire—a popula-tion on the make, in search of a new life cut off from the past, itself long banished, though never wholly overcome, in the new world.

Film noir served for me and many women of my generation as a form of documentary reportage on the lives of our parents. Shown daily on *Million Dollar Movie*, these black-and-white lenses into the 1930s and 1940s, years of our parents youth about which they were militantly silent, cued us to their hairstyles, clothing, and home and work lives. Isolated snapshots of my parents—my mother and her sisters posing as pin-ups on tar beach, my father in cut-off sweatshirt tramping across the blankets of Brighton Beach—accrued narrative heft in the convoluted plots of these films. I understood why they could never speak about the past; it was simply too dangerous. The black Bakelite telephones, the white Venetian blinds, the curved Studebaker windshields, the brass Zippo lighters, the mirrors and doorways and hats presented a menacing world of the mundane. In her memoir of her middle-class girlhood in 1950s St. Louis, Charlotte Nekola details how she and her girlfriends attempted to live out Ida Lupino's sinister travails.[21] I too have never quite shaken this sense of film noir; no matter how wacky and contrived the plot, the films speak truths; they offer designs for living. This is precisely what Adorno was railing against and what James found so useful about popular culture. These films operate fantastically to give the feel of the real, but they also catalogue the pulpy back story that is the real America.

Black & White & Noir offers a historical and theoretical overview of the noir sensibility, expressed almost daily during the late 1990s in the pages of the *New York Times*, on Hollywood screens, in fashion, and in the cultural fascination with lurid murder trials involving white women and black men, from the case of trailer-trash mom fatale Susan Smith to that involving Brentwood confidential—O. J. Simpson's white Bronco, Bruno Maglis, and the bungled police work of the LAPD. At the MAC cosmetics counter you can buy a dark purple lipstick called "film noir"; at Pottery Barn you can purchase a black *Dial M for Murder* telephone (the dialer, however, is actually a touch tone); stiletto heels are once again available from Gucci and Manolo Blahnik, not just fetish stores; and since Quentin Tarantino's *Pulp Fiction* simultaneously resurrected John Travolta and film noir in 1994, even sugary Carly Simon got into the act; she reappeared imitating a femme fatale in her album *Film Noir*, which was used as the theme music for the American Movie Classics marathon film noir series that year.[22] As Andrew Sarris recently commented, "Everything is noir—try finding something blanc! . . . Every film is a film noir now. . . ."[23] Literary noir, from its heyday between the 1930s and 1950s, has been institutionalized with the publication of the Library of America anthology, but it also has generated a neo-noir genre of memoir, such as James Ellroy's gripping memoir of his mother's 1958 murder, *My Dark Places*, and literary trash, such as Joyce Carol Oates coming out as Rosamond Smith with the publication of *Starr Bright Will Be With You Soon*.[24] Even that Pillsbury doughboy Garrison Keillor and the jaundiced suburbanite John Updike have their noir alter-egos: Guy Noir and Beck Noir, respectively. The "effetto noir" even reached as far as the mountain town of Trento in the Italian Alps where an exhibition of films, comics, pulp fiction, and clothing was held in Summer 2000. The many forms noir has taken—movies, photos, novels—are valences of the changing racial and class makeup of urban America.[25] In the midst of Nixon's presidency, film noir's resurrection in 1974 by Roman Polanski in *Chinatown*, with its textbook screenplay by Robert Towne, captured the ways in which government intrigue, legal trials, and congressional hearings surround popular culture. The postwar moment of noir was dominated by HUAC hearings, the Army-McCarthy hearings, and Smith Act trials; the second flowering of noir coincided with Watergate, with its significant missing eighteen minutes of tape, the Vietnam War (yet another generation of traumatized veterans), the Chicago Seven trial, among many others, and, in a terribly personal way for Polanski, Charles Manson's trial for the murder of Sharon Tate, Polanski's pregnant wife, and her guests.

Film noir, rather than reflecting these changes, in my view, prefigures them, encodes them, and makes them intelligible. Cultural sensations coalesce around the spectacles of crime in part due to the conventions film noir provides; it's a template. American political hegemony being assured, at least in retrospect, since the end of the Great War meant that as an empire the nation barely registered an external world. Of course, this is an exaggeration; numerous wars fought in Europe and Asia, as well as the pervasiveness of cold war brinksmanship, meant fears of foreign aggression were matched by military force. However, the national imagination remained fixed within interior landscapes; the terror of nuclear attack was personalized as each schoolchild was trained to "duck and cover" in the event of an attack, for instance, despite everyone's knowledge—gleaned from sci-fi movies as well as John Hersey's *Hirsohima*—that we'd all be vaporized instantly. In his argument about the rise of "imagined communities" of national identification, Benedict Anderson links the daily reading of the newspaper to monumental structures of capitalist nation building. The pervasive dailiness of the newspaper—its ability to appear every day on one's doorstep or to precipitate a daily walk to the newspaper stand—and structure each morning's activity singularly but communally is part of the mundane accession to nationalism. Anderson is not too interested in what is in the paper; however, Mikhail Bakhtin and Walter Benjamin, writing in the 1930s, considered the contents of the feuilleton—the endless accounts of murder, suicide, assault, and scandal—to be a central feature of modern social experience. The fact of their presence alters ideas about literary culture.

Film noir's obsessive return to the scene of the crime anticipates how ideas of guilt about America's violent history would emerge as crucial facets of twentieth-century politics. My girlhood fascination with my parents' past secrets was also an attempt to pry loose the mask covering the nation's brutal history. Growing up in the 1950s, if one were at all sensitive to the messages flowing over the airwaves, left one perpetually ill at ease. You knew things were wrong, even if it was unclear what that might be, no matter how insulated you were in your modern suburban house, as I was by the middle of the decade. The film noirs on your television set confirmed it. But I was watching the equivalent of reruns. These films had foreshadowed the anxieties I felt, intimately aware as I was with a father working in the defense industry, of impending destruction. Like fortunetellers, film noirs predicted the nation's future.

This is a book about film that barely mentions them. At once film and feminist theory, American cultural history, literary criticism, photography study, and political analysis, *Black & White & Noir* reconsiders the cultural politics of the 1980s and 1990s by tracing a hidden stream in 1930s and 1940s popular and leftist (often overlapping) cultures that has recently resurfaced. If one reads the credits of Hollywood B-movies of the 1940s and 1950s, it appears HUAC was right: American movies were plying the minds of average citizens with critiques of capitalism. Between August 26, 1927 (the executions of Sacco and Vanzetti), and June 19, 1953 (the executions of Julius and Ethel Rosenberg), left-wing culture permeated popular American life. The Depression ushered in a wave of working-class agitation, and World War II propelled a massive Popular Front to fight fascism; during this brief quarter century, movements to challenge state and corporate violence seemed, if not triumphant, at least legitimate. However, like the bombings of Hiroshima and Nagasaki to end World War II, the two acts of state violence against immigrant left-wing working-class people lurk as residual horrors.

Black & White & Noir offers an interdisciplinary cultural history of twentieth-century America through episodic readings of films, photographs, and literature—a history of the myriad detritus floating beyond the borders of acceptable scholarship. Tracing the dark edges of trash lurking amid our postwar political unconscious, this book views pulp as prefigurative, a kind of political theory of America's problematic democracy disguised as cheap melodrama, with origins in two submerged aspects of American modernity: the contradiction of slaveholding in a democracy and the suppression of working-class organizing. Violence is at the core of both of these strands. Noir—emerging out of German Expressionism and pulp fiction, among other sources—normalizes horror by deflecting it from the public arena into the private home. Politics in twentieth-century America becomes pulp fiction; or, more accurately, pulp fiction leads the way in matters political. A generation was raised on the dichotomous popular cultural images television offered in Ozzie and Harriet, on the one hand, and the reruns of Ida Lupino and other B-movie stars, on the other. The Nelson's neat, spacious, modern home was supposed to signal a radical break from war, fascism, and the Depression, but the ghosts around Ricky were interference from that earlier program. The dark side of 1950s culture was silently indebted to the cultural politics of the 1930s. Today's political imagination is haunted by all forms of our everyday trash, from the spent uranium bomb casings littering Kosovo to Monica Lewinsky's literary tastes, from the tons of debris from the destroyed Twin Towers to Arabic flight-training manuals. My central premise is that modernity in America is structured around two poles, each working to suppress a hidden history of state violence: racial codings (hence the black-and-white motif) and class melodrama (hence the recourse to noir sentimentality and nostalgia). These in turn are revealed in the pulpy silhouettes of the femme fatale—the dark lady who glows in the bright key lighting of B-movies.

Part I, "Black," begins just as noir makes the big time. If John Huston's *Maltese Falcon* (1941) signaled the emergence of this new sensibility, shifting Humphrey Bogart's role from the thuggish gangster in *Bullets or Ballots* (1938) toward the morally complex detective figure of Sam Spade because of the introduction of a new term—the "femme fatale," seductress and betrayer—then the war-time photographs of Esther Bubley charted what happened to Mary Astor's Brigid O'Shaughnessy. Chapter 1, "Already Framed," examines unrecognized precursors to film noir in the work Esther Bubley did for Roy Stryker's Office of War Information (OWI). Her photography projects in Washington, D.C. rooming houses and across bus and train stations throughout the country found a nation of solitary, determined, dreamy, rootless women. Bubley, one of the last photographers hired by the Farm Security Administration (FSA), stayed on when the department became the OWI. She continued to train her camera on the disrupted lives women experienced during and after the war. On her long bus trip across the Midwest and South during the war years, her images of women alone and of segregated waiting rooms revealed a dark underside of the war that would find its way into noir. After the war, she worked for corporations such as Standard Oil, TWA, and the pharmaceutical company Ciba, continuing to take disturbing images while under their sponsorship. Her troubling images belie the consensus forming around postwar corporate liberalism. Her haunting photograph of a lone woman waiting to pick up a sailor in a Washington, D.C., bar, like Marion Post Wolcott's defiant shot of two couples drinking rum and Coke in a juke joint, push the 1930s images of ruined, yet noble, womanhood into the terrain of noir.

The lone woman surviving the city, like Lutie Johnson in Anne Petry's novel *The Street*, are also relocated daughters of the Depression's "Migrant Mothers." Set in geographical and social motion by World War II, they end up singing in a *Road House* (like Ida Lupino) or looming up *Out of the Past* (like Jane Greer), packing a pistol if they are white. But if they are black, like Lutie, they find themselves cleaning these bad girls' rooms. Chapter 2, "Domestic Labor," looks at the racialized sexuality of the maid in pulp fiction and film noir in order to examine how African-American women's left-wing literary culture fed into, yet transformed, the stereotypes of black female sexuality. Writing in the 1940s and 1950s, Petry and Gwendolyn Brooks pick up the femme noire to revise her depiction in that classic melodrama, Fanny Hurst's *Imitation of Life*. Each considers how race, ethnicity, and class are detected on the female body, especially those of various fatal moms of 1930s to 1950s popular fiction, such as *Mildred Pierce*.

Chapter 3, "Double Cross," reads Richard Wright's 1953 novel, *The Outsider*, as a film noir. Reversing many film noirs that "rip their stories from the headlines," Wright lifts dozens of plots and scenes from the movies he saw in late 1940s Paris. Moreover, the 1952 rewriting of his own life story in Ralph Ellison's *Invisible Man* (resulting in the National Book Award for Fiction) spurred Wright's own revenge plot. Both novels owe much to 1930s detective fiction and 1940s film noirs' unconscious charting of the changing racial make-up of postwar cities, the absent presence in their depictions of urban space. These two African-American authors used the genre's conventions to expose the Communist Party's racism, in much the same way as other left-wing writers had used the gangster story to expose capitalism's exploitation of workers. They rewrite the passing narrative into one of amnesia and changed identities and pulp America's racial melodrama (and the theme of the "tragic mulatto") through noir.

Where part 1 maps noir across the wretched spaces where a restless population dwelled—waiting rooms, hotel rooms, kitchens—part 2 ties noir to a nostalgia for America's past. "White" returns to some overlooked sources for noir from the 1930s—Farm Security Administration photography, labor iconography, and radical social workers' accounts of Depression privation. Chapters 4, 5, and 6 address how pulp modernity is expressed through pictures of rural white poverty, nostalgia for the heroic "working stiff" of proletarian culture, and literary investigations of prostitution and domestic chaos, respectively. Quite paradoxically, representing the pockets of 1930s poverty paved the way for the homogenous 1950s, enabling an amassing of a white urban middle-class culture by offering it images of what it wasn't. Chapter 4, "Blanc Noir," begins with *Fargo*, the Coen brothers inversion of film noir and its city locales, to argue that America became a modern mass nation not during 1920s modernism—marked by its gleaming skyscrapers and efficient assembly lines—but later, during the 1930s, when an urban, middle-class audience could consume images of white rural poverty—a dystopian pastoralism—through the mass media.

Chapter 5, "Melodrama/Male Dramas," considers how the tradition of labor documentary is suffused with melodrama (especially 1930s proletarian melodramas of the unemployed "working stiff") to express working-class masculinity. This historical investigation turns to two recent labor documentaries—*Roger & Me* and *American Dream*. Each film demonstrates how so-called postindustrial labor relations in which corporations must become "lean and mean" mimic the sleek muscular working-class body of the idealized proletarian man. At the same time, unemployed workers slacken because the new labor solidarity requires hiring media consultants rather than picketing to counter corporate hegemony. This feminized labor force takes up noir melodrama to narrate its story.

Chapter 6, "Not 'Just the Facts, Ma'am'," reads the history of debates about welfare through the social work novels written in the 1930s and 1940s by Caroline Slade. Slade's female social workers investigate the deviant bodies of poor white women to show the deep connection between pulp aesthetics and left-wing politics in the United States. These social workers resembled detectives; however both their gender and their relation to the state meant they had little autonomy. Instead Slade's social workers mirrored the many women reporters, like Martha Gellhorn, who had toured the nation and the world documenting the crises of war, fascism, and the Depression. This reportage and fiction often verged on a tabloid noir. It was cleaned up in the layouts of *Life* but splayed across pages of *PM*. Margaret Bourke-White's first assignment in the town of New Deal, Montana, (in *Life*'s first issue) sanitized the sensational photojournalism of Weegee, both of which, like Slade's novels, wrap class conflict in racialized sexual perversions.

Part Three: "Noir" muses on how the ominous trappings of women's daily lives that circulated in film noir coalesced into feminism. Chapter 7, "Barbara Stanwyck's Anklet," connects the case-hardened steel persona of the femme fatale to the various solid objects surrounding and enclosing her. How to dress and accessorize the femme fatale? Phyllis Dietrichson descends her staircase in anklet and spiked slippers; Thelma Jordan stands in District Attorney Cleve Marshall's doorway in her black pumps. Stanwyck's iconic poses in this footwear, as well as in her black shades or with her black Bakelite telephone, are accessories to the crime of female desire. The chapter analyzes how gender creates difference in and through objects by tracing philosophical, political, and psychoanalytic discussions of footwear. Objects tell stories. In the 1960s, when feminists argued against women's position as sex objects, demanding subjectivity, objects acquired a lousy reputation. But in commodity culture, as Marx suggested, they have something to say. Film noir highlights their sinister nature as consumer goods meant for women's use.

The concluding chapters argue that just as 1950s popular culture refers unconsciously to 1930s political culture, recent popular political culture gestures continually to noir. This section pulps postwar America by linking aspects of culture not usually thought of as pulpy—documentary (with its serious attempt to expose crises) and avant-garde (with its communal, visionary ecstacies) and literary fiction, especially its middle-brow magical realism—to this pattern of deflecting racial horror and class tension onto scenes of privacy. Chapter 8, "Medium Uncool," shows how indebted second-wave feminism was to the 16mm black-and-white movie culture of the 1960s. It finds in women's experimental cinema made during the Vietnam War an uncanny domesticity akin to film noir's unsettling post–World War II views of household objects and the city. Chapter 9, "Mapping Noir," concludes the book with a trip through recent women's fiction and a history of literary "dark ladies." It describes how American fiction has performed political theory through sensational narratives. The two chapters thus draw a larger picture of postwar American suppression of the Left within various strains of popular political culture, explaining, in part, why Hollywood bankrolled "neo-retro-noirs" in the 1990s.

Black & White & Noir risks appearing eclectic and incoherent. Yet, precisely because the book ranges among seemingly disparate fields of inquiry, it demonstrates the wild totality possible through interdisciplinary work. Only by stepping out of bounds, like the doomed characters in a film noir, can one link film noir to FSA photography or to social workers' reports, or investigate Richard Wright's debt to film noir. Just as a prism's many facets refracts white light into the full range of colors—ROYGBIV—the chapters of this book break apart the constituent elements within, behind, and emerging from noir. By arguing episodically for the presence of a noir sensibility—a pulp politics—throughout twentieth-century America, I improvise a method for theorizing its peculiar modernism, not as seamless grand narrative, nor as tightly focused case study, but as the chaotic repetition of the familiar. The title plays on the various forms of black-and-white circulating in modern culture—newspapers, pulp fiction, photographs, B-movies, 1950s TV, underground films—and, of course, indexes the racial system superintending American life. Symbolically, there is a connection. This book frames it; that's what noir is all about.

PART I

BLACK

ROOMS AND RAGE

CHAPTER I

ALREADY FRAMED: ESTHER BUBLEY INVENTS NOIR

ROOMING HOUSES

There comes a moment in many film noirs when the bad girl emerges snarling with anger as she ensnares the dimwitted doomed guy. The appropriately named Ann Savage turns on hapless, guilty Tom Neal in *Detour*, her face transformed from forlorn innocence after he picks her up hitchhiking into vicious rage when she reveals to him that she recognizes his clothes and car as belonging to another man, the dead one Neal has dumped along the highway. Jane Greer, dressed like a nun, turns on Robert Mitchum in the final moment of *Out of the Past* after she kills her gangster lover Kirk Douglas, leaving Mitchum dead and framed for a number of murders. So too Barbara Stanwyck in *Double Indemnity* sneers at Fred McMurray when he starts getting cold feet about their plans to murder her husband. By the time she appears in *The File on Thelma Jordan*, Stanwyck can turn on her former pimp with such fury she blinds him with a cigarette lighter. Gloria Grahame laughs at Jack Palance when he slaps her face in *Sudden Fear*, reducing him to her sex toy after she threatens to alert his rich wife, Joan Crawford, that he is already married. Lizabeth Scott in *Too Late for Tears* reveals her greedy murderous desire for the cash hurled mistakenly into the

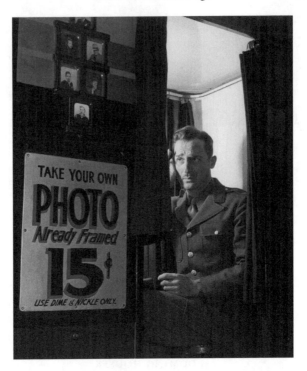

FIGURE 2. Esther Bubley, "A picture-taking machine in the lobby at the United Nations service center," December 1943.

convertible she and her husband drive. She viciously gets rid of one man after another until she lands in Mexico alone with the money. These scenes repeat themselves again and again as if it is not enough that the women's morbid sexuality already marks them as bad. They must also mutate into animals. Simone Simon in *Cat People* literally turns into a seething black leopard stalking her competition, her husband's assistant, and killing her psychiatrist after he kisses her. This early noir horror film sets the image of sexual allure as animality. Because it is literalized, we never see Simone Simon's face transform; it is her body, which is never actually seen either. Instead, we hear the rustle of her paws amid the leaves, see the shadow of her form, discover the slashes of her claws. Good girl "Kansas" in *Phantom Lady* dresses up as a femme fatale to get drummer Elisha Cook Jr. to admit to seeing the elusive woman in the hat accompanying her boss. When she goes with him to the after hours jam session, she lures him with her orgasmic responses to his drum solo. The image of the woman turning into wild beast is a code for the impossible: to see the moment of female orgasm. Its terrifying ability to alter the woman's face is perhaps what these moments of vituperation are really about. Rather than the laugh of the Medusa, we see her fury at men's irrelevance.

This view of triumphant female rage—refusing to look pleasing, to be the soothing and demure helpmate—inevitably results in death. Both she and the man are doomed, but for a tiny instant her desire and its expression have trumped social conventions about femininity. We watch Jean Wallace in Joseph H. Lewis's *The Big Combo* as her lover Richard Conte slowly goes down on her. The camera remains focused on her face as it fractures following her orgasm. By this time when the genre had entered its baroque period, with films as different as Robert Aldrich's *Kiss Me Deadly* (1955) or Samuel Fuller's *The Naked Kiss* (1963), the moments of female rage—when Lily Carver points her gun at Ralph Meeker's Mike Hammer and begs "Kiss me, Mike" or when Kelly grabs the phone receiver and beats Grant to death after she discovers his pedophilia, repeating and mirroring the first scene where she beats her pimp with a leather handbag—had entered the realm of domestic sit-com camp. During the mid-1940s, however, these scenes still had the air of tragedy clinging to them because they revealed anxieties circulating within the culture about women's wartime mobility and participation in heavy industry. Women's seething rage could burst forth without logical antecedent; it's somewhat confusing to the man why the femme fatale explodes at the moment she does. The plot motivation is never quite enough to account for it; only her unpredictable and invisible sexuality explains it. A mystery to the ordinary men attracted to these women, it is always transparent to the women who meet them; yet, knowing who they are, the women rarely condemn their demonic sisters. As Gloria Grahame insists in *The Big Heat*, "We're sisters under our minks."

This dangerous autonomy, visualized in the snarl that comes invariably at the moment when the female takes control of the man and the situation, indexes the changing position of women accelerated by the Second World War. Women had experienced a different kind of mobilization during the 1940s when many left poorly paying

27

jobs as domestics or clerks in search of more lucrative employment in factories and in federal government offices. Many of these women ended up living in rooming houses full of other single women with whom they shared meals and chores and movie dates. Marjory Collins's April 1943 shot of women massing a downtown block for an evening movie documents a female takeover of urban space, one that Giuliana Bruno revealed had occurred in Italy during the rise of fascism and throughout the war.[1] Crowds of "Thursday night shoppers [stand] in a line outside a movie theatre" in Baltimore, Maryland, as neon flashes above them a huge exclamatory: NEW.[2] Louis Faurer's photograph of working women waiting for a bus on Broadway before a poster advertising a Barbara Stanwyck movie (clearly misdated as 1948, because the movie is the 1950 film *No Man of Her Own*) details how women could move through the city at night dressed much like the actress (in that film she assumes the identity of a dead woman she befriended on the train to San Francisco just before it wrecks). In 1948, the Kinsey Report had opened up discussions of Americans' sex lives. As Andrea Fisher observes in her ground-breaking look at the women photographers working in the FSA/OWI, "[T]hese images from the 1940s . . . cast suspicion on their promise of a visual presence, their fascinations turn on an offering of sexuality."[3] That offering could be had, in part, because women could live alone, occupying single rooms. If the film noir femme fatale rarely possessed this kind of domestic isolation—she's usually a kept woman—her snarl set her apart from proper domesticity. She didn't need to work a job, like the women flocking to war work, but she was their sister nevertheless.

Photographer Esther Bubley was among the last members of the extraordinary crew of artists hired by Roy Stryker to document government programs aimed at ameliorating poverty during the Depression and, when the nation entered World War II, to record the efforts undertaken by citizens to support national defense. Hired as a negative cutter, Bubley stayed on after the Farm Security Administration had become the Office of War Information. Her large body of work focused on these uprooted working women. Bubley tracked the private lives of young women, such as her sister Enid, who lived in boarding houses or in a series of furnished apartments, as Esther and her other sister, Claire, did, while they worked government jobs. Her many photographs, intimate moments of pri-

FIGURE 3. Marjory Collins, "Thursday night shoppers in a line outside a movie theatre." Baltimore, Md., April 1943.

FIGURE 4. Louis Faurer, "Barbara Stanwyck Movie Poster, Broadway NYC, 1948." Miriam and Ira D. Wallach Division of Art, Prints and Photographs, The New York Public Library. Astor, Lennox and Tilden Foundations. Silver gelatin print. Permission by David Ferber.

vacy—daydreaming out a window, napping on a couch, thumbing a magazine, arranging personal objects on a dresser—offer a sense of stasis, of lives held in abeyance waiting alone for an uncertain future. In her most famous image, captioned, "Girl sitting alone in the Sea Grill, a bar and restaurant, waiting for a pickup," Bubley anticipated the signature icons surrounding the femme fatale: a lone woman sits at the end of long booth, a glass of beer almost empty, smoking, framed by Venetian blinds. Behind them the night is black save for the neon letters above her; but a man's head is visible outside the window behind her, peering at her back. She waits under surveillance, explaining: " I come in here pretty often, sometimes alone, mostly with another girl, we drink beer, and talk, and of course we keep our eyes open you'd be surprised at how often nice, lonesome, soldiers ask Sue, the waitress to introduce them to us."[4] Like Ella Raines in *Phantom Lady*, who sits night after night watching bartender Andrew Tombes Jr. until she finally follows him through the dark streets one night aggressively chasing him, not for companionship but for information, Bubley's girl also "keeps her eyes open" for men. In her impassive availability, she signals her desire; yet hers is a figure in relative repose, arms crossed, not in defiance but resignation. For the young women in the rooming houses and bars of Washington, D.C., in 1943, nightlife is spent usually alone or in the company of other lonely women; they wait, but they are free. The sequence of pictures from the Sea Grill contains some of the most detailed captions written by Bubley. They constitute a pulp narrative about how to pick up soldiers. One image notes a "Girl and a soldier came into the Sea Grill separately, but are developing a beautiful friendship."[5] Another zooms in on "A slightly inebriated couple at the Sea Grill."[6] These women, as Bubley makes clear, are poised in a strange contradiction. Alone and mobile, they are free from family scrutiny and control; yet their availability is limited by the absence of men who have deserted this and other urban spaces for war.

Hints of lesbian desire appear everywhere in Bubley's images as the women curl up together to read or listen to the radio, but the overriding sense is of a deep malaise. All dressed up and nowhere to go, these women wait—for men. No wonder the films made immediately upon the war's conclusion feature a new brutal kind of female sexual aggression. Phyllis Dietrichson in *Double Indemnity* doesn't

FIGURE 5. Esther Bubley, "Girl sitting alone in the Sea grill, a bar and restaurant waiting for a pickup. 'I come in here pretty often, sometimes alone, mostly with another girl, we drink beer, and talk, and of course we keep our eyes open you'd be surprised at how often nice, lonesome, soldiers ask the waitress to introduce them to us.' " Washington, D.C., April 1943.

just await Walter Neff after he arrives at her bungalow door to sell her an insurance policy. She shows up later at his door, hair coiffed and perfumed in sweater and slacks, asking for a drink. Although she is housed in a tidy bungalow complete with step-daughter, husband, and maid, and the year of the film's action is 1938—before the war had even started in Europe—thus seeming to have little in common with Bubley's sisters and their roommates, she too appears poised for something to happen. As does her step-daughter, Lola, whom we find playing Chinese checkers a few nights later with Phyllis when Neff shows up to have Mr. Deitrichson sign the insurance policy, biding her time until she can go downtown to meet her boyfriend, Nino Zachetti. After her father's death, Lola moves into her own apartment: "Four walls and you just sit and look at them," as Neff characterizes it. Filmed in 1943, the movie locates these two women—the murderous stepmother and the grieving, alienated daughter—who live out a solitary female existence, dependent upon, yet divorced from, men.

Although the rooming houses Bubley was documenting seemed wholesome enough in 1943, the rooming house remains, in fiction, film, and art, a sinister place filled with wild women and brutal men. Cornell Woolrich's novel (which became the Stanwyck film *No Man of Her Own*) *I Married a Dead Man* tracks Helen Georgesson as "she climbed the rooming-house stairs like a puppet dangling from slack strings. A light bracketed against the wall, drooping upside-down like a withered tulip in its bell-shaped shade of scalloped glass, cast a smoky yellow glow. A carpet-strip ground to the semblance of decayed veg-etable-matter, all pattern, all color, long erased, adhered to the middle of the stairs, like a form of pollen or fungus encrustation."[7] This dreary space, home to the rejected, pregnant nineteen-year-old girl becomes an iconic zone of danger and defeat; Gloria Grahame, her face hideously scarred when her gangster lover scalds her with hot coffee, holes up in tough cop Glenn Ford's room in Fritz Lang's 1953 film, *The Big Heat*. In Robert Siodmak's *The Killers*, Burt Lancaster (Swede) awaits his murderers in his small dark room with stoic calm; double-crossed by a woman, he has simply given up the will to live. More recently, the Coen brothers made the hotel where *Barton Fink* suffered Hollywood writer's block a central character in their parodic, moody film noir. Ed and Nancy Keinholz's *Pedicord Apt.*, an installation in the Weisman Art Museum in Minneapolis, reconstructs a seedy 1940s rooming house, letting us enter its claustrophobic hallway and eaves-drop on the domestic melodramas behind each grim door. Just those sorts of doors had been the actual inspiration for one of the greatest works of twentieth-century America fiction. Living in and managing the rundown hotel his family owned, Nathanael West watched its long-term residents who lived out a desperation during the Depression. They became the basis—along with a cache of real letters he was given—for his brilliant dissection of transience, *Miss Lonelyhearts*.

What distinguishes Bubley's images of the rooming-house young women from Helen Georgesson or *Miss Lonelyhearts*, for that mat-

ter, is the way her camera has opened the doors finding behind each
rather clean, well-lighted spaces often cluttered with friends, magazines, pictures from home, and drying hand laundry. These women
have made this zone of violent transience homelike, inviting, quite
unlike the noir vision of enclosure. In the typical film, a woman (or
man) is trapped in the rooming house, like Tom Neal and Ann Savage in the apartment they share in Los Angeles; its walls close in
upon the inhabitants, whose only escape are endless cigarettes and
cheap booze. The opening sequence of Jean-Pierre Melville's hom-
age to American film noir, *Le Samourai*, begins in the dark room
where Alain Delon lies absolutely still on his bed. The slow pan from
one desolate object to another tracks a bleak existence enlivened
only by his pet bird. The noir rooming house barely provides cover
much less shelter; it is a space of waiting and death. These were the
places New York crime photographer Weegee (Arthur Fellig) fre-
quented in his work as freelance photographer for a number of daily
newspapers during the 1930s and as staff photographer for *PM* in the
early 1940s. Weegee's tabloid images of murder and accident victims, or of apprehended criminals, always held an aura of intimacy
about them; he knew his subjects, hanging out with them in the
Bowery restaurant Sammy's. Bubley's rooming-house images seek
to portray another side of transience, one that might make single life
possible for middle-class women. But they shade into discomfort
with the dullness attendant upon the working life. Margaret Bourke-
White, on assignment for the first issue of *Life*, photographed the
men and women filling up the transient housing of New Deal, Montana, as they built the Columbia River dams. These pictures of hard-
drinking men, women, and even children suggest an unsavory element to the search for employment. Weegee's images make nighttime New York look like a lurid zone crawling with lowlifes, cops,
and high-society dames. However, Bubley shows a more middle-
class world, a world of sisters and friends who carefully wash their
nylons every night in preparation for work the next day. These
women might have been the spinster aunts of a generation before.
However, they are not at home. Instead they circulate within the
rooming house entertaining men or at the bars on the lookout for
soldiers or just lie together dreamily listening to the radio. Unlike
Woolrich's Helen, who finds an envelope tucked under her door
containing a five-dollar bill and a one-way railroad ticket back to her

FIGURE 6. Esther Bubley, "Listening to a murder mystery on the radio in a boarding house room." Washington, D.C., Jan. 1943.

hometown San Francisco, Bubley's rooming-house women have settled in, even if they would eventually leave for acceptable marriages.

At the same time, however, there is a darker side to the rooming-house pictures. Bubley frames many of the images through open doorways. She finds the woman staring out the window, or reflected in her bureau mirror. These solitary women, dislodged in their lodging house, languorous, in limbo, which, while not filled with incipient dangers, like those awaiting Gloria Grahame in *The Big Heat* for turning on the gang, suggest at once a radical dis-ease and a stubborn revelry within their solitude. In picture after picture, women are caught sleeping while a card game goes on in the background; they sit alone smoking while listening to the radio. Beautiful rebellious Pearl Ginsburg "refused to have her boarding house rent raised;" yet she too sits alone on her bed staring pensively, averting her eyes from the camera.[8]

34

FIGURE 7. Esther Bubley, Washington, D.C., 1943.

FIGURE 8. Case-hardened and hard-boiled Barbara Stanwyck stands behind Fred McMurray's door in *Double Indemnity* (d. Billy Wilder, 1944).

Each of these scenes reactivates the gangster movie sequence of the hole-up, when, on the lam or in the midst of gang warfare, a group of men, reconstituted as a family (think of Michael Corleone being instructed by his elders in how to make a sauce in *The Godfather*), huddle together waiting out the heat. In other images, glanced from the hallways into rooms with doors left open while a man visits, the deep focus hints at the possibility of a sexuality central to noir.[9] In one of Bubley's images, a single hall light glows behind two partial silhouettes of a man and a woman who stand talking in the darkened foreground. Between them and framing the woman's face is a sliver of her lighted bedroom glimpsed through the open doorway. Here erotic lighting clashes with the codes of respectability enshrined by the open door. This 1943 image anticipates a scene from *Double Indemnity* in which Phyllis stands behind Walter's open door hiding from Barton Keyes. In the shot, the door itself separates the two, who are starkly-lit: Neff stands against his dark apartment; Phyllis against the spot-lit hallway. Mystery and eroticism are performed within the space of iconic objects—open doors and light fixtures—Bubley had scrutinized. In another of her photographs, two women lounge together—one dreamily staring into space, the other smiling warily at her—on a bed separated by a bare light bulb that burns between them casting deep shadows across their faces. Is this seduction? It's faintly in the air, especially as the eye travels up between the two women's faces to the bare bulb encircled by a halo of wire from the missing shade and the Degas print of a nude woman reading taped to the wall above it. Again, the bare bulb and the line of the door on the far edge of the picture reinforce the curve of the barred bed frame, all details of desire.

Another photograph of two women together, which Bubley captioned "Women gossiping in a drugstore over Cokes. Washington D.C., 1943," places the women, again lit from behind, conspiratorially together across a wooden table. Smoke hangs in the air between them as one woman partially covers her mouth seeming to gesture behind her with her hand while speaking to her rapt friend. Only the paper cup and the women's heavy coats keep this from looking like a much seedier bar. These interior shots by Bubley all conspire to define a sense of enclosure and desperation, even as they portray daily mundane spaces and activities: women sitting together or alone talking on the phone, listening to the radio, playing cards, writing a

FIGURE 9a. Esther Bubley, "Pearl Ginsburg refused to have her boarding house rent raised." Washington, D.C., Jan. 1943.

FIGURE 9b. Esther Bubley, Washington, D.C., 1943.

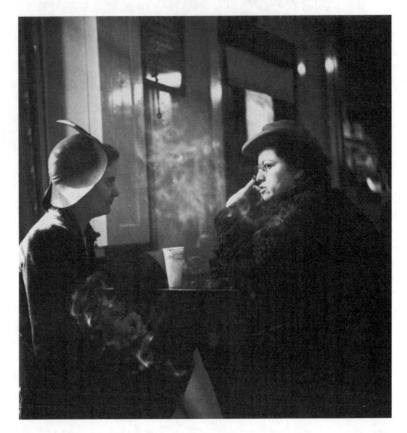

FIGURE 10. Esther Bubley, "Women gossiping in a drug store over Cokes." Washington, D.C., 1943.

letter. These often grim moments are supplemented by the occasionally tense, intimate visits by men. Even with the front across the oceans, the war takes its toll.

Bubley's photographic portraits of single working women living in rooming houses or picking men up at bars, included a series of women working at their government and industry jobs. At the Western Union telegraph office, women are shown operating all manner of the machinery of communications. Miss Ethel Wakefield sits at a PBX board; Miss Genie Lee Neal reads perforated tape; Miss Helen Ringwals works with pneumatic tubes; Muriel Pare commands the switchboard.[10] These images of serious and competent young women, almost all of whom Bubley identifies as "Miss," in control of the inner workings of the system wiring the nation together during a time of war, became staples of film noir iconography. The repeated presence of telephones and telegraphs in so many films, and the important role these devices play in the plots, signal, like the empty dark highways or train tracks crucial to so many of these films as well, a new sense of women's mobility, freedom, and power through their essential labor for the war effort. Women like Kathie Moffet in *Out of the Past* call the boss when the caper collapses; women like Leona Stevenson in *Sorry, Wrong Number* rely on the telephone to protect them; women like Vera in *Detour* die of strangulation by a telephone cord. Bubley's work among these young women in Washington, D.C., incarnated the iconography so central to film noir's sense of dislocation: the lonely aggressive female who can adroitly use a series of mundane objects—telephones, cigarette lighters, radios—with deadly results and who inhabits and works in a world full of others like her. Bubley's photographs remained largely unpublished during and after the war years, unusual for the project whose purpose was to broadly underscore a national sense of purpose. Her disturbing intimations of female eroticism, authority, and autonomy were perhaps too unsettling. Nevertheless, looking at the photographs now, it seems clear that she was inventing the icons of female pulp modernism—on the one hand, a kind of sleepwalking existence of endless sexual deferral; on the other, eventual economic self-sufficiency.

Bubley's rooming-house photographs oscillate between varied images of the nondomestic domicile, the house that is not a home, the uncanny. One aspect derived from half a century of pictures of Bowery flophouses, like those Alfred Stieglitz found in 1892 at Five Points, which became the basis for the one Lillian Gish inhabits in D. W. Griffith's *Musketeers of Pig Alley* (1912), and that Weegee was splashing across the New York papers every day. His two solo exhibits at the left-wing Photo League were entitled *Murder Is My Business.*[11] The other developed from wholesome images of young female co-eds lounging in college dormitories flooding many mass-circulation magazines.[12] While she was in Washington, D.C., Bubley's other projects included following the lives of students at Woodrow Wilson High School, who were busy decorating the gym for the prom, checking new fashions, and hanging around the cafeteria. These images of stable middle-class normalcy, coupled with a

39

FIGURE 11. Esther Bubley, "Miss Helen Ringwals works with the pneumatic tubes through which messages are sent to branches in other parts of the city for delivery." Washington, D.C., June 1943.

FIGURE 12. (*Opposite page top*) Esther Bubley, boarding house, Washington, D.C., 1943.

FIGURE 13. (*Opposite page bottom*) Claire Trevor on display for Dennis O'Keefe in *Raw Deal* (d. Anthony Mann, 1948).

series of photographs of GIs sightseeing in the nation's capitol, stressed that the nation was, like the well-appointed home, still a safe haven; they helped allay fears of enemy invasions.

ROAD TRIPS

Rooming houses offer temporary solace and privacy for the city's poor or unattached workers. The rural version is the motel, the inn, or the roadhouse, whose utilitarian rooms allow anonymous bodies temporary rest after a long day on the road. The opening shot of the Coen brother's *Blood Simple* (1984) plays on the classic noir scene of the couple driving through a rainy night, stopping at the neon sign calling their restless bodies to "Dew Drop Inn." The noir sensibility is based both on the black-and-white aesthetics of cities and on the open stretches of gray asphalt, telephone wires looping along their shoulders, fleeing them.[13] But as with so much of the noir effect, it had origins in earlier movements. During the late 1930s, a number of women published book-length sagas about their travels among the world's downtrodden. Women photographers were mobilized during the Depression years to take their cameras with them on the road in search of "the trouble I've seen," as Martha Gellhorn called her book-length reportage. Reversing the plaint of the blues song, Gellhorn and, even more insistently, photographers such as Margaret Bourke-White, working for *Life* magazine, and Dorothea Lange, working for the FSA, sought to make sure everybody'd seen the trouble they'd seen. Bubley's photographs of her bus trip throughout the midwestern and southern United States are part of this tradition. In fact, Bubley cited Margaret Bourke-White's 1936 *Life* cover spread on New Deal, Montana, as inspiring her to become a photographer.[14] Like them, she recorded a nation of women beaten down by or making do with whatever raw deal they'd cut.

In many ways, the "bus story," as she called her assignments, made Bubley's career as a photographer.[15] Although Bubley had worked briefly for *Vogue* during their busy pre-Christmas season in 1940, she left New York to return to Washington, D.C., for a job at the National Archives in early 1941, where she took pictures of her sisters' rooming house. A word from her supervisor to Roy Stryker landed her a spot in the darkroom at the OWI lab, and thus

Stryker licensed her study of single women, which became part of the file even though it had not been formally assigned. After he left the OWI, Stryker hired Bubley to work on the huge Standard Oil of New Jersey project he was coordinating, and she became known for her industrial photography and worked not only for "slicks," such as *Redbook, Life,* and *Ladies Home Journal,* but for numerous corporations, including TWA, Ciba, and Pepsi.

Writers, such as Ruth Gruber, Ella Winter, and Anna Louise Strong, had marked out the entire globe for inspection. Offering politically observant versions of traditional women's travel narratives, these women found other women in Soviet Russia or on the Long March through Hunan Province who were shock-workers and soldiers. British writer Rosita Forbes detailed her excursions among *Women Called Wild* with sensational stories of sex slave markets in Arabia, Stakhanovite women window washers in Leningrad, women opium addicts in Java, Foreign Legion camp followers in Morocco, and prostitutes in the " 'Waste Spaces' between 'Buenos Aires' and 'Shanghai' " in Algiers: in short, the usual salacious Orientalism found traditionally in these.[16] But like her left-wing sisters, Rosita Forbes embarks on her journey as a participant observer, one of the wild women who lurk the jungles of Yucatan disguised as cheetahs. It appears from Forbes's telling that "cat people" can be found the world over, not just in the "delicious" novel she cites entitled *Lady Into Fox.*

Women on the road through slave markets and harems, through China and the Soviet Union, through bus terminals and rooming houses, were called "wild." Those who recorded what they found often did so with a kind of uninhibited mania, even as they might abhor what they found. Going on the road in search of misery, hoping to expose and thus to ameliorate it, was one of the effects of 1930s movements' goals.[17] Of course, it was also part of American self-mythologizing, from Huck Finn's "lightin' out for the territories" to Horace Greeley's call to "go west, young man"; now the automobile and burgeoning highway system made it possible for most anyone, not just rebellious boys. Commenting on her road trip through the nation in 1947, Simone de Beauvoir notes "the gas stations, roads, hotels, and solitary inns . . . these things are profoundly part of America. The landscapes of the Far West [she was] driving through exist essentially for the sake of tourists." De Beauvoir distains the way in which the stark landscape has been transformed because of tourism; yet she herself, like so many, participates in the experience of national space via the automobile. She revels in it: "Night is falling; it has fallen," she comments as if narrating a film noir, "A luminous wheel turns in the darkened sky: a hotel sign" looms up from the desolate highway connecting Las Vegas to Los Angeles promising "a martini and a hearty dinner. . . . We've still got four hours on the road."[18] Amazement at the vast spaces of this country give way to a sense of claustrophobia as de Beauvoir boards a bus to travel through the South observing Jim Crow first hand.

Esther Bubley had already made this trip in 1943 for the OWI, whose photographers, she explained to Tony Van Witsen, "did the war effort. They did shipbuilding and I did buses. I traveled through the country riding on a bus."[19] Another FSA/OWI photographer, Marion Post Wolcott, shot the gleaming silent snowed-in streets of Woodstock, Vermont, in March 1940, the halo glow of the streetlight sanctifying this zone of peaceful America. Wolcott also commented visually on Jim Crow. Her October 1939 photograph is captioned: "Negro man entering movie theater 'colored' entrance. Belzoni, Mississippi, in the Delta area." Its stark shadows indicate the distinctions between black and white, the sign pointing to "Colored Entrance" just one of many crowding the side of the building. Two years later, she was making portraits of blacks and whites in the Florida Glades relaxing at their "juke joints." In one photo, two young black men stare sullenly at her camera, beer cans on the table between them and an advertisement for Cobbs Creek whiskey featuring a white bespectacled judge slamming his gavel to declare "judged *mild* 43 million times!" In another, two young white couples drunk on whiskey and Cokes (the empty pint of whiskey lies on its side between them) lean hotly into each other under a hand-painted sign announcing "Rooms/ By-Nite or Week/ Ask - at - Bar." These images play on the disjunctures between the efforts of self-presentation and those of documentary disclosure, on the one hand, and on the secrets kept hiding behind images of America's economic recovery, on the other. Within a year, neither peaceful Vermont nor steamy south Florida would resemble itself; war altered everything. Wolcott's attention to architecture exposed racial tensions that Bubley found in the restless yet drowsy women living in "a waiting room."[20]

Like Wolcott, Bubley subtly notes the discrepancies racism fosters between blacks and whites during a time of national mobilization.

FIGURE 14.
Marion Post
Wolcott, "Two
couples in a booth
in a juke joint."
Near Moorehaven,
Florida, 1939.

FIGURE 15. Esther Bubley, "A girl who is waiting between buses in the ladies'
lounge at 4 AM in the Greyhound bus terminal." Chicago, Ill., Sept. 1943.

Her trip began by heading through Pennsylvania to the Midwest. She is attentive, as she was in the Sea Grill, to evolving sexual dynamics opened up by the war. Her pictures of young women sleeping in bus stations across America detail the tedium of commercial transport—"a nation of zombies."[21] In Chicago, she finds "A girl who is waiting between buses in the ladies' lounge at 4AM in the Greyhound bus terminal."[22] Stretched out on a wooden bench, her purse strap linked around her arm, shoes on the black-and-white linoleum below her feet, she dozes after reading the newspaper opened on her small suitcase. These women, coiled in exhaustion, are, as curator Andrea Fisher notes, open to inspection; yet, lost in sleep, they maintain their dignity. They are wholly isolated even as they are on public display. This sense of separation is powerfully conveyed in one image of a young woman wearing a tailored suit getting off a bus in the middle of an empty field. Self-contained, she strides off through the brush, her clutch purse firmly locked under her arm, but it is impossible to see where she is headed.[23]

FIGURE 16. Esther Bubley, "Girls sleeping in the waiting room of the Union station." Washington, D.C., March 1943.

FIGURE 17. Esther Bubley, "A girl getting off the Macon bound Greyhound bus in Georgia. Passengers can get off at any place they wish along the road." Sept. 1943.

The world of the bus is also set apart, maintaining its own ecology. Sleeping women are curled up against wooden booths everywhere in Pittsburgh and Indianapolis and Cincinnati and Louisville bus terminals. They are living along the highways with their families in converted gas stations left empty because of wartime gasoline rations, leaving the place, as the sign in front announces: "Closed Nothing For-Sale."[24] Noting the items available to travelers in the Chicago Greyhound bus terminal's ladies' restroom, she finds a culture and commerce of daily life on the road: "Items ranging from soap and nail polish to soda for upset stomachs may be rented from the maid on duty, who owns her own stock. Her business is usually

47

FIGURE 18. Esther Bubley, "Bus passengers in the Greyhound bus terminal's ladies' restroom. Items ranging from soap and nail polish to soda for upset stomachs may be rented from the maid on duty, who owns her own stock. Her business is usually brisk." Chicago, Ill., Sept. 1943.

very brisk."[25] Bubley, like many FSA/OWI photographers, was an inveterate list maker; objects fascinated her.[26] Walker Evans surveyed the belongings of the three tenant families he and James Agee had documented in *Let Us Now Praise Famous Men*; Bubley depicted the shelves and dressers of the women in the Washington, D.C., rooming house.

These images, glanced from her bus window or stolen in waiting rooms or disclosed as she followed bus drivers and charwomen into their rooms, reveal a nation on the move yet strangely caught, stuck in limbo. In one caption of a picture of bus driver Clem Carson, Bubley lists the contents of his suitcase: "a cigarette package with

48

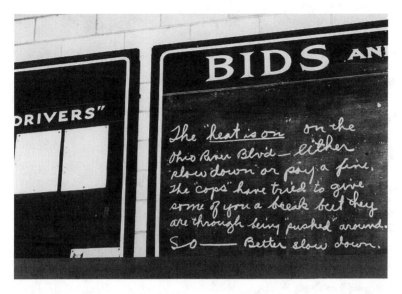

FIGURE 19. Esther Bubley, "A warning on a blackboard in the drivers' room of the Greyhound garage." Pittsburgh, Penn., Sept. 1943.

one cigarette, a pay sheet signed by the dispatcher, a flashlight, extra batteries, cash fare pad, form for cutting transfers, 1 look magazine, 1 Pic magazine, 1 small can shaving powder, 1 baggage crank, 1 knapkin [sic], shaving lotion, razor, shaving cream, work gloves, baggage checks, comb, 1 black address book, envelopes, trip reports, hair tonic, two packs of gum, name plate, whiskey ration card, pliers, screw driver, soap, pencil, 1 red address book, bus schedules, towel, 3 handkerchiefs, toothbrush, 2 pairs sun glasses, a washcloth, 1 shoestring, ammonia inhalant, ticket clamps, witness pads, company rule book, tarriff [sic] sheet, shirt, tie, socks and underwear, old pay sheets, and 1 cockroach with which buses are frequently infested. This was removed."[27] It's a Whitmanesque catalogue singing of the modern body electric. Driver "Bud" Carson lived at the Southern Hotel in Columbus, Ohio, explaining how he and another driver doubled up in the room; then he revealed to Bubley his anger that he had received a "checker's" report accusing him of smoking and eating a candy bar and stopping too long at a rest stop. The mundane intimacy of this list and of the items kept for women passengers by the restroom attendants was part of the Office of War Information's attempt to demonstrate a quality of the everyday to workers' and travelers' lives during the war.

Bubley, like most of Roy Stryker's field photographers, had a wry sense of humor and was ever on the look out for contradictions. She included a synopsis of "Us on a Bus," the novel-in-progress by a driver who detailed how he bought a bottle and nipple and milk for a young mother only to be told he'd make a good father; a soldier who jumped up and "loudly announced to the world . . . 'Memphis is God's country' "; an old lady who "unscrewed a thermos jug and took a drink explaining to the public in general that she was a frequent traveler from Texas to Nashville, that she like to drink when she liked it"; and many young women on the lookout for, or being hustled by, soldiers.[28] Her picture of "an eating place near the Greyhound bus stop" in New Bedford, Pennsylvania, shows a giant coffee pot that serves as the café.[29] This emblem, like those de Beauvoir stopped at a few years after the war, "exist[s] only for the tourist and

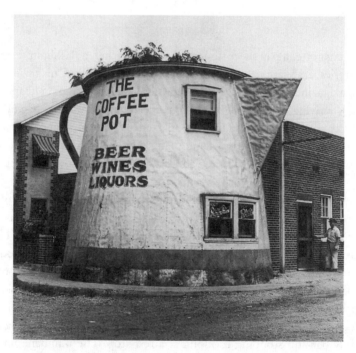

FIGURE 20. Esther Bubley, "An eating place near the Greyhound bus stop." New Bedford, Penn., Sept. 1943.

because of the tourist," according to de Beauvoir's assessment;[30] however, Bubley places it firmly within a landscape of work—the bus driver's job necessitates stops for the passengers' comforts, who, like one woman, is on her way to Nebraska to study nursing—and housing shortages. The café is connected to a home and serves, like the gas station-turned-house or the bus itself, as a reconstituted family living space. It domesticates the vast and savage emptiness of the nation's landscape; it's cozy in its hokey absurdity.

These images, like the rooming-house pictures, preserve a sense of continuity, even as they track endless mobility, by emphasizing everyday life. When Bubley went on the road to photograph Standard Oil workers while working for Roy Stryker after the war, she kept a diary that listed objects and their associated activities, images she intended to record. Running down the page for the week of January 22–26, 1948, they read as a protofeminist poem about women's invisible, intimate labor:

Beating rug	scrubbing porch
canning	vacuuming
washing windows	wheeling baby
on Ladder	bubbling baby
cooking	baking
~~canning~~	gardening
hang out wash	painting screen door
waxing floor	piano lesson
sewing	defrosting refrig
mending	waxing floor
taking children out	painting sashes
dishes	making aprons
feeding older kids	
ironing	
dressing child	
cooking meal	
putting child to bed (story)	

Her accounting includes the names of the Texas women whom she had photographed, as well as the hours they spent doing each of their various tasks. The focus on women's domestic labor, performed within the suburbs springing up around Standard Oil's

Texas refineries, contrasts with the images Bubley had been recording in Washington, D.C., of single, urban women operating the machinery of communications. This bus trip uncovered a new stability and predictability to women's daily lives.

Yet it was the same year Hollywood was churning out *Raw Deal*, *Kiss the Blood Off My Hands*, *Road House*, *They Live by Night*, and *The Lady from Shanghai* among many more that featured tough women fleeing domesticity and traveling in pursuit of pleasure and cash. In fact, the images from Texas are unsettling. The houses crammed together, dwarfed by enormous television antennas, are far less hospitable than the gas stations, waiting rooms, or coffee-pot café. By the end of the year, Bubley was living her own domestic noir melodrama. In November, she was busily working a job at Doylestown, Pennsylvania, shooting enough for her to underscore that she "used 2 cases bulbs" on Wednesday, November 10, 1948. The next day, she recounts the following entry: "Doylestown— worked all day—Ed [Locke, her husband] called—sounded very sorry for himself—also drunk—I got sorry for him too but I don't like being pushed around. Garage .75 Br. L. D. 3.50."[31] Throughout the next year, her journals record a series of jobs—including the amazing *Ladies Home Journal* assignment series on mental illness— and the dollar amount she had given Ed with notations that he was drunk again. Her 1950 passport, issued under the name Esther Bubley Locke, has a handwritten line crossed through her married name.

Even before then, Bubley's eye had already differentiated a postwar aesthetic from the kinds of socially concerned documentary images taken only a few years earlier. Where Wolcott records the lonely climb by a single dignified man up the colored-only stairs of a Mississippi movie house in 1939, Bubley suggests that the war had altered the racial landscape considerably. Her shots of the Memphis bus station, with their pointed focus on the signs designating "White Waiting Room" dominating the frame above masses of black and white men and women crowding onto the waiting buses, stage a sense of frenetic activity. The bodies mix together, jamming their way forward to the open bus door, and tell a story of conflict and change rather than the enduring legacy of Jim Crow. Certainly she includes a stark image of the "Colored Waiting Room" sign found in Rome, Georgia, which she captioned with damning simplicity: "A sign at the Greyhound bus station." But there is something about

FIGURE 21. Esther Bubley, "Waiting for a bus." Memphis, Tenn., Sept. 1943.

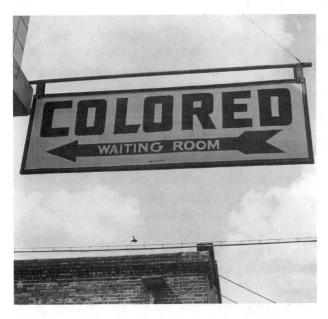

FIGURE 22. Esther Bubley, "A sign at the Greyhound bus station." Rome, Ga., Sept. 1943.

the composition, with the phone wires running just below the sign, connecting the brick building behind it to the rest of the world that offers a sense of impending change. Where the pictures of the South taken by Dorothea Lange, Walker Evans, and Margaret Bourke-White challenged the nation with the images of an enduring racial caste system little distinguished from that of Reconstruction, despite the automobiles occasionally found lining the streets, Bubley's bus trip limns a glimpse of the nascent civil rights movement in the sheer physical movement of a restless population.

MENTAL ASYLUMS

Shortly after her Texas assignment, Bubley was offered a number of assignments for *Ladies Home Journal*. *LHJ*, like the Italian *Enciclopedia delle Donne* which could be bought monthly at newspaper stands, was designed in part to facilitate the rise into middle-class suburbs of a postwar rural and urban working-class population in the United States. (In Italy, its job was to help teach peasants and laborers to become urbanized national citizens of the new democracy.) With popular fiction by such middle-brow writers as John Marquand and extensive hints on fashion, homemaking, gardening, as well as features on marriage and childrearing, it also included political commentary and art criticism. In the April 1949 issue, Esther Bubley's photographs illustrated a serious examination answering "What *Is* Mental Illness?" The special and general features sections include an essay by Eleanor Roosevelt, a reproduction of El Greco's *Virgin with Saints*, a discussion of "American and Un-American Social Security," advice on moving "From School to Job," and on "Making Marriage Work," as well as a "Diary of Domesticity." Bubley's photograph of a young schizophrenic woman "being treated with electric shock" depicts a pained woman in hospital dress hunched over and covering her face with her hands. Behind her, framing her, is a large window crisscrossed with many panes suggesting bars. Off to her side and behind her sits another patient staring out another window; her hand also covers her face. "Mrs. Templeton—that's not her real name, of course—is not unusual." She is one of the 3,000 women admitted annually for "involutional melancholia, an emotional illness to which women in the change of life are particularly susceptible," which "shock and hormone treatments have proved

FIGURE 23. Esther Bubley, "Paranoid Schizophrenic," from *Ladies Home Journal* (March–June, 1949). Property of Jean B. Bubley.

tremendously fast and powerful in treating," claims author Joan Younger.[32] The image is chilling; a cropped version, with just the girl in the foreground, became a standard depiction of schizophrenia in psychiatry textbooks.[33]

It is the image Hitchcock uses to conclude his noir "docudrama," *The Wrong Man*. After finally being cleared, Manny (Henry Fonda) visits his wife Rose (Vera Miles) in the mental hospital where she retreats from the tensions accruing from his arrest, trial, and conviction. Her final comment to him: "That's fine for you," contradicts any sense of a Hollywood happy ending. Hitchcock had meticulously researched this film, making sure that the Queens and Manhattan locations were accurate, even visiting Riker's Island jail to observe how inmates carry their bedding to their cells. It seems logical that he would have found an authentic image to portray Rose's descent into madness so he could avoid the Hollywood clichés of "the snake pit" imagery of insanity.[34] Bubley's image of a schizophrenic woman codified film noir iconography. The caption for Bubley's photograph asserts, "She is being treated with electric shock and there is hope for her recovery," but her gestures, like Rose's comment, suggest otherwise. Bubley's image, like that of Hitchcock, lends a caveat to this hopeful scenario, exposing the

55

potential detours of danger and desire sending anyone veering off the road.[35]

Because of the *Ladies Home Journal* article, Bubley worked again in mental hospitals documenting the effectiveness of Ciba Pharmaceuticals's antischizophrenia drug Serpasil. Her work appeared in a promotional booklet for the drug that lauded its benign effectiveness. Bubley's before and after photographs of a young black schizophrenic woman who "displayed marked denudative tendencies" show the positive effects of this "drug which the Indians had claimed for centuries could aid the mentally ill." In the top picture, a solitary naked black woman kneels on her stripped bed, her head pressing down on the mattress ticking. The contrasting bottom image, just one day after her first injection, shows her sitting up in a made bed in striped pajamas drinking a glass of water with a prim white nurse looking on. In this image, the nurse stands in a flood of sunshine coming in the room through an open window; however, the top photograph includes only the bed partially in dark shadow.[36] It is an eerie vision of induced normalcy. Even under contract to promote Serpasil, Bubley managed to disturb the images and cast noir overtones across them.

In their attention to the enclosed spaces of solitary women living in institutions with others, these photographs extend the projects she had begun in Washington, D.C., and continued in Texas as she tracked the daily work routine of Standard Oil workers' wives. Like the images shot for the federal government and big industry, they have a disturbing element of celebration for capitalism and conformity, even as they also hint at rebellion just below the surface. One set of photographs from March 1949 focused on the emerging new technology of television and concentrated on "TV Antenna," "TV FAMILY," "TV Home," "Parent TV." These images tracked a further move into the confines of a claustrophobic domesticity in the postwar period. An undated set of contacts, entitled "Black Star Girls," suggests this refashioned domesticity was an on-going interest. These pictures of B-girls taking bubble baths or standing on a bathroom scale, range across their possessions—spiked heels and baby dolls. Perhaps they figured as the back story to the *Ladies Home Journal* feature "How America Lives" that Bubley also worked on during the late 1940s. To some extent, these and the 1949 assignment for the "Profile of Youth" series continue her OWI project on Woodrow Wilson High School as they focus on the lives of five high-school girls from Maine's "potato empire"—three are "still hanging on the thin edge: Phyllis Donaghue, whose lumpy exterior covers some driving dreams; Leona Pryor, a dynamic young beauty with a restless urge; and Loretta Lannigan, a little 'nobody' who can't make up her mind what she wants to do." Bubley "personally found more interesting the struggle of the children who were determined to stay in high school no matter what odds were against them, [so she had] thrown in two more stories—the story of Dorothy Lynch and Muriel Breuer, both of whom are working their way through high school . . . the only possible ticket to the outside world. All are in the lower third of their class."[37] These girls present a new generation of young women whose lives, despite the postwar

FIGURE 24. Esther Bubley, "A boarding house rule forbids men guests to come into girls' rooms and vice versa." Washington, D.C., Jan. 1943.

FIGURE 25. Esther Bubley, "Riding on a street car." Washington, D.C., March 1943.

prosperity, seemed headed for trouble, or at least boredom, without the possibility of escape from small-town life. The opportunities for sex and anonymity provided young women by the Venetian blinds in the Sea Grill have collapsed into grueling tasks, like those of the oil workers' wives, alleviated by television. No wonder involutional melancholia was epidemic.

Bubley framed the changing experiences of young women between the onset of the United States's entry into the Second World War and the nation's emergence as a world power by concentrating on the melodramas of daily life. Her pictures, made for the federal government and major corporations—both intent on advertising and marketing their triumphant goods and services, perhaps reflecting her own life's experiences, focused on a certain unmistakable darkness "behind Washington's marble fronts."[38] These girls, with names straight out of Hollywood's B-movies— Loretta, Leona, Phyllis—were already framed, their faces about to break into a raging snarl at any moment. After all, they were featured in a *Ladies Home Journal* "profile of youth" article called "Teen-Age Cruelty" as examples of "poison personality girls," like "the super- sophisticate" who "wears black whenever possible, likes lots of jew- elry, uses a cigarette holder," and is "too utterly bored by every- thing."[39] Notwithstanding her surname, Esther Bubley could be counted on to photograph lives already framed by the boredom, routine, restrictions, and despair that was lurking everywhere across a nation supposedly teeming with frenzied war (and postwar) pro- duction. Someone who worked constantly, with "a pride of craft,"[40] and was an avid movie-goer, she also spent time in a Brooklyn box- ing gym working out, after a visit to it on assignment convinced her this was the solution to the backaches she suffered carrying around her equipment on her 5'4" frame.[41] Like her own refashioning of her body during an era when women did not work on their biceps, her images of seductive women alone in bars, of single women on the road, of anguished women isolated in asylums, of bitchy girls claw- ing their way out of small towns belied America's postwar vision of femininity. Her photographs had already framed the femme fatale.

CHAPTER 2

DOMESTIC LABOR: FILM NOIR, PROLETARIAN LITERATURE, AND BLACK WOMEN'S FICTION

On the trail of the missing Kathie Moffett, private investigator Jeff Bailey begins Uptown, in a Harlem nightclub, by interviewing Kathy's maid, Eunice. In this minor scene in Jacques Tourneur's *Out of the Past* (1947), Bailey enters the smoke-hazed, jazz-filled club and is escorted by the maitre d' to a table with two couples; he asks which woman worked for Kathie. Bailey seems at ease in the club; like many private eyes, he's used to interacting with African Americans, and after one couple leaves for the dance floor, he inquires about Kathie. Elegant and sly, Eunice says she has no idea where she went, Miami perhaps—she got some vaccinations and took off. Bailey buys the table a round of drinks and leaves, commenting, in his detective voice-over narrative that you don't get vaccinated to go to Florida. Kathie took off to Mexico. James Naremore describes this scene and others like it depicting encounters between beautiful, sophisticated black women and the white detectives in film noirs as crucial to the noir hero's/detective's "aura of 'cool' . . . his essential hipness," because the integrated nightclub is an iconic transgressive location within film noir.[1] As Kathie's maid, Eunice served a dark woman *but* she is herself a black woman; moreover, her visual position between two men—one white, the other black—is critical to understanding the different complexion of the femme fatale.

Coded through dress, lighting, and mise-en-scène as a femme fatale in her own right, Eunice is Kathie's aura—another type of literal femme noire. The dark lady of film noir is a woman with a past, a kept woman who performs no useful function other than sex. Her body is available, draped in mink and diamonds, for display and desire. She is free to meet men at night or in the afternoon because she is unencumbered by the usual trappings of domesticity. She is free in part because she has a housekeeper to clean up after a long night of drinking, to fix the drinks and make the coffee, to help her dress. The "aura of cool" blacks impart to the white detective occurs through a transference: as authentic bearers of alienation, African Americans are, in Richard Wright's term, the original outsiders. Both the white detective and the white woman he pursues acquire their abilities to pass into the underworld through their encounters with and knowledge of darkness found beyond conventional work and marriage (both of which, because of slavery's legacy, have been denied to African Americans). Like the "authenticity" of the original possessing an "aura," according to Walter Benjamin, Eunice stands before Bailey as the "prerequisite" of another woman he has never seen.[2] Eunice holds no metaphoric status as femme noire. She embodies it. In this, she resembles Benjamin's notion of the "original" work of art, which remains fixed within "tradition," while its copies, endlessly available, are mobile and potentially destabilizing.[3] She vibrates sexuality—a sign hanging around black women's necks since they unwillingly arrived shackled together on this continent— and thus allows us to know Kathie through her. Yet Eunice resists Bailey; she is straightforward in her lie, and Bailey can see through her because she is the original woman of the dark. She points up Kathie's double duplicity. The white femme fatale has the potential to disturb the "tradition" of racism, especially its economic and sexual effects. However, her rupture with conventional white femininity is limited because, as a "mistress," she still remains dependent on this tradition.

While Eunice never reappears in the film, her presence hovers behind the white femme fatale in this and many film noirs. Out on a date in Harlem, dressed as Billie Holiday did in the 1940s—upswept hair coiffed with a veil of white camellias, black dress accented with

FIGURE 26. Theresa Harris (Eunice) on a date in Harlem dressed like Billie Holiday in *Out of the Past* (d. Jacques Tourneur, 1947).

white trim—Eunice, stylish and independent, assuredly resists a white man's authority; she defends herself and her former boss in a gesture of female solidarity, which extends to her look. The two women are erotic cross-dressers, as the white femme fatale will inevitably wear the clothes of the torch singer and the maid may acquire her boss's hand-me-downs. Her deception parallels the deceit embodied by the object of desire, in this case femme fatale Kathie Moffett. Eunice's loyalty is to her employer, whom she knows has had a rough time with men. Presumably, as a single woman kept by those same men, Kathie doesn't require too much work from her. When Eunice aids Kathie, it's an isolated incident within the film. Yet, in Max Ophuls' *The Reckless Moment* (1949), Lucia Harper's (Joan Bennett) black maid Sybil (Frances Williams) appears as a central figure in her boss's cover-up.[4] Like many domestic melodramas that rely on the household presence of a maid, Sybil helps Lucia, who hides evidence (a body) that her daughter has killed a blackmailing gigolo. In so doing, she also allows Lucia access to an underworld and its erotics. In this film, as in the classic melodramatic vehicle in which a black maid's domesticity facilitates a white woman's business, *Imitation of Life* (1934, 1959), the maid participates in the maintenance of middle-class white family economic order, helping to support it when there is no man around, and acts as confessor for the white woman she serves.[5] The black maid, like the detective or the femme fatale, by occupation, slides between two worlds. As a black woman in racially segregated America, she lives on the margins of white America; as a servant to the bourgeoisie, she inhabits the bedrooms of the white middle class. As entertainer, cook, and servant, the black woman is rarely the center of the action in film noir (see Jean-Pierre Melville's *Le Samourai* (1967) with an impassive Alain Delon as the hitman for a post–civil rights and French exception to this), but her presence appears necessary to the complex postwar sexual and racial dynamics that film noirs track by linking domestic melodrama to hard-boiled proletarian culture.

What kind of work does the maid perform in film noir? Her service to the femme noire, as an overt femme noire, is more complex than simply that of the loyal employee in Hollywood melodrama. Her ability to understand and function within alien worlds makes her more of an equal to the female protagonist; yet she does little more than protect her, lying and covering up for the white woman. Because the dark lady of film noir is a rebellious white woman— glowingly white in her initial key-lit scenes—the black domestic worker of film noir crystallized racial and class issues raised by the Left during the 1930s when domestic labor debates resurfaced after disappearing with Charlotte Perkins Gilman's powerful 1903 tract *Women and Economics*. She shows up the bourgeois house as little more than a brothel whose sole purpose—now that even the housewife is freed from housework and childcare—is sexual and reproductive. Racial erotics, tracked throughout the 1930s in reportage, poetry, and short fiction, became the focus of postwar novels by black women. Ann Petry's *The Street* (1947) and Gwendolyn Brook's *Maud Martha* (1953), two novels by authors connected to the Left, were both published during the heyday of Hollywood's film noirs. Like the films' concerns with the new kinds of social relations forged during the Depression and World War II, each locates black women's labor within proletarian literary culture by linking domestic melodrama to female Bildungsroman. Each also revises the image of the black domestic from mammy to maid, recasting a symbol of antebellum racial hierarchies into an urbanized form of labor.[6]

As a popular medium, albeit often in its "B" form, postwar film noir began to visualize many of the issues lurking within proletarian literature—city life, the organization of work, social mobility, cross-class desire. Noir films borrowed 1930s proletarian narratives, themselves hybrid revisions of socialist realism and domestic fiction. They also generated new literary concerns. *The Street* owes much to Stephen Crane's *Maggie, Girl of the Streets* and American naturalism, but it also taps fears haunting Jacques Tourneur's *Cat People*.[7] Gwendolyn Brooks structures *Maud Martha* like the jazz orchestrating film noir as she revises a coming-of-age story to reveal why the black femme fatale cannot be visualized in racist America. Alan Wald and Michael Denning have recently argued that the radical novel, or the cultural front in American literature, exceeded the bounds of 1930s proletarian culture.[8] For many writers, especially black writers, the themes and concerns central to 1930s fiction—the experience of collective subjectivity within social relations formed by economic and racial stratification—appeared after the Depression had ended. *Invisible Man* is a 1930s novel, even if it didn't appear until 1952; so too is Margaret Walker's *Jubilee*, begun in the 1930s and completed in the 1960s.[9]

Focusing on the difficulties black women faced in supporting themselves and their families, analyzing the racial and sexual dynamics of black domestic workers in white women's households, these two novels deepened the domestic labor debates central to women in the American Left. They pushed the discussion beyond analyzing one's own housework as a "double burden" for the working woman employed outside the home to consider what it meant to maintain two homes—one's own and another's of a different class, race, and neighborhood.[10] This contradiction became a focus of Toni Morrison's first novel (set during the 1940s) *The Bluest Eye*. Pauline Breedlove travels between the white family, doting on the blonde daughter of her employer, and her own, where she ignores her dark-skinned daughter Pecola (whose names echoes that of Peola in *Imitation of Life*) with tragic consequences. Richard Wright's *12 Million Black Voices* graphically displays the social differences between the maid's workplace kitchen and her own. In a two-page spread, pictures of the dank kitchenette are contrasted with the uniformed maid in a sparkling kitchen. This image of a black mother tending white children is among the only recognition of a black woman's labor by Wright whose first-person plural nar-

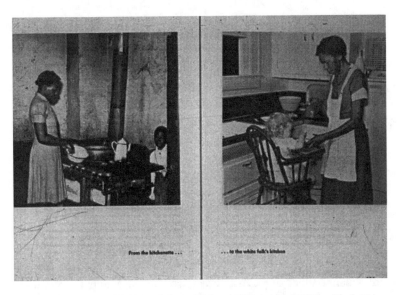

FIGURE 27. Two-page spread from Richard Wright, *12 Million Black Voices* (1941). Left: Russell Lee, "Mother and Son." Chicago, Ill. Right: Marion Post [Wolcott], "Maid." Georgia.

rative "we" does not include women who are pointedly spoken of as "our women." Nevertheless, the racial dimensions of domestic labor had been an on-going concern of writers throughout the 1930s; the pages of the *Crisis*, the *New Masses*, and the *Daily Worker*, among countless little journals sponsored by the Communist Party, explored black women's double life under white supremacy and capitalism; but these were often works of short reportage, poetry, or short fiction. They never attained the recognition that a novel did.[11] For instance, Belle Traub "Discovered: A Modern Slave Block!" and interviewed one of the many black women lined up on the street corners of major cities waiting for day work as a domestic during the 1930s. Mrs. Rose Johnson described her day as follows: "I get up at six each morning. Get breakfast for my three children. Wash the dishes, fix sandwich lunch for them, and send them off to school. Then comes a bit of family work. All this, before coming out on the block . . . and then to stand around on a street corner for hours waiting" for the same work in another woman's house.[12] Ella Baker and Marvel Cooke went underground to detail the workings of "The Bronx Slave Market" in the *Crisis*. Here, on Jerome Avenue, black women line up waiting for day

65

work within the mostly Jewish households of the neighborhood. "Paradoxically," they note, "the crash of 1929 brought to the domestic labor market a new employer class. The lower middle-class housewife, who, having dreamed of the luxury of a maid, found opportunity staring her in the face in the form a Negro women pressed to the wall by poverty, starvation, and discrimination."[13] The work appears especially onerous, for in addition to the usual window washing, scrubbing, laundry, dusting, turning of mattresses, and chasing off the wandering hands of the son, to wash dishes Orthodox Jews required "a different dishcloth for everything they cook. For instance, they ha[d] one for 'milk' pots in which dairy dishes are cooked, another for glasses, another for vegetable pots, another for meat pots, and so on," according to their informant Millie Jones. As late as 1940, Louise Mitchell decried the "Slave Markets" where "Negro women wait[ed] for employers to come to the street corner auction blocks to bargain for their labor."[14] The authors advocate self-organization among the women, castigating "organized labor's limited concept of exploitation, which permits it to fight vigorously to secure itself against evil, yet passively or actively aids and abets the ruthless destruction of Negroes," and citing the hopeful signs of an "embryonic labor union . . . in the Simpson avenue 'mart' . . . [where for] the recent Jewish holiday, habitués of the 'mart' actually demanded and refused to work for less than thirty-five cents an hour."[15] While the strains between black workers and Jewish petit bourgeois entails a legacy of anti-Semitism and racism lurking within the *Crisis* exposé, the description of the housework, with the exception of the extra dishwashing for Orthodox Jews, is typical, with the white woman expecting immense labor—weekly window washing for instance—from the black woman for a pittance—five dollars a week and carfare. Millie Jones lost her position when she took Sunday off because her boyfriend was visiting.

Gwendolyn Brooks's "Hattie Scott," one of the residents of *A Street in Bronzeville* (1945) also resists her employer's demands on her time to pursue her own desire. Nora, "a butter-colored maid with the hair on the 'riney' side" and resident of Marita Bonner's "Frye Street" in Chicago rejects her lover Sam when she decides to enroll in City College to study law at night, only to die of pneumonia brought on by exhaustion. But Hattie Scott daringly seeks pleasure with a black man, leaving the white woman and night school behind.[16]

> If she don't hurry up and let me out of here.
> Keeps pilin' up stuff for me to do.
> I ain't goin' to finish that ironin.'
> She got another think comin.' Hey, you
> Whatcha mean talkin' about cleanin' silver?
> It's eight o'clock now, you fool.
> I'm leavin.' Got somethin' interestin' on my mind.
> Don't mean night school.[17]

Again, petty domestic chores—polishing silver, for instance—interfere with the speakers' sexuality and romance. The title of the poem, "the date," suggests that Hattie Scott plans not only to make love, "somethin' interestin' on my mind," but to go out in public (perhaps to a nightclub like Eunice) first. As the "Queen of the Blues" sings, the point of domestic labor in a white woman's kitchen is to support the man she loves and get his loving in return: "I was good to my daddy. / Gave him all my dough / . . . Scrubbed hard in them white folks' / Kitchens / Till my knees was rusty / And so" (58). This story is repeated almost verbatim by Lutie Johnson in Petry's terrifying novel *The Street*. Lutie abruptly leaves domestic service when she learns her husband is living with another woman. She eventually becomes a nightclub singer in the Harlem club owned by the gangster Junto, who expects to pimp for her. As historian Jacqueline Jones points out, during the Depression, "it was the entertainment field that fueled the dreams of black girls who yearn[ed] for a life's work of glamour and triumph" as nightclubs, radios, and records featured the voices of Billie Holiday, Bessie Smith, Ella Fitzgerald, Lena Horne, and others.[18]

This plot trajectory, from domestic work to entertainment to prostitution, was typical: "A young girl from North Carolina came to New York City in 1936. Unable to find work in a respected capacity, she sought domestic work. Here, her relations with her employer were not entirely moral, but at least raised her income. Finally domestic work becoming odious, was forgotten, and another prostitute was created."[19] The link between domestic labor and prostitution—sexualizing housework and racializing sex work—is central to the image of the femme fatale's maid who can keep the house of a woman not known for her domestic virtues because she, too, exchanges her body for pay. Lutie Johnson runs up against this continually as a live-in maid in Lyme, Connecticut. Overhearing conversations among her employer, Mrs. Chandler, and other women friends, neighbors, and relatives, Lutie learns that these women fear her as an attractive, young (and therefore obviously sexually available) black woman: they all assume she is a "whore." "Apparently," she realizes, "it was an automatic reaction of white people—if a girl was colored and fairly young, why, it stood to reason she had to be . a prostitute."[20] Chester Himes inadvertently endorses this connection between young black maids and prostitution, discussing his work as a hotel bellhop in Cleveland during the 1930s, he recalls: "Black women were easy to pick up and made exciting bedmates; maids were the easiest and good-looking whores were the hardest."[21] This continual sexualizing of the young black female body in the employ of white middle-class families is directly connected, as Himes notes, to the history of slavery, which made the bodies of black women available to the white master to, in the words of Frederick Douglass, "make a gratification of their wicked desires profitable as well as pleasurable."[22] Moreover, it shrouds the sex work of the white housewife, whose livelihood as a legal prostitute is covered by displacing it onto the maid.

Jacqueline Jones points out that for the black woman, the "forces that shaped the institution of human bondage in the American South endured, albeit in altered form, long after the last slave embraced freedom . . . [as she] toiled . . . in the kitchen of a Chicago white woman" (3). During the Depression, urban black women's labor was restricted to domestic work and laundry work; even during World War II, when factory jobs opened up, they were janitorial. Seeking to expose this, the *Daily Worker* routinely decried women's work, especially domestic labor, as slavery, seeing even female industrial workers as "slaves" whose bodies were being destroyed by brutal work.[23] A typical page lists the following headlines: "Rubber Workers Paid $2 Daily for Slavery," "High Maternity Death Rate Under U.S. Slavery," "Women Slave in Steel Mill."[24] In this they echoed the complaints of Bessie Smith's 1928 "Washwoman's Blues": "All day long I'm slavin' / All day long I'm bustin suds . . . just to make my livelihood . . . rather be a scullion / cookin in some white folks' yard / . . . wouldn't have to work so hard."[25] Historian Phyllis Palmer finds that in the South "service was a job for slaves. After emancipation that imagery of service remained intact. White Americans," moreover, "were trained in or learned from the southern models after the Civil War, and northern beliefs in the housewife's duty to supervise labor meshed with southern beliefs in leisured ladyhood."[26] Thus black womanhood was associated with domestic service, or slavery, while white women were seen as supervisors of domestic labor, not as workers themselves.[27]

This continues a curious history of the use of "slavery" as a metaphor for wage labor. As historian David Roediger notes, in antebellum America, "[t]o be a slave, even a white slave, was to be associated with degradation. Genteel factory women who rejected the term knew this, and knew that slavery implied sexual exploitation as well. To be a slave also implied a connection with blackness."[28] During the Depression decade, the American Communist Party portrayed workers as strong virile examples of democratic men; the image of the robust factory worker standing tall in interracial brotherhood against he forces of decayed, effeminate capitalism appeared in prints, poems, novels, and essays.[29] So it appears surprising that the *Daily Worker* relies on the imagery of slavery to describe workers, but not so strange when one realizes that these workers are female. Moreover, among female workers, racial differences still encoded the black woman as a slave, while her more revolutionary white sister has understood "that we have a government of murderous bandits, parasites and oppressors" and thus could excoriate her black sister as insufficiently politicized. For instance, Fannie Austin exhorted:

> Negro working women! When you go to look for a job you find it very hard to get, and, when you do get it, you only obtain ten or twelve dollars for a big week of *slavery*. You are very much oppressed and exploited for a little nothing and you are looked upon by the bosses as *not human*. You are handled by the exploiting parasites as if you are *sold to them*. They hire and fire you any time they feel like it. Are you going to let those fat-bellied bosses fool and *enslave* you forever? Are you going to be pressed down and stepped upon forever—or are you going to unite with your white working women sisters in struggle, in

battle against the capitalist oppressive system—against the *wage slave, lynching system?* Negro and white women workers!

she concludes, should join the Communist Party: "Show your solidarity, show your strength! don't sleep—wake up!"[30]

These metaphors of the slave mart and the slave block to describe domestic labor and women's work in industrial labor indicate the long history of invalidating women's labor by sexualizing it as reproductive labor, differentiating women workers from those members of the "producing classes."[31] Presidential candidate Al Gore's use of the term "working families" called forth this ambivalence about the nature of work and class conflict within America.[32] On the one hand, trying to appeal to the so-called gender gap, "working families" feminizes labor as service done on behalf of family, (all work is thus domestic labor); on the other hand, by insisting, as Gore did in late August 2000 to a rally of workers, that they needed to ask "which side are you on?" he signaled an association with the tradition of masculine workers fighting the boss. The next line of Florence Reece's, 1930s song answers: "you either are a union *man* or a scab for D. H. Blair."[33]

The dynamics between the white female employer and the black maid cannot be seen as merely about economics. As Baker and Cooke note, domestic work barely registers as labor by union organizers; its location in the privacy of the home and the intimate nature of the work—cooking, cleaning, caring for children—blurs the lines between workplace and home. Domestic workers might organize (as they did) across households, but that still did not alter the private day-to-day engagement with the employing woman who is often home alone with the maid.[34] Lutie notes the bizarre change that occurs in her dealings with Mrs. Chandler, who often confided in her when the two were alone, even chatting amiably on the train down to New York "about some story being played up in the newspaper, about clothes or some moving picture. But when the train pulled into Grand Central, the wall was suddenly there. . . . There was a firm note of dismissal in her voice so that the other passengers pouring off the train turned to watch the rich young woman and her colored maid; a tone of voice that made people stop to hear just when it was that the maid was to report back for work. Because the voice unmistakably established the relation between the blond young woman and the brown young woman" (51). Trudier Harris points out that "[i]n moving from her home to that of the white woman, the black woman connects two racially and spatially distinct worlds in one direction—she goes into the white world."[35] Lutie's public train travels with Mrs. Chandler back into New York City imply a reversal of this racial/spatial direction; it is this threat to the white woman's social location that must be contained. Yet this is the awkward intimacy film noir broaches as it revises domestic melodrama to enable a new kind of pulp modernism embodied within unencumbered female aggression and sexuality.

Lutie had noticed that the tensions over sexuality were racial not class based, as the young white women hired to serve meals at the Chandlers never became the object of women's jealousy or men's desire, nor did they receive the intimate outpourings or the cast-off clothes of the white woman employer. In public, the blonde woman oversaw the brown one; employer controlled employee. In private, Lutie fed the bored bridge club a ladies lunch and watched Mrs. Chandler kiss a friend's husband on her couch. In fact, she watched Mr. Chandler watch her watching Mrs. Chandler. The two women were intimately connected. Of course, the history of the British novel is a history of tales of domestic labor. From *Clarissa* to *Jane Eyre*, the domestic novel recorded the plight of the serving girl whose isolation in a large, empty household sparks gothic stories of lust, terror, and surrender through letters and diaries. For eighteenth- and nineteenth-century British novelists, the consolidation of the bourgeoisie could best be tracked through the travails of the female domestic servant, governess, or teacher alone in the home of a wealthy man. Her body and her bedroom became the intimate locus of desire driving the narrative.[36] What Petry had done was to take the American version, which racialized the class conflict of the domestic novel, and use pulp fiction to modernize the naturalistic settings of urban horror so that the nightclub and the train station replaced the attic and the cellar, thus moving gothic domestic settings into sleazy noir public spaces.

With the exception of the insistence on interracial solidarity among black and white women's auxiliary workers in steel mills, auto plants, and rubber works celebrated by the Communist Party as a vital aspect of its antiracist work, in popular culture, black and white women were routinely portrayed interacting only in private through domestic service: a white woman employed a black woman to tend her children and fix her meals and clean her home and laundry.[37] In Fannie Hurst's novel, *Imitation of Life*, this intimacy is reinforced by the different kinds of work the two women perform: Bea pounds the pavement drumming up orders for maple syrup; Delilah turns the extra syrup into candies to be sold, eventually becoming the basis for B. Pullman enterprises. In the 1959 Douglas Sirk version, the white mother Lora's career as actress and singer takes her out at night. Annie, the black mother and Lora's maid, stays home and supports her two families. Through the perfect waffles she makes, first for her two charges—her daughter, Sarah Jane, and Lora's daughter, Susie—and then for an ever-expanding public, she eventually runs a domestic business, while Lora lives the high life of celebrity. Not only is there a connection in the political unconscious linking domestic service to prostitution through the bedroom and living room couch, this connection is transmitted by staging entertaining and performing as housework. Sarah Jane's passing eventually leads her to "imitate" in a debased form (as nightclub singer) Lora's imitative profession (as actress), as Lora's house begins to resemble a stage set.[38]

In the film version of *Mildred Pierce* (1947), Mildred (Joan Crawford) relies on Lottie, her black maid (Butterfly McQueen), to expand Mildred's pie-baking expertise into a booming business, primarily as domestic servant but also as her assistant.[39] However, once Mildred makes it, Ida (the tough white woman who first hired Mildred as a waitress) replaces Butterfly McQueen as a sidekick. In James. M. Cain's novel, the lower-middle-class women of Glendale understand that service, whether as domestic or waitress, is essentially prostitution. When Mildred finally confesses to her neighbor, Mrs. Gessler, that she has taken an unspecified job, her cynical neighbor quips: "I hope you picked a five-dollar house. You're too young for the two-dollar trade." Mildred provides the details that she is a waitress, to which Mrs. Gessler comments: "It rhymes up the same way," something Mildred quickly learns as she hustles tips from businessmen who run their hands up her legs.[40] As a single woman, the femme fatale employer offers a kind of solace from the sexual harassment of sons and husbands. The two dark ladies are alone together, sometimes conspiratorially, as the maid becomes protective of her employer and the employer needs the maid's confidence.

In the melodramatic noir film version of *Mildred Pierce*, Eve Arden plays this sidekick role, and it is clearly meant to be understood as a lesbian role: the lover and consort of an increasingly butch Mildred, who moves from waitress to freelance pie maker to restauranteur, eventually owning a string of franchises and, in the process, like Lora, conspicuously upgrading her house. Thus she has converted domestic labor into a small business by moving domestic functions out of the house and making public her private acts of fixing drinks, meals, and desserts previously done for her family. Lutie also moves out of her home into a nightlife offer by the Junto Bar and Grill on her street corner when her causal singing along with the jukebox lands her an audition with Boots Smith's band. But, as she has already surmised from her neighbor, the madam Mrs. Hedges's, offer to fix her up with a white man, "on this damn street you're supposed to want to earn a little extra money sleeping around nights" (84). As usual, there's more to the job than fronting the band. After accidentally killing Boots, who pimps for Junto, and his white bankrollers, who run everything in Harlem, Lutie ends up on the lam. She had tried to get money off Boots to hire a lawyer to pry her son from the child welfare agency, where he was taken for mail fraud. She surmises that Bud's life would be better off in reform school, because as a murderer she'd lose custody anyway. Finding herself thinking and acting like a criminal, she rifles Boots' wallet for money, hides her bloodied gloves, takes the stairs rather than the elevator down from the apartment, and heads for Penn Station. There, she buys a one-way ticket to Chicago, where she could disappear, slide into the anonymity of the Southside, maybe get a job singing at a nightclub, hustling drinks.

Lutie's poverty and race have sent her on the trajectory prepared for her by the jealous wives of Lyme, Connecticut; she's on the way to being the femme fatale of film noir. Yet, as a black woman, all she can hope for is the bit part as her maid, the one who covers her trail, helps cover up her crime, backs up her alibi, sings her torch song. The black femme fatale cannot be visualized within film; she is not going to be discovered in Chicago and end up packing a road house as Ida Lupino's Lily in Jean Negulesco's *Road House* did. Her presence remains located aurally in recordings of blueswomen's voices. Ultimately, however, she finds her way into these novels. We can watch Mildred Pierce and Lucia Harper, as overly devoted mothers of noir melodrama, cover up crimes committed by their ungrateful daughters. Both depend on the domestic servants they employ to get them out of a jam; but no one can come to Lutie's or her son's aid; nor can she expect to be picked up from the two-bit bar where she might end up singing in Chicago to star in a *Road House* (1948).

The classic femme fatale, Ann Savage in *Detour* (1945) for instance, moves from the street to the bedroom. She ensnares the doomed noir hero first by her freedom to move alone through the urban landscape, then by her outspoken desire for sex, and finally by her dead body. The femme fatale possesses a power offered by the street that is never available to the maternal woman of postwar Hollywood films who has planted herself in the kitchen. The domestic white woman appears to be denied erotic power because her function is solely reproductive. However, her domestic servant, as Lutie learned, produces an economy out of the invisible reproduction of the home.[41] Living at her work site, having a bedroom in her employer's house, resexualizes the reproductive labor of housework. The maid turns into an object of desire who appears as mobile as the femme fatale pacing the sidewalks nightly, like Ella Raines in *Phantom Lady* (1944). Because she is from elsewhere and will eventually also return there, she too has a double life, one never of interest overtly to her employers but nevertheless hanging as a veil between them. She cannot be wholly owned. As free labor, rather than wife, she is able to dismiss herself. Even if "The *Mistress* terminates the *interview*, Mildred," as Mrs. Forrester reminds Mildred Pierce when she comes for the job of housekeeper, the "servant" can always take off: "Mrs. Pierce, if you don't mind. And I'm terminating it" (43). Mildred's assertion suggests her connection as a servant to black women. In Langston Hughes's "Madam" series, Alberta K. Johnson declares: "My name is Johnson— / Madam Alberta K. // I do cooking. / Day's work, too! /Alberta K. Johnson— / *Madam* to you."[42] Each may end up running her own business. "The Madam stands for business." Usually, however, as Lutie Johnson discovers, except for work in a laundry or prostitution, no other employment is open to a black woman, even though Lutie manages to land an underpaid civil servant's job that allows her to move to the disastrous street.

Mildred Pierce, as a self-sacrificing suburban mother and a respectable white woman, can scoff at the haughty Mrs. Forrester, herself a kept woman recently installed as the second wife of her wealthy husband. A black maid, even if she too were a self-sacrificing mother as Lutie is, is subject to suspicions about her sexuality, and her job possibilities are far more limited than even Mildred's. Baker and Cooke correctly called the Jerome Avenue "mart" a slave block because domestic work recalls, as Phyllis Palmer notes, antebellum racial and sexual divisions of labor. Myra Page's *Gathering Storm* (1932), a novel about the Gastonia, North Carolina, textile mills strike, tracks the tripartite class and racial divisions in the milltown of Greenville. In it, Martha Morgan dies fighting off a rape by "that young massa" Elbert Haines. Her family is murdered and lynched after her fiancé avenges her death.[43] Page's novel directly links the Gastonia strike to the Scottsboro case and makes clear the remnants of white supremacy in the South, with black workers living as tenants on the plantation and with black female servants at the mercy of white men. Because a domestic servant lives in a bedroom of her employer's house, her intimate connection with daily life reinforces her sexuality. While the image of maternal labor seems at odds with sexuality, when that labor is performed by another, it opens the domestic to exploitation and fantasy. She is at once maternal and sexually available. Moreover, she also makes her female employer sexually available as she frees her employer from domestic drudgery. For the single, white female employer, the black domestic becomes the surrogate mother. She allows the white woman access to the streets where she can conduct business and have affairs.

In Fannie Hurst's *Imitation of Life*, Delilah moves into Bea Pullman's house, freeing Bea to spend days hawking maple syrup up and down the Atlantic City boardwalk, using her dead husband's business cards announcing simply "B. Pullman."[44] Delilah tends Bea's ailing father and her infant daughter as she cares for her own daughter, Peola. She cooks, cleans, takes them for walks, then gives Bea nightly backrubs. Eventually, her cooking skills become the basis for Bea's business success. Like the train car whose name Bea assumed with marriage and whose porters were organized into the most powerful black union, "[s]o it was from a going household of Delilah and three babies that Bea plugged every morning into the territory for the day."[45] Bea walks the boardwalk, "with her vigorous, honed-down contours," as an anomaly, "a woman salesman" (78). In *The Reckless Moment*, Frances Williams stays home tending the children while Joan Bennett, left alone to manage her family when her husband gets a commission overseas, travels to downtown Los Angeles from their Balboa Island beach house. She wanders the streets trying to borrow money from pawn brokers and loan sharks for the blackmailer hounding her murderess daughter. Walking the streets is an essential element of the white femme fatale's deadly eroticism, as is her "honed-down" phallic presence.[46] She may end up in the bedroom (or more typically the living room couch) of her doomed lover, but she got there by stepping out of the bounds of home. By contrast, the black domestic alters the contours of the white bourgeois home, making it into a fit home when her employer is a single mother, co-conspiring with her single, white woman employer, and becoming the object of sexual desire when her "mistress" has a husband.

Gwendolyn Brooks directly takes on this erotic "epistemology" in the chapter of *Maud Martha* bitingly entitled "the self-solace."[47] In horror, Maud Martha watches as Miss Ingram, the white woman salesman of beauty products, tires to sell Maud's beautician, Sonia Johnson, a new product line for "dark complexions," including a lipstick called "Black Beauty" (279). Critic James Smethurst notes that Brooks's ambivalence about popular culture, including products that remake African-American women's physique advertised daily in the black newspaper *Chicago Defender*, reflects Brooks's engagement in a debate within the 1930s black Left about the relationship of the masses to popular culture, which had altered from the Third Period to the Popular Front.[48] Where Langston Hughes, unlike Richard Wright, found in American popular culture the possibility of a jazzy voice to indict its racism, Brooks's sensitivity to gender exploitation made her far more skeptical of its subversive potential. For instance, when Maud Martha and her husbnd, Paul, travel to downtown Chicago to see a movie at the World Playhouse and find themselves "the only colored people here," it's clear that American popular culture is racially restrictive. Not everyone is part of the masses supposedly participating in mass culture (214). Lutie Johnson discerns the emptiness of the Chandler's lives, "learn[s] all about Country Living," by skimming "the pages of the fat sleek magazines . . . *Vogue, Town and Country, Harper's Bazaar, House and Garden, House Beautiful*" (50). Maud Martha's disdain for Miss Ingram's failure to discern black differences—"in the 'Negro group' there were complexions whiter than her own, and other complex-ions, brown, tan, yellow, cream"—grows into raw fury at her casual racism (279). Complaining of her working conditions, which force her into "walking the streets" in all kinds of weather, the saleswoman comments, quite unconsciously, "I work like a nigger to make a few pennies. A few lousy pennies." (280–1). Even when targeted for black women, mass-marketed beauty, offered in movies, magazine, and make-up, excludes and ultimately degrades them.

Like the private battles between white female employers and black domestics, this rare interaction between a white woman and black women occurs over work. Again, the work is about intimacy: here, refashioning the body; there, the home. The white woman walks the streets, but it's not Jerome Avenue and she's not in search of a "slave" to bring home to do her housework. In this case, she enters a black businesswoman's shop as supplicant. In a role rever-sal, she must please the black woman. Mrs. Johnson notes that some black beauticians were "glad to have the whites at their mercy, if only for a few moments. They made them crawl. Then they applied the whiplash. Then they sent the poor creatures off–with no orders. Then they laughed and laughed and laughed, a terrible laughter" (278). Their job as beauticians to redo black women's hair was now vengefully aimed at refashioning the white woman into a "poor crea-ture" dependent upon them for her economic survival. Is Miss Ingram reasserting her racial superiority by referring to herself as a nigger before these two dignified black women? Or is she seeking to align herself with them in a misguided attempt to name herself a "slave"? For Maud Martha, the answer is clear; the woman is a racist and should be called on the carpet for insulting Sonia Johnson in her own shop. However, Mrs. Johnson declares: "Now 'nigger,' for instance, means to them something bad, or slavey-like, or low. They don't mean anything against me. I'm a Negro, not a 'nigger.' " (283). Sonia Johnson's assertion of racial pride misses the echoes of the nineteenth-century mill girls' refusal to be called "wage slaves" that Maud Martha clearly discerns. Just because streetwalkers were also called "white slaves" doesn't excuse Miss Ingram's reimposition of racial superiority (especially if it comes through an invocation of gender solidarity).

Smethurst argues that during the 1930s, African-American poets were engaged in a project of reclaiming folkloric images of the black

masses that could bridge rural southern and urban northern vernacu-
lars. To some degree, the figure of the domestic servant in the novels and films I describe is connected to this ambivalent location
within and outside of modern political economy and commodity
culture. For Lutie, domestic service opens a pastoral zone skewed by
racism and loneliness. It ultimately destroys her own family when
she must live with the white family on their tree-lined street. For
Page's Martha Morgan, domestic service differs little from slavery.
For Baker and Cooke, the women on the slave blocks of northern
cities link domestic service in the urban industrialized north to servitude in the antebellum south. Bea Pullman's marketing scheme for
her sweets business is to photograph Delilah as a stereotypical
mammy; her big breakthrough comes when she dresses her in white
toque and apron to cook waffles in her boardwalk stall. Joan Crawford puts Butterfly McQueen to work on her pies in Glendale, California, just as Vivien Leigh had relied on her to midwife Olivia de
Havilland's baby a few years before in *Gone with the Wind* (1939). In
the novel, the maid Lettie, like Ida and Mildred, is white, so that
when Veda discovers Mildred's uniform hidden in her closet and
insists Lettie wear it when she accompanies her two charges to the
swimming pool, it confirms Mildred's connection to service and her
potentially aggressive sexuality but maintains her whiteness. Lettie
takes the girls to the pool daily to flirt with the lifeguard. But when
Butterfly McQueen (as Lottie) is seen wearing Mildred's clothes, it
suggests another trajectory: like Marlene Dietrich emerging in
blonde wig from the gorilla costume in the "Hot Voodoo" number
of *Blond Venus* (1932), it points up the camouflage of racialized sexuality. Underneath the costume of blackness—gorilla suit and
voodoo, uniform and domestic service—lurks a white movie star,
whose value is in maintaining racial purity (and so the bourgeois
home). Lutie takes pride in never wearing any of the hand-me-
downs she receives from Mrs. Chandler that were "Designed for
Country Living," sending them instead to her father's girlfriend to
be worn "nightly in the gin mill at the corner of Seventh Avenue and
110th Street" (50). These Connecticut clothes serve as a kind of drag
to stabilize white bourgeois femininity. Luties's revenge against her
employer lies in revealing their function by ripping them out of their
context as benign charity and placing them in a site of transgressive
pleasure. The idea that Butterfly McQueen could support Joan

Crawford's shoulder pads adds comic relief, but it also undercuts Mildred by linking her to servitude, destabilizing her value as broad-shouldered star.

In both versions of *Mildred Pierce*, Veda's shame that her mother wears a uniform in public is deflected by forcing the maid, hired to help Mildred take care of her growing pie business, to appear as a servant. Crawford's voice-over narration begins by intoning that her life had been little more than service, wearing an apron forever cooking, cleaning, baking. "I was always in the kitchen. It felt as though I'd been born in a kitchen and lived there all my life. . ." But the crucial distinction is over the public display of her service, which connects her to Lottie. In Ramona Lowe's devastating rebuttal to *Imitation of Life*, "The Woman in the Window," a short story published in the Urban League's journal, *Opportunity*, Mrs. Jackson endures the humiliation of publicly dressing as "Aunt Jemima . . . a ol' Southern mammy" (the very image of Delilah Bea had concocted to help sell her maple sugar candies) to fry chicken in the window of a restaurant of the same name. Mrs. Jackson, like Mildred Pierce, cannot hide her uniform from her children, who discover her one day while walking home from school and are shamed when the white kids call her "nigger." Mrs. Jackson lets her children know that "[s]ome work's dignified 'n' some ain' so dignified. But it all got t' be done. My work's cookin' 'n' there ain' nothin' wrong with that." Like Maud Martha, she insists on confronting white racism: *"'N' son, doan you never let me see you run no more when a body say nigger. You turn roun' 'n' give 'm such a thrashin' they woan never forget."*[49]

As David Roediger and Lauren Berlant point out, questions of labor, racialized as they are in American history, are always questions of citizenship.[50] During the 1930s, membership in the Communist Party, or at least, as Michael Denning has argued, allegiance to the Popular Front, became a vehicle for a group of "plebeians," European immigrants, and southern migrants and their first-generation urban children to participate, albeit oppositionally, in American culture.[51] Film noirs, based so often on fiction from the 1930s, visualized this racial and class dynamic. Central to the femme fatale's position as a mobile figure on the landscape was the Depression and the War and the shifts in populations and work opportunities it provided women. This is, in part, what allows Lutie Johnson to disappear to Chicago—the massive migrations of African Americans to industrial cities, coupled with her essential anonymity. She is an "invisible (wo)man."[52] Within the film noirs of the 1940s, like many of the 1930s novels, there lurks a figure of questionable race or ethnicity—Mexican, Spanish, Italian, Jewish, Greek—dark, but never black, who moves near the femme fatale. The femme fatale, like Kathie Moffett, can establish an identification with her beautiful maid, Eunice, because she has no place within bourgeois domesticity; yet her visual presence in popular culture is overdetermined.

Gwendolyn Brooks's two volumes of poems from the 1940s and her 1953 novel, *Maud Martha*, all conclude with the end of World War II and its ambivalent effect on black Americans caught within the racist United States. Maud Martha notes the returning soldiers parading maimed, but alive, in contrast to "the Negro press (on whose front pages beamed the usual representations of womanly Beauty, pale and pompadoured) [which] carried the stories of the latest of the Georgia and Mississippi lynchings"(321). Brooks expressly links color stratification within the black community to the racist lynchings of black Americans by whites. This is the violent underpinning of America tracked by film noirs, many of which were made by left-wing directors from fiction by left-wing writers. Kathie could flee to Acapulco; Lutie only makes it to Chicago, where, like Maud Martha, she'll find her "type is not a Foxy Cat favorite," her "color" also acts "like a wall" (Brooks 223, 229). What appears to adhere to the surface of the black woman's body in popular culture is "the plight of the black woman (which is, precisely, a problem of nonrecognition)."[53] In postwar Jim Crow America, she cannot be seen; thus her narrative might be sung or written, but not filmed.

When Eunice resists Jeff Bailey's entreaties to help him find Kathie, she underscores, through her deceit, a loyalty that Kathie will inevitably betray. The white femme noire double crosses white men because she can get away with it; she's never had to clean up her own mess. Lutie Johnson and Maud Martha, keen observers of their cities' grimy streets, recognize her type immediately; they've seen her, read about her, even worked for her, many times before. Perhaps she sings in dives in Harlem or Chicago's Southside along with Ida Lupino. But they also would recognize Eunice out on a date, like Hattie Scott or Lutie or the other "[y]oung women coming home from work—dirty, tired, depressed—[who] looked forward to the moment when they would change their clothes and head toward the gracious spaciousness of the Junto . . . because they couldn't bear to look what they could see of the future smack in the face while listening to radios or trying or read an evening paper" (144–45). Like the radio and the newspaper, proletarian literature and film noir, in part, also dimly outlined their unrecorded stories. Once again, these dark visions of mid-century America provided a template for sketching an alternative to either Betty Crocker or Aunt Jemima. Lutie and Maud Martha know exactly what happens to the femme noire; she gets out anyway she can.

CHAPTER 3

DOUBLE CROSS: WRI(GH)TING
AS THE OUTSIDER

THE NOVEL AS FILM NOIR

Most film noirs began first as text—novels, short stories, plays or scripts, screenplays, treatments—but as soon as they appeared, they began generating prose. Just as the films depended on the kinky nighttime police shots of *PM* photographer Weegee, whose book *Naked City* became the basis for Jules Dassin's film of the same name,[1] or the eerie bus ride series from Esther Bubley's OWI assignment, so too did they generate new photographic obsessions in Robert Frank's and Diane Arbus's street photography that captured in a single frame what the films took an hour and a half to spell out: America was a nation of loners and misfits. The films also created new works of prose. Much popular 1930s fiction included hard-boiled, tough-guy detective and police procedural novels—often written by those connected with left-wing literary radicalism.[2] These were part of an emerging pulp literature that, with the paperback revolution, crossed the boundaries of respectable literature and sleaze. What is one to make of Pocket Book's 1941 edition of Emile Zola's *Nana* with its lurid cover of a torch singer in a transparent white dress? Its back-cover blurb declared, "she squandered fortunes, ruined lives with sublime contempt and abandon—yet her last disease-ridden days were spent in squalor and oblivion." Is this art or trash?

Moreover, many 1930s novels, such as Ralph Ellison's *Invisible Man*, didn't get published, or even written, until long after the decade was over. Vicissitudes of politics and culture kept these works out of print. Richard Wright's wildly popular and disturbing sociological roman noir *Native Son* launched his career as literary superstar; however, its popularity and his political disillusionment with the United States and with communism took its toll on his ability to get another novel into print. He was traveling and living in France, Spain, and Africa, participating in black expatriate political culture in each place, writing some of his best work. But it was nonfiction, and in the minds of mid-century literati, this was second-class material. As Georgia O'Keeffe would later comment about the "city men" of the late 1920s and early 1930s: "They talked so often of writing the Great American Novel—the Great American Play—the Great American Poetry."[3] O'Keeffe was definitely not speaking about literary radicals, much less black intellectuals, but the sentiment against nonfiction prevailed in all quarters. It would not be until James Agee smashed the boundaries of narrative, fiction and nonfiction alike, that reportage/journalism/memoir would achieve critical stature, but this happened in the 1960s, decades after he had written and published *Let Us Now Praise Famous Men*. Wright's struggle with himself over the scope of his second novel plays itself out in the ultimate form it assumed. Full of violent battles, the narrative of *The Outsider* enacts a contest with itself over its own philosophical and aesthetic legitimacy by recreating iconic visuals from film noirs.[4] Much as the 1943 zoot suit riots in Los Angeles had pitted hip Latino teenagers against uniformed sailors, *The Outsider* plays out its internal and external conflicts through dueling styles. In Wright's case, literary style, like fashion, signals political and philosophical affiliations that set its user apart from dominant culture as it advertises its subcultural allegiance. Subcultural style, according to Birmingham Center critics Angela McRobbie and Dick Hebdige, describing a theory of British punk style, visually maps class and ethnic and gender clashes of Thatcherite Britain onto the bodies of its victims.[5] Richard Wright's novel falling into the midst of McCarthyite America—it was published just months before the Rosenbergs were executed—exhibits how literary style also maps racial and political conflict.

BLACK & WHITE AND NOIR

This chapter reads Richard Wright's second novel, *The Outsider*, as a literary version of film noir—a reversal, in more ways than one, because, for the most part, film noirs began as prose. Much has been written on the spider women who gleam white as snow in their low key-lit frames and in turn frame guys who should know better—but don't; or on the visual style that foregrounds negative space. But practically nothing has been written on the "blackness of blackness," the racial codes of these films.[6] Typically, film noirs picture lower middle-class WASP horror. Set in Los Angeles, the garden suburb revealed as hell, many film noirs look back to New York or sometimes Chicago, as places apart, zones of difference, where a man could lose his identity and pick up another for a small price. Within the standard plot—a regular guy works a regular job (say he sells insurance like Fred McMurray playing Walter Neff in *Double Indemnity*), gets hooked by an evil woman (say she wears an anklet like Barbara Stanwyck playing Phyllis Dietrichson), and commits murder—maybe gets away with it—but then she's got something on him, so, most likely, he kills her; but she gets him anyway, because there's another guy (say he's a cop or investigator like Edward G. Robinson playing Barton Keyes), who's a pal, likes him too much, can't see the forest for the trees because "He's close, too close"—"Closer than you know, Walter."

Within that dark woods also lurks a minor character—usually a gangster, but sometimes a hot-headed youth, always coded ethnically: dark, with names that are Greek or Italian or Spanish or Jewish, who is out of place in the world of daylight, preferring to slide out from behind thick shrubbery or stand on corners late at night for a secret rendezvous. This character has something on the guy, and on the spider woman, and often on her "other"—the innocent maiden who stumbles into the plot when she falls for the doomed guy. He is not central to the plot, but he is always there. And because he is, and because of what he becomes in the late phases of the style (*Touch of Evil* and *Crimson Kimono*) and in its second (*Chinatown*) and now third reincarnation (*Devil in a Blue Dress*), and because, in America, the play of light and dark, as Toni Morrison reminds us, is always about race relations, these films, which barely feature black faces, signify race and its meaning within postwar American urban imagination.

84

Richard Wright took this cinematic variation on melodrama, inverted it, and pushed its implications to the limit—outside it really. He did so, because, in true noir style, it provided a means to "take care" of three "problems": racism in the United States, the Communist Party of the United States (CPUSA), and his literary protégé-turned-rival Ralph Ellison. The plot of *The Outsider* trails Cross Damon, a brainy and well-read black postal worker from Chicago's Southside, on the lam for numerous murders, theft, and fraud. Fortuitous accidents and clever aliases land him among New York's circle of Communist Party intellectuals, where he commits still more murders until finally caught by the tenacious hunchbacked district attorney, Ely Houston. "A crime story in a newspaper evokes a sense of excitement far beyond the meaning of the banal crime described, a meaning which, in turn, conjures up, for inexplicable reason, its emotion equivalent in a totally different setting and possessing a completely contrary meaning," wrote Wright.[7] Michel Fabre notes that Wright's first story, "Suspicion," based on the "gothic detective stories" found in pulp periodicals, was a rewriting of an Edgar Allan Poe tale, and that both "The Man Who Lived Underground" and "The Man Who Killed a Shadow," like *Native Son*, were based on Wright's perusal of true crime reports.[8] Margaret Walker recounts how she clipped the news items from the *Chicago Tribune* on the Robert Nixon case and sent them to Wright after he left for New York.[9] Wright was always on the lookout for intriguing stories to probe the absurdities and horrors of the racial system governing America. His friends contributed anecdotes. For instance, sometime during the mid-1940s, the city of San Francisco was terrorized by a serial rapist, a light-skinned black man who targeted white women. After the man was arrested, tried, convicted, and sentenced to the die in the gas chamber, a police officer got interested in the case of "Green Gloves," as he was known, and discovered he was actually white.

Knowing Wright's interest in this kind of twisted plot, psychologist Horace Cayton wrote a long detailed account of the case, which included a deep Oedipal fixation—because his mother had routinely punished him by saying she would send him back to "the black people"—and intense rage at Negroes. Eventually, "something happens (mothers death or violent argument with her) which . . . causes him great emotional distress . . . he falls into fancicy [sic]" and concocts a "history" that his father had been lynched by white racists who accused him falsely of raping a white woman. Thus he decided to seek revenge on them as a black man by himself raping white women. He refused to acknowledge that he was not black, going to his death as "a Negro rather than undo the great harm which he had done the Negro community," which had endured a vicious race-baiting mayoral election, police sweeps of thousands of young black men who "were put in jail and lost their jobs," and a near race riot. Along with the story, Cayton even supplies a title: "You could call it 'Black Blood' or 'The Man Who Turned Black' or facetiously, 'Mind over Matter' or 'What Ho!, The Oedipus.' Seriously I hope the plot interests you. I will send you all of the material I have on it if it does. It might fit into your series like 'The Man who lived underground.' "[10] Cayton knew that Wright relished true stories on which to base his fiction, partly because Wright felt he was inventing a realist tradition for African-American literary history.[11]

Fabre's careful tracing of Wright's earliest literary sources begins with a perusal of the crime pages of the Memphis *Commercial Appeal* and *Flynn's Detective Weekly*, but he notes in passing, one need also look at more than these "gothic detective stories," because "the weekly billings of the Strand, the Majestic or Loew's Palace could be checked with profit to map Wright's early movie culture" (13). Moreover, Wright's education in Parisian existentialism, after his 1946 expatriation, also included "other domains of true aesthetic expression, films in particular," running twenty-four hours at the Cinematheque.[12] Going to the movies is a central pastime for both Bigger Thomas and Cross Damon, who spies among Gil and Eva Blount's belongings and finds in her diary that she too spent her time in postwar Paris watching American movies: "a horrible gangster film with a tense, melodramatic atmosphere" (*The Outsider*, 209). By 1951, Wright had written the screenplay for (and even acted in) a film version of *Native Son*. This immersion in movie culture and true-crime plots, spurred by the rave reviews of *Invisible Man*, unleashed a flood of prose between February and May 1952, that became the 650-page manuscript of *The Outsider*.

For the most part, *The Outsider* is viewed as a failed novel; the reviews neatly clipped and collected for Wright repeatedly refer to it as a sloppy "melodrama."[13] While this feminizing epithet is bad enough, the critics often go on to compare Wright's novel to cheesy pulp fiction reminiscent of Mickey Spillane.[14] It is characterized as a "thriller," "a surrealistic cops-and-robbers story," "a cheap drugstore whodunit."[15] Perhaps the most galling of the reviews were those that directly linked the novel to Ellison's as did the critic for the *Nation*. So too did Granville Hicks, writing in the Sunday *New York Times Book Review* on March 22, 1953, and Harvey Curtus Webster in the April 6, 1953, *New Leader*. What scholarly criticism has been written tries to salvage Wright's name by discussing, as many of the original reviewers did (with sneers), its Dostoevskian nihilism, or Kirkegaardian dread, or Christian existentialism, or Freudian psychoanalysis, and of course his disillusionment with communism, to deflect attention from its awkward trashiness. In fact, the novel fits perfectly within the contours of what James Naremore, quoting Graham Greene, calls "blood melodrama," a modernist "interest in popular stories about violence and sexual love."[16] So it is not surprising that Fabre reads it as a "novel of ideas disguised as a melodrama" (*Quest*, 367). However, Wright's contemporary reviewers relished the novel for what it displayed about him. "His almost psychopathic lust for violence," wrote the reviewer for *Jet*, " his story becomes as completely phony and unreal as a cheap drugstore whodunit."[17] Whodunit, indeed. Wright is out for vengeance and not just against the Party and the nation he felt had so betrayed him.

His rivalry with Ellison, whose *Invisible Man* is the mirrored backdrop for the novel, becomes a second frame for the plot. In a letter to Ellen Wright written a few weeks before its publication, Ellison asks her to "[t]ell Dick that I hope that I haven't let him down since it is the best I could do."[18] Still anxious about his status in relation to Wright, Ellison appears as supplicant.[19] However, within a year a radical reversal of fortunes would occur. At the bottom of a long typed letter, dated January 21, 1953, the last one it seems that Ellison sent Wright, in which he notes "I will be right at the bookstore on the 18th [the scheduled date of its release] to get a look at *The Outsider*," is a handwritten addition: "Perhaps you've heard by now that lightning struck me, leaving me standing amazed with the 1952 National Book Award for Fiction."[20] No more letters from Ellison, who had had a long and voluble history of letter-writing to his former patron, exist in Yale University's Beinecke Library files, as if the lightning that had left Ellison standing had taken its toll on Wright. Wright had predicted according to Ellison's recounting that "Negroes will not like it [*The Outsider*]," to which Ellison had reassured him that Roy Ottley, who had been "going around discussing me as simply 'a disciple of Dick Wright's'," and Ben Burns in *Jet* hadn't liked *Invisible Man* either; but this could hardly offer solace to Wright who was clearly anxious about his reputation.[21] Ellison's long discussion of Chester Himes's new 1948 novel in many ways prefigures the criticisms that would be lodged against Wright's novel. "I believe," he remarks, "that when one writes of politics one is called upon to do more than cull a few terms from *Materialism and Empro-criticism* [sic] and scatter them dialoguewise between episodes of a cops and robbers plot."[22]

Despite claiming that "the hard-boiled stance and its monosyllabic utterance" of stripped down 1930s prose could not work for an African-American writer steeped in the "alive language" of the blues, the dozens, and gospel preachings, Ellison brilliantly employs the genre's first-person narration to tell his noir tale of descent.[23] More-over, his letters to Wright read like a series of revenge plots in which a group of disaffected former gang members bicker among them-selves. They are filled with jousts lodged at the insider world of estranged African-American [former] communists, as if a constant battle to be on top required vigilance about what one said or did in each other's company. Noting that Chester Himes had not been to see him, Ellison speculates, "Could he fear that I might put him in *my* book?" After all, he notes "The character referred to as 'Ellsworth' who argued with Lee concerning the material character of certain class divisions of the Negro family, actually refers to me and a conversation I had with Chester last year."[24] "The Party boys around Harlem," including Abner Berry, who "wrote an attack in *The Worker*, calling me the standard names and saying that I had 'sold out' in writing *Invisible Man*" simply confirmed Ellison's and Wright's understanding of the CPUSA as another gang.[25] It could only have enraged Wright to find an article entitled, "Native Doesn't Live Here," which complained that "While Wright sits out the threat of totalitarianism in Paris, an abler U.S. Negro novelist sees the prob-lem of his race differently. Says Ralph (Invisible Man) Ellison: 'It's a big wonderful country.' "[26] Maybe so, if you win the National Book Award. However, in his biographical remarks, Wright describes his novel about an outsider, not an invisible man, as a response to the cold war. "The message to the West 'the game is up.' "[27]

While Cross Damon does not narrate his story retrospectively, the novel has, as Wright wrote his agent Paul Reynolds, "four murders, a suicide, an ambush murder, which ought to be enough blood. There is a kind of love story in it, but rather a dark and tortured one" (quoted in *Quest*, 366). The early drafts of *The Outsider*, however, indicate that Wright began the book by writing it as a first-person testimonial: "Wherever possible, I shall present facts, documents, rather than my own words to substantiate this record, for that is what it is: a record." Using this device that was so prevalent in the film noirs he was attempting to reshoot in prose, his narrator reveals that instead of being underground, he is speaking from "beneath the water-line of this city." Like so many film noirs, the hero of this earlier draft is a disillusioned veteran, "here in this damp cell . . . sit[ting], brood[ing] and think[ing]" in his ship's brig.[28] Wright's original idea for the novel came from a story he had followed about a black soldier who faced court martial for refusing to go to the front. To his General Court Martial Order Number 20 issued by Headquarters 69 Infantry Division 4th Signal Battalion April 5, 1945, Corporal John Jones had simply declared himself, "Not guilty please." Wright also notes another case of a soldier court martialed for not guarding mail bags in 1946. These apparent acts of defiance against the United States Armed Forces intrigued Wright as he struggled to find a story to fit his proposed title "Cornering a Man" during the mid-1940s.[29] A would-be author, asking Wright's help and advice, grasps the difficulties ahead for anyone wanting to take on World War II: "I know by now that nothing—nothing is as dead as World War 2—any phase of it. Not even pulp magazines will touch it. I've check [sic] many sources of information in the publishing field on that point and the consensus of opinion is that not even a Tolstoy could sell a ms. on it. . . . If one wrote of WW3—a nice juicy, red-baiting, witch-hunting job dripping with blood from Communists' heads on pikes—ah—that's magic; *that* would certainly sell."[30]

Not even pulp magazines would touch the Second World War directly; however, both Wright and Ellison used the conventions of pulp to dissect race, postwar America, and the CPUSA, including the pseudophilosophy conveyed in long speeches that is also one hallmark of the more literary forms of the genre. In the final pages of *The Maltese Falcon*, for instance, Sam Spade explains to the back-stabbing Bridget, the woman he loves, why he has to turn her in. It is long lesson in the credo and ethics of living private eye: "Listen, this isn't a damned bit of good. You'll never understand me, but I'll try once more and then we'll give it up. Listen . . .," he says before listing the attributes of a PI that make him both someone with no use for the police yet someone with a moral stance.[31] Like Poe's detective Dupin a century before them, Sam Spade and Philip Marlowe and the other noir detectives dismiss the police and the DAs who prosecute and investigate criminals as inept cogs in the wheel of a corrupt system; yet they share their work. Occasionally the DA crosses over, as does Wendell Corey after he falls for Barbara Stanwyck in *The File on Thelma Jordan*, or he is too close to the frame, as is insurance claims investigator Barton Keyes in *Double Indemnity*. So, in *The Outsider*, DA Ely Houston, a man "crammed with guilty knowledge," solves the murder cases because as a hunchback he lives in the shadows of normal life too; but, because of this, he fails to see that Cross actually committed them.[32]

The formula for noir—guilt, knowledge, desire, deceit, vengeance, a past weighing heavily on the present, and a lone man, an outsider, who, like DA Ely Houston, is "crammed with guilty knowledge"— provides a frame for understanding African-American experience.[33] As Houston tells Cross AKA Addison Jordan AKA Lionel Lane, paraphrasing W. E. B. Du Bois: "Negroes as they enter our culture, are going to inherit the problems we have, but with a difference. They are outsiders and they are going to *know* that they have these problems. They are going to be self-conscious; they are going to be gifted with double vision, for being Negroes, they are going to be both *inside* and *outside* of our culture at the same time. . . . They will become psychological men . . .; they will be centers of knowing" (129). Wright's position as the foremost African-American literary figure of the mid-twentieth century, a center of knowing, who remained outside of his nation's borders, embodies the identity he has cast for Houston.[34] Cross agrees, relishing in the delicious irony that he is talking to a white DA as a black fugitive—a man presumed dead who has just gotten away with murder—a man "haunted" by desire, "desire for desire": "I desire desire, he told himself. . . . And then there came to his mind the memory of the many sultry, smoky nights when he had been drunk with his friends in cheap dives and seen girls like this (25)." Du Bois had argued that Booker T. Washington's program for advancing the race amounted to a suppression of desire: "Mr. Washington distinctly asks that black people give up, at least for the present, three things,—

First political power,
Second, insistence on civil rights,
Third, higher education of Negro youth."[35]

After setting off this list like a poem or chant, he goes on to note the peculiar characteristic of racist logic. Without some sense that "spiritual strivings" will be fulfilled, any African-American citizen "must more and more brood over the red past and the creeping, crooked present, until it grasps a gospel of revolt and revenge and throws its new-found energies athwart the current of advance." (80) The African-American condition of "double consciousness . . . ever a twoness" provides an understanding of social and psychological, historical and private, political and individual subjectivities (2). Richard Wright had traced his own version of the great migration in *Black Boy*, his poetic account *12 Million Black Voices* and his introduction to *Black Metropolis* explored how his personal story was part of a mass history. "The problem of the twentieth century is the problem of the color-line" depicted in film noirs in the stark black-and-white Venetian blind slats crossing the faces of the femme fatale and her doomed fall guy. African Americans already lived the noir world, guilt and betrayal the central theme of their American experience.[36]

Nelson Algren had characterized *Native Son* as a "threat . . . a personal threat. . . . I don't think any white person could read it without being either frightened or angry at the end." Algren went on to detail how the novel should be read: "It's the best detective story I ever read. It can be read like somebody'd read *Serenade* also—just for reading a tough book. But *Serenade* is tough for the sake of being tough, just as Poe is full of horror for its own sake. Moreover *Serenade* ends so damn cold, yours ends warmly. It could be read for its sociology much more convincingly than *Studs Lonigan*. And it's readable as a political novel as well. I read it as a horror story, and kept going on that to the end, where he's alright [sic]. Then I realised [sic] that it was, above the other things, to be read as an humanitarian work." Algren understood just how significant linking racism to horror and detection—to the "tough" writing of James T. Farrell and James M. Cain—was to evincing the proper emotional response in America's readers: "It's the first book I ever came on wherein gruesomeness served a social purpose . . . simply to scare whites into thinking about Negroes."[37] Where Farrell, following Dashiell Hammett in *Red Harvest*, had relied on tough-guy prose, though without the detective per se, to expose the rottenness of lower-middle-class white society, Wright retrieved the horror story and connected it to the crime plot to lay bare the psychology and social pathology of racism. Wright's unraveling of Bigger's "lava-like waves of cultural hunger which reside in the souls of the slow moving men who walk the streets!" was designed to show Bigger *"just as white America had been taught to expect him."*[38] Racism was a racket corrupting everyone in its orbit—black and white, businessman and Communist.

Yet Wright had been severely criticized for this by Ben Davis in *The Daily Worker*. Wright penned a long response to Mike Gold that ends with a direct comment to Davis, who wrote that in keeping with International Labor Defense (ILD) policy, Bigger should have pleaded not guilty to his crimes: "Ben, all of us who live in the world today and want peace, bread, and freedom are *guilty!* Bigger was *guilty* because he wanted to live. The Germans who work in Underground Germany are *guilty!* The French workers who conspire for peace are *guilty!* The English worker who is against Chamberlain is *guilty!* The American who fights for democracy is *guilty!* You see, Ben I'm using guilt in a much deeper and more suggestive sense than you suspect. Today the world is *guilty!* With the doom of fascism hanging over our heads, we are all *guilty* if we want to live!"[39] If *Native Son*, written while Wright was an active member of the CPUSA, was all about investigating guilt, *The Outsider*, written after his disillusionment, was predicated on the refusal of guilt: 'Because in my heart . . . I'm . . . I felt . . . I'm *innocent*. . . . That's what made the horror," Cross finally tells the District Attorney (440). Refusing to acknowledge, much less accept, the guilt of crime and desire makes Cross Damon an outlaw more despised than Bigger Thomas, who claims his guilt because he wanted to live. But Wright ends *The Outsider* on another note: "He was dead." In this Cross Damon follows Eva Blount, who commits suicide to escape the clutches of the Party, which would "destroy" her because she was "guilty not because of what I've done, but because of what I know" (209). It is knowledge itself that is dangerous in the noir world of American race relations.

DETECTING RACE

In her stunning 1929 novella, *Passing*, Nella Larsen uses the devices of popular pulp fiction and true detective stories collected in 1920s

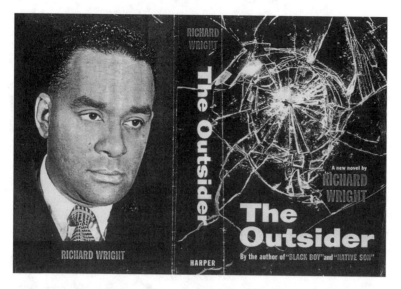

FIGURE 28. Book jacket from first editon of Richard Wright, *The Outsider* (1953).

dime periodicals like *Black Mask* to retell the classic African-American tale of the tragic mulatto.[40] Since William Wells Brown's 1853 novel, *Clotel*, and especially after the 1896 *Plessy v. Ferguson* decision, racial confusion and its detection have been a central theme in American literature, allowing writers as diverse as Mark Twain and Charles Chestnutt to expose the mysteries of racial categorization that persisted in Jim Crow America. For instance, Melville's "Benito Cereno," anticipating Twain's *Pudd'nhead Wilson*, turns on the problem of race and investigation. And, like Poe's "Purloined Letter," the solution to the mutiny lies in plain sight—but because race codes knowledge so powerfully in American imagination, Amaso Delano can barely detect it. *Passing* updates these nineteenth-century narratives and makes clear that urban life (like *The Outsider*, the novel moves between Chicago and New York) provides further opportunities to transfigure the African-American self. Passing, Clare hides in plain sight of her husband; even her former friend Irene, the "race woman," is not above passing when she needs to escape the hot, dirty streets of downtown Chicago in August to the airy tearoom atop the Drayton Hotel.

The Chicago of Wright's *The Outsider* by contrast is a snow-covered, wind-blown tundra, frozen and icy, the whiteness of its winter setting off Cross Damon from his environment, even as he himself has set himself off from his community. This is a community of betrayed women—his mother, his wife, his lover, a prostitute—and of well-meaning coworkers who sort mail during the night shift at the post office. Wright sets the scene of an urban wilderness, of neon staining the dirty snow, of smoky bars smelling of old whiskey, as Cross listens to his friends chide his "quadruple A program" "*Alcohol. Abortions. Automobiles.* And *alimony*" (3). FDR's Triple A program had been "plowed under" in defeat. Like so many doomed guys haunting noir, Cross is mired in the residues of the Depression, trying to extricate himself from a past that includes a series of women who want things from him he can't provide. Plagued by his inability to control these scheming women—and underestimating their ability to work the system of sex and money exchange—Cross tries to appease first one, then other, of his women: women once desired, who now represent stale legacies, desire's fulfillment. He knows very well that there is always a morning after.

Cross's entanglements with women, his debt, his dislocation set the stage for the noir plot. Double-crossing, two-timing, drinking and self-pity characterize the noir hero—Walter Neff in *Double Indemnity*, Wendell Corey in *The File on Thelma Jordan* are just two classic examples—white-collar workers bored with their routines, drinking too much, caught up in the machinations of women—wives, lovers—who need (or sometimes have) money, their masculinity eclipsed by their desire for these scheming female bodies. Wright describes a woman Cross meets slinging hamburgers at a lunch stand by focusing on "her sloping hips . . . her plump arms, her protruding breasts, the gently curving shape of her legs, and the width of her buttocks." In "the bluish haze of tobacco smoke" this girl becomes "woman as body of woman"—pure physicality, and dangerous too . . . "an intractable bitch" (24).[41] In the white city, what begins in desire ends in death—the only end for desire—as the novel begins with dread and ends with decision.[42]

In its African-American retelling, the noir city appears covered with snow and ice—a white out. In *Passing*, Irene (perhaps) murders Clare in the midst of a terrible snow storm; Cross gets away with tossing Joe's murdered body out a cheap hotel window when it lands in a snow drift. Ellison's invisible man, almost killed making "optic white" at Liberty Paints, wanders Harlem's snow-covered streets until he collapses. Where the white noir hero lurks the black night streets of steamy (or more often rainy and foggy) cities; the black noir figure is alone in a bleached landscape devoid of color, his body in constant contrast. The *blanc* world in which Cross Damon lives is no asphalt jungle—more like Siberia. The heart of darkness for an African American is frozen—white as a snow-covered pavement, as a blonde's neckline. It is a city simultaneously full and empty, affording the possibility of invisibility and of chance encounters. Cross Damon, like Melville's Captain Ahab, must confront the horror at the vacuum, the cipher, of whiteness itself.

Like Ellison's invisible man, Cross Damon changes names throughout the novel. Supposedly dying in a fiery train wreck, only to be resurrected as anybody riding a train to New York, Cross reverses the usual drift west. These noir noirs travel north or east, fugitives in search of a presumed freedom. Cross takes the name Addison Jordan when he introduces himself to the radical sleeping-car porter and the hunchback DA who ponders black psychology whom he meets on the train east, then renames himself Lionel Lane to enter the Party. As one who feels a form of outsiderness, his deformed body leaving him a man alone, living behind a kind of veil, Ely Houston, like the detective in *Laura*, lives on the edge of crime, obsessed with its logic and its possibilities. We know he will return. Chance meetings on a train, as in Hitchcock's 1951 *Strangers on a Train*, set the plot in motion for many of these movies. In *No Man of Her Own*, the film version of Cornell Woolrich's novel *I Married a Dead Man*, Barbara Stanwyck, pregnant and deserted on her way to California in pursuit of her lover, survives a train wreck and assumes the identity of a wealthy young wife sitting near her because she has slipped on her wedding ring.

In the classic noir world, the femme fatale—almost always a gleaming blonde hiding a dark past and a cold heart—is coded as noir. She is dark, despite her blonde hair, because of her steaming sexuality. Often, as in *Out of the Past*, she is opposed to the peaches-and-cream blonde whose all-American wholesomeness dims her sexuality. Because the femme fatale moves in the night world, the border world of the underground, she uses her sexuality to acquire wealth, power, and control. She has contacts with the dark ethnically marked men of crime; she figures in the equations of gangsters and mobsters, sings in their nightclubs—like Rita Hayworth in *Gilda*, or Lauren Bacall in *The Big Sleep* or Lizabeth Scott in *Dark City*—gambles in their Mexican casinos—like Jane Greer in *Out of the Past* or Lizabeth Scott in *Too Late for Tears*—and, of course packs a pistol. In Richard Wright's inversion of film noir, white women offer black men the transgressive power of the femme fatale.[43] Like the femme fatale, she is desirable because she is trapped. Jenny, the Chicago prostitute, and Eva, the abstract expressionist in New York, are caught by systems controlling their desire; pimps and brothels, on the one hand, and the CPUSA, on the other, resemble the gangster world. However, these women are truly victims, not scheming, two-timing bitches. These roles Wright reserves for black women. In an early draft of *The Outsider*, Jenny tells Cross her story—and it's straight out of James M. Cain and Horace McCoy: "I got into trouble with a boy and had an abortion. . . . You wouldn't think it, but 'til two years ago, I didn't know where babies came from. . . . I ran off and came to Chicago. The first week I worked in a Greek café; like a dope, I went out with the Greek. He raped me. Sounds crazy, hunh? . . . I want to go to California." To which Cross can only respond: "Movies?"[44] But, as Maud Martha and Lutie Johnson know, running off to Hollywood to star in the movies was not an option for the black women Cross encounters; their roles are circumscribed by race to that of the loyal maid. Recognizing this, however, does not make Cross sympathetic; instead it infuriates him because he is dependent on these same women. Despite the greater obstacles within black women's lives, the nasty femme noire role is appropriated for the black women in Cross Damon's life: his wife, who will never question the circumstances of his death because she can cash in his insurance policy and thus walk away with the house and car paid up and some cash; his lover, who uses her pregnancy and her threats of statutory rape to blackmail Cross into marrying her or paying her off; the "bitch" at the lunch counter who turns her back on Cross. Cross's vengeance against these women paradoxically raises them to central billing.

Cross Damon's rage against black women, like everything else in this novel, is exaggerated, over the top. Cross cannot decide where he stands with these women whom he at once desires and detests. First expressed so acutely in *Native Son*, Wright's fictional violations of African-American women occur in the "white city." The access Chicago provides to white women's sexuality inexorably pushes Wright's African-American men to transgress the racial divide in American culture; crossing the color line violates the spatial and sexual order of America, and cities foster this circulation. Where film noirs recognize the threat of urban white women's mobile sexuality to the middle-class family, Wright also understands how it destabilizes Jim Crow social conventions as well. Knowing beforehand of her betrayal, the white noir hero still cannot resist the enticements of the white femme fatale; his revenge is doubled because he is betrayed and because he knows it. Like the femme fatale, Cross is a knowing betrayer, but of black women as well as white men. His rage is turned on them because they know the nature of his betrayal—desire for the white woman's body. This desire sends America into its pulpy modernity. In Ellison's novel, the crazed veteran warns the young invisible man on the bus north to New York not to seek symbolic freedom in a "dance with a white woman" (136). In phrasing his warning, he admonishes the boy to "learn to look beneath the surface" (137). Racial differences appear only skin deep; however, their imbrication in virtually every aspect of American life, from sexuality to economics, makes them profoundly significant. The fact of depth—that the surface masks hidden, profound, secret, truths—is central to noir sensibility. That not everything can be immediately discerned at first sight became the basis for Ellison's play on invisibility, for Wright's use of the outsider, for Larsen's anatomy of passing. The obsession with racial differences and their subsequent confusions in postwar urban America left DA Ely Houston "wonder[ing] why [he] couldn't detect this feeling of the outsider in the Negroes [he] met" (133). Detecting race—seeing the passing woman as a black woman, as Clare's husband finally does at Irene's Christmas party, or seeing nothing but a black man, as everybody does who meets Ellison's invisible man— is the standard American plot. Like film noir, it always results in catastrophe.

GOING UNDERGROUND

B-movies gave American left-wing writers a venue to reveal the underside of American consumerism and postwar homogeneity.

They pried open the inside of the bungalows in Los Angeles, the crooked deals in the DA's office—"The Story on Page One," as the title of one of the (mercifully) rare Clifford Odets directorial efforts declares—as sources for the noir world that was hiding in plain sight. John Dos Passos and Kenneth Fearing used the bizarre quirks of American news headlines to fill their chronicles of twentieth-century America, commenting by citation on the perversities of daily life. Wright, following his close friend, Ellison—answering Ellison, upping the ante—took the headlines he found in the *Herald* and, using the pulpy plots of postwar true crime and film noir to shape his memory, rewrote his Communist Party story, his city-life story, and turned a genre that Ben Maddow and other Party members had used to expose capitalism to unmask racism in the CPUSA.[45] Chance run-ins with agents from the past, deals and double deals, assumed names, amnesia, changed identities, undercover meetings, overheard conversations, innuendo, loyalty, and treachery: all are the fantastic plot twists and series of coincidences at the heart of noir. They were also aspects of the secret world, the noir world of the CPUSA, traced deftly by Ellison and turned utterly campy by Wright. The Party, especially as Cross Damon encounters it in New York, begins to resemble the numbers racket that novelist Ira Wolfert had detailed in his 1943 novel *Tucker's People*, which became the source for Abraham Polonsky's *Force of Evil* (1948). It constitutes an alternative, double cross, an underground organization that defies, yet duplicates, the legitimate one on the surface.[46]

When the invisible man first travels with Brother Jack to meet Emma at the skyscraper Chthonian, he notes the "uncanny sense of familiarity" about the soundproof elevator, the doorman, the bronze door knocker, and, most tellingly, the "smartly dressed woman . . . a clip of blazing diamonds on her dress . . . her perfumed softness. . . . I had somehow been through it all before. I couldn't decide if it were from watching some similar scene in the movies, from books I'd read, or from some recurrent but deeply buried dream" (260). For the invisible man, the dream quality of popular fiction and film becomes the central trope describing the increasingly surreal aspects of his situation, even though he reminds us on the first page of his narrative that he is "not a spook like those who haunted Edgar Allan Poe; nor . . . one of your Hollywood-movie ectoplasms" (7). Ellison seems drawn, despite himself, to the very hard-boiled scenarios he claimed to eschew for the "alive" African-American vernacular. But Wright, whose first story was a rewrite of Poe, self-consciously responds to Ellison's call with dozens of scenes from those same Poe stories and Hollywood movies. Cross Damon, already a dead man in contrast to Ellison's invisible man who's still waiting underground, acts out the plots of any number of the "spook" films he saw in "the consoling shadows of movie houses" where he spent time working out the details of his disappearance and new life (140).

The "party" to which Cross Damon is invited—like the one at Emma's, and like any gangster organization featured in noir night-club scenes—offers a complete world equipped with its own logic, its own structure, its own language. As a counterinstitution, it can offer Cross a new name, a new identity, a new residency in the down-town underground of Greenwich Village. Where (white, often Jew-ish) left-wing writers had used the intricacies of criminal enterprises to expose capitalism as the gangster underworld, Wright and Ellison flipped the genre and used it to decry the underworld of the CPUSA, as the counter-institution that mirrors society but is even more ruthless, particularly in its betrayal of African Americans.[47] In the 1940s film noirs spilling into Paris after the wartime embargo was lifted—such as *Criss Cross, The Killers, Out of the Past,* and the gang-ster movies of the 1930s Wright had watched in Chicago, home of Al Capone, "where every 3 A.M. corner looks hired"—gangsters know not only how the system works, but how to work it as well.[48] Armed with a theory of capitalism and a disciplined organization, this is also how the CPUSA operates in these two novels. The gangster world is an urban phenomenon, born in the poor, ethnic ghettoes to coun-teract the traumas of U.S. capitalism and discrimination, paradoxi-cally by taking advantage of the negative model they afforded peas-ant immigrants. This is the essentially American story behind the rise and fall of Little Caesar (with Jewish Edward G. Robinson playing Italian Rico Bandello), Scarface (with Jewish Paul Muni playing Ital-ian Tony Camonte), and that totally Irish Public Enemy (Jimmy Cagney as Tommy Powers) which Francis Ford Coppola revived so magisterially in *The Godfather.* In many ways, during the 1930s, the CPUSA resembled this organizational model as well, comprised of close-knit neighborhood- or workplace- (which usually meant eth-nically-) based units that ironically provided an alternative entry into American culture.

The picture of the Communist Party that Wright paints, like that offered by Ellison, is one of venal deception and raw exploitation. When it needed a black face, the CPUSA was willing to take on a stranger and provide a new identity. But should that stranger question the discipline required of him, he would be left dangling—offered up to rivals, including the police, to protect the organization. Mark Naison claims that despite Harlem Section leader James Ford's antipathy toward him, Wright's status as a Party "influential" meant he was protected from severe discipline by "cultural commissar" V. J. Jerome and others.[49] Naison's reading of Wright's two "Party-inspired" works finds them at odds with official lines about black-white relationships and about class alignments among African Americans during the 1930s. This picture of openness was certainly not the one offered by Wright in his testimonial "I Tried to Be a Communist" and far from the portrait of CPUSA dishonesty animating *The Outsider*. The excesses of betrayal by the CPUSA's leadership—mirrored in the excesses of violence Cross revels in, Gil Blount's abasement of Bob Hunter, his seduction of Eva, his blatant use of Damon, Hilton's insinuations to Houston, Blimin's revelations to Eva—become the excuses for Cross's series of murders. Once Cross was officially declared dead, he lived under an assumed identity, gleaned from a tombstone, a technique he learned from newspaper reports about "underground Communists" (145). Where changing names for African Americans might represent deassimilation, a refusal of a past that had obliterated their past, assuming an Anglicanized name, meant, for the immigrant Jews in the Party a chance to assimilate and forget Europe.

Cross also found an organization that could give him access to American culture, not its democratic and egalitarian aspects but rather its seamy and pulpy history. He had found an organization premised on vengeance, betrayal, and lies that freed him to act on his theory that "Maybe man is nothing in particular. . . . May not human life on this earth be a kind of frozen fear of man at what he could possibly be?" (135–6). As a "god [that failed?]," he could commit his series of murders, fall for the white girl, and converse with his nemesis Houston, listening attentively as the D.A. recounted how the double murder of the Communist Party leader Blount and the tellingly named fascist, Herndon (after Angel Herndon who was a cause célèbre for the ILD), were the act of a third man, an outsider,

FIGURE 29. Richard Widmark (Henry Fabian) on the run from Greek gangsters through the ruined streets of postwar London in *Night and the City* (d. Jules Dassin, 1950).

like Cross Damon, like himself. This is what the noir city offered Wright, a space to transgress proper form, including literary form. The postwar city is a ruined zone full of gangsters seeking revenge, in which the lone man who tries to beat them at their own game— like Richard Widmark's Harry Fabian in Jules Dassin's 1950 *Night and the City*—will be tracked down and murdered at dawn because the entire underworld has been mobilized. Pursuit paradoxically afforded Cross Damon an odd freedom.

Toward the end of the novel, Houston increasingly takes on the noir hero's role, tracking Cross Damon as Damon flees his pursuers. Like the gangster's underworld business practices and the CPUSA, structured as a hierarchy, with many layers of subordinates beholden to the boss or central committee, whose power is total, a big city DA's office also operates by intimidation and psychological threat. Where the gang or the CPUSA is a total system that requires a discipline impossible to the noir hero, ironically the New York Distract Attorney's office provides Houston the kind of independent operation necessary for his type. He can maneuver within its confines, finally eliciting a deathbed confession from Cross; but Cross had not escaped the relentless organization—it covered the city and like his life "it was . . . horrible" because it always worked as a system (440). Like the gangster whose Tommy gun shoots up both his rivals and the symbols of legit society, spraying bullets across storefronts and billboards, Wright's pen had become a weapon turned at once against himself, his personal rival (Ellison), the CPUSA, and the system of American racism. A decade before finishing *The Outsider*, he had written critic Mike Gold that "we must use our pens to beat down this wall behind which people are hiding from reality . . . our pens must be cruel towards ourselves. Our pens must become a lash. . . . If some are hurt in this fray, then ship them behind the lines; let them take ether!"[50] Writing as an outsider, from exile, was possible because American culture permeated Wright's world. Its crimes, its movies, its racism, relentlessly followed him across the ocean. Like the noir detective, he was obsessed with the sleaze spreading across the nation, hidden yet quite obviously there. Wright's noir city, a dreamlike city of memory, pried open the workings of two submerged cultures in the United States, African-American intellectual circles and the CPUSA. These two arenas were seemingly off limits to American popular culture and mutually sustained by tense antagonisms; yet, paradoxically, they inspired much pulp fiction in the 1940s and 1950s, such as Chester Himes's *If He Hollers, Let Him Go*, Ed Lacy's *Lead with Your Left*, Ira Wolfert's *Tucker's People*, and A. I. Bezzerides's *Thieves' Market*, the later two themselves inspiring two great film noirs, *Force of Evil* and *Thieves' Highway*. Left-wing pulp truths about American politics were found in the phantasm of the city and its underworld. The city noir and the city of noirs posed a challenge to postwar American middle-class prosperity and racial consensus, revealing the shades of violence still walking the mean streets.

PART 2

WHITE

WORK AND MEMORY

BLANC NOIR: RURAL PULP AND DOCUMENTARY MODERNISM

CON/FRONTING NATIONAL CULTURE

In the wake of the 1995 bombing of the Alfred P. Murrah Federal Building in Oklahoma City, the popular media echoed the sentiments of the city's residents—This sort of thing doesn't happen here; maybe in New York or Los Angeles, but not here in the heartland. Mirroring a belief that the large cities of America are somehow un-American—filled as they are with the poor, minorities, immigrants, gays, and artists—which fueled the defunding and depopulation of urban centers during the three decades between 1960 and 1990, this idea of America's heart as rural, untainted by the ills of the other half, persisted in the American imagination, even when New York, Chicago, and Detroit were centers of commerce, industry, and capital.[1] In the national imagination, America dreams itself as essentially pastoral; the center city cannot hold. Now viewed, an absent space ringed and crossed by expressways zooming suburbanites in and out of their jobs, its emptiness a sign of dangers inherited from the past, the city resembles the nightmare of postwar ruin caught in Jules Dassin's *Night and the City*.[2]

The week following the Oklahoma City bombing coincided with the closing of an important show of documentary photographs at

New York's International Center for Photography. Two exhibits—one of Dorothea Lange's photographs from 1930s through the 1960s, and the other of Joseph Rodriguez's recent multimedia documentary of East Los Angeles gang members' lives—etched divisions not only temporal, but spatial, and ultimately ideological as well. Critic Sarah Boxer contrasted Lange's depictions of noble suffering rural poor (women), whose demeanor spoke of dignified defeat, to the glaring hostility emanating from the stances of Rodriguez's urban (male) gang poseurs.[3] Rodriguez's show included long textual passages by his subjects, the room assaulted the viewers with a wall of sound as gangsta rap pulsed within. For Boxer, the gaping divide between these two shows exposed the limits of the documentary project today. It no longer holds a place in the public imagination, not merely because both observers and photographic subjects are such savvy image mongers, but primarily because, as she says, nothing is to be done for these defiant poor who refuse the pose of noble defeat and seem to aggressively challenge the viewer. (This despite the statistics indicating that many of the faces on the walls were those of the dead—victims of gang warfare and police brutality, of disease and disaster.) Lange had worked for the Farm Security Administration, which used her and others' photographs to persuade the nation of the need for drastic efforts to overcome the devastation of the Depression and the Dust Bowl. Amelioration, a central conceit of documentary, implies the *New York Times* critic, only works for some documentary subjects, not all. Why? To trace how Boxer can assert documentary's failure today to effect change, it is necessary, I believe to go back to the 1930s and follow the contours of its spectacular success.

This chapter examines the residue of documentary rhetoric clinging to various artifacts of noir popular culture in America. But it also looks at the ways in which documentaries during the 1930s—which condition everything we know of the documentary since then—were encrusted with the pulp of fiction. A national popular culture developed from the intermingling of documentary forms and popular (front) sensibilities, most spectacularly through the images of poor rural Americans—the migrant farmers forced off their land who hit the roads West, occasionally banded together huddling in Hoovervilles to share meager wares, or lined up to join work teams digging ditches and building the dams and bridges sponsored by the

Works Progress/Projects Administration (WPA). This image of rural poverty—defeated Southern whites (and occasionally blacks) stalwartly moving across the ruined landscape—provided the content for tens of thousands of photographs coming from the Farm Security Administration (FSA) project, a number of important documentary films funded by the Resettlement Administration (RA), and millions of words in pamphlets, novels, and book-length accounts of the devastation. These government-sponsored visual and literary records covered those left behind in America's quest for modernity. Ironically, this mournful retrospective of a people dispossessed, wandering in "An American Exodus," as Paul Schuster Taylor and Dorothea Lange called it, provided the substance for a modern national public culture that has lasted to this day. In the shock that terrorism happens in the "heartland" of Oklahoma City, we heard again a version of this national fantasy—that good, pure, innocent victims of social and natural catastrophes only reside out there, somewhere recognizable as America's wide open spaces.[4] The terror of city life makes those places outside the centers of media (New York and Los Angeles) or culture (Boston and San Francisco) or industry (Chicago and Detroit) appear at once more American and less violent, as if the two terms were not intimately united.[5]

Joel and Ethan Coen's blanc noir *Fargo* (1996), like their first feature *Blood Simple* (1984), troubles this image of rural purity. Playing with Karl Marx's characterization of "the idiocy of rural life," and with the sensational noir journalism of Truman Capote's *In Cold Blood*, these neo-noirs focus relentlessly on the seeming emptiness and stasis of the mid-American landscape. Roads cut through vast expanses of uniform flatland covered by prairie or snow that resist efforts to alter them. Motels, bars, even giant statues of Paul Bunyan and his blue ox Babe cannot change what Michael Lesy called the "Wisconsin Deathtrip" of small-town life. In fact, even the city itself, gleaming glass-encased Minneapolis, sitting uneasily on the open land, like Oz shimmering just beyond the poppy fields, fails to effect any changes on the horrors of rural homogeneity. However, the two films also track the ways in which the rural is suffused with a modern urban sensibility; in fact, it is a creation of it and, in turn, helps to produce it. Like Marx, Capote, and Lesy, the Coens produce a vision of the rural gothic from the safety of urban zones: Minneapolis, where they come from; Hollywood, where they work.

What *Fargo* instructs us about is the very disingenuousness of claims to an anti-urban rural space. If modern urban centers like Minneapolis or Oklahoma City can turn themselves into Fargo and become far-gone zones outside contemporary culture, it is only because the image of the heartland, as a pastoral space exempt from urban crime, violence, and social upheaval, has been thoroughly appropriated by residents of these urban centers.

In characterizing middle America as a zone apart, both the cynics in the media centers of New York and Los Angeles and the naïve dwellers of the heartland, the residents of Oklahoma City, like Frances McDormand's intrepid pregnant cop from Brainerd, Minnesota, add a melodramatic dimension to the tragic deaths. Oklahoma City's residents become a premodern people, living close to the land, despite highrises, televisions, and freeways. The rural is ever imagined as the last outpost of American exceptionalism where the histories of land development and industrial labor are denied and repressed. Thus it is somehow more disturbing for the countryside—or for cities that define themselves as rural spaces, as the heartland—to face economic or political or social crises, because modern culture dreams the heartland as the site of unalienated labor and pastoral bliss. The rural, which signifies the last zone of an original white protestant culture in America, is supposed to be an antidote to the problems of modern urban life, with its racial and ethnic minorities, its poverty, grit, and crime, but this very dichotonmy is itself a profoundly modern notion.

Imaging 1930s rural poverty and its devastation paradoxically brought a respite from the traumas of urbanization—a crisis that foregrounded labor unrest, immigration, black migration, and the sense that WASP hegemony had been severely dislodged by the 1930s. The images of tenant farmers surveying their dried-out garden patches from tar-paper sheds provided a familiar narrative through which to mediate the enormous economic and social upheavals following the in wake of the Depression. This tale resonated equally well with such diverse groups as the Communist Party's Popular Front, corporate liberals, New Dealers, and nostalgic populists. By contrast, the image of an urban underworld linked America to a decayed European modernity. The United States, reinvented as a modern industrial space, could ill afford its isolation from global politics; but rural poverty contained within it a vision of democratic vistas from the past—the tenants seemed lifted from another era, as writers such as James Agee "praise" the subtle beauties of kerosene lamplight and the pleasures of a late-night trip to an out-house—even if it were littered with human wreckage.[6]

An earlier documentary impulse, also tied to social reform, ferreted out poverty lurking behind the cities' tenement doors in reeking rooms stuffed full of dark people working day and night in airless spaces. These uses of documentary—to expose poverty and filth in urban America—reminded Americans that New York was little better than the London of the 1840s recorded by Henry Mayhew and Charles Dickens, or the Manchester where Friedrich Engels earned his living and then described in *The Condition of the Working Class in England*. Those nineteenth-century documentaries could rely on first-hand testimony and newspaper accounts to convey the horrors of the industrial town. The invention of the mercury flash brought Jacob Riis into the squalid tenements of the Lower East Side of New York to reveal "how the other half lives."[7] This "other half," ethnic and poor, did not possess the true faces of America; they were foreigners, "street gypsies," as Riis called them. However, by the 1930s, the one-third of a nation—ill housed, ill clad, ill nourished—imaged by the FSA and *Life* photographers would assume a thoroughly American visage. Even the grotesques Margaret Bourke-White pictured in her book *You Have Seen Their Faces* looked disturbingly American, its "pure products" as William Carlos Williams called them: their lives, like their gaunt faces, molded by the contours of this continent's physical geography; its plains and rivers. Documentary rhetoric in the 1930s reworked the form into a vehicle for creating a national popular culture, securing the city, or letting it languish, as grist for pulp fiction, a space apart from the location of political truth, until Hollywood returned to the city in the postwar years with film noir.

Thus I am tracing three divergent but intimately linked exchanges in the 1930s public imagination that set the ground for the film noirs of the 1940s and 1950s: the links between documentary rhetoric and popular imagery; those separating rural from urban America; and the one superintending femininity and masculinity. Left-wing film scriptwriters and directors brought documentary rhetoric, made possible by technology and necessary for ideology—e.g., mobile camera, voice-over narration, melodramatic stories—into the pulp-fiction films of the 1940s and 1950s.[8] At the same time, the Popular Front

FIGURE 30. Dorothea Lange, "Destitute pea-pick-ers in California, a thirty-two year old mother of seven children." Nipomo, Calif., 1936 [Migrant Mother].

refigured Jefferson's yeoman farmers who had been denied the fruits of democracy by forces of nature and capitalism into a virile working class, and thus knit the Left into a nation drained by economic depression. Each helped to create a corporate- and government-sponsored public sphere.

It is virtually impossible to hear the word "Depression" and not conjure up Lange's iconic "Migrant Mother." Conversely, seeing the image of maternal suffering signifies Depression: ever after a woman holding a near-naked infant and surrounded by vacant-eyed children will sum up human catastrophe.[9] This feminized and rural picture of privation is barely balanced by the more masculinized image linking the Depression to the urban breadline Lange offered America in "White Angel Breadline" in 1933. This powerful rhetorical slippage between image and word is central to my contention that documentary photography, its overabundance, meant that the images circulating of rural poverty escaped no one's view. During the 1930s, over 77,000 photographs were made by the FSA, now held in the Library of Congress; popular phototextual magazines such as *Life*, whose first printing of 380,000 reached 650,000 readers by the seventh week, were widely distributed. America became a modern nation, in a sense, through nostalgia, but its view backward could not find a rosy past in the hollowed out children of migrant mothers.

Images of American rural poverty, especially white rural poverty, worked to convey a national identification with New Deal projects, and thus worked to achieve a coherent picture of America, by foregrounding want and the tenacious efforts of people of the land, often photographed as solitary figures, alone against the elements, to survive with dignity. The images of individual faces, of unique bodies, served to knit together a national public culture through conventional devices of heroic portraiture, landscape, and still life. Looking at privation, at the heart of darkness within the American dream, undid, by avoiding, the xenophobic and regionalist mentalities of an earlier era, precisely because these migrant poor people were neither urban nor ethnic. America became modern, became a mass society, by looking at those whose lives had escaped modernity.

TRUTH-TELLING AND POPULAR MEMORY

In his 1942 Yenan Talks on art and literature, Mao Zedong took time off from the Long March to consider the role of art in the revolution. His prescription for good art was simple yet fraught with the contradictions he sought continually to bring into relief. Art must both "expose" and "extol": first disgorge the horror of oppression, then sing the possibilities of liberation. This was a distillation of the aesthetic platform of the Popular Front, the broad-based coalition forged by the Communist Party to combat fascism. Ironically, Mao's dualism has structured virtually all contemporary political rhetoric about culture from both the Right and the Left (think of the National Endowment for the Arts debacle or the panic generated by gangsta-rap lyrics, on the one hand, and the uproar among gays and lesbians over *Silence of the Lambs* or *Basic Instinct*, on the other) precisely because variations on Popular Front culture remain dominant. They provide the basis of much fretting over positive images and role models and declaiming over the loss of innocence in America's heartland. The didacticism Mao called for assumed art's instrumentality; it is supposed to *do* something. Mao thus rejects the modernist sensibility claiming "l'art pour l'art." However, the effects of the Popular Front, of which Mao's Yenan Talks are a cogent summation, were paradoxically thoroughly modern.

This call for purposefulness, for useful art, which appears so utilitarian, so modern, if not modernist, slips into an antimodern sentimentality when its form is documentary whose explicit purpose is rhetorical. Documentary seeks to convince you that what you see is what you get: the truth. In truth-telling, or in posing as truth tellers, documentaries, however, appeal to raw emotion. Their often naked and direct calls for our engagement are blatant and disturbing. Documentaries are always a bit unseemly. They come about because someone has crossed the line of decorum—snapping pictures of the worst moments, cruelest situations, most extreme events—snatching a bit of another's miserable life and parading it for all to see. It is this perversity that is so fascinating and so disturbing, and that evokes from even the most nostalgic documentary project a pulp modernist effect.

Usually what we consider documentary seems far removed from popular culture. Yet the interpenetration of the two forms has a long-standing history, made most explicit in the 1930s when various technological and economic changes made possible the widespread dissemination of images for practically nothing.[10] In a segment of the PBS series *American Cinema*, B-movie director Joseph H. Lewis (*Gun Crazy*, *The Big Combo*, and other great trashy noirs) noted that the techniques of film noir—mobile camera, location shooting, night-for-night shooting—were the direct result of technical innovations brought about by World War II and the experiences film directors had shooting military footage for night reconnaissance with lightweight 16 mm cameras and new faster film stocks invented during the war. What he failed to mention, however, was a further connection to the documentary expression of the 1930s (as William Stott called it) in the many screenplays written by left-wing proletarian writers, such as *Force of Evil*, Abraham Polonsky's 1948 film of Ira Wolfert's novel, *Tucker's People*; or *Theives' Highway*, Jules Dassin's 1949 film of A. I. Bezzerides's novel *Theives' Market*; or *Body and Soul*, Robert Rossen's 1947 film from Abraham Polonsky's screenplay.

Film noir, that quintessential pulp-fictional style, relied on documentary rhetoric and methods. These, in turn, resulted from new technologies, most spectacularly the ability to print photo and text on the same page and the push to blend short story and journalism in reportage. John Steinbeck's 1939 best-seller, *The Grapes of Wrath*, began as a piece of reportage on California migrant workers written in 1936, which was reprinted in 1937 as a pamphlet to accompany Dorothea Lange's FSA photographs. Richard Wright's publisher, Viking, rushed *12 Million Black Voices* into print after the success of *Native Son*. Wright's poetic documentary text was culled from his personal experience, as well as fieldwork and archival research conducted by the Good Shepherd Community Center in Chicago and accompanied by a selection of FSA photos chosen by Edwin Rosskam. Wright's 1940 novel, *Native Son*, followed a sensational murder trial reported daily by the Chicago papers and clipped for Wright by the young poet and WPA writer Margaret Walker.[11]

These borrowings back and forth between documentary and fiction and, among proletarian and pulp fictions, crossed genders as well. Not only were proletarian writers connected by style and politics to "tough-guy writers," but women's proletarian fiction, because it saw sexuality as central to female experience, reworked romance. Hope Hale Davis remembers writing *True Stories* serialized "confessions" during the 1930s to make ends meet and appeal directly to working-class women by inserting political messages into the softcore pulp.[12] Occasionally women authors were castigated for inserting "smutty vulgar sex stories" or "pornography" into what should have been wholesome tales of proletarian struggle.[13] The commingling of genders, genres, and forms is central to the cultural coworking of 1930s documentary and Hollywood films. Documentary images circulate a rhetoric of truth that has powerfully shaped our ideas about public life, political action, and popular culture by relying on, yet denying, sentiment. The rhetoric of truth so important to documentary is didactic—documentary tells the truth for a purpose; it has become the means to bring previously forgotten men and women into view by objectifying their faces and provoking their political subjectivity. Because its mode of truth-telling so conforms to Mao's "expose and extol" thesis, it is also the prevailing aesthetic for much popular culture.

PULPING NATURAL HISTORY

In a famous piece of rhetorical analysis, Kenneth Burke parses a speech by Franklin D. Roosevelt, who declares to his audience: "You are farmers. I am a farmer too." Burke describes the powerful rhetorical gesture FDR has made by inserting himself—upper-class New Yorker—into the frame of reference of his listeners by invoking a commonality between worlds so vastly separated as to constitute two nations.[14] FDR's design to slip into a rural, even pastoral, ideal in order to persuade his listeners of his sincerity so that he might form a united front with them is part of a long history that reinvents the nostalgic rural past from the vantage of spoiled urbanized present as a response to changing economic and social formations. In the summer of 2001, President George W. Bush enacted his own version of pastoralism when he moved to his ranch in Crawford, Texas, during August to pursue his "working vacation" chainsawing brush, dubbed "Home to the Heartland." Early in Raymond Williams's magnificent study of the changing relations between "the country and the city," he posits the image of the escalator, moving ever backward. This endless retreat seeks to account for the moment when rural bliss was first deformed by the hand of man, leading inexorably to decline from a long lost Edenic past. He cites a few lines from George Crabbe's 1783 poem, "The Village":

> No longer truth, though shown in verse, disdain
> But own the Village Life a life of pain.
> By such examples taught, I paint the Cot
> As Truth will paint it, and as Bards will not.

Williams describes Crabbe's bold move away from a tradition of pastoralism, which revered the country as untouched and Edenic, toward a new realism, a realism that is also pulp fiction, in which the truth of rural life—a life of toil and pain, of exploitation—becomes the basis for a new poetics of truth: a documentary rhetoric.[15] Williams brilliantly shows that although the rural is supposed to be a place modernity, and thus capitalism, left behind, the very ways culture imagines this space apart is precisely a product of the same developments supposedly alien to country life. The idea that rural people are outside modernity is itself a modern notion—one that provides an antidote to the problems of modern life: economic crises, urban decay, and so forth—generated through the images constructed by urbanites. "I'm goin' up the country . . . where the water tastes like wine," sang San Francisco band Canned Heat in 1967. Thus the country is both always idealized as the untouched zone and yet, within modern culture, is also painted as the site of truth, a truth found in the detailed documentary exposition of the labor and expropriation attendant upon making the country seem a space apart from capitalism. FDR and George W. Bush, both from East Coast patrician families, can claim to be farmers because they have access to a history of images of rural life drawn by those far removed from it. Dorothea Lange may have begun her documentary career walking the streets of San Francisco, shooting the disgruntled men she found waiting for work or protesting its exploitations, but the project that hired her to photograph poverty was the *Farm* Security Administration. What the government needed to persuade mostly urban middle-class Americans to support the New Deal were not images of a dangerous urban army of the poor; instead it reclaimed the vanishing land and its way of life as its core subject. While many relief programs targeted the urban poor, the documentary projects generated by and for the New Deal envisioned the United States as a series of rural regions inhabited by a folk population fast disappearing because of the forces of nature itself.

A desire to trace the prehistory of the dust bowl led Pare Lorentz to invest his 1936 documentary *The Plow That Broke the Plains* with a vision of natural forces at war with social and economic developments; his film was an act of preservation, even as it tracked the disappearance of topsoil blown off by incessant winds and excessive machinery. Lorentz left the investigation of faces to the still photographers. His two films—criticized by *Plow's* left-wing cinematographers Leo Hurwitz, Paul Strand, and Ralph Steiner for leaving out the human dimension and so the politics of land abuse and labor exploitation—exposed the larger ecological impact of wind, sun, and rain on the great central plains of the American continent. Shortsighted irrigation projects resulted in land damage, but profits, cities, and war—all human inventions—were destroying the land's capacity to renew itself. Lorentz's film, made through financing by the FSA and Resettlement Administration (RA), was meant to help various extension agents devise plans for alternative land use and convince local populations to implement them. Rural offices, however, bristled at the depiction of Texas as a barren zone and sought to have *Plow* suppressed.

A year later, Lorentz's vision of water covering over two thirds of the continent also submerged human faces into a saga of rain, floods, and erosion. In *The River* (1937), however, a solution worked by government agencies seemed likely to succeed. The great dams of the Tennessee Valley Authority (TVA) were among the most popular New Deal projects, employing thousands and bringing visible evidence of modernity—huge modernist structures of reinforced concrete—to the heart of rural America. Lorentz's majestic view of the American continent stressed its openness. The heartland was meant to remain empty; wind, sun, rain would never be vanquished. The scene of a demurely dressed woman, wearing a clean white apron and heels, bravely sweeping her porch steps as her baby sits amid the rising sand dunes forming around an abandoned plow called into question the hospitality of this continent a hundred years after European settlers pushed West. It is also a rare glimpse at the human figure stranded within this immense and barren landscape.

This image, like Lange's stark portrait, "Woman of the High Plains, Texas Panhandle, June 1938," offers a stoic, even heroic, refusal to succumb to natural forces. In these pictures, mothers still sweep and worry about their children even as the land around them threatens to swallow them up. In her attention to the "social scene of our time," Lange was limning the rhetoric of documentary visually. A few years later, in a catalogue put together by Ansel Adams for the 1940 San Francisco World's Fair, Lange verbally defined the genre:

Documentary photography records the social scene of our time. It mirrors the present and documents for the future. Its focus is man in his relation to mankind. It records his customs at work, at war, at play, or his round of activities through twenty-four hours of the day, the cycle of the seasons, or the span of a life. . . . It is concerned with methods of work and the dependence of workmen on each other and on their employers. It is pre-eminently suited to build a record of change. Advancing technology raises standards of living, creates unemployment, changes the face of cities and of the agricultural landscape. The evidence of these trends—the simultaneous existence of past, present, and portent of the future—is conspicuous in old and new forms, old and new customs, on every hand. . . . Documentary photography invites and needs participation by amateurs as well as by professionals. Only through the interested work of amateurs who choose themes and follow them can documentation by the camera of our age and our complex society be intimate, pervasive, and adequate.[16]

In her call for repetitive cycles chronicling changes over time—a day, a year, a life—and her assertion that amateurs as well as professionals record the simultaneous existence of past, present, and future, Lange was explicitly linking documentary photography to history. She saw in documentary the ability to link the residues of the past and of nature to the technologies of the present. In fact, it was through this technology—amateur photography, undertaken by those trained through reading *Life* magazine and seeing Hollywood films—that an image of America as a nation would emerge. Lange's 1940 manifesto also points to the ways in which the great FSA and *Life* photographers who produced "photo-textual books" during the Depression decade were responding to competing currents already traced by Hollywood.[17] Still and moving images, documentary and pulp genres, infected each other; they required each other in much the same way as rural imagery fed urban ideals. Those capturing the heartland were not its native sons or daughters. Images of rural poverty and collective labor—especially those staged to fulfill a national fantasy—eased the traumas of the Depression, insuring a troubled nation that neither poverty nor collectivity were threats to American political culture; rather they were signs of its permanence.

FINDING FARGO

Tensions embracing the dark and comic sides of the Depression, that is, anxieties brought up by urban ethnicity and rural poverty, continue to haunt popular culture as the discourse surrounding the Oklahoma City bombing shows. A modern urban center such as Oklahoma City can define itself as the heartland through the legacy of 1930s documentary rhetoric. Because of the ravages, grotesques,

FIGURE 31. Two-page layout from a cover story photo-essay on New Deal, Montana, in the first issue of *Life*, Margaret Bourke-White (November 1936). Note photo duplication.

and stoicism imaged by Lange, Bourke-White, and Evans, we believe it is somehow more disturbing for the countryside to face social, economic, and political upheavals. The heartland, repository of pastoral simplicity, site of documentary truth, not poetic invention, escapes the pulp fiction of urban life, even if cities with populations of more than a million can be found there.

After the Second World War, film noir reimagined the city—this time that quintessentially Western city, destination of the displaced tenant farmers from Oklahoma and Arkansas, sunny Los Angeles—as a dire, claustrophobic space where the individual will always be subsumed by the machinations of the larger immoral network of crime, guilt, and complicity.[18] These visions of terror erupting anywhere, coming after the revelations of the Holocaust and the destruction of European Jewry, were written and directed by the very same (often left-wing Jewish) artists who helped forge a countervision of proletarian resistance in the organization of violent ethnic gangsters, on the one hand, or the muscled shoulders standing in class-conscious solidarity, on the other. These left-wing visions of the machinery of urban solidarity never entered the popular imagination the way that those of rural privation had. However, as the Depression leaked into war preparation, and mobility seemed more purposeful—not dislocation, but mobilization—a new vision of a female urban space emerged. Dorothy Arzner's 1940 parody of Busby Berkeley's 1930s musicals, *Dance, Girl, Dance*, with a screenplay by literary radical Tess Slesinger, traces the darker side of chorus-line work. Sexual exploitation and objectification, competition not cooperation among the girls on the line, commodification and mechanization of a creative process, are both embraced and blown wide open in the ironic, darkly cynical tale of Maureen O'Hara's portrayal of ballet dancer Judy as burlesque "stooge" for Lucille Ball's "Tiger Lily White," a performer with "oomph." This noir musical rehearsed the divisions between documentary and pulp, rural and urban, popular and elite, and presaged the powerful bad girls of film noir.

By war's end, both the city and women's bodies had become sinister but intriguing again, filled with hidden vices and dangers lurking around each curve. The perils of an alien urban landscape and modern America had been temporarily allayed by images of rural poverty in 1930s documentaries, but they had never really gone away. James Agee's ventriloquized ruminations on Annie Mae Gudger's sexuality formed a pulp fiction out of the lives of these impoverished tenant women. Yet, almost immediately, even the more radical visions of those working for the FSA were tamed. Within a few years of Lange's "Migrant Mother" image of rural poverty and need, FSA photography head, Roy Stryker, was directing his photographers to find more wholesome images in the kitchens and clinics of Pie Town, New Mexico, and the new suburban Greenbelts that welcome the Joads at the end of Hollywood's *Grapes of Wrath*. Roy Stryker's job, now that the New Deal projects were in place, was not to convince middle-class Americans of the need and privation driving New Deal programs but instead to demonstrate their successful transformation of the face of rural poverty into a horn of plenty. One reason Agee and Evans's book, with pictures shot in 1936, was such a failure when it finally appeared in 1941 was that on the eve of America's entry into World War II, Stryker was directing photographer Jack Delano to gather "autumn pictures . . . cornfields, pumpkins . . . emphasize the idea of abundance—the 'horn of plenty'—and pour maple syrup over it."[19] The brief moment when rural poverty could be seen and spoken of in polite company was over; however, it was precisely its fact and its visibility that forged an American national identity with the rural heartland as a central icon of authenticity.[20]

The image of the blown-out, plowed-out family whose integrity was destroyed by weather, technology, and monetary policies was in stark contrast to both Hollywood's violent underworld and the working-class family whose burly rippling musculature would valiantly march forward into a new future free from hunger and exploitation promoted by the Communist Party USA. The images of wreckage and disaster won out within historical memory. Hugo Gellert's *New Masses* cartoons of muscled workers are just that, caricatures. The heroic face masks Hollywood's noir nightmare of anomie and alienation that quickly reappeared after the War. Properly modern American tragedies, like proper Americans, did not dwell in the corrupt mire of the modern cities made up of aliens whose ethnicity could be marked by Hollywood—as gangsters and B-girls—but remained unnoticed by the government documentaries. The subjects of 1930s documentaries were the last remnants of a rural order of dignity and pride and hard work, which, white or black, had its roots in the soil of the Midwest or the South. The endurance of the suffering tenants caught by Evans and Lange and the contorted figures of privation snatched by Bourke-White appear full repositories of truth despite the distorted, staged, rearranged, and posed elements of each image. Because each says "I am truthful," these visual accounts of an ever-receding past hold power over our present imaginations and memories. They do so through their content—their straightforward presentation of space, objects, people, and form—their black-and-white simplicity, purity of line, depth of field. These images serve as the backdrop for film noir, which relocated the probing camera's eye from the emptying land to the corrupt city, tracking the sons and daughters of those migrant mothers after they returned from war to settle into the supposedly comfortable bungalows lining the Los Angeles hills. Documentary's power still forms our vision, as the media continue to "expose and extol" both the political truths and pulp fictions of postmodern America by dividing the country from the city, even if it is called Fargo.

CHAPTER 5

MELODRAMA/MALE DRAMA: THE SENTIMENTAL CONTRACT OF AMERICAN LABOR FILMS

LABOR'S MELODRAMA

"Do not ask me to write of the strike and the terror. I am on a battlefield. . . . But I hunch over the typewriter and behind the smoke, the days whirl, confused as dreams," declared the young Tillie Lerner (Olsen) during the 1934 San Francisco general strike.[1] In this classic example of reportage, the division between observation and participation, between fact and fantasy, has broken down. "I am on a battlefield," not merely as a war correspondent but as one of the combatants. In Florence Reece's ballad trumpeting the news of the 1934 Kentucky coal strikes in bloody Harlan County, one must decide "Which Side Are You On?": "if you go to Harlan County / there is no neutral there, you'll either be a union man / or a thug for J. H. Blair."[2] The labor struggles of the 1930s had clearly defined battle lines, and everyone sympathetic to workers knew which side was right; yet the engaged writer, knowing she was on a battlefield, was left "behind the smoke . . . confused as dreams" by her double duty—to march and to type. Contemporary labor documentaries owe much to the literary genre of reportage, especially as practiced in the 1930s by committed journalists and worker correspondents. This form collapses distinctions between reader and participant by placing the observer/writer in the midst of the action as it happens; and because the two poles are clearly marked—you either are a union man or a thug—sentiment lodges on the side of labor. Florence Reece and the other balladeers could march *and* sing, but writers eventually left the line to tell the story. By leaving the line, the writer momentarily escaped the conflict, confusing her class allegiance; however, an either/or situation demands that both reporter and reader must choose sides within a dichotomous class structure. In reportage, documenters serve not only to witness, but to fight, like Frederick Douglass, who stresses that his indoctrination into the "hell of slavery" began when he recognized his role as "a witness and a participant" and ended only after he battled the overseer Covey, vowing never to be whipped again.

During the 1930s, many writers forged these sentimental contracts as they journeyed in search of "the trouble" befalling a nation suffering through extreme economic crisis.[3] In many ways, reportage mediated the feminized stance of the novelist—whether male or female, the writer was viewed by the Left as effete, bourgeois—and that of the hard-boiled reporter, as tough masculine worker, because these writers did not simply report from the sidelines; they put their bodies on the line. In modern times, radical intellectuals often have romanticized the industrial worker as the authentic vehicle of revolution. Moving into workers' homes to march with them became a standard activity of radical journalists following the strikes in coal, rubber, and steel during the 1930s. For instance, in 1934, a young Smith College graduate, Harriet Woodbridge, writing as Lauren Gilfillan, traveled to the coal fields of western Pennsylvania to report on the strikes there. She entered the struggle only to be reminded that she was an outsider. *I Went to Pit College* described her position as radical journalist within a mining community, riven by rival unions, political enmity, class conflict, and racial, ethnic, and religious divisions, which at least coalesced around a mutual suspicion of outsiders, especially those sporting linen dresses. Her book, widely reviewed and often denounced as sentimental tripe and a melodramatic portrayal of middle-class feminine thrill-seeking, was also praised for a willingness to bare herself as a voyeur and explore these class confusions, as it provided a vivid portrait of a community torn apart by labor strife.[4] Reportage, "in no way content simply to depict facts," risked sentimentality, according to Georg Lukács, because it "does indeed appeal to our feelings, both in its depiction of the facts and in the call to action."[5] Too much investment in one side of the battle, too much detail, a fetishistic "portrayal" of the victims of capitalism, however, got in the way of clear-sighted "scientific" analyses of the prevailing economic and political crisis. Because it opens the way for tears, reportage treads a fine political line, locating sentiment in the house of labor.

Sentimentality emerges in eighteenth-century England under curious and contradictory conditions. On the one hand, discussions about the proper use of tears were linked to a long history of antirational conservatism, starting with the embarrassingly sentimentalized male philosophers, such as Edmund Burke, resisting the Enlightenment revolutions in France. Claudia Johnson argues persuasively that "the welfare of the nation and the tearfulness of private citizens—actual as well as fictional—were understood in the 1790s to be urgently interconnected."[6] I would add that this was no less true of the 1990s. On the other hand, the rise of the bourgeois state required a break with the teary-eyed men who maintained a chivalric honor unnecessary under a new democratic regime. Men's tears are throwbacks to an era when the spectacle of men crying could be understood as part of the workings of an aristocratic order of "sentimentality [under which] the prestige of suffering belongs to men" (17). Within the culture of middle-class sensibilities, women became the vessels of feelings. The new forms of gendered subjectivity developing within bourgeois culture, feminist literary historians such as Nancy Armstrong, Cathy Davidson, and Jane Tompkins argue, require the "cultural work" of women's sentimentality to establish the modern subject, a being drenched in emotion and encased in privacy during the age of revolution and after. Sentiment became private because its public expression threatened social order. According to Raymond Williams, what Burke resisted was the incursion of the rational state into zones previously cordoned off as civil society. Emotions publicly displayed by citizens of a democracy led to the frightening spectacle of mobs and masses in the streets.[7] Bourgeois culture thus contained sentimentality within women's domain. Its leakage into "the methods of science" appropriate to journalism,[8] especially in the service of that most melodramatic public staging—the strike—threatened to undo political authority. That would seem a good thing if one's goals, like those of the literary radicals of the 1930s, were to overthrow a failed capitalism.

However, in the rhetoric of both the Left and modernism, bourgeois culture as a whole had taken on the sentimentalized characteristics of feminized, aristocratic decadence—an image repeated in IWW iconography, socialist cartoons, Thorsten Veblen's *Theory of the Leisure Class*, communist pamphlets, modernist manifestoes, and even in Teddy Roosevelt's speeches.[9] Only the heroic workers (or modernist poets, but that's another story) standing shoulder-to-shoulder in solidarity could break with sentimentality and usher in a new world. The working stiff, like the freelancing detective and the mobile femme fatale, offers a tough resistance to the decay of modern life. This picture of masculine triumph had its own sentimental logic that also dates from the eighteenth century. "The first great tribune of the industrial proletariat," William Cobbett, declared, according to Raymond Williams, collective action to be "a movement of the *people's* own," a concerted response to the "masters [who] combine against them," leaving them barely able to feed themselves and their families (*Culture and Society*, 3, 17). If a strike provides a stirring, emotionally-saturated, political tableau, its visual economy owing much to melodrama, where the forces of good and evil are decisively separate, that is because since the late eighteenth century, the working class has been cast in heroic and victimized poses.[10]

In twentieth-century America, the most powerful icons of this dual image of the working class have been found within the traditions of the documentary photography inaugurated by Lewis Hine. Hine's 1932 children's book, a photographic record called *Men at Work*, subtitled "Photographic Studies of Modern Men and Machines," offers a vision of labor poles apart from his earlier images of children dwarfed by massive looms. This volume carefully integrates the male body into the machinery of modern construction (many of the images are from Hine's on-location photographs of the Empire State Building rising from the streets of Manhattan as it was built). The scale of the masculine body establishes the size of the machine it works. Some of the "men of courage, skill, daring and imagination" are "heroes," says Hine paraphrasing Marx in his introduction, "the spirit of industry." Heroes because "cities do not build themselves; machines do not make machines. . . . [R]eal men make and direct them."[11] Hine shoots individual men intimately curled over and around their tools, but he also provides a vision of collective labor in shots showing how modern work requires cooperation among many men on the job.[12] This highly erotic, actually homoerotic, vision of men and machinery became a staple of documentary, culminating in Robert Flaherty's 1941 *Louisiana Story*, where the arrival of the enormous oil derrick moves the young boy to explore the world of machinery as he had once covered the natural landscape. The boy, embraced (literally) by this all-male world, ultimately integrates nature and machine and his body in the penultimate shot as he curls himself around the "christmas tree," the capped oil pipes, left standing in the bayou. Flaherty's film was hardly a left-wing celebration of machinery and labor; Standard Oil footed the bill for this "fantasy," as Flaherty referred to it.

Hine's 1932 photographs initiated a visual rhetoric of sentimentality that cloaked workers bodies and gigantic machinery in a celebration of the collective labors required to build America. In this, his images were visual updates of Melville's ecstatic whale-rendering scenes in *Moby-Dick*. This new sentimentality contrasted with Hine's earlier portraits of America's working victims suffering under capitalism's brutality. The recourse to sentiment among labor's documenters is tied to confusing gender codes, which have historically dictated who can and who cannot cry, and to conflicting class and national allegiances, which also involve delegating the proper expression of sentiment. Modern national allegiance requires tears—one need only watch any athletic segment or any commercial during NBC's broadcast of the 1996 or 2000 Olympics to get a shorthand lesson in the centrality of tears to national identity. We watch as athletes cry in victory or sob in defeat; we cry with them at home, our living rooms linked mysteriously through the flowing tears. Like nations, class formations, precisely because they require imaginative communities linked through ideas and sentiments, resemble these emotion-laden fantasies. Class codings can be made invisible with proper grooming and elocution, so says Henry Higgins to Elizabeth Doolittle in *My Fair Lady*, because unlike sexual or racial differences, they are not inscribed on the bodies' surfaces. For this reason, class is a slippery analytic category, even among feminists otherwise sensitive to nuanced gender, sexual, and racial differences. In the differing views of Burke and

Cobbett, workers combined, either sinisterly as a mass or rationally as a class, in response to the workings of the capitalist state, a state formed in the interests of one class, the bourgeoisie, in part by cordoning off sentiment. This is also why the rhetoric of sentimentality—so crucial to modern national and class formations—still circulates within labor documentaries, even those questioning the form of documentary itself.

ROGER & ME(N)

In differing ways, Michael Moore's *Roger & Me* (1989) and Barbara Kopple's *American Dream* (1990) tap this long-standing tradition of figuring class conflict through gendered discourses of sentimentality.[13] *Roger & Me*, ever ironic about documentary, General Motors, and government policies that favor corporate greed over human need, cannot escape its heritage. In the 1930s, Hugo Gellert, a cartoonist for the left-wing journal *New Masses*, illustrated a selection of writings from Karl Marx's *Capital* with his drawings of solidly muscled workers.[14] The butt of in-jokes within the Left, these heroic figments of radical imagination were fantasies of excessive virility.[15] A strong working class could overcome both the crisis of capitalism and the malaise the lost generation was suffering after the First World War. A heavy load to bear—making the revolution and saving American masculinity at once—this construction of the manly worker occluded a vision of the working-class woman, who, in Gellert's drawings, bulge with hefts of muscle and a muscled breast nourishing her buffed-out baby boy, the kind of "revolutionary girl" celebrated in proletarian poems by such forgotten poets as H. H. Lewis. By contrast the bourgeoisie was a feminized and decadent class: corpulent men stuffed into top hats and tails, like the banker on the Monopoly game, sucking the vitality from the labor of others; or desiccated spinsters whose dried up lives were doomed to disappear once the new working-class family took possession of its rightful place.

It was a ludicrous picture then, when at least a quarter of the work force was female. In the 1980s, it should have been trotted out only as parody; yet *Roger & Me* returns to these stock types with a straight face to cast its saga of deindustrialization. Almost all the scenes with women target the lavish lifestyles of the rich and infamous of Flint, Michigan, and feature chiffon-dressed women sound-

FIGURE 32. Hugo Gellert, "Primary Accumulation," from *Karl Marx 'Capital' in Lithographs* (1934).

FIGURE 33 Hugo Gellert, "The Working Day," from *Karl Marx 'Capital' in Lithographs* (1934).

ing like Marie Antoinette before the revolution. The one exception—the lonely rabbit breeder whose uncanny pragmatism (pets or meat) seems demented at best, vicious at worst—clearly survives outside the economy of contemporary American late capitalist relations. She is a holdover from another era and another place, perhaps the mountains of Kentucky from which many autoworkers migrated during and after the Second World War, like a character out of Harriet Arnow's 1954 novel, *The Dollmaker*, devastated by city life and industrial work discipline.[16] Moore is drawn to this odd woman; she reappears as the star of his short sequel, *Pets or Meat: The Return to Flint* (1993), which also aired on PBS stations.[17]

Sentimentality requires a hero, just as melodrama demands clearly defined sides. Moore is a contemporary (anti-)hero, a goofy guy who has shed his class origins just barely because his skills lie in intellectual labor—the production of words and images—not the backbreaking assembly work of his father's generation.[18] His film unveils "an anti-aesthetics of failure in contemporary documentary,"[19] an absence that looms large in this story of contemporary labor: no strikes; no "men at work." What *Roger & Me* finds instead is lack: the lack of union militancy; the lack of work, as thousands of autoworkers have been laid off; the lack of industry, as plants close and move their operations overseas. Flint, Michigan, stands as an emblem of militant union organizing; site of the 1936 sit-down strike, the most effective use of the strategy in American history, whose stirring images of men curled amid their tools and machinery asleep on the shop floor galvanized generations of organizers. Josephine Herbst had caught this scene, connecting it to the rise of "the worker-writer," when she closes her 1939 novel, *Rope of Gold*, with a striking autoworker penning his autobiography.[20] As a fantasy melding industry with aesthetics, like a bridge girder or a poured concrete dam, this quintessential modernist figure—an idle worker sprawled across the plant floor recording the details of the strike for the *Daily Worker*—has no place in a deindustrializing economy. Even the sitdown strike is ineffective against plant closures. The story has shifted elsewhere to the corporate and financial boardrooms where the flows of capital not productivity (which requires bodies) are key to profits.

Without the bodies of workers at their machines or the masses on the picket line, Moore's saga comes down to a lone quest for an elusive figure, General Motors CEO Roger Smith. Smith's continual absence is one more hole in the fabric of American industry; a boss can no longer be embodied either. The rotund cigar-smoking capitalist who lorded over a semifeudal "industrial valley" has also been displaced.[21] For example, in the new world order of virtual strikebreaking, to combat striking unions at Detroit's two largest newspapers, *The Detroit News* and *The Detroit Free Press* no longer needed to hire thugs. They set up home pages on the World Wide Web denouncing union tactics on the picket lines and praising those who cross the lines, including stories about the terrific food served to those who show up for work.[22] Moore fails to get close to the real boss—Roger Smith—so he goes for the cheap shot, the vacuous country club wives of Chevy's middle managers who declare Flint a wonderful city and wonder why everyone is complaining.

If the CEO cannot be located, neither can the worker; he is neither on the picket line nor on the assembly line. Charlie Chaplin's working-tramp represented the modern anti-hero of labor—dwarfed by the machine, encompassed by the masses. The counterpart to the Tramp's incorporation into the machine of capital is Chaplin's wonderful overhead crane shot, which offers a visual joke on working-class unity as the Tramp, after picking up a red flag that has fallen off the back of a carriage, unknowingly leads a demonstration of protesting workers only to find himself beaten and jailed by the police. Instead, Moore finds his postmodern worker-tramp in Ben Hamper, a contemporary Midwestern worker-writer, in the tradition of Jack Conroy, the "rivethead" whose column had previously appeared in Moore's alternative newspaper, *The Flint Voice*, now a novelist. Hamper explains, while aimlessly shooting hoops, that he was laid off with a medical disability because he had cracked up on the shop floor. He feels like a fraud compared to the women he met in the hospital—suicidal and depressed—whose mental illnesses were somehow more real, caused as they were by domestic, personal troubles. The public world of work is not supposed to cause mental breakdowns, but without the masses to provide a collective shelter for the worker, his psyche becomes as fragile as a housewife's.[23] Moore empathizes with his high-school buddy; they share history, each with a middle-aged, working-class inelegance that has no place, despite their new roles as intellectuals, circulating language and images.[24]

Moore's film, picked up and distributed by Time-Warner, sparked a major debate within corporate boardrooms and across business and industry pages;[25] his wry humor showed up GM as callous, the Flint Chamber of Commerce and Mayor's Office in the pockets of GM, and a citizenry suffering from delusions and privation so extreme that "recovery" appears unlikely.[26] Moreover, his decision to tamper with history, revising chronology to suit his narrative, caused a minor stir.[27] Moore's recourse to staged melodrama—placing Ronald Reagan in Flint in the midst of the shut down—gave ammunition to GM, which wanted to defuse the film's effects.[28] But Moore's manipulations came from a long tradition of documentary filmmaking. As he remarked: "With nonfiction, you have no idea when you go out to shoot what's going to happen, and you have to figure it all out once you're in the editing room."[29] Dziga Vertov's scissors cutting celluloid in *Man With a Movie Camera* had foregrounded the editing process as crucial to *Kino-Pravda*—a job requiring the hands of his female assistant editor, Yelizaveta Svilova. With absence—no jobs, no organization, no boss—as capital flows elsewhere and workers sit idle, its central feature, Moore's postmodern portrait of labor still rests on the prehistory of modern male worker's melodramas, embodied by the two forces—Roger, endlessly beyond the camera, and M(oor)e, endlessly performing for it.[30]

SPAM'S HOME

American Dream follows Kopple's magisterial view of worker solidarity in *Harlan County, USA* (1976) with a darker vision of the contradictions and complexities of contemporary union organizing in the heartland. Despite the ostensibly amiable atmosphere of Garrison Keillor's Lake Woebegone, Austin, Minnesota's, Hormel plant, and the efforts of meat packers at Local P-9 of the United Food and Commercial Workers (UFCW) to maintain union solidarity, *American Dream* presents a wretched scene. Anticipating the gruesomeness of *Fargo*, it lends bloody Harlan County a nostalgic glow. Kopple's complex gesture in *American Dream* traces the present conditions for union militancy in a typically Midwestern industry—hog processing—during this era of multinational corporate flight; its story of the multiple forces working at odds complicates the melodrama of union men vs. scabs staged in *Harlan County, USA*. The 1984–85 strike against the Hormel plant dramatized how the arena has been complicated with a proliferating cast whose allegiances and identities are not so easily coded as good or bad. This corrective seems in part a response to critiques of her earlier film as overly humanistic; perhaps deindustrialization forces another cinema as much as another politics.

American Dream begins with shots of the hog kill room, which Kopple was able to film with a hidden camera by posing as a New

York high-school student doing a report on the meat industry. The process of turning pigs into bacon is dangerous and disgusting work; the work site and work process, which are not central to the film's story, focusing as it does on the intricacies of local and international organizing, bargaining, and the strike and its aftermath, establishes the source of the action. If the establishing shot of the typing pool on the bottom floor of the Pacific All-Risk Insurance Company in *Double Indemnity* reminds us of the repetitive boredom of white-collar office work that contributes to film noir, the assembly line at Hormel presents pure horror and exploitation. In the brief encapsulated history the film provides, we hear Reagan's "off-the-cuff" remark about the economy: "I'm prepared to tell you it's a hell of a mess." Jesse Jackson then tells a packed crowd in 1986, "[W]hat Selma was to the civil rights movement, Austin is to the movement for workers' rights." The scene shifts two years earlier and follows two men past a playground where children swing and climb and slide to the front door of a large house where the wife of a Hormel executive lectures the men to be grateful they now receive $8.75 an hour: "When we were your age . . ." she begins, but the men cut her off: "Give us a fair shake, like you got." Although a town like Austin represses its class structure, visible evidence lies everywhere. In Austin, 22,000 people live in "a little world by ourselves," Hormel counsel Nyberg explains, echoing the boosterism found at the town's border: "Enjoy Austin, where the good life is here to stay." To some extent this civic hype rings true; as the Hormel promotional film Kopple inserts into hers outlines, the social contract the corporation struck with its workers decades ago guaranteed good wages, lifetime benefits, and profit sharing. But the ragged years of recession, corporate mergers, and wholesale assault on unions fostered by Reagan's administration have taken their toll. "Let us live in our house," pleads one woman stuffing envelops at the union hall, "our $32,000 house." The company that makes that quintessential American product, SPAM, staple of United States Army K-rations during World War II, now expresses "the mood of the industry," as CEO Knowlton declares; despite record 29.5 million dollar profits in 1984, Hormel workers receive a 23 percent wage cut.

Thus the stage is set for the nightmare to unfold; a dark romance Kopple scripts around the struggle of a "new family," as the striking P-9ers describe their changed relationships to each other and to their formerly paternalistic employer, to come to terms with the betrayal by the new "father," Jay Hormel, son of the corporation founder who instituted the "social consciousness" of the company. But the real battle in Kopple's eyes involves a conflict waged by outsiders, distant cousins arriving to contest the company's will: on the one hand, Ray Rodgers, New Yorker and vegetarian head of Corporate Campaign whose successful national boycott of J. P. Stevens Co. finally resulted in union recognition in many southern textile plants; and, on the other, Lewie Andersen, hard-bitten vice-president of UFCW, former hog butcher and tough negotiator, who has finally accepted the UFCW's strategy of across-the-board contracts to bring up the wage floor in nonunion meat-packing plants. These giants battle on a grand scale for the hearts and minds of the P-9ers; their personalities are so charismatic that they seem to be determining the action, sweeping the quieter, restrained Minnesotans along with them. Yet the determination of the strikers and their families is the real story: they keep on with the strike even after P-9 has been decertified by the UFCW; they keep gaining support from unions around the country even after the AFL-CIO, America's central union organization, discourages its affiliates from offering solidarity; they keep showing up at the picket lines even after the National Guard has been called out and some local members defy the strike. Playing out against the bleak snow-covered landscape is the new "American dream" of community and family and their fracture, with brother turned against brother, another civil war with the inevitable result.[31]

Kopple's fascination with grand melodramatic historical epics owes as much to D. W. Griffith as the fragile voice of Hazel Dickens's ballads in *Harlan County, U.S.A.*; but in Austin the heroes are less pure and villains less obvious, if more devious. Unlike the coal miners' strike in Kentucky, where "you either are a union man or a thug for D. H. Blair," the complexities of fighting on three fronts—against the corporation, against the state, and against the union's international—complicate the dichotomized narration of melodrama. However, this multiplying set of powerful forces allied against the tiny P-9 local does not automatically call up greater sympathy for the strikers. Instead, those who gave up and crossed the picket line in the face of community censure invoke the rhetoric of sentimentality. Shedding tears is central to the labor documentary—

Lawrence Jones's martyred body and his mother's wailing marked the turning point for the United Mine Workers in *Harlan County, U.S.A.*—but in *American Dream* it is the scabs who mourn themselves as outcasts. The question is: Do we care about these crying men?

American Dream had its public debut in Minneapolis (following its premiere in Austin) as a fundraiser for the Pittston miners' strike. The stage was crowded with Kopple, Senator Paul Wellstone, author of the Replacement Worker Bill barring the hiring of permanent replacements for strikers, and striking miners from Pittstown, West Virginia, as well as the remaining striking P-9ers, still out of work yet offering donations to the strikers in West Virginia. The entire audience was moved to tears by the spectacle of solidarity, suggesting that Kopple's interpretation of the dream came from a textured vision of class in contemporary America as deeply contradictory and overdetermined. Many local union activists and P-9 supporters, however, condemned the film; they felt it to be a betrayal for failing to capture the culture that grew during the strike. Her conclusions question P-9's tactics, even blame them for losing the strike; but evidence to the contrary remained on the cutting room floor. (Actually unused footage for *American Dream* is housed in University of Wisconsin's archives.) The picture is complicated because the politics is complex, but also because the profound shift in the economy has dislodged the melodramatic form of this battlefield and its representation.

An inheritance from the CPUSA's 1930s Popular Front attempt to meld communists (overwhelmingly urban and immigrant and Jewish) into the People, the sentimental invocation of "family," "movement," "community," and "culture" can insidiously repress conflicts and differences within America's class and racial structure. In 1938, General Secretary of the CPUSA Earl Browder outlined *The People's Front* as a program whose "first consideration in promoting new forces is to find native Americans" to lead its organizations, because the Communist Party was "destined to carry on and complete the work begun by Tom Paine, George Washington, Thomas Jefferson, and Abraham Lincoln."[32] To an extent, *Harlan County, USA* participated in this "archaic aesthetic," as Jesse Lemisch calls it,[33] and Kopple received a series of critiques for her "conventional" portrayal of social events from a position of "knowledge" available to the outsider.[34] The postmodern condition of labor in the 1980s demanded another sort of story; Kopple responds by exaggerating the rhetoric of sentimentality until its claims collapse. Kopple manipulates the codes of sentimentality to the point that our tears seem to merge the viewer with the scabs and against the strikers.

This direction comes in part because the situation in Austin, unlike that in Harlan County, is multiply fractured. Kopple may just be doing her job as a documentary filmmaker by presenting a comprehensive picture of strikers, scabs, and international representatives; or she may be paying a debt to the many locals and internationals that contributed funding for the film; or she may be attempting to enter the action, much as she did in Harlan County, at the picket line, by witnessing the sense of emptiness and hostility of those who break ranks. In Kentucky, her presence at the daily "sunrise revivals" became a factor in the escalating violence during the strike. At times it appeared that Kopple's crew egged on the scabs and company goons; at others, the camera clearly helped avert violence. In Austin, when she shows the scabbing P-9ers (the P-10ers, as they were derisively called) crying as they decide to cross their union's picket line, Kopple would seem to be siding with their unpopular decision. Yet the scene is filled with bathos, its emotional timbre highly suspect as the men cry on cue about how hard it is when you can't feed your family. Their tears are supposed to elicit our sympathy; but clearly their actions do not. Which side are we, the viewers, supposed to be on?

Unlike me, most critics of the film—such as Peter Rachleff, who wrote *Hard-Pressed in the Heartland* in part to counter Kopple's Academy Award–winning portrait of the Hormel strike—consider Kopple a sell-out because she provides a forum for these men, who from the first worked hand-in-hand with the UFCW leadership to undermine the strike and now run the trusteeship union that replaced P-9.[35] Rachleff refers to the local treasurer, John Williams, as her "star" because he gets so much screen time to anguish over his actions.[36] Maintaining a nostalgia for working-class authenticity and community characteristic of America's Left since the Popular Front, Rachleff fails to register the squeamishly maudlin and trite picture being painted. Kopple is relying on the left-wing conventions of picturing the scab as feminized (a scab, like a thug, is not a union *man*) that would seem to reinforce Rachleff's position, but the men's tears are powerful visual cues calling forth audience sympathies. So the picture is confusing, but this seems to be precisely the point: in the era of deindustrialization, it is not so easy to distinguish the union man from the scab.

While the strikers are presented as full of conviction—perhaps a bit naïve in their faith in Ray Rodgers—they are still proud and angry folks, even if their militance includes media-savvy campaigns. The scabs snivel about their lost manhood and the betrayal they feel: they hate to cross a line; the union has driven them to it. Lewie Andersen may steal the screen with his hard-nosed cynicism about P-9, but the UFCW comes off as retrograde and suspect, especially after UFCW President Wynn storms into a meeting shouting that he will make the P-9 local sign the contract: "[A]ll it takes is a few good men, oh and some women too," he nods to "the little lady there with the camera." Perhaps because Kopple's style is so consistently illusionistic—she appears to offer a pure vision of the struggle in Harlan County and a balanced version of the strike in Austin—the excesses in *American Dream* don't read as critique; but I think they should—not necessarily of the P-10ers but of the aesthetics and politics lodged in the sentimental itself as much as in the paradox of union politics in deindustrializing America.

Although correcting Kopple's film served as one impetus for both of the book-length accounts of the Hormel strike, neither does more than mention Kopple's presence in Austin.[37] Her authority is implicitly challenged by the reports of these partisan insiders who were active in the support systems—either Corporate Campaign (Hardy Green) or Twin Cities Support for P-9 (Peter Rachleff); Kopple remained an outsider. Falling for the charismatic Lewie Andersen, she failed to see the transformative effects the strike had on the lives of the union members and their families as she had in *Harlan County*. This transformation from alienated labor to a "movement culture" requires the creation of the alternative "prefigurative" institutions through which working people can galvanize into a collective agent for social and economic change.[38] To understand this process, outsiders need to get inside the homes, churches, and meeting halls of the strikers, but Kopple's up-close-and-personal moments more often come between her and the P-10ers or Andersen. Rachleff provides a prehistory of P-9 through analyses of its earlier incarnation in a consumer and producer union, which had achieved wall-to-wall unionization in Austin during the 1930s, establishing the base for the militancy and solidarity of the 1984–85 strike, the first against Hormel in fifty-two years. The two books also explain the changes in the meat-packing industry as a whole since the 1970s and in the contracts at Hormel that led Hormel to slash wages by 23 percent after promising to maintain them. What had been a locally owned, paternalistic company in a homogenous town in southern Minnesota became a lean and mean corporation with national and international subsidiaries linked to other major corporations during the era of mergers and buy-outs. Kopple fails to give this kind of background from the point of view of Austin; instead of letting the strikers speak, as she had in Harlan, where old-timers recounted the bloody days of the 1930s strikes for her through memories, songs, and photographs, she leaves it to Andersen to fill in the background.

Rachleff accuses Kopple of turning the P-9ers into "victims" rather than seeing them as victimized by the collusion of business unionism, state and local police, and corporate conglomerates, all working in tandem to destroy a renegade local that had taken on enormous symbolic significance in the antiunion climate of Reagan's America. Yet the only ones to appear as victims, in the classic melodramatic sense, are the "P-10ers" who sob before the camera after deciding to cross their union's picket line: "A person takes a lot of pride in being a breadwinner," says Ron Bergstrom. Since the eighteenth century, sentimentality, argues Robert Markley, has served as a "theatrics of virtue" for the display of feminized emotions; within the sentimental, the "passive victim" is always female, and it is up to the sensitive male to sympathize with her.[39] This is a class politics of bourgeois affects, thus hardly the virile profile of labor militancy so crucial to left-wing romance; the P-10ers vamp as hero(in)es. Kopple positions her camera with the men who do cross the line and, with them, gets barraged with insults from neighbors, friends, even brothers, such as R. G. Bergstrom, who is a firm supporter of the strike. He lives outside Austin on a 4 3/4-acre farm with his wife and three kids and explains that he goes to the picket line to watch his brother cross it as much as to perform strike duty. R. G.'s brother, Ron Bergstrom, by contrast, has accepted the logic of Hormel and 1980s corporate concessions for workers: "If you want a job," he tells Kopple, "you're going to have to take it." Ron Bergstrom becomes one of the original seven local members to return to work after twenty weeks on strike. In a telling scene later on, these seven watch themselves crossing the picket line and being jeered on the television news that evening: "The minute we crossed that line," remarks one, "we left them, left that organization."

POLITICAL TEARS

Because the union itself, Hormel's policies, and the subsequent reconstructions of the events have turned on the familial make-up of the town, its work force, and its organizations, the act of scabbing is more than a betrayal of a lifetime of working-class upbringing and consciousness; it is also a divorce, a disownment, a severance of all family ties. These men have placed themselves outside the gates of the city when they reenter the factory gates. Their overly melodramatic responses to their own acts fail to exculpate them however: they may have been forced by circumstances to return, yet the circumstances are outdated, based on an ideal of the male breadwinner providing fully for his family. In both working-class and middle-class American homes, the family wage has failed to provide adequately since the 1970s. These men are victims as much of a passé vision of masculinity as of an outmoded form of unionism that is apparently ineffective against vicious corporations, although they do all right for themselves. Lewie Andersen has predicted from the start that the P-9 strike will fail, and it appears—though not so clearly in the film as in the written accounts of the strike—that the UFCW has actually worked to ensure failure, in part by courting these few dissident critics of the Corporate Campaign. In a reversal of fortune reminiscent of melodrama, these men assume leadership of the local after it is put into trusteeship.

If the P-10ers are pathetic, even bathetic, the P-9ers occasionally appear misguided. Lacking strategy, lacking a program, they are a bit too smitten with the New Age self-esteem assertiveness-training mentality that Ray Rodgers trumpets with quotations from Bruce Springsteen. Yet when one of the women leaves the "war department" (the office in the union hall for strike committee meetings) after a meeting with Lewie Andersen, she explains, "I want a union for the 1980s." The strikers are trying to explain to Andersen that something more than wages is at stake in this strike. In part, they have bought Ray Rodgers's theory that traditional organizing tactics are ineffective under current corporate structures with easy flows of capital allowing quick relocation. Unions must use intensive media campaigns to dishonor companies by targeting investors and stockholders. More important, however, is the alteration of the community's social fabric. P-9 President Jim Guyette and many others describe how the union hall became a "fun place to be" where people "did what they liked to do," fixing cars, carpentry, cooking, in an informal bartering economy set up during the strike. Vying for the power inherent in its sentimental invocation, they claim that "a whole new family" was formed through their union activism. This is especially true of the women's support network, which both Hardy and Rachleff contend accounts for the widespread "movement culture" P-9 was able to create. That Austin is an extremely homogenous and insular small town with a paternalistic company that stably employed generations contributed to the ease with which a "new family" could be formed within and through the union, but it also explains the sense of betrayal the Hormel workers felt at the concessions demanded of them by both the company and the UFCW, which set the stage for rupturing Local P-9. But this (women's) story does not grab Kopple as it did in Harlan County; she's watching the men cry this time.

This feel of intimacy is a modern feature characterizing both oral history and documentary. Kopple had moved in with the miners' families in Harlan County. Her attendance at meetings and on the picket lines and road blocks happened because of her connections with the strikers, even though she came from the outside. The presence of her camera became central to some of the action that happened. When Kopple is asked by the coal company thug for her press pass after she comes up to him with camera and tape recorder to ascertain his opinion of the strike, she turns the question on him, demanding to see his identification. They come to a testy truce, after each refuses to produce these documents of identity. The camera watches as he turns his pick-up truck around and leaves, averting violence. When a miner's wife pulls a revolver from her bodice, she directly addresses the camera, daring her viewers to judge how violence escalates. The media contribute to its eruption, heightening the rhetoric and action of the strikers, even as it may rein in its actual expression. The camera's presence sometimes provokes confrontation and violence, as when the armed thugs single out the camera as if it were a body to be beaten. Like the infamous scene in *The Battle of Chile*, in which cameraman Leonardo Henricksen filmed his own murder at the hands of Pinochet's army, this scene suggests that despite a legacy of bloody confrontations, the filmmaker's presence may be provoking violence. However, Lawrence Jones's death occurs off-screen, leaving us to wonder whether he might still be alive if the crew had ventured out that morning. Instead, Kopple films the emotion of the funeral, lingering on Jones's mother's anguished cries, tracking her collapsing body as it is carried from the church. The raw feeling spilling out inappropriately for public consumption accentuates the keenly divided world of victims—strikers—and tyrants—mine owners and their goons.

Watching *Harlan County, USA* still moves me to tears, despite my recognition of the discourses of sentimentality at work; the carved worn-down faces of the old timers and the incredible youth and poverty of the others, the violence and fear, the haunting ballads pull at the heart strings just as any tearjerker out of Hollywood might. Yet the tough talking women, the humorous encounter between the miner picketing the Wall Street offices of Brookside's parent corporation and the New York City cop comparing benefits, wages, and working conditions, the old miners—black and white—suffering from black lung joking that, although when they entered the mines each day they were different colors, when they left they were all "soul brothers" temper the pathos with humor. It gives *Harlan County, USA* the feel of solidarity. The escalating crisis and its violence are offset by the heady sense of power gained through collective actions. The sheer brutality of the labor miners perform pales compared to the degree to which companies will go to keep workers from improving their lives. In the United States, in the mid-1970s, citizens who worked full time in a major industry still lived without plumbing, without heat, in rickety shacks. Mines are not metaphors for hell; they are hell. Despite her obvious differences as a young, single New York Jew with a camera, she entered the privacy of the miners' lives. Unlike Lauren Gilfillan's more ambivalent attempt in 1934, Kopple's move had opened a hidden world of exploitation to public view and garnered tremendous support for the mineworkers. A strike still looked noble in 1976, especially when it was clear which side one was on.

American Dream, unlike *Harlan County*, slips the veil of sentimentality over the wrong faces. When Peter Rachleff refers to the

P-10ers as the "stars" of Kopple's film, is it because they get too much screen time? Or is it because they get to explain their decision more fully than those who remain on the line? Or because in their explanation, they resort to emotional outbursts of tears, rather than the anger expressed by R. G. Bergstrom at his brother's betrayal, and so appear conventionally sympathetic? Kopple's grim tone, set early in the film and accentuated by the bleak, blanc noir, Minnesota winterscapes of Austin, the tacky interiors of meeting rooms and negotiating suites in hotels, the gruesome images from inside the Hormel plant, offer none of the elevating and alleviating humor, hope, warmth, or sarcasm that occasionally lightened *Harlan County, USA*. The miners' pineboard shacks nestled in the hollows of West Virginia conveyed the picturesque, aestheticizing poverty in a way that James Agee deplored, even as he lyricized the perfect symmetry of the tenants' housing he found in Hale County, Alabama, in *Let Us Now Praise Famous Men*.[40] Nothing of the sort exists in Austin, a tidy middle American town of postwar tract housing. The spirit of possibility following the democratization of the United Mine Workers is also missing from *American Dream*. It seems the dream of solidarity is over too—another casualty of Reaganomics. If Moore undermined the heroic male worker through satire, Kopple finished off his image as the one who will lead us from the brutality of capitalism through united movements of militant solidarity. The American dream of the 1930s Left, that the male working class holds the keys to revolution, rests on modernist economic relations and their melodramatic stagings. It served as the background for the dilemmas of the noir hero caught in a cruel and overdetermined world ruled by rank corruption and uncontrollable desire. The film noirs of the 1940s and 1950s appeared as cynical antidotes to both the melodramatic romance of the 1930s working stiff and the nostalgic portrait of the 1930s migrant mother. But the power of genre is such that labor's sentimental contract persists. Kopple undercuts the rhetoric of the labor documentary by thoroughly inscribing the sentimental. Obsessively observing the contract to the letter, she uses men's tears against their modern origins to tell a postmodern tale still unfolding around us.

CHAPTER 6

NOT "JUST THE FACTS, MA'AM": SOCIAL WORKERS AS PRIVATE EYES

INVESTIGATING RACKETS

The urban underworld of noir always includes a woman with a past who pulls the man into the orbit of crime. We know these images: Barbara Stanwyck's anklet and cat glasses in *Double Indemnity* snare Fred McMurray; Rita Hayworth's black sheath and gloves in *Gilda* destroy Glenn Ford; Ava Gardner's flowing black hair and diamond necklace choke Burt Lancaster in *The Killers*. But how did these troubling women get there? How did they land in a world of gang kingpins and petty thieves, hapless working stiffs looking for a break and cynical detectives seeking the facts? In the classic noir narrative of male criminality and male investigation, this question is never posed. It is simply a given, a verity, like the palm trees lining Hollywood Boulevard, themselves hardly native, but so tall they seem to have grown from time immemorial. In a draft of *The Outsider*, Cross Damon learns that Jenny, the Chicago prostitute he helps, is headed for California, dreaming of a career in the movies. Her background as pregnant runaway who undergoes an abortion, then becomes rape victim, and finally a prostitute suggests she is headed West to disaster, not discovery. This chapter delves into a few possible sources for the story of Jenny and her fatal sisters, sources found in the files of the female counterpart to the private eye, another appendage of the state (even Philip Marlowe works sometimes as investigator for the DA's office), the social worker. Often an attaché of the court and sometimes child-protective investigator for the District Attorney, the social worker operates as the state's prying eye.

The 1930s and 1940s detectives were independent operators. They may have started with a partner, as do Philip Marlowe in *The Maltese Falcon* or Jeff Bailey in *Out of the Past*. But, conveniently, the partners always die, leaving the private eye free of the institutional structures of the bureaucratic workplace; he has no bosses, coworkers, or employees. However, his investigations into the homes of rich and poor alike are enabled by his quasilegal connections both to crime and the courts (but always in competition with the police). The femme fatale also moves alone among this dangerous world of men. Her upward mobility made possible because of her sexual debasement or her willingness to debase men sexually. Like the detective, she's stepped outside of the domestic frame, though she may inevitably become part of another frame-up snaring the detective. As an enigma, she works against the male detective's desire to get to the bottom of the case, to zero in on "just the facts." The detective, no matter how cynical he appears, is committed to the facts. He uncovers corruption because he is unattached, free to circulate. No such status is available for the female truth-seeker. In the noir world, she is by definition corrupt if she is on her own. An unknown and unknowable, she is false, a double-crosser, so even if she is after the goods, they will elude her. However, during the 1930s, a large number of women began to investigate, looking for truths. They worked for the state and its agencies as the profession of social work became central to ameliorating the effects of the Depression. Middle-class women's access to poor women's homes occurred through a supervisory effort to protect children's welfare during a decade of unprecedented attention to poverty's effect on children. Like the dick, the social worker has multiple allegiances; but unlike him, she is not free to work as a private eye—her eyes are resolutely public. Representing at once morals and the state, she condemns faulty mothering, violent fathers, greedy degenerate girls, and delinquent boys, even as she works to help them. Still, she shares with the nihilist detective a belief that there is no way out of the "racket": the system that produces poor women produces her too.

In 1930s crime films or hard-boiled novels, gangsters called *Little Caesar*, *Public Enemy*, or *Scarface*, on the one hand, and detectives named Sam Spade or Philip Marlowe (both played by Humphrey Bogart), on the other, circulate within seedy urban spaces. These genres of crime invariably feature male activities—accession through the criminal ladder in urban ghettoes to "top of the world" before inevitable death, or lonely battles with the corrupt world of police and petty crooks in not-so-sunny California that take place in masculine spaces—cars, gambling halls, jails, dusty offices—by small men who ultimately get snared by seductive, two-timing women. It's certain that these deadly women will appear from *Out of the Past*. But one rarely learns how they became so brutal. Horace McCoy's chilling 1935 novel, *They Shoot Horses, Don't They?*, offers clues about their origins in a parallel, feminized, world of deadly competition. A retrospective tale, narrated by a condemned murderer, it explains how Robert Syverten came to shoot his marathon dance partner Gloria Bailey. As Syverten awaits his death sentence, his first-person monologue details how he met Gloria (another aspiring Hollywood bit player), decided to join in her pursuit of the dance marathon prize, and finally acquiesced to her desired suicide by shooting her in the head, just as he had witnessed his grandfather put a lame horse out of its misery as a boy back in the rural Midwest. Gloria, cynical and taciturn, increasingly despairs as the two dance their way through days and nights of derby racing, Lindy hopping, and polishing the big apple, under the scrutiny of a loyal audience until the Mothers' League and the cops disrupt the action. His deadly private act, and the state's public murder, provide a vehicle for Gloria's story to unfold. But the court records do not reveal her narrative. Because she falls outside of conventional femininity, the state and its guardians of morality have no access to her experience. Only her killer knows what has driven her to beg him to pull the trigger.

"You—goddam—whore!" shrieks Mrs. Higby, president of the Mothers' League for Good Morals, after Gloria Bailey, on the dance floor for more than a month, challenges her authority to dictate what constitutes proper behavior for poor women. "You ought to be in a reform school!" continues the frustrated Mrs. Higby. Seven hundred sixty-three hours into the dance marathon, the leaders of the Mothers' League arrive at the Santa Monica pier dancehall to condemn the "low and degrading" contest.[1] The women announce their intention to pressure the city to end the marathon unless the promoters disqualify a visibly pregnant woman and renege on an advertised promise to marry a couple on the dance floor; the women invoke "our duty to keep our city clean"(130). The battle-ax—derived from Carrie Nation's efforts to control male drinking through social housekeeping—is a stock image of nineteenth-century domestic melodrama, a staple of silent film, including the original scenario for D. W. Griffith's classic *Intolerance* and his two-reeler, *The Mother and the Law*.[2] In it, a young woman dressed in rags defiantly resists the guardians of state morality trying to rescue her child from poverty and abuse by declaring her an unfit mother. By the late 1930s, popular culture was full of parodies of these types—think of Claire Trevor (as the prostitute Dallas) and Thomas Mitchell (as drunkard Doc Boone) being hounded out of town by the wizened members of the Ladies' Law and Order League in John Ford's *Stagecoach*, among many examples.

But unlike Dallas, who silently leaves Tombstone on the stage, Gloria unleashes her anger at Mrs. Higby: "Your Morals League and your goddam women's clubs filled with meddlesome old bitches who haven't had a lay in twenty years. Why don't you old dames go out and buy a lay once in a while?" Gloria has seen her share of moral mothers: "While you two noble characters are here doing your duty by some people you don't know, your daughters are probably in some guy's apartment, their clothes off, getting drunk. . . . You drive 'em away from home with your goddam lectures on purity and decency, and you're too busy meddling around to teach 'em the facts of life." Gloria lands the last word of this argument. She speaks from experience as marathon dancer, Hollywood extra, and reform school runaway: "I was in one once. . . . [T]here was a dame just like you in charge. She was a lesbian" (131–34). Gloria Bailey, depressed and exhausted, speaks for all the lone bad girls who, having fled violent, abusive homes, end up on the street corners of Cincinnati or the breadlines in St. Paul—or in Hollywood looking for a big break.[3] This heated exchange crystallizes essential elements about the modern interdependence of poor women's sexuality and middle-class women's professionalization. Because class is structural, each social position can only be understood in relationship to the other. Through designating the female body as mother or whore or lesbian within spaces cordoned off from, yet contained within, the state, these structures become legible within personal stories.[4] The Mothers' League investigates and polices the marathon as a scene of a crime—after all, an accused murderer was arrested on the dance floor—that is especially troublesome for women.

"I feel that this investigation may help in some manner. / I do hope it may. / I am now making a very general statement as a beginning." Thus concludes Muriel Rukeyser's "Statement: Philippa Allen," a section of her long poem, "Book of the Dead," in *U.S. 1.*[5] Philippa Allen, a social worker who offered key testimony to the congressional hearings on silicosis, a lung disease contracted by the 2,000 workers on the Gauley Tunnel in West Virginia, is cited by Rukeyser as among "the many investigators and writers who made this poem possible" (146). Recognizing the special expertise and patience of Philippa Allen, whose casework sent her hitchhiking back and forth across Gauley Bridge tracking the effects of disease on the families—white and black—living in towns named Alloy, Vanetta, and Gamoca, Rukeyser insisted, "Poetry could extend the document" (149). In this, Rukeyser was herself extending the genres from reportage and fiction to poetry that used social workers' cases as the basis for literature—a practice Henry Street Settlement House leader Helen Hall had used in her collaboration with writer Clinch Calkins, who had turned case histories from the settlement house into literary narratives in order to detail the horrors of unemployment for a broader audience, providing fodder for sensational and political fiction.[6]

Caroline Slade, described in the jacket blurb of her fourth novel as "a reformed social worker" whose fiction was derived from her cases as an attaché of a children's court and an investigator for a district attorney, was the first executive secretary of the Saratoga (N.Y.) County Board of Child Welfare before lobbying in Albany, New York, for state protective legislation for women and children. The five novels she wrote during the 1940s feature intriguing portraits of the failure of one aspect or another of the social welfare system. These thinly disguised case studies elaborate the stories of child prostitution that Slade recounted almost verbatim in her scandalous first novel, *Sterile Sun* (1936).[7] Her 1940s novels serve as diatribes against the failures of Aid to Dependent Children (ADC) and other relief programs to address the poverty and violence endemic to unemployed Depression-era workers by focusing on the intimate family arrangements that very often result in child prostitution. These five novels (*The Triumph of Willie Pond*, *Job's House*, *Margaret*, *Mrs. Party's House*, *Lilly Crackell*) contrast a politically astute social worker, who fights the courts and welfare bureaucrats by arguing that they should take a more systemic view of delinquency, with a savvy delinquent girl who ends up in the social worker's caseload after she is caught in "the business." Social workers in Slade's novels, no matter how empathetic, such as Mrs. Sleight and Miss Southard—dressed in real silk stockings and tailored suits—cannot help but condemn the vermin-infested cramped households they enter in their efforts to aid poor mothers and children. They are emblems of respectability, representatives of the state. Yet, as professional women, they too are suspect. As Gloria says, they are "lesbians." While they fault the slack housekeeping of their charges as moral defect, their sexuality is questioned by the families they investigate and by the authorities to which they report.

In the middle of Philippa Allen's testimony, a congressman interrupts: "You found the people of West Virginia very happy to pick you up on the highway, did you not?" Allen, like the many young girls who end up in reform schools, is picked up on open road. Her age, her class, and her profession protect her body; people "are delightfully obliging," all asking, "What can be done?" (15). Allen's authority as a representative of the state may help them, so they protect her. Like doctors and journalists, her mobility and expertise as a "reality definer" mean she can speak on their behalf and get their story out.[8] Stories of crime and detection, including corporate "rackets," as Congressman Marcantonio calls them, often feature first-person narration (*U.S. 1*, 57). Thoroughly modern in their literary influences and in their juridical ones as well, first-person accounts, whether testimony or confession, counter the official paperwork in police files and social workers' case records. They are immediate, getting at what the bland machinery of the state cannot convey through its carbon copies. Yet both the detective and the social worker (and the scholar, if you follow the trail far enough) do not merely record data. Their files are filled with judgments about the characters, gleaned from the appearance, speech, dress, and so forth of those under investigation; these judgments, of guilt or innocence, deserving or undeserving poverty, determine state action.

Miss Allen may come in for congressional approbation for getting picked up on the highway, but she never felt in danger as a pick up. Girls hitching alone, however, are usually not so well protected. Fleeing a family so poor it has farmed her out as a servant to a better-off couple, fourteen-year-old Sue, one protagonist of Slade's *Sterile Sun*, hits the road. She takes the money she has earned having sex with her employer's husband and an old man who was the couple's gardener and runs away to survive on her own. Picked up on the highway by a traveling salesman, Sue keeps running away from fleabag hotels and fancy whorehouses until she ends up in "the business" alone on skid row. No one will listen to poor girls' stories, or rather no one will believe them. If they are on the road thumbing or walking the streets, they must be looking for it. After all, they are just "goddam whores" so deserve what they get. The kindness of strangers leads this girl to an opium den (white slavery is an incessant theme in Slade's novels). She escapes to a skid row hotel, where she dies from a botched self-induced abortion because she doesn't seek help from the two older prostitutes who befriend her.

Sue's story is told in three parts: a run-on flood of her girlish words, which is picked up by her two friends in Allie's tough tale and Winkie's sad delusions. Each woman explains how she came to the seedy upstate New York town—maybe Albany or Troy—as a young teen, entered "the business," got into trouble with the law, and then, in the case of hard-bitten Allie and sentimental Winkie, watched Sue die. Like Robert Syverten's story in *They Shoot Horses, Don't They?*, *Sterile Sun* too is a recounting from the grave, shading into roman noir. It became a textbook in social work classrooms because it vacates the bland and moralistic voice of the case report by giving voice directly to the girls. Caseworkers' reports, typically no more than a few paragraphs, judge these delinquent girls by using the language of social science fact-finding. Even so, some measure of "voice" comes through. For instance, feminist historian Linda Gordon provides details of one case: Susan, an incest victim of her father and her mother's boarder/lover and brothers, who, along with her younger sisters, was removed from her home, while all the male members were never charged with a crime and allowed to remain living at home. In her case history, Susan's story, a mixture of self-contempt and defiance, reads like the fictional Sue's. "I was always a whore," Susan concludes. Her social worker's prose and the actions she takes to remove Susan concur.[9]

STREAM-OF-CONSCIENCE

Sterile Sun eliminates investigative interpretation and offers the girls' cogent analysis of the sexual economy of poverty directly. Sue begins her story: "I am a prostitute the Judge said to me young lady if you keep on going the way you're going now you will be nothing but a common prostitute so I kept on and I am only us girls don't call it that we call it doing business. I do business on the street now and we all get good and mad if anyone calls us like whores and prostitutes" (15–16). Allie's narrative begins, "Sure, I'm a goddamn sonofabitch whore, I get what money I have selling myself to men" (95). Winkie starts her story, "This is a wicked business for a girl to be in, I bet I get out of it just as quick as I got enough money in the bank. When I think about how I am a dirty whore I get cold all over me, my heart gets to going fast I get choked up, I got to get out of this business and live decent and respectable" (121). In essence, each of these girls elaborates Susan's declaration into a profoundly social theory of justice, religion, work, and the state. Self-pity and self-loathing are tempered with pride; without the moralistic intercession of the caseworker's commentary, the girls' insights become political.[10] Gordon points out that during the Depression, child protection workers and social welfare agencies came to believe that "the children of the poor were by definition neglected"(152). However, this increasing awareness of poverty as a primary cause of child neglect and abuse did not necessarily result in a greater sensitivity to gender and sexual inequalities in girls' and women's lives. These daughters (and sometimes mothers) know things neither the Mothers' League nor social workers can imagine. Thus Slade's novels are essentially instructional manuals in the political economy of "sexual delinquency."[11]

For example, Slade's 1946 novel, *Margaret*, hailed on its cover as "a novel of profound significance to every mother," fills in the girls' stories Slade ventriloquized without analysis or commentary in *Sterile Sun* and only sketchily outlined in her second and best-known novel, *The Triumph of Willie Pond*.[12] Invariably, deficient mothers are the problem: one might be too lax, a slovenly woman who loves her children too much and cannot refrain from bearing them endlessly; another is too restrictive, a withdrawn woman suffering her husband's beatings and failing to protect her daughters from male violence. In either case, the precocious daughter, such as Mary Pond, knows (and knows she knows) more than her mother: "I don't like you talking that way, Mary. If you know things you ought to pertend you didn't. A girl your age," complains her mother.[13] Mary quickly discovers she can make money when the rest of the family cannot and becomes embroiled in a prostitution ring organized by an older girl. One of the things all the wayward daughters know—they go to school and have access to a world of objects (like the toothbrush Ruby wins in class, in Martha Gellhorn's *Trouble I've Seen*)—is that their families are lacking: the food is dreadful, the clothes ragged, their mothers affectless, naïvely allowing the official women of the state to enter and pass judgment on their lives.[14] These poorer younger cousins of Daisy Miller and Lily Bart, both insufficiently mothered American daughters brought low by society's censure, are subjected to society's professionalized embodiment, the social worker, who, as high society does, exercises pervasive control over these wayward daughters.

In the social-worker novel, adolescent girls discern the social order more keenly than others: "They don't own us, do they?" demands Mary Pond. "Coming in here all the time! . . . They just walk right in . . . coming in our house. Bossing us around"(29). The mothers are dependent: "But they give us relief. We couldn't get by without the Welfare." The daughters see instead that "they get paid for it! They all've got swell clothes and cars . . . and wear real silk stockings"(30). Still these modern representatives of the modern state—who often appear as enemies of the poor women they aid— challenge the far more censorious moral judgments of the courts and police by intervening (invisibly) for the girls. Nevertheless the daughters are deemed incorrigible, or the household deemed unable to nurture them. Social workers, with names like Mrs. Sleight or Miss Southard, oversee their detention in reform school. It is for their own good, of course, even though the girls' attachments to their mothers—a crucial (antimodern) aspect of immigrant working-class families—is profound. In her study, Gordon cites a 1927–28 Boston Children's Aid Association Annual Report that acknowledges the agency's failure to save a delinquent girl from her mother: "Born out of wedlock, her first ten years spent with an immoral mother who lived in a wretched tenement in a poor district

. . . thirteen-year-old Jane who came to us from one of our courts as
a delinquent child . . . proved to be untruthful, restless, never happy.
She had great affection for her mother and was determined to be
with her although she knew the kind of life she was living. Several
times she ran away to her, and to the vicious old neighborhood
which she seemed to love. . . . We believe the chief factors in our failure were the bad home background, strong affection for a mother
she knew to be immoral" (135–36). In the rationalist view of social
welfare, knowledge (and morals) should trump affection. That it
doesn't is Slade's central point.

Slade knew firsthand the dilemma facing social workers. In her
various capacities, she observed the devastation of poverty and the
failures of state solutions to child neglect. She witnessed the double
standard that let wealthy male pedophiles off while jailing their
young poor prey. She was among the earliest left-wing critics of Aid
to Dependent Children (ADC).[15] She gave up social work for novel
writing out of frustration with the welfare system. She hoped to
effect changes through broadening her appeal to a reading public
primed by 1930s literary radicalism.[16] Still her novels resort to every
stereotype circulating within popular culture to portray both young
female delinquency and social reformers' officiousness. Why? In
part, she is a turgid and plodding writer who cannot creatively
maneuver around the conventions of the genre. Moreover, these are
cautionary tales and as such fall deeply within the melodramatic
imagination. They are designed, as Ruth Blodgett writing for the
Book-of-the-Month Club News noted, to instill in readers "a burning
responsibility to insist such dreadful living conditions must not continue in our post-war world."[17] There is more to it. Slade's lesson,
particularly in *Margaret*, is a modern, Foucaldian one: unless the
courts and social workers intervene early to protect children from
brutal beatings, overwork, and poverty, their environment will
inevitably turn them into incorrigible delinquents; children must
learn to internalize proper behavior. Mrs. Sleight discovers the
depths of depraved delinquency when she meets Margaret, who has
been pimping for a ring of pedophiles. Grown weary of sex with
their ringleader, Pinky, Margaret lures her upstairs-neighbor friend
Sophie to the men's apartment; twelve-year-old Sophie slips into
madness when she is raped and beaten by Skinny, the fat sadist who
bankrolls the ring. As the social worker overseeing Sophie's family,

Mrs. Sleight is assigned to Margaret's case. But she has met her match; thus she argues with the judge that preemptive moves to protect children are essential to avoid their degradation by adults. He argues firmly for the rule of law that limits court intervention until after a crime has been committed. Poverty is not criminal in capitalist America; however, poor girls' solution to it—sex for money—is. It is only after the fact that something can be done about child molestation, and then only to the girls who are now criminals; the rich men are never found much less charged.

This pedagogical aspect of Slade's 1940s novels may have been a reaction to reviews of her 1936 book, *Sterile Sun*, many of which rebuked her for offering no solutions. Comparing her novel to Gellhorn's series of four bleak novellas gleaned from her work for the Federal Emergency Relief Administration, *The Survey* decried the "bitterness of her hatred of society" and Slade's failure to "lift the banner of faith that would lead on to social action."[18] Yet social action—a favorite of radicals, liberals, and New Dealers—is precisely what Slade engaged in as a fiction writer. Faith in society was not going to solve these girls' problems. Slade's years as a social worker had taught her that already. These girls' Depression stories are about survival and desire (for sweets or stockings); deprivation sets the stage for "sexual delinquency." The first time these eleven-, twelve-, fourteen-year-old girls have sex, it is with men older than their fathers. Always it is excruciatingly painful; each bleeds profusely, screams, passes out, withdraws, and (with the exception of Sophie, who regresses to mute fear, and her defiant sister Mary, who squeals on Margaret) keeps quiet, then returns because the scared, furious, or guilty man pays her well—fifty cents, a dollar, even a fiver.

In these novels, the girls are not only matter-of-fact about the exchange of sex for money, they are remarkably savvy about the welfare and legal systems. Even as the older ones pimp for the younger girls, they share whatever knowledge they have gleaned from experience and rumor whenever they get together—in the makeshift whore houses where they work or the jail cells and reformatories where they end up in custody. The girls learn to tell sympathetic social workers how sorry they are and remind their case workers how much they miss their dead mothers. These scams, along with the enlightened treatment the girls receive—coaching in proper hygiene and housekeeping, learning "useful" skills, like waiting tables (though the *Daily Worker* reports this line of work as little better than slavery) instead of the water hoses and ice baths used in the past to cure girls of their sexual depravity—turn the social workers into fools, easily duped and mocked by these worldly wise girls. Yet social workers were not entirely naïve. The important journal of social commentary, *Midmonthly Survey*, ran a regular column—later collected into a series of pamphlets—entitled "Ask Miss Bailey," offering caseworkers practical advice on problematic clients: the ones who refused a CCC (Civilian Conservation Corps) job, bought a car instead of food, went to the movies too often, indulged a sweet tooth, or, more sinisterly, had daughters who earned extra money from unknown sources to buy themselves silk stockings. Miss Bailey's approach was soundly ridiculed within the pages of *Social Work Today*, the left-wing journal of the radical social work movement. She might be well meaning when she allows relief families "the fifteen-cent motion picture, the permanent wave and the family dog," but she is hopelessly ineffectual, blaming bourgeois mores rather than capitalism itself, for caseworkers' difficulties with clients. The editors note, "the gain in social insight afforded the relief worker is highly questionable."[19]

The author of the Miss Bailey columns and Slade's reviewer in *The Survey*, Gertrude Springer, claims, "there wasn't a thing the matter with the Ponds but poverty."[20] Unlike Slade, she believes that relief work can make a difference: "social workers never come out very well in Mrs. Slade's books," however, "they are less the villains of this piece [*Lilly Crackell*] than the victims of the same social stupidity that blighted Lilly," she concedes.[21] Slade offered a more nuanced view of the social worker—one in line with left-wing critiques of poverty. *The Triumph of Willie Pond*, praised by James T. Farrell and Diana Trilling, received a rave review from *Social Work Today*: "to say every single social worker in the United States ought to read it is to do it injustice;" it should be read not out of "professional *obligation*" but as "one of the high points of his [sic] reading experience. Willie Pond is your client. You know him right away."[22] Yet Slade was still working within the social-worker story—the tale of how better-educated, better-dressed women fronting for a repressive state apparatus intrude upon the lives and homes of the poor, condemning the defective mothering that fails to maintain proper order.

Vanguard Press, publisher of Farrell's somewhat risqué novels, printed disclaimers about the content of Slade's books. In a terse preface, Vanguard Press warned readers that it was issuing *Sterile Sun* "in a special edition, the sale of which is limited to physicians, psychiatrists, sociologists, social workers, educators and other persons having a professional interest in the psychology of adolescence." Ruth Blodgett worried that "some doubtless will read this [Margaret's] story out of the same morbid curiosity with which they read of sex crimes in the tabloids."[23] Seeking to distance Slade's fiction from the tabloids, Vanguard publisher Jim Henle enlisted the Reverend John Howard Melish to write an introduction to *Sterile Sun* justifying its publication for "professionals." The book "should not be placed on the shelves of a public library for young people with a pornographic urge to read," he exhorts (11). The pornographic urge to read among young people, like their delinquency, is in part caused by adults procuring children and enticing them with gin, candy, money, even books. But it is also part of their modern psychosexual make-up. With the Depression and War over, "the social evil . . . juvenile delinquency," notes Blodgett, "is one of our increasing concerns."

In fact, Reverend Melish goes so far as to compare *Sterile Sun* to Joyce's *Ulysses*, a book he, as an expert, "hate[s]." Nevertheless, he assures readers that hateful as its subject may be, *Sterile Sun*, like *Ulysses*, is serious art. The comparison may seem bizarre—an obscure tale resembling the Number One novel, a pulpy exposé comparable to high modernism? Yet *Sterile Sun* owes much to *Ulysses*.[24] In a short note written to the *New Masses* in 1929, novelist Josephine Herbst explained that female literary radicals, rather than rejecting modernist stream-of-consciousness for socialist realism, were seeking to write like "Marcel Proust, and maybe Balzac."[25] These literary radicals extended modernist narrative experiments to American workers and the poor. Slade, like Joyce, gives voices to loose women, a stream-of-conscience novel, a case report as stream-of-consciousness. Like the illegal copies of *Ulysses* that Herbst and her husband, John Herrmann, carried back from Europe, *Sterile Sun* is a rarity.[26]

All of Slade's novels include a scene in which the errant girl rages against the invasions—and the moral censure accompanying them—of the social worker into their private lives. Miss Bailey's relief work-

ers notes these outbursts as well: " 'She's a stubborn, ungrateful, little piece who ought to have a good spanking,' snapped the home
worker. . . . A too-tight coat and black-cotton stockings were, it
seemed, at the bottom of fourteen-year-old Carrie's rebellion. . . .
'They're perfectly good stockings, and she ought to be grateful she
has any kind of coat at all. Instead she fights me every inch of the
way. Says I'm just a dumb old maid. She's getting the family turned
against me,' " complained one.[27] Interrogations are routine in casework, but they often reveal more about the lack of the social
worker's knowledge than information about child abuse. The children are working under a code of honor to each other (or fear of
each other) that social workers, unlike detectives, cannot fathom. As
middle-class women, no matter how extensive their education, they
are limited in their mobility and access to the depths of social
depravity. But they may also be realists, unlike the cynically idealist
private eye, understanding the limits of their power to change the
situations they confront. In *Sterile Sun*, Sue describes her social
worker as "a old maid I could guess that because I see how much she
didn't know about things she kept saying to me dear and dear child
and then she tried to make me tell what I done she said to me dear
child have you had intercourse—no of course that—no I mean have
you slept with a man or a boy—well I mean not only slept but you
know—that is—she acted so funny I had to try and not laugh right
in her face but I told her no ma'am I never did because I promised
Mr. Smith I never would tell and I never did" (16–17). The detective
always knows when he's being lied to; he has ways to get to the bottom of the story. The social worker, although she too may know
she's being lied to, can do little about it. She is dealing with a child
who is labeled a criminal but is really a victim.

For instance, Carmen Sternwood, the younger daughter of General Sternwood, Marlowe's employer in Raymond Chandler's *The
Big Sleep*, is drugged and photographed naked by the pornographic
bookseller Arthur Gwynn Geiger. She too is a child of insufficient
mothering. Sternwood is a widower who had his children late in life.
Carmen's wealth protects her from predatory men who offer poor
girls fifty cents for sex, but it makes her an easy mark for blackmail.
Her gambling debts and drug habit further deplete her desiccated
father, who spends his days dozing in his orchid hothouse. Marlowe
oversees Carmen in ways that social workers can never protect their

young cases. Carmen has the sheen of money. Marlowe has the power of a badge (and a gun); he is both within and above the state. A bachelor is not the same as an old maid, a widower not the same as a single mother (and obviously money talks). The PI is employed secretly to rescue an errant daughter, even if she is a murderer, and bring her home. But the state sends the social worker to officially investigate the home life of a delinquent girl already in its charge because her home cannot shelter her.[28] When her mother is found, she is found wanting. In these situations, the state is a meddling force with overarching powers to steal one's children away. Social workers become enforcers in a state-sanctioned protection racket, especially when they perform their mid-monthly surveys. One of the first questions Miss Bailey answers, "Are Relief Workers Police-women?" is resolutely negative: "With the woman 'living in sin' with the lodger. The worker's concern with the lodger is only his economic status in the family." Yet, quoting a supervisor, Miss Bailey opines, "I don't know whether we are policemen or not. . . . We try not to be, though I suspect that the public would support us in a high moralistic stand."[29]

Poverty, particularly among single mothers and their children, is always cause for suspicion. Ruby, the relief girl Gellhorn found, was lured into prostitution with promises of money for roller skates, candy, the canned peaches her mother cherishes, and even a tube of toothpaste. Eventually removed from her home, she is placed under court supervision. Eleven years old, she cannot gauge the time away from her mother when she arrives weeks later to inform Ruby that she cannot take her home: "They say I'm not fit to keep you. They say I should have known what you were doing, and if I didn't then I'm not a good mother" ("Ruby," 172). Mrs. Mayer leaves Ruby literally in the clutches of the warden Miss Mayfield, walking off in the wrong direction from home, now a lone woman on the street. In Ann Petry's *The Street* (1946), Lutie Johnson's son, Bub, is paid by her crazed building superintendent to steal mail. She also loses her child to state custody. After Bub is placed in the children's shelter when he is found home alone, Lutie immediately assumes her son will "graduate from reform school into DannemoraSingSing."[30] Bub has absorbed his mother's worries over money; left alone while she works days in an office and nights as a singer, he too is insufficiently mothered. When she ventures to the shelter to see

Bub, Lutie is struck by the huddled-over bodies of black and white women—foreigners mostly—waiting to see their kids. Lutie's poverty, not race, transforms her and all these "waiting women" into "animals" (409). Lutie eventually abandons Bub to this brick institution after she murders the pimp she has approached for money to pay a lawyer. Reasoning "the Court wouldn't parole him in her care either, because she was no longer a fit person to bring him up," she buys a one-way ticket to Chicago, leaving Bub to survive alone (433).

Lutie's terrible logic, that it is better to abandon her son to the institutions of the state than to try to fight for him, is based on her experience as a foster mother and a black woman. Harlem nightclub singer, single mother—Lutie's life appears a cliché: she's black, she's bad, her son criminal. Thus, in rebellion, Lutie refuses to allow Bub to know himself through this narrative: the son of what racist social convention deemed she was—a violent, slutty mother. Racism adds another dimension to the poor mother's dilemma.[31] For instance, the mother in Marita Bonner's 1935 story, "The Whipping," inadvertently kills her son Bennie after spending three nights in jail for slugging her relief worker, who promises "an investigator" will check on her story—"no food, no coal, the water frozen, the pipes burst."[32] Lizabeth cannot run away from the women's reformatory, where she has been placed after hitting Bennie. Her unsuccessful attempts to find relief for her son and mother send her into a rage, and hunger blurs her judgment. She takes it out on her son: "Bad character! Keep her! the court decided"(77). The streets of Chicago or Harlem, or seedy upstate towns, invariably result in violence. Poverty kills in many forms: black, single mothers find themselves unable to get relief; white families, those deserving poor who do get relief, are demeaned by inspection and supervision. In these narratives, the welfare and court system is at once overzealous in monitoring its white clients and utterly apathetic to black women's needs. In all cases, once the women or children encounter authority, the family is doomed. The ever-practical Miss Bailey assures us that a relief worker's job is to provide food, clothing, and shelter, not to club slovenly housekeepers into cleaning up their smelly, bug-infested houses or punish those who don't.[33] These fictions from the 1930s and 1940s suggest the facts are otherwise.[34]

WHAT FILM NOIR KNOWS . . . ABOUT WELFARE

Half a century later, in 1996, when President Clinton promised to "end welfare as we know it," he indulged in his now legendary parsing of the English language. He was not going to end welfare *tout court*, just welfare as we know it. But no one questioned whether we as a nation actually did know it, either experientially or theoretically. Certainly, speculation ran to what the new configuration would look like, but little attention was paid to its history as detailed by Caroline Slade and Miss Bailey, not to mention Marita Bonner or Ann Petry. What is the welfare we know? Is it the Social Security Act of 1935, the 1944 GI Bill of Rights, the Interstate Highway Act of 1956, all of which have been enormously successful in alleviating poverty through pensions, education, health insurance, and subsidies for construction and jobs, and most of which have benefited white male workers and their families? No. Welfare is a program that enables welfare queens to drive Cadillacs, as Ronald Reagan once asserted. It is a devious tool pathologizing the black family, as Daniel Patrick Moynihan once implied, the root cause of the "culture of poverty," which could not be alleviated even when Lyndon Johnson declared a "war on poverty."[35] In short, under the reign of Cadillac queens, lodged in the pathological family and culture, welfare, as we know, is about greedy, slothful women and their delinquent, possibly illegitimate, children, no matter how much Miss Bailey had argued otherwise.

Welfare as we know it is feminized, localized in decaying urban housing projects or in shabby trailer parks, hardly visible in the expansive American university system, the ten-lane highways crisscrossing the continent, or the tree-lined suburbs ringing our cities that are the legacy of postwar social investments. These strategic investments were made to help the millions of returning World War II veterans reenter civilian life—a process understood to be fraught with the enormous "problems of homecoming" that required the same massive federal intervention to stave off the potential chaos, violence, and dangers facing the men, their families, and the nation as had the Depression.[36] The 1940s problem of homecoming, like that of 1930s unemployment, was debated endlessly among "experts" and in the pages of such diverse publications as *Reader's Digest* and *The New Yorker*. Like the concern for girls' delinquency during the 1920s and 1930s, it too became the subtext of much post-war popular culture. Addressing the problem of homecoming became a way to remasculinize, in Susan Jeffords's term, welfare.

For instance, like many film noirs of the mid-1940s, *The Blue Dahlia* focuses on the strains three returning World War II veterans face as they reenter civilian life. Set in Los Angeles, the film contrasts the bright exteriors of sunny Southern California with the gloomy reality of shell shock, unemployment, war wounds, and psychic estrangement GIs faced on homecoming: Buzz (William Bendix) suffers whenever he hears "monkey music." The hot jazz screaming from radios, jukeboxes, and nightclubs makes the steel plate in his head vibrate, leading him to violence and amnesia. After Johnny (Alan Ladd) confronts his two-timing party-girl wife who has taken up with a Hollywood club owner, he's accused of her murder. The men react violently to the incursion of black America, or its "monkey" music, into the all-white bars and homes of suburbia, and to the parallel excursion of married women into the workforce and onto the dance floors that occurred while they were away at war. Through their own detective work, Buzz, Johnny, and their buddy, George, are eventually cleared of the crime (and Johnny gets a new girl [Veronica Lake]) setting up the possibility of a smooth future. But the scenario of adultery, murder, amnesia, and bar brawls conveyed a distinctive uneasiness about these "heroes."[37]

The plight of the returning GI had been seen as a "problem" years before the War ended. Scores of local newspapers featured articles headlined, "Vets Seen as Big Problem." The pages of social work journals and social psychology studies within the Research Branch, Information and Education Division of the United States Army, and other federal agencies fretted about the massive influx of young men into an America now booming with war production.[38] These GIs had left a far different America—one reeling from a decade of depression, which forced the first unified federal welfare programs to secure Social Security and unemployment insurance, as well as provide "relief " for poor, unemployed urban families and displaced rural farmers. During the 1930s, welfare was understood as a response to a crisis—as a defense against social disarray, anarchy, and fascism, and as relief from privation. By the time the United States entered the Second World War, welfare was officially trumpeted as national defense.

War meant an improved economy, but social welfare advocates, especially those on the Left, warned against the possible dependence on a heated up war economy as a substitute for a system to combat perennial unemployment. They viewed the WPA, which had been cut back throughout the 1930s by probusiness forces in Congress, as the only solution to maintain full peacetime employment. Discussions about welfare during the depression years of the 1930s stressed images of relief and recovery. The crisis was understood as temporary, and only federal intervention could provide the necessary aid to those in need. Roosevelt's New Deal goal was "freedom from want." The language of aid, relief, and recovery made the welfare recipient seem a foreigner in her own land—a refugee, a disaster victim—and the sheer magnitude of the crisis required military-style intervention. As the crisis in Europe and Asia made war inevitable, and U.S. involvement seemed only a matter of time, the discourse on welfare shifted considerably. Welfare became an aspect of national defense and security. The forces of fascism would best be staved off through social security, unemployment insurance, and, most important, full employment, especially for youth whose delinquency was increasingly seen as incipient fascist behavior. The communist-oriented journal *Social Work Today* praised the report in the *Annals of the American Association of Political and Social Sciences* special issue, "Prospects for Youth," which linked child welfare to democracy. It favorably quoted Aubry Williams's comment that "government responsibility for youth has as its primary basis the fundamental democratic principle of equal opportunity for all."[39] At least among left-wing social workers and political scientists, government welfare programs were indispensable for assuring a democratic nation. Only guaranteed work could eliminate the disparities in income that spelled the end of freedom. In this era of the Hitler-Stalin Pact, left-wing social workers also characterized welfare as "the first line of national defense" against Roosevelt's stepped up war production and its incipient militarized economy.[40] Gwen Barclay called for "Welfare, Not Warfare," and Henry Doliner proposed full employment "In Answer to War Hysteria."[41] However, when the Communist Party had shifted its line about the war, after Germany's invasion of the USSR, a new department had been added to the journal: "Social Work and Defense," with headlines declaring "Social Work: 'A Defense Industry.' "[42]

Once the United States entered the war, this left-wing discourse became more widespread. Not only communists insisted that welfare was necessary to the defense of democracy, the armed forces did too. Welfare served the national defense by insuring a supply of well-nourished and healthy young men, by aiding in the mobilization of all citizens into war work, whether as soldiers or civilians, by providing childcare to working mothers, housing to relocated defense industry workers, and education and recreation for young people who were the nation's future soldiers and workers. Through its association with defense, welfare would "give soldiers something to fight for as well as with."[43] The shift from defense to war, according to the November 1940 Executive Order authorizing the Office of Defense Health and Welfare Service, meant the "obligation to provide the basic social services in wartime rests with the Government." Federal responsibility for "Family Security" was part of the "Defense Activities" of the Federal Security Agency. Welfare demanded national mobilization, and mobilization required national welfare: first to defend the nation, then to win the war. As a social worker in Slade's 1943 novel, remarks: "Roosevelt said a while ago that undernourishment was one factor in the cause of illiteracy, and when he discovered that over four hundred thousand men have been refused by our Army for being illiterate, poor feeding comes out into the light and becomes a national issue."[44]

In addition, with the rise of ADC during the 1930s and 1940s, the threat of delinquency—black and Chicano urban men hanging on street corners in zoot suits and sexual promiscuity by white women out walking the streets to defense jobs—emerged as a national concern for welfare workers and civic leaders. War and the Depression, it was felt, had unhinged American morality and the cachet of a uniform—whether of a "cult" member's zoot suit[45] or of the Armed Forces' draftees and enlisted men—meant young women were swooning: "juvenile delinquency is on the up-and-up and Children's courts can't stop it. You can't help what war does—poor people getting a lot of money to spend and women working out instead of at home," remarked one of Slade's fictional social workers.[46] The focus on delinquency, especially new sexual mores among urban youth, appeared as a return to nineteenth-century social welfare concerns. Yet, as Eliot Ness reported to the National Conference of Social Workers, the 1941 Social Protection Program to "reduce venereal disease hazards to those in the armed forces . . . and to rehabilitate women and girls . . . exposed to prostitution and promiscuity" was part of the Federal Security Agency.[47] *Lilly Crackell* tracked the changing concerns of social welfare caseworkers, family and juvenile courts, charity agencies, and federal and state welfare programs, following the life of a wayward girl as she matures through successive pregnancies into the mother of four sons bound for war. The novel's end finds a group of social workers paradoxically worrying that with the booming war economy they will be the ones who end up unemployed. They worry too about "what the men will be like after they've seen so much blood and killing."[48]

DEFENDING A NATION

As social workers were reading Slade's withering dissection of welfare's history, they were already dealing with the next "national issue," returning veterans like George, Buzz, and Johnny. Like Hollywood, social welfare discourse avoided reference to the massive death and destruction of the war. At most, veterans might suffer "postcombat jitters" or "battle dreams."[49] The real "Big Problem" with veterans was that they would flood the job market sparking postwar recession. Again, a welfare program conceived as yet another essential aspect of security and freedom, the 1944 Servicemen's Readjustment Act (GI Bill of Rights) launched the most extensive health, education, housing, and jobs program in U.S. history; it was aimed at reintegrating men trained in armed combat into a world with little semblance to the one they had left. Social work journals, echoing national agencies, outlined the concerns as follows: guys returning who had not worked before the war, guys returning to new families and wives they barely knew, guys expected to return to their homes as dutiful sons. They'd seen Paris, and much, much worse. Local newspapers were exhorted to stop running headlines stressing the problems vets posed to the newly recovered, newly relieved economy and start broadcasting the federal resources available to them. To further secure the peace and insure that the vets troubled by the Blue Dahlia would become solid citizens, not aging juvenile delinquents, the Servicemen's Readjustment Act expanded the 1934 Federal Housing Authority program guaranteeing mortgage insurance and offered stipends for higher

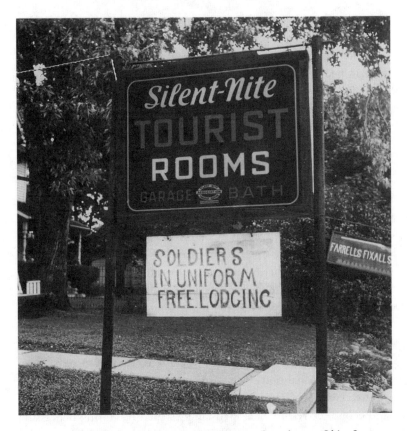

FIGURE 34. Esther Bubley, "A sign." Washington Courthouse, Ohio, September 1943.

education and job training. Along with the Interstate Highway Act (1956), these social welfare programs for building a postwar middle class (by 1946, for the first time in U.S. history, more than 50 percent of Americans lived in their own homes) masked massive welfare expenditures to the upwardly mobile new residents of suburbia as cold-war defense spending. Throughout the mid-twentieth century, welfare expenditures were considered crucial to national security. In the 1930s, they maintained democracy and freedom (not to mention capitalism) through relief, especially through Aid to Dependent Children (precursor to today's Aid to Families with Dependent Children [AFDC]). Then during World War II, they helped defend the nation. Finally, during the cold war, they functioned to secure the peace. In short, welfare was not just a women's issue as welfare rights activists in the 1960s asserted.

Relief, freedom, security, defense: the large-scale fulfillment of human needs was obviously a task for the federal government, one intimately connected to the economic and military goals of American stability and democracy. In the wake of postwar neo-domesticity, what became understood as welfare returned to earlier constructions of mother's aid, even when President Johnson launched the War on Poverty, again invoking the military metaphor to achieve the goal FDR's Vice-President Henry A. Wallace outlined in 1942: "freedom from want." The language of welfare returned to dependence as AFDC with its suggestion of weakness, both personal and political, dominated welfare debates. The feminization of welfare insured its demise as "a national issue" to be addressed positively and shifted its visibility from heroic efforts to preserve democracy to shameful handouts to the undeserving. Since the 1960s, as the picture of poverty appeared increasingly nonwhite and the cities emptied of well-paying jobs, leaving the only laissez-faire capitalist enterprise—drug dealing—in their place, welfare became localized within deteriorating neighborhoods. By the 1980s, what had once been touted as national defense became personal dependence. The shift resurrects ideas of deviancy and delinquency, not as temporary social and economic results of altered family structures during depression and war, but as the inevitable result of the perennial culture of dependence fostered by "the chains of welfare," as Representative Bill Archer called it.[50] In a classic Orwellian move, freedom (from want) now became a prison.

Welfare as we know it means AFDC the incarnation of 1930s relief programs, among them ADC, itself a federally instituted program building on early twentieth-century "mothers' pensions," which repeated late nineteenth-century charity work by the "friendly visitor."[51] Early twentieth-century social welfare workers responded to "sex delinquency" among girls by inspecting the households of their poor mothers. In 1972, welfare rights activist Johnnie Tillmon proclaimed "welfare is a women's issue," forcing feminism to address poverty, but also indicting a policy that cordons poor mothers off as a "cancer," the "undeserving poor." Responding to Moynihan's characterization of the "black matriarchy," she noted, "AFDC is like a supersexist marriage. You trade in *a* man for *the* man."[52] The 1990s attacks on welfare again castigated poor women, immigrants, and racial minorities, whose opportunities to partake of the economic boom are severely limited by lack of affordable housing, transportation, childcare, and education—the same issues plaguing the nation's security and defense in the 1930s and 1940s. It is as if the entire nation suffers Buzz's amnesia as we forget the mid-century history of welfare. When these same problems threatened white men's ability to serve as breadwinners or as soldiers, they became "national issues," not of dependency, but of freedom and security. The crises Buzz and other GIs faced surfaced in film noirs through the exposure of the rotten world faced with existential resignation by the lone hero. Welfare mothers never were so exalted in their degradation. Instead, they were marginalized within the social-worker novels and case reports as unfit, incapable of dealing either with their corrupted daughters or their curious social workers.

ON THE CASE

Caroline Slade was a woman obsessed, you might say. Like Raymond Chandler or Erle Stanley Gardner or their detectives who return again and again to the scene of the crime, Slade couldn't stop worrying her story of pregnant teens, child prostitutes, inept mothers, acidic welfare workers, and the sad, strange spaces they inhabit—filthy apartments, stuffy courtrooms, fumigated reformatories. Her 1948 novel, *Mrs. Party's House*, tells the life story of a "madame." It begins with a psychiatric social worker's naïve comments about how "society keeps you in the business," to which Mrs. Party replies to the contrary that she has found her "call" (3). *Mrs. Party's House* offers a history of government, legal, journalistic, welfare, and economic investments in prostitution. Mrs. Party is party to the system that periodically mobilizes against her whores: first the officials come to call as patrons, then they sit in judgment from the bench.[53] *Lilly Crackell*, Slade's sequel to *Willie Pond*, traces the many generations of Crackells, labeled "bad" by city elders, who become the clients of the newly established Board of Child Welfare's "executive secretary, typist, case worker, bookkeeper, cleaning woman, and general factotum," Miss Ethel Stalling (161). Following the story of Lilly, impregnated by a rich boy at age fourteen, through the births of her five "bastards," the novel is about Miss Stalling's attempts to rationalize child welfare—and so move it away from its moralistic refusal to aid "unwed mothers"—to provide emergency relief for all children. The novel begins in the aftermath of the First World War and ends with the Japanese bombing of Pearl Harbor. As poverty, malnourishment, and illiteracy become issues of national defense, the focus of child welfare shifts from policing the "wayward girls and immoral women" to nourishing the boys who will fight overseas.[54]

It is only when the class dimensions of the state come into full relief (so to speak), that is, appear detached from female sexuality, that Ethel Stallings allows herself to ask questions of a larger systemic nature. Yet she shies away from the inevitable conclusions. She's not a communist; still "she was forced to ask herself: 'Why should some people be so destitute?' And then: 'Why should there be so many poor in a land capable of supporting many more than are already living upon it?' And then: 'Why should there be any poor?' And at last: 'Why should there be a large group of people living upon the poor?' " (586). The last questions answers itself: " 'The truth is, I live upon the lives of hungry, cold, poverty-stricken people; their misfortunes make possible my good job. . . . Why, my own income rests upon the backs of the poor!" Miss Stallings's realization that she is "one of the poor" horrifies her because she knows what poverty looks like, having made her living closely monitoring it. " 'Social workers and people on relief should be hand in hand, demanding—' " she muses (587). Miss Stallings cannot go on with her analysis, because, like Mrs. Party, the establishment whore, she has always submitted to the powers controlling her job—judges, wealthy board members, supervisors—who might fire her at any time.

Philippa Allen believed her investigations made while hitching across Gauley Bridge would "help in some manner" to alleviate the suffering caused by silicosis. Unlike Miss Bailey, she viewed social work as a cause in the struggle against capitalist exploitation; yet she believed in its premises—investigate and report. Her optimism that a sympathetic ear found in high places (Congress, court) would effect change, however, mirrors Miss Bailey's homespun belief in the merits of relief work. It helps. Another Miss Bailey, Gloria, perhaps her client once, dancing endlessly, failed to find relief. For her, there was no escaping capitalism's daily derby race to weed out the weak; nothing could help her; she had already been "reformed." In the obsessive way that Marlowe returns to Geiger's shady house, each time finding new evidence and culprits, Slade returns again and again to the scene of her crime—the "two hundred years or more of tight reins and poor laws and power over giving out relief," and how "we've set this relief business apart . . . never considered it in relation to the whole" (*Lilly*, 601). She finds no relief but much to reform, though it is not necessarily delinquent girls. These awkward, ungainly novels *do* consider this relief business "in relation to the whole"—from the monologues of prostitutes, to the case reports of bad girls and good girls gone astray, to the musings of officious social workers and their radical critics—offering tantalizing clues to unravel the larger racket of capitalism that was the subject of so many film noirs.

I too have been tracking down clues, pillaging files of New York State Family Service offices in search of Caroline Slade née Beach, born 1886 in Minneapolis, died 1975 in Saratoga Springs. I have unearthed her novels from dusty library stacks (last checked out in 1954) or in dank used bookstores, the pages yellow, brittle; her prose old fashioned, but her tales amazingly current. I have searched the New York archives. I have listened to a distant relative recount her genealogy.[55] Sergeant Friday of television's *Dragnet* demanded, "the facts, ma'am, just the facts," but he did so with a deadpan flourish. The private eye, like the novelist and the professor, knows that reconstructing the crime requires elaborating—through observation, investigation, narration—the secrets of private lives. My mother remembers the dread her mother felt before a relief worker's visit. Like Carolyn Steedman, who watched her mother humiliated by a house visitor and vowed never to endure this herself, my mother got a college degree and, briefly, a job as a caseworker.[56] These stories of poor women's encounters with the state and its face—an educated woman: social worker (Slade, my mother) or teacher (Steedman, myself)—shadow me too. It is not just the facts that need investigating, as film noir knows, but the investigators themselves.

PART 3

NOIR
HOUSEHOLD OBJECTS

CHAPTER 7

BARBARA STANWYCK'S ANKLET

FETISH, ICON, SYMBOL?

"That's life. Whichever way you turn, fate sticks out a foot to trip you," moans Tom Neal into his half-full coffee mug as he begins his grisly tale in *Detour*. In the noir world, where lowly objects assume large proportions, that foot is bound to be shod. This chapter considers the plight, or more properly, the power of objects. To redeem the object, I argue that, compared to the subject, it has gotten an unjustifiably bad rap. Film noir achieves its identifying texture from an array of formulaic images, plots, locations, visual styles, and objects—cigarette lighters, car windshields, doorways, Venetian blinds, and, the focus of this chapter, shoes. Investigating shoes as essential elements of noir's cultural work salvages these lost objects, making it clear that the abject state of objecthood holds compelling authority within psychic and social formations. There can be no subjects without objects.

Why, from Karl Marx and Vincent Van Gogh in the nineteenth century through Martin Heidegger, Charlie Chaplin, and Walker Evans in the twentieth, have men tracked aesthetic value, social standing, and the meaning of labor through the boots of workers; while women, following Sigmund Freud's consideration of the shoe

as fetish object, have understood shoes to signal freedom and con-
straint—at once powerful symbols of mobility and icons of and for
desire? I speak of two modes of desire: for the commodity itself,
objects of use—products, "equipment," as Heidegger called them—
no matter how apparently excessive; and within its representation in
paintings, photographs, films, novels, and advertisements. These, as
Jacques Derrida goes to great lengths to point out, are not the same
thing; yet because of the oddity of this particular object, an object in
need of another for it to be put to proper use, desire doubles back
on itself, collapsing differences between materiality and representation because the "shoes are always open to the unconscious of the
other."[1]

The shoe as emblem of death and icon of sex collapses within the
tawdry mise-en-scène of film noir. When femme fatale Phyllis Dietrichson (Barbara Stanwyck) descends the stairway to meet insurance
salesman Walter Neff (Fred McMurray) in Billy Wilder's 1944 film
Double Indemnity, the camera lovingly focuses on her gleaming
white legs, feet sheathed in puffy high-heeled mules; above one
drapes a gold anklet. Moments later, seated crosslegged before Neff,
Phyllis waves her foot ostentatiously in his face, distracting him
enough that he mentions the "nice anklet you've got there." She
removes her foot and straightens up primly; but the scene evokes the
power of the woman's foot to control a man. The anklet, no matter
how thin its gold chain appears, is always one-half of the shackles
that snare him. Cinderella got her prince because only she among all
his subjects could fit into the tiny glass slipper styled for her by her
fairy godmother. The anklet, that piece of jewelry adorning one leg,
at the bottom of the body rather than the top, calling the eyes to
travel down the length of the body and fix on one foot, foregrounds
the fetishistic quality of women's footwear, especially, as in the case
of Cinderella as well, the isolated, single bare foot and its adorn-
ment. Cinderella got her prince; Stanwyck's golden snare leaves Neff
a man silently walking home alone after murdering her husband. He
hears no sounds, not even his footsteps: "It was the walk of a dead
man," he recalls. Derrida points out the important differences
between a pair of shoes and a single one: the pair, useful, regular and
normal, a heterosexual couple; the lone shoe, perverse, bisexual,
destabilizing.[2]

The iconic pan from the floor up to the star's face tells us every-

thing we need to know of her character.[3] So that, for instance, when
the camera, with Cornel Wilde, first gazes at Ida Lupino draping one
shoeless bare leg over the boss's desk before traveling up to a close-
up of her face in the 1948 film noir *Road House*, we know that
despite whatever nasty banter ensues, they will eventually become
lovers. Wilde moves across the room toward the desk dividing them
watching Lupino smoke and play solitaire and picks up her shoe—a
platform sandal, designed to replicate Stanwyck's anklet and open-
toed mule, displaying "toe cleavage" and a bound ankle.[4] She
snatches it from him and hides it behind her back as one would any
intimate article found lying about in plain sight. Ida Lupino's shoe
is out there in a public display so raw she might as well have been
naked before his and our eyes. Worse, her naked display is not only
of her sex, but of his as well. The single shoe "combines in a system
the two types of object defined by Freud: elongated, solid or firm on
one surface, hollow or concave on the other." Shoes, for Freud, like
"a whole number of dream-symbols are bisexual and can relate to
the male or female genitals, according to the context."[5] Hollywood's Hays production code forbade nudity and other overt representations of sex, sending directors and cinematographers to
search out legible covert symbols. Like Walter Neff, they knew
where to look. After all, as Wendy Lesser points out, a far different
Stanwyck had already tripped up a man a few years before snagging
Fred McMurray. In Preston Sturges's wonderful 1941 screwball
comedy *The Lady Eve*, Stanwyck surveys the ocean liner dining room
through her compact mirror—which makes a tiny movie screen—
and comments, like a knowing critic, on the various types of women
eyeing the oblivious herpetologist Henry Fonda, who's been "up
the Amazon" researching snakes. As he passes before her, she sticks
her foot out to trip him into her lap, snagging him.[6]

For women in the movies, especially postwar B-movies, shoes,
most likely high-heeled pumps, clatter methodically along the hard
concrete sidewalks. They sing a chorus combining vulnerability—
she cannot run too fast in them—and menace—her relentless
approach or retreat signal her ever-presence. They tap the cobble-
stones like armor, like weapons. In Jacques Tourneur's 1942 *Cat
People*, Serbian designer Irene (Simone Simon) pursues her American rival, the wholesome "new kind of other woman" Alice, through
a Central Park tunnel at night. The camera pans from one set of

black pumps to another. As the clicking magnifies and echoes within the space and the sounds merge, Alice is overtaken with a terror that lifts only when she is startled by an oncoming bus that she boards even though it takes her back the wrong way. *Phantom Lady*'s Kansas (Ella Raines) threatens bartender (Andrew Tombes Jr.) by following him after sitting immobile night after night in his bar. Her slender trench-coated figure waits for him under the streetlight, and again we see only her black pumps swiftly pursuing him through the night, their rhythm matching the man step for step. By all logic, high-heeled women should not constitute a threat: but they do. Critic Farah Jasmine Griffin recalls hearing that her Aunt Eartha fought back when her second husband tried to hit her, striking him on "the head with one of her tan stilettos. . . . [She] never understood high heels to be an impediment to women's safety."[7] The opening shot of the British noir film *Yield to the Night* follows Mary as she paces across a square and into an alleyway; clicking heels foreshadow the gun shots she will unload into her lover's girlfriend that land her in prison, where she gets religion and repents. The opening sequence of *Caged* (1950) shows Marie (Eleanor Parker) seated in the paddy wagon among an assortment of jaded prostitutes; her demure and plain flats set her apart from them. However, by the time she is released on parole, she has been transformed. She signals her "new" life outside, on the streets, by entering a car full of men and crossing her legs so that her high heels are visible and her knee available for fondling. The black high-heeled pump was an essential element of postwar working women's attire. She doesn't find God; instead she seeks cold cash, this being a very American noir.

These examples from classic film noirs (or their 1960s British variation) contrast with Van Gogh's invocation of work boots as signs of poverty; they speak of women's aggressive mobility in postwar urban spaces. The physical movement and sexual predation available to women emerge visually from their shapely legs and aurally from the sound of their heels beating the pavement. They walk the streets—streetwalkers—turning public spaces relentlessly into scenes of crime and themselves into objects of desire. As streetwalkers, their shoes are also useful; they work/walk the pavement nightly. However, the icon of the high-heeled pump rarely registers as working apparel. It is a marker of sexual violation and allure, not labor. Yet an economy of desire is always first an economy, a point exaggerated to absurdity in Samuel Fuller's 1964 noir spoof *The Naked Kiss*, in which prostitute Kelly (Constance Towers) beats her pimp by pummeling him with her rigid black patent leather purse while standing over him in stilettos to retrieve the money he owes her. She then disappears into small-town America to enter her new life as a nurse for disabled children, only to discover that she cannot escape corruption: in Grantville, cops pimp for the brothel across the river, and the leading citizen and philanthropist is a pedophile. To protect the young women and girls of Grantville, Kelly beats the local madame with her stiff black leather purse and kills the pervert with his black Bakelite telephone receiver (both repeating her shoes, one in its material, the other in its form), only to end up in jail when her pimp presses charges for assault—the shoe was prologue.

In his discussion of "Fetishism," Freud puts it quite simply: "I announce that the fetish is a substitute for the penis. . . . To put it more plainly: the fetish," he continues, "is a substitute for the woman's (the mother's) penis that the little boy once believed in and—for reasons familiar to us—does not want to give up."[8] The fetish, as the simultaneous sign of disavowal (of woman's castration) and attachment (to the fantasy of the female phallus), is often connected to this contradiction through its partial nature. Thus the single foot or the single shoe—seen first from below as the child looks up at the vagina—suits at once "both the disavowal and the affirmation of the castration."[9] As a synecdoche, the fetish is at once too much and not enough, anticipatory and remainder. "The fetish, like a 'screen memory', represents this phase [a submerged and forgotten phase of sexual development] and is thus a remnant and precipitate of it."[10] "What is substituted for the sexual object," says Freud in "Three Essays on Sexuality," "is some part of the body (such as the foot or hair) which is in general very inappropriate for sexual purposes, or some inanimate object which bears an assignable relation to the person whom it replaces and preferably to that person's sexuality (e.g., a piece of clothing or underlinen). Such substitutes are with some justice likened to the fetishes in which savages believe that their gods are embodied."[11] Thus the shoe, which, like the foot that holds power "as an age-old sexual symbol which occurs even in mythology," is a "corresponding symbol of the *female* genitals."[12] Age-old and savage, the fetish is antimodern.

Possession and disavowal overvalue the fetish as a relic of an image of plenty destroyed, never quite admitted, and so reinvested with god-like power. Freud's description of the fetish locates the trauma of castration within the "little boy" and presents the fetish object as *his* substitute. Gilles Deleuze remarks that as "the last object he saw as a child before becoming aware of the missing penis (a shoe, for example). . . [t]he fetish is . . . not a symbol at all, but as it were a frozen, arrested, two-dimensional image, a photograph to which one returns repeatedly to exorcise the dangerous conse-quences of movement, the harmful discoveries that result from exploration."[13] Deleuze distinguishes between the object and its representation. The fetish is a photograph, frozen and arrested; yet the photograph, as Roland Barthes mournfully insists in *Camera Lucida*, is a melancholic object, par excellence.

Can women fetishize shoes? Or is it instead shoes that stir desire, turning the woman herself into fetish? As phallic mother substitute, the fetish, like the phallic mother, presents the girl an ambivalent homosexual identification with the female phallus as a woman's gen-italia. It circulates, but just barely. The shoe, as Freud admits in "On Dreams," especially the high heel, is both phallus and its lack. As such, it fulfills Victor Turner's definition of a ritual symbol. These incorporate contradictory social practices: "symbols are social facts, 'collective representations,' " he says in *The Forest of Symbols*, that are "multireferential," at once "sensory" and "ideological," whose "empirical properties" include "(1) condensation; (2) unification of disparate meanings in a single symbolic form; (3) polarization of meaning."[14] Rather than being immobile—frozen, as Deleuze calls the fetish—shoes as "social facts" are in constant flux. The shoe and the pair of shoes have almost nothing in common, no matter how redundant (but of course not, they're different) the two are. Hence freedom and death, sex and labor, accessory and necessity, object and symbol: magic, a mysterious thing. "Yes yes, we're magicians," assures Vladimir as he and Estragon struggle to get Estragon's boots on in *Waiting for Godot*.[15]

As lowly objects, abject objects, shoes remain as reminders, remainders of death. The lone shoe lying in the middle of a street following the shooting of German SDS leader Rudi Dutschke is a melancholy memento; its photograph part of the collective archive of 1968 and the German Autumn that followed.[16] The piles of shoes lining the railroad tracks of Auschwitz that appear in Alain Resnais's

Night and Fog, like the recent catalogue of photographs of articles of clothing, mostly shoes—remains of the men slaughtered and buried at Srebenica during the Bosnian War—are monuments of horror, reminders of the destruction of twentieth-century genocides. Articles meant to take the wear and tear of daily use, shoes remain in tact after other personal effects, and with them, their owners, have disintegrated, disappeared. "The Still Life as a Personal Object," from which Meyer Schapiro argues with Martin Heidegger over a pair of shoes, are the very shoes, as Derrida notes, left behind in the flight from the soil still clinging to one's work boots for an urban exile. *Nature Morte*, indeed, death follows their footsteps.[17] Shoes, as symbolic objects themselves, travel across three fundamental planes of human experience: work, sex, death.

"A MAGICAL OBJECT"

"The fetishism of commodities has its origin . . . in the peculiar social character of the labour that produces them," Marx wrote. "It is value, rather, that converts every product into a social hieroglyphic."[18] His example of this oxymoronic process of collective indecipherability goes as follows: "When I state that coats or *boots* stand in a relation to linen, because it is the universal incarnation of abstract human labour, the absurdity of the statement is self-evident. Nevertheless, when producers of coats and *boots* compare those articles with linen, or, what is the same thing, with gold or silver, as the universal equivalent, they express the relation between their own private labour and the collective labour of society in the same form." It is this "fantastic form," this "mist-enveloped region," this "mysterious thing" that fetishizes the commodity, separating it from its use-value as a product of human labor into an abstract value of exchange equivalent to all others and masking the "social character of the labour that produces them."[19] Walter Benjamin notes that Karl Korsch pushed Marx's insight into the fetishism of commodities to account generally for "human self-alienation . . . [b]y revealing *all* economic categories to be mere fragments of one great fetish."[20] As a religious practice, "fetishism seem[s] to appear only among peoples who have already attained to a certain degree of civilization."[21] In those "mist enveloped regions of the religious world" where "the productions of the human brain

FIGURE 35. Vincent Van Gogh, *Les Soulieres* (1886).

appear as independent beings endowed with life, and entering into relation with one another and the human race" fetishism emerges as a transition after totemism (72).

Relying on the same primitivist ideas animating Freud's work on the fetish, Marx also views its power as suspiciously ancient.[22] It depends, according to Marx's story of *Robinson Crusoe*, on circulation, that is, on alienation and the division of labor, and on consumption, the appropriation and incorporation of objects as values. Thus commodities carry within them, and thus within capitalism, the residue of the past. In a characteristic gesture, Benjamin, quoting Theodor Wiesengrund Adorno, describes the fetishized commodity as a "phantasmagoria," creating "a consumer item in which there is no longer anything that is supposed to remind us how it came into being. It becomes a magical object, insofar as the labor stored up in it comes to seem supernatural and sacred at the very moment when it can no longer be recognized as labor."[23] Again, anxiety about the non-Western, primitive, irrational basis of fetishism—"we're magicians"—the commodity and its consumer, like the fetish and its worshipper, are suspiciously feminized, or at least as emasculated as Gogo and Didi.

Unpacking his library, Benjamin notes the peculiar fascination with ownership that certain items produce for consumers within bourgeois culture. These items, like books or shoes, are those that can form a "collection," and collections produce "collectors" for whom "ownership is the most intimate relationship that one can have to objects."[24] Collections, like genres, operate on the principle of repetition with a difference, as every item resembles its other yet must be distinct at the same time. In his dissection of bourgeois living room objects, in "Paris, Capital of the Nineteenth Century," Benjamin discerned the origins of detective fiction as a genre that required objects, collected idiosyncratically by their owners, to provide clues, traces of evidence. The generic formula depended on the generic nature of the objects surveyed—every parlor has a chair, but what kind? Is it upholstered and draped by antimacassars or wooden, etc.? Susan Stewart calls this "the total aestheticization of use value."[25] For Stewart, this aspect of collecting acts to annihilate history; however, a shoe collection must always retain its historicity—that is the trap of fashion, it's of a moment, au courant. The collector acts like a criminal in his relentless pursuit of the missing items, rare editions, and so forth. "Every passion borders on the chaotic, but the collector's passion borders on the chaos of memories" such that "the life of the collector [is] a dialectical tension between the poles of disorder and order" (60). Within a commodity fetishistic culture, then, ownership becomes both a sickness and its cure. Furthermore, collectors oscillate between stasis—one needs some place to put the objects collected—and movement. Travel is essential to collecting: Benjamin remarks that he made his "most memorable purchases on trips, as a transient. Property and possession belong to the tactical sphere. Collectors are people with a tactical instinct; their experience teaches them that when they capture a strange city, the smallest antique shop can be a fortress, the most remote stationery store a key position" (63). In short, the collector is always one who walks; she needs a good pair of shoes.

Calling Benjamin our greatest theorist of the object, critic Douglas Mao argues that the "feeling of regard for the physical object as object—as not-self, as not-subject, as most helpless and will-less of entities, but also as fragment of Being, as solidity, as otherness in its most resilient opacity—seems a peculiarly twentieth-century malady or revelation . . . one of the minor trademarks" of modernism.[26] For Mao, the object and desire for it cannot resemble the fetish and fetishism as charted by either Marx or Freud, despite Benjamin's obvious reliance on their sources. Suggesting that "solid objects" were under siege as the concrete and particular gave way to vast abstract systematizing of science, Mao sees a melancholy rescue of the object in the Anglo-American high modernist writers, such as Virginia Woolf. Orlando's feat of Restoration consumption in redecorating the ancestral home is matched when, as a modernist poet, she drives to the department store in pursuit of various household necessities, including "boy's boots, bath salts, sardines," only to be foiled by the plethora of stuff spilling across the aisles she glances as the elevator lifts her from floor to floor of loaded counters. Orlando, however, rather than dispute seems to confirm, even in her choice of words, Marx: "In the eighteenth century, we knew how everything was done; but here I rise though the air; I listen to voices in America; I see men flying—but how it's done, I can't even begin to wonder. So my belief in magic returns."[27] All this magic; yet she fails to return with any of her shopping list items—so many products, incommensurate things. Woolf implies that for the modern woman commodities are interchangeable and inconsequential; but Woolf's modern woman is educated, a woman of privilege, striding purposefully through time and space, even if her mansion has become a museum.

OTHER SMALL OBJECTS

In *The Gold Rush* (1925), Charlie Chaplin's Tramp cooks and serves himself his boiled boot to fend off starvation in the Klondike. His careful dissection of the boot, picking each hobnail out as a finely-trained waiter might debone a trout, and precise twirling of the laces into a mound of spaghetti calls forth the animal quality of shoes— made of leather, absorbing the odors of the feet (one aspect that makes them so likely to become a fetish according to Freud)—and thus close to edible; yet their proximity to the filthy ground, their sweaty smells make them unappealing, disgusting. Chaplin had his boots constructed from licorice—sometimes called shoe-leather— and thus ate them with relish. In the section of *The Arcades Project* on the Saint-Simonians, Walter Benjamin quotes from a "revealing" Leon Halevy poem, "La Chaussure":

> This people, whose head and hand you fear,
> Must march, must march—no halting!
> It's when you stop their steps
> They notice the holes in their shoes.[28]

They notice the holes in their shoes only when they have time to contemplate their poverty, that is, when they no longer even have work and thus become a curious kind of excess, the detritus of capitalism. This impoverished proletariat, presocialist and anarchic, like the Tramp, as Roland Barthes calls him, is "still hungry . . . expressing the humiliated condition of the worker."[29] Work boots full of holes have no use. They no longer can be considered "equipment," in Heidegger's sense, and, like their unemployed wearers, signify a miserable supplement to their lack. Those gone to extremes—forced to eat their own shoes, self-devouring and empty—are useless as either producers or consumers within capitalism.

> Of shoes: ordinary work shoes may be called 'typical'; only if you remember that old Sunday shoes, tennis sneakers, high tennis shoes, sandals, moccasins, bare feet, and even boots, are not at all rarely used: it should be known, too, that there are many kinds of further, personal treatment of shoes. Mainly, this: Many men, by no means all, like to cut holes through the uppers for foot-spread and for ventilation: and in this they differ a good deal between utility and art. You seldom see purely utilitarian slashes: even the bluntest of these are liable to be patterned a little more than mere use requires: on the other hand, some shoes have been worked on with a wonderful amount of patience and studiousness toward a kind of beauty, taking the memory of an ordinary sandal for a model, and greatly elaborating and improving it. I have seen shoes so beautifully worked in this way that their durability was greatly reduced.[30]

James Agee's treatise on the clothing of the tenant farmers of Hale County, Alabama, like his "counter-spy" Walker Evans's

FIGURE 36. Walker Evans, "Boots." Hale County, Ala. (1936).

photographs of George Gudger's Sunday shoes drying before the "altar" of the decorated fireplace, or his work boots airing in the sun, refute Agee's call to avoid considering their book as art. Still they cannot help themselves: Agee compares the blues of the farmer's overalls and workshirts to "the blues of Cezanne" (267); Evans quotes Van Gogh's peasant boots. Each emphasizes the beauty of objects so thoroughly tied to use-value, yet conveying the most private longings for aesthetics. Agee writes:

> There is great pleasure in a sockless and sweated foot in the fitted leathers of a shoe made of most simple roundnesses and squarings and flats, of dark brown raw thick leathers nailed, and sewn coarsely to one another in courses and patterns of doubled and tripled seams, and such throughout that like many other small objects they have great massiveness and repose and are, as the houses and overalls are, and the feet and legs of the women, who go barefooted so much, fine pieces of architecture. . . . They are worn out like animals to a certain

ancient stage and chance of money at which a man buys a new pair; then, just as old sunday shoes do, they become the inheritance of a wife. (270)

These clay-encrusted objects placed symmetrically before the fireplace are emblems of labor, of poverty, and they are symbols of the essential uniqueness and dignity the reporters find in the lives of America's forgotten. "Clay is worked into the substance of the uppers and a loose dust of clay lies over them. . . . The shoes are worn for work" (270). Shoes carry within them the traces of the struggle to survive. Carved up, they are heavy with the grind of fieldwork; they are vessels of pain. Yet, like a wife, they are open, they exist to receive: a sweaty foot in fitted leather.

According to Swedenborg, shoes signify a "lowly nature," at once "humble and despicable." Men's shoes, claims Gertrude Jobes, served as "ancient means of binding a contract," because the removal of the shoe meant "loss of legal rights," which corresponds

FIGURE 37. Dorothea Lange, "The commodities on the counter represent two week's allotment for four people. Photograph made in FSA distributing station for emergency grants of food and clothing to destitute agricultural workers." Bakersfield, Calif., Nov. 1938.

to religious interdictions against wearing shoes in sacred places as they possess "contagion from the secular."[31] Yet Jean Servier "observes that 'to walk shod is to take possession of the ground.' "[32] These images of land and its ownership entrust the shoe with powers at once menial and imperial. The workingman's shoe carries the earth in its ancient creases and thus remembers labor and its equipment. In their iconic usage, the work shoe becomes attached to lowly peasant labor in the fields; whether Heidegger registers Van Gogh's boots as belonging to the farmer's wife (or, as Schapiro insists, as "clearly" the painter's own), we know they must be read as figuring some form of abject masculinity. As Agee points out, women's work shoes began as men's, only becoming their wives' (or daughters' or mothers'-in-law) possessions after they were near disintegration. This becomes clear in two of Evans's photographs where women are shown wearing shoes—the family portrait of the Woodses in which Miss Molly wears a battered pair of boots and the picture of Margaret Ricketts washing dishes in an old pair of men's shoes. The destination of worn boots means that they are not firmly latched to masculinity—or that the masculinity to which they are attached is hardly secure; it is the province of "humble" men tied to the earth; their movement is toward dissolution—the eventual wearing away of the leather soles, but not before they have been transferred onto women's feet—sunk even lower. Heidegger relied on Van Gogh's paintings of peasant shoes as a secondary, rather than immediate, way to consider the movement from equipment (as a pure useful thing) to its apprehension in the truth of an artwork. Tellingly, Heidegger reads Van Gogh's shoes as belonging to the farmer's wife—hand-me-downs, already-used, second-hand equipment, leftovers.

According to Joseph Kockelman's rendering, those shoes evoke for Heidegger a loneliness and rugged tenacity of earth and the "wordless joy of having once more withstood want" through the endless repetition of wearying field work.[33] This "heavy pathos of the primordial and earthy" denied what for art historian Meyer Schapiro was the central point of Van Gogh's paintings—that the still life objects were the *artist's* personal belongings—his self representation.[34] Work shoes symbolized the labor of the artist. Heidegger frequently referred to shoes and shoemakers as exemplary of being in a world in which materials and labor create meaning.[35] In

FIGURE 38. Hugo Gellert, "Money, or the Circulation of Commodities," from *Karl Marx 'Capital' in Lithographs*, 1934.

short, workingmen's boots—as useful products—and shoemakers— producers of use-values par excellence—aestheticize, even romanti- cize, human drudgery as survival. Hence Van Gogh's multiple returns to this readily available subject. In one of the remarkable moments in Art Spiegelman's *Maus*, Vladek describes how he sur- vived liquidation by claiming to know how to repair boots, thus securing himself a source of income by fixing a guard's broken sole. Without any skills, except hustling and a good memory, Vladek lands a position in the shoe shop and earns enough to bribe various capos into transferring his wife Anja into a barracks near him in Birkenau. Ever practical, not only does he describe the story to Artie, he draws a picture for his son, showing how to repair a boot.[36]

What all this thingness of equipment and beauty of utility and earthy broken shoes and so forth have in common is a remarkably consistent image of the peasants' shoes and the toiling shoemaker as central icons of heroic survival, of noble yet lowly subsistence, of a beauty and truth to be found in the very scraped bottoms of the filthy boots that trudge the heavy furrows to bring forth the meager means of human subsistence, to establish the ground for mid-twentieth-century philosophical musings on death, art, time, work, and being. Left-wing cartoonist Hugo Gellert also quoted Van Gogh's shoes for his illustration of Karl Marx's explanation of the "circulation of commodities" in his illustrated edition of *Capital* because shoes connect the laborer to the earth, and to toil and deprivation. They show the shoemaker as a craftsman who transforms raw materials—leather, itself an organic material—into a useful item. Like evocations of the land and rural life, as antidotes to industrialism (or even as evocations of productive work in general), these images of solidity, earthiness, and use are sentimental; left-wing iconography of labor, on the one hand, fascist icons of soil, on the other, would redeem a bereft manhood. Men's work boots reek of hard labor; and while Agee and Evans revered this, Preston Sturges was mocking it in his satire of proletarian social realism, *Sullivan's Travels*: Joel McRae ends up on a chain gang after his shoes, in which his servant has hidden his ID, are stolen by a tramp in a flophouse.

But enough with the heavy trod of hobnails and creaky mud-encrusted leather! Yes, men's boots and shoes evidence the nobility of soil and the grind of stoop labor. Shoes, even men's work shoes, also have other uses; they signal other kinds of labor. In the 1950s, Nikita Khrushchev banged on the United Nations table with his hefty black Oxford, declaring "We will bury you!" His denunciation of American capitalism—made in New York City, capital of capital, was a reminder of his peasant origins; yet the shoes were resolutely corporate in their anonymity. Van Gogh and Agee and Evans evoked the individuality of the work shoe, molded by years of wear to the foot; but the black leather Oxford was meant, like the Organization Man who wore it, to fit in and disappear. The opening shots of Alfred Hitchcock's *Strangers on a Train* (1951) track the rushing commuters' shoes crisscrossing up and down the aisle until they come to rest when Bruno (Robert Walker) and Guy (Farley Granger) bump into each other, two men outside the corporate economy (as wealthy gay man and tennis player, respectively) who wear more distinctive footwear. In Robert Aldrich's *Kiss Me Deadly*, another 1950s thriller that explicitly refers to the Soviet nuclear threat, Mike Hammer (Ralph Meeker) is able to discern the killers who have gotten hold of the "great whatsit" by recognizing their two-toned wingtips, a distinctive sign of precarious masculinity.[37]

6″ WITH ANKLE STRAP

Women's shoes, especially those meant for dress-up, are so much more useful; even Mrs. Gudger put on "[b]lack lowheeled slippers with strapped insteps and single buttons" on Saturday, market day at Cookstown.[38] The work they do is invisible as work; yet they too point to sites of labor. For Agee, shoes are cunts—the worn leather molded to the sweated bare foot, and none more surely convey terror and desire than the spiked high heel—*vagina dentata*. Mrs. Gudger's demure flats hint, with their straps and buttons, at the sexual intimacy connected to the removal of shoes. A *New York Times* article pictured a Tristan Webber sandal, with four-inch tapered heel featuring spikes protruding from the instep strap, the heel, and the ankle strap; over the image was the caption: "Shoe or weapon?"[39] Pierre Silber's advertisement for a $35 six-inch spike, available in sizes 6–14, offers a woman's shoe destined for a transgendered foot walking across skin, not pavement.[40] The stiff black pump of 1940s film noirs operated as a bullet case, sheathing the woman's foot and hardening it against the concrete pavement she traversed in her search for desire and power.

The woman's shoe as weapon begins Fuller's campy film noir *The Naked Kiss*, but it is also a pivotal scene in Herbert Biberman's 1953 left-wing labor film, *Salt of the Earth*. In this saga about a New Mexico miners' strike and the increasing activism of the miners' wives, Esperanza (Rosaura Revueltas), wife of macho strike leader Ramon, breaks free from her husband and children to join the women who have taken over the picket line after a Taft-Hartley injunction prohibits the men from marching. Handing her newborn infant to a stunned Ramon when the sheriff's deputies draw their guns at the women, Esperanza "stops for a second, slips off her right shoe [as deputy] Vance knocks the other woman down, pulls his revolver from his holster. Esperanza whacks him over the wrist with her shoe, knocking the weapon out of his hand."[41] Esperanza joins the women's group and forcefully helps lead the strike, leaving Ramon to take over the domestic chores. This labor melodrama, made during the height of McCarthyism by blacklisted actors, screenwriters, and directors, condenses many left-wing feminist and labor ideals in this one scene, which taps into latent fears of female autonomy. After this episode, Esperanza, still wearing her demure flats, is rarely home as housewife; she carts her kids to the picket line or else leaves them with Ramon to feed.

Shoes facilitate women's social mobility. In *Salt of the Earth*, a simple flat bests a gun, averting violence; but a hooker's spiked heel can almost kill a man, as Constance Towers demonstrates. So we arrive at the third "meaning" of the shoe—as symbols of travel, especially the journey to freedom, and/or death—an abstraction that cannot be seen despite its objectification.[42] Dorothy skips her way along the yellow brick road protected by the ruby slippers, which will eventually transport her home when she clicks their heels. The shoes transfer their power from one body to another, as they are themselves transferred from the Wicked Witch's shriveled feet onto Dorothy's, precipitating the journey and the ensuing struggle to possess them. The ruby slippers are very powerful, as Glenda surmises; yet their power is clearly gendered: no man seems interested in them.

This lavish 1939 MGM musical signaling the end of the Depression anticipated the ubiquitous sound of the femme fatale's heels. These postwar emblems of women's newly acquired sexual freedom, in turn, became powerful indexes for female fantasies of escape during the 1950s. Twice in Sandra Cisneros prose poem *The House on Mango Street* (1983), the narrator, Esperanza, astutely notes her sexual vulnerability as a girl on the verge of adolescence, a child of Mexican immigrants living on the edges of urban poverty. Both of these moments occur through her recognition of her unsettled footing within her world. This footing, literalized in the form of shoes, oscillates between a clunky 1950s girlhood, epitomized by bulbous saddle shoes, those sturdy markers of practicality bought by Depression-era mothers to last a whole school year, worn to the fancy party for which Esperanza is dressed in a new frock. Her ceremonial coming out—a dance with her uncle—is thus forever marred by the twin signs of poverty and gawkiness. No party shoes accessorize this dress. Esperanza has glimpsed the power of impractical shoes when she and her friends try on a few discarded pairs of dyed high heels and wobble around the block eliciting catcalls from the men and boys hanging on the street corners. Thrilled and terrified by their newly acquired swaying hips, the girls toss the heels as soon as they discover that men now see them as sexually desirable. With these two scenes, two crucial aspects of modern female footware are represented: that class position is instantly recognizable by looking at the soles of all folk, and that women's desires are tied to their (in)ability to move within them. Ultimately, Esperanza dreams of leaving the confines of Mango Street, changing her name to Ze Ze the X and possessing a house of her own emptied of all furnishings save blank paper and a pair of shoes neatly stored by her bedside.[43]

Women's decorative shoes, especially high heels, like Cinderella's glass slippers and Esperanza's yellow heels, reveal female sexuality. They become weapons and as such also convey those attracted/attached to them toward danger, even death. Women appear vulnerable in these wobbly unstable objects, but they elevate themselves to greater heights, commandeering space through the constant clattering of their heels on the hard surfaces of city streets and work places (whether office buildings or bedrooms). As objects of desire for both men (who, unlike the aristocracy of sixteenth century, now only watch them) and women (who can both watch and wear them), these icons also slide across genders. They lead inevitably to death. Not the inexorable, slow death of decay, but rather a sudden, violent death.[44] "These boots are made for walking," sang Nancy Sinatra in her thigh-high white boots, "and one of these days they're gonna walk all over you." Through work or sex, shoes journey to death; but the path they take, at least partially, runs through freedom. Pursuit is dangerous, but it's better than bondage. The broken feet of aristocratic Chinese women curtailed their movement, forcing them to take small mincing and painful steps unless carried. Shoes move us across space; desire for mobility leads us to death. When Marlene Dietrich kicks off her heels to follow Gary Cooper across the sands of *Morocco*, is it desire or death that propels her? She'll never make it barefoot, yet she grabs the camp followers' recalcitrant goat and walks on out of the screen. In the Hans Christian Andersen fairy tale, the Little Mermaid, pursuing her desire for her beloved prince, succumbs to a witch's brew that allows her to silently walk on legs as sharp as knives piercing her body, only to be left mute and alone. In "The Red Shoes," a young girl's desire for shiny red shoes, inappropriately worn to church and funerals, leads to her being controlled by her independent red shoes. Try as she might to take off the perpetually

moving shoes, they remained fast on her feet, dancing her freneti-
cally past the coffin of the old woman who had cared for her. Only
when an executioner chops off her feet, leaving her crippled, can
she stop dancing and repent her vanity. Broken in spirit, like the Little Mermaid, she dies blessed, another terrifying story of female lust
set in motion, then crippled, by footwear.

Carolyn Steedman recalls a recurring dream she had as a child of
a woman in a New Look coat entering a doorway, her severe black
pumps clicking along the bleak, postwar London sidewalk just out
of young Carolyn's reach. Steedman's mediation on "the politics of
envy" dictating the terms of her mother's brutal life's landscape
depended upon a thorough understanding of the connection
between female mobility and clothing. Buy a good pair of pumps, a
New Look coat, a smart suit, and a working-class woman, skillfully
shedding her accent, could transform her destiny.[45] Leaving her ratty
Lancashire mill town for the precarious possibilities open in London
during the Depression, Steedman's mother used her sexuality to
secure another future for herself and her two daughters. Fundamental to her mobility—spatial and class—was her ability to wear the
proper articles of clothing appropriate to her desires. The trajectory
from Lancashire to London depended on learning how to move in
the smart pumps of postwar women's autonomy. Like the many
femme fatales in film noir who traverse the dark city streets of San
Francisco, New York, and Los Angeles in search of power, pleasure,
and money, Steedman's postwar London mother knew how to dress
for success.[46]

Success for the young middle-class girl growing up in this postwar world was mapped out, as Charlotte Nekola remarks in her
memoir, *Dream House*, by "the progression from childhood to full
womanhood . . . Mary Janes to flats to pumps with a small tasteful
heel, and finally to the realm of pure sex and authority, 'spike' heels."
Remembering an incident when she moved her "convertible" strap
on her Sunday dress-up Mary Janes so that her girlish shoe would
magically appear as a mature flat, Nekola describes how this gesture
"instantly transformed [her], now a sinful Cinderella with some new
shoes of big-girl life."[47] However, when she showed her mother her
magnificent maturity, she was enraged by her disapproval. Like the
old woman who tries to steer Karen from the red shoes, Nekola's
mother insists Charlotte keep the strap tightly fixed around her

instep, maintaining the freedom of her "native girlhood" as long as possible (49). Cisneros's Esperanza and her girlfriends had quickly retreated from "Cinderella" to their native girlhood after their triumphant "tee-tottering" in the "lemon shoes and the red shoes and the shoes that used to be white but are now pale blue" cast-offs of the family of little feet because the threat of their sexual allure—men were suddenly whistling, offering each a dollar for a kiss—would inevitably lead to dangers—sex, pregnancy, marriage (40). Or worse: Barbara Stanwyck's anklet and heels, her cigarette and whiskey, her cat glasses and gun would indeed turn you into a femme fatale—murderous, deadly, and doomed to die in a hail of bullets.

Growing up in the 1950s, many young girls studied these films, found on late-night television, as documentaries of lives our parents might have lived, if not for the fortunes of free education from City College and the GI Bill enabling the installation of the nuclear family in the suburb. Office of War Information photographer Esther Bubley had recorded actual noir women who rode midnight buses and trains across the country in search of war work, residing in rooming houses along the way. Her bus trip throughout the Midwest and the South undertaken in 1943 took her to bus stations where she photographed single women sleeping on benches waiting for the 5 A.M. to Memphis, their black pumps dangling from their swollen feet. These intimate images of migrant women, solitary and vulnerable, hint at a fleeting return to innocence forever gone with war mobilization.

Bubley's single working women in transit during World War II presaged the "evil women [who] were women of psychological difficulties . . . who lived entirely in scenes of blood, murder, suicide, and physical and psychiatric violence of all kinds. Barbara Stanwyck's career . . . [was] built on the portrayal of this type of gangster woman." These women's crime films were so popular, noted one of American popular culture's critic C. L. R. James's female informants, who was "a sensitive and well-read observer," because, according to her, "they are the only performances that seem to be *real*."[48] Quoting documentary photography and dramatizing the pleasures, powers, and terrors of women's new-found mobility, made visually and aurally explicit in the erotic high-heeled slippers and anklet of Phyllis Dietrichson in *Double Indemnity*, the relentless clatter of

Kansas's black pumps in *Phantom Lady*, and Kelly's vicious spiked heels in *The Naked Kiss*, film noir turns women into magicians. If commodities could speak the secrets therein, they might tell us just what a woman wants—Shoes! Wedgies, platforms, sandals, thongs, mules, flats, pumps, loafers, heels, slingbacks, sneakers, and don't even start on the boots.

CHAPTER 8

MEDIUM UNCOOL: AVANT-GARDE FILM AND UNCANNY FEMINISM

"THE MOVIES ARE A REVOLUTION" (TAYLOR MEAD)

In his examination of the uncanny, Freud teases out the definition of the sensation accruing when "everything . . . ought to have remained hidden and secret, . . . yet comes to light."[1] The uncanny, that which is most familiar suddenly estranged, manifests itself in a curious dance between repression and recurrence. In chapter 7, I investigated the gendered residue clinging to the worn shoes repeating themselves iconically throughout modern culture. In this chapter, I offer a microhistory of the interconnections—both literal, in the form of personal relations, and theoretical, in the form of shared ideas—between early radical feminism in the United States and 1960s avant-garde film culture. Each bears an uncanny relation to American popular culture and its pulpy politics by examining what "ought to have been concealed but which has nevertheless come to light" through the intense personal self scrutiny that was a hallmark of both the avant-garde and feminism (148). Microhistories of local events, movements, and cultures form a central component of the new scholarship on women. Seeking a method that avoids globalizing assumptions drawn from relatively limited data, microhistories assert the authority of the local to explain how theory becomes activated and experienced. This is not simply an academic claim that "Small is Beautiful" or an exhortation to "Think Globally, Act Locally" but rather an attempt to understand how superstructural processes of cultural production and political organizing create what Raymond Williams calls "lived experience" through "structures of feeling."[2] Western Marxism since Antonio Gramsci locates culture as a site for struggle, in part, because of the unprecedented capital tied to it. Thus organizing countercultures is a hallmark of late capitalism because "an immense and inflationary issuing of superstructural credit; a universal abandonment of the referential gold standard; an extraordinary printing up of ever more devalued signifiers" unleashed "social energies" that built new movements, including radical feminism and the avant-garde.[3]

My argument is that the movement for women's liberation in the United States, which exploded within the New Left and captured the attention of the mainstream media in 1968, owed much of its rhetoric and practice to postwar avant-garde film, which, in turn, was indebted—albeit oppositionally—to America's pulp modernism. These two movements would appear to have nothing in common with the pulp fiction, government documentary, and Hollywood B-movies I have been discussing throughout this book. However, even in this cultural and political realm seemingly cut off from popular pulp, the same process by which cultural form anticipates political action is at work. Revealing the seamy underside of postwar America occurred across a wide spectrum of film cultures. The very repetitive nature of this exposure hints at feminism's uncanny investment in rescripting domestic melodrama, especially when staged during wartime, by bringing its noir elements "to light."

Because it is an uncanny one, this story of American feminism, film, and the long 1968 requires the kind of doubled and crisscrossed narrative technique of film noir.[4] Jay Boyer declares "you will never read the novel you might like to" about the 1960s because "there is no way to say it."[5] The 1960s defy verbal representation—or rather narrative—because words fail; image and sound—helicopter blades chopping the air over Vietnam and urban America, rock 'n' roll, nightly body counts from the battles at home and in the jungles of Southeast Asia—are what remain. Todd Gitlin offers a more verbose but essentially similar point: "the years 1967, 1968, 1969, and 1970 were a cyclone in a wind tunnel. . . . When history comes off the leash, when reality appears illusory and illusions take on lives of their own, the novelist loses the platform on which imagination builds its plausible appearances. . . . Reality was reckless, and so there is the temptation to dismiss it—say with the cliché of compilation, snippets of pure spectacle, in the style of a ticker tape or a clunky documentary:"[6] He goes on to reel off the following list:

> draft card burnings . . . the Pentagon . . . Stop the Draft Week . . . the Tet offensive . . . the McCarthy campaign . . . Johnson decides not to run for another term . . . Martin Luther King killed . . . Columbia buildings occupied . . . Paris . . . Prague . . . trips to Hanoi . . . Robert Kennedy killed . . . Democratic Convention riots . . . hundreds of students massacred in Mexico City . . . Miss America protest . . . Nixon elected . . . deserters, flights to Canada and Sweden, mutinies, "fragging" in Vietnam . . . Eldridge Cleaver underground . . . San Francisco State, Berkeley, Stanford, Harvard, etc., etc., besieged . . . People's Park . . . police shootouts with Black Panthers . . . student, freak, black, homosexual riots . . . SDS splits . . . Woodstock . . . women's consciousness-raising . . . the Chicago Conspiracy trial . . . Charles Manson . . . Altamont . . . My Lai . . . Weatherman bombs . . . Cambodia . . . Kent State . . . Jackson State . . . a fatal bombing in Madison . . . trials, bombings, fires, agents provocateurs, and the grand abstractions, "resistance," "liberation," "revolution," "repression"—to name only some of what was swirling."[7]

Of this long litany, two entries interest me: Miss America and women's consciousness-raising with "clunky documentary," his visual metaphor describing the whole rapturous horrible vortex, providing the means to suture the images. Like a clunky documentary edited together from a stockpile of found footage, I compile images from multiple sources of feminist film culture in 1968.

First Reel:
1967 *Bonnie and Clyde* (Faye Dunaway)
1968 *Rosemary's Baby* (Mia Farrow), *Barbarella* (Jane Fonda), *Funny Girl* (Barbra Streisand), *Vixen*, *Night of the Living Dead*

1969 *Butch Cassidy and the Sundance Kid, They Shoot Horses, Don't They?* (Jane Fonda), *Easy Rider, Midnight Cowboy, Once Upon a Time in the West* (Claudia Cardinale), *Medium Cool*

Like the long eighteenth century, which stretches for British cultural historians from 1660 to 1832—Restoration to the Reform Act—1968 is not so much a year as an era.[8] Gitlin runs 1967, 1968, 1969, and 1970 together in his tale of the white male New Left. The long 1968 for United States feminism and film stretches from 1965 to 1972, from Gunvor Nelson's and Dorothy Wiley's *Schmeerguntz* to the founding of Women Make Movies. However, one can always push the inaugurating moment back further and further.[9] Samuel Fuller's *Naked Kiss* was released in 1964, a year after *Griswold v. Connecticut*, the Supreme Court case opening the way for widespread distribution of contraception, including the newly available birth control pills. It, along with Grace Metalious's pulpy yet political novel *Peyton Place* (1963), unveiled the simmering desire and rage beneath the prim hedges clipped by small-town American women. Going back a few more years, Shirley Clarke's 1960 film of Jack Gelber's off-Broadway play, *The Connection*, was banned on grounds of obscenity by the motion picture division of the New York State Board of Regents. As I have been arguing, Clarke's exposé of an urban underworld owes its debt to Hollywood B-movies, which in an uncanny turn, like its antithesis the American avant-garde, could trace their lineage to Maya Deren's 1943 experimental noir exploration of the domestic uncanny, *Meshes of the Afternoon*.

By 1975, when Chantal Akermann released her beautiful and unsettling probe of noir domesticity, *Jeanne Dielmann, 23 Quai du Commerce, 1080 Bruxelles*, the whole picture of feminist work in film had changed: Laura Mulvey's influential article, "Visual Pleasure and Narrative Cinema," signalled the shift. It contributed to what became the emergence of feminist film theory as a discipline by substituting a rigorous semiotics for a simplistic sociological approach to women and film. ("Visual Pleasure and Narrative Cinema" being in some sense Laura Mulvey's answer to Molly Haskell's *From Reverence to Rape* (1974), this British Marxist-feminist Lacanian analysis of the system of desire paralleled the deft theorizing of female subjectivity in *Psychoanalysis and Feminism*, Juliet Mitchell's rib at

American feminists' anti-Freudian bent, exemplified by Phyllis Chesler's *Women and Madness.*) Women Make Movies supplemented New Day Films and Third World Newsreel as sources of women's documentaries and expanded to include independent films challenging Canyon Cinema and Filmmakers' Co-op by only distributing women's films. Thus by the mid-1970s, feminist film practice was firmly institutionalized, spanning filmmaking collectives, narrative, documentary, and experimental films, distribution companies, film festivals, journals, and women's studies courses, which tracked "images of women" in Hollywood and European art cinemas or sought to recover lost women's visions by unearthing the feminist subversion of Ida Lupino or Dorothy Arzner.

Three tendencies can be traced in United States film practices of the long 1968: New Hollywood, a commercial response to the end of the studios and the rise of television (filmmaking as industrial production); new documentary, tracking issues within New Left politics (filmmaking as collective activity); the Underground, celebrating the counterculture (filmmaking as individual art/craft, personal vision). Paralleling this, feminist cultural politics move against female stereotypes—e.g., Miss America (and in so doing get into view through the news media), document the politics and history of women and women's struggle—e.g., Newsreel's *The Woman's Film* (and in so doing challenge the news media), and experiment with visions of femininity—e.g., the personal films of Marie Mencken, Carolee Schneemann, Gunvor Nelson, and others (and in so doing detail domesticity—its bliss and horror—the daily life of a woman artist, often an artist's wife outside of the media). Like the projectionist in Robert Coover's "Phantom of the Movie Palace," who splices films, projecting two and three at a time, canting the projector at crazy angles to gather all of film's history into one monument, I need at least three screens for this exhibit on feminist film practice: one confronts popular culture, especially its pulpy aspects, a concern for radical women since at least the 1930s, but taking on greater urgency in the 1960s; another documents an alternative female culture, a concern for women artists since the 1920s, but assuming new political guises in the 1960s; a third builds an apparatus, both scholarly and institutional (journals, courses, distribution companies, festivals, etc.), for its dissemination. Sometimes the images fuse in lap dissolves, sometimes they run separately at competing venues.

Second Reel:

1964 Obscenity cases ban *Scorpio Rising* and *Flaming Creatures* (connected to the "clean-up" of New York for the World's Fair)

1965 NEA and state arts boards funded; 428 university film courses offered in the United States

1967 AFI established; *Cineaste* founded

1967 Marshall McLuhan's *Mechanical Bride* reprinted

1968 *Un Chien Andalou* (1929) first screened in the United States

1968 Hannah Arendt biography of Walter Benjamin published in *The New Yorker*

"THE PUBLICITY OF THE PRIVATE"
(ROLAND BARTHES)

Roland Barthes describes photography's impact as effecting a vast inversion of two reigning terms within modern culture—private/public—by relentlessly bringing the daily and personal into public view, on the one hand, and pushing the historic and political into daily life, on the other. "[T]he age of Photography corresponds precisely to the explosion of the private into the public, or rather into the creation of a new social value, which is the publicity of the private: the private is consumed as such, publicly."[10] An uncanny refashioning of the snapshot, the news photo, the official portrait, the wedding picture, each a specific genre with a discrete function, meant they began to merge. Faces and bodies become at once strange and familiar. Barthes is talking about still photography, with its fetishistic quality of a memento mori, at once sacred and disposable in its common place around the homes of the modern working and middle classes. But moving images, especially in the television age of the 1960s, the age of home movies, assume aspects of this eeriness, as if the images coming from the blue light of the television or flickering across a living room screen in eight millimeter conveyed "spirits and ghosts."[11]

Stan Brakhage's "amateur" films—home movies of his family life scratched over by hand—Jack Smith's "Baudelarian" films of friends camping in his apartment, and Jonas Mekas's diary films all bring into public view highly erotic, private fantasies of seeing.

Despite fairly wide distribution (in 1965 Mekas estimated that in New York, more than forty venues screened non-Hollywood films), these early films of the New American Cinema, routinely became the object of state censorship. They pushed into view a personal cinema—accomplished with minimal funds, cheap equipment, no crew, and committed to celebrating the particular, idiosyncratic visions of its maker—"a way shaped . . . by an ever-increasing knowledge of historical aesthetics AND, as is of primary importance, a being true to my senses in all my experiencing of the present," declares Brakhage. In the summer of 1961, twenty-five New York film artists, known as The Group, published their "First Statement of the New American Cinema Group," declaring "official cinema all over the world . . . morally corrupt, esthetically obsolete, thematically superficial, tempermentally boring . . . we know what needs to be destroyed," they continued, "and what we stand for . . . our rebellion against the old, official, corrupt and pretensious is primarily an ethical one. We are concerned with Man . . . with what is happening to Man."[12] Published in Jonas Mekas's journal, The Group signaled that, just as *Cahiers du Cinema* was the organ of the Nouvelle Vague, *Film Culture* gave voice to the New American Cinema.

Film Culture itself is like a family album—hand-typed letters and taped conversations—in which the personal and private lives of "troublemakers and beatniks" form the public documents of a new age (Aquarius begins in 1962) and art. Shirley Clarke (along with Mekas and the others in The Group) figured "there must be 40 or 50 others like me in the country, with a desire for self-expression and no urge to move to Hollywood and make soap opera."[13] One such filmmaker, Stan Brakhage, was living and making films in the Colorado Rockies. In a letter to his daughter's principal, after Myrrena's body odor had become a topic of concern to the Rollinsville Elementary School, Brakhage cites his own "life's work, as a film artist, [which] particularly qualifies me to search out and create thru the finest qualities of human vision" in his refusal to be shamed into bathing Myrrena, if she is not so inclined.[14] This letter appears with a selection of Brakhage's correspondence in *Film Culture*. By decade's end, in his "Defense of the 'Amateur' Filmmaker," Brakhage summarizes the move from private to public as New American Cinema became institutionalized: "I have

FIGURE 39. Kenneth Anger, *Scorpio Rising* (1963). Museum of Modern Art Film Stills Archive.

been making films for over 15 years now. . . . Mostly I have worked without title in NO collaboration with others—I have worked alone and at home, on films of seemingly NO commercial value . . . 'at home' with a medium I love, making films I care for as surely as I as a father care for my children. As these 'home movies' have come to be valued, have grown into public life, I as the maker of them have come to be called a 'professional,' an 'artist' and an 'amateur.' "[15]

Preceeding Brakhage's correspondence in this issue of *Film Culture* is an interview with Kenneth Anger about *Kustom Kar Kommando* and the first screening of *Scorpio Rising* after Anger had won its censorship case. "What *Scorpio* represents is me cluing in to popular American culture after having been away for eight years . . . living in France." His luscious, idiosyncratic observations of American male homoerotic subcultures obsessed with cars and motor bikes became a documentary: "I don't see the difference between a symbol and a thing: its the same."[16] Anger, who grew up in Hollywood and would use his early experience in his wild excursion into *Hollywood Babylon*, found the sugary lyrics of early 1960s pop songs menacingly strange; blue velvet was scarier than black leather. For Anger, the icons of working-class American male popular culture—cars, motorbikes, leather jackets—all of which suggested a deeply homoerotic attachment to certain objects were intimately tied to popular music's ironic send-up of heterosexual romance. Anger understood what Adorno never quite got, or more aptly never quite got over: America is the modern uncanny often found in pulp.

Anger's "cluing in to popular American culture," like Brakhage's "being true to [his] senses" formed the central tenets of 1960s arts and politics—expose the weirdness of normality and express the dailiness of wild originality. One can find versions of these declarations everywhere, as in Carolee Schneemann's "Notebooks" for "Round House," her Happening created for the July 1967 International Congress on Dialectics of Liberation. Her notes range among thoughts on quantum physics, the Vietnam War, casual meetings with friends, ideas for the piece: "Happening as basic psycho-social guerilla life-fare," she quips. Then, "expose exposure demystification yes get rid of old deadly mysteries women *our genital and our pronoun* new mysteries waiting for us get it all out tell and show"

```
the waitress. . . . . . . . . . . . . . . . . . . . .?
the airline. . . . . . . . . . . . . . . . . . . . . . . . . . . . . . . ?
the heiress. . . . . . . . . . . . . . . . . . . .?
the hostage. . . . . . . . . . . . . . . . . . ?
the steward. . . . . . . . . . . . . . . . . . . . . ?
HOSTESS STEWARDESS. . . . .!17
```

As in her early 1967 five-screen film/performance, "Snows," which she described as "a work based on Vietnam atrocity images," Schneemann's nude body was central to the politics of her art.[18] In 1960s America, according to Schneemann, both Vietnam and

Woman are known through airing "atrocity images" and the struggle against the devastation of each entailed reclaiming those images. In her next piece, "Naked Action Lecture," Schneemann discusses the "Istory" of her work while dressing and undressing. It asked the questions: "Can an artist be an art istorian? Can an art istorian be a naked woman? Does a woman have intellectual authority? Can she have public authority while naked and speaking? Was the content of the lecture less appreciable when she was naked? What multiple levels of uneasiness, pleasure, curiosity, erotic fascination, acceptance or rejection were activated in an audience?"[19] For the woman "amateur," cluing in to popular culture and being true to her senses required a public display of her body, the nude female body—always object of art, retrieved into subjectivity—"to bridge the conventionally public/private areas of experience."[20] By collapsing subject and object—art work and art historian—into one, Schneemann foregrounded her body as a battleground. Other women artists focussed instead on the role the image apparatus itself played in both constructing and violating privacy.

Third Reel:

1966 Charlotte Moorman arrested in New York for performing "TV Bra" with Nam June Paik

1966 *Chelsea Girls* cannot be screened at the Cannes Film Festival because it requires two projectors

1967 "New Documents" at Museum of Modern Art

1967 *Portrait of Jason*

These last two 1967 events—Jason camping at the New York Film Festival and the Jewish Giant hanging in the Museum of Modern Art (MOMA)—are crucial installments of my tale of feminism, film, and 1968. Each brought the mundane quality of daily life into weird relief by forcing spectators to look carefully at what was usually ignored, avoided, and repressed. As the only female founding member of The Group, Shirley Clarke made her reputation through the avant-garde narrative films *A Cool World* and *The Connection*, which explored African-American and drug cultures. When she created the self-mocking cinema vérité film *Portrait of Jason*, she declared the result "a portrait of a guy who is both a genius and a bore."[21] Like Diane Arbus's photographs, it forced viewers to confront their

FIGURE 40. Shirley Clarke, *Portrait of Jason* (1967). Museum of Modern Art Film Stills Archive.

investments in voyeurism because each accorded the objects of her camera's gaze some element of subjectivity. Each woman—wealthy intellectual New York Jewish Bohemian—defiantly took her camera into the urban underworld of men and forged a new kind of intimate documentary: Arbus as a street photographer; Clarke in her "fictional documents" of various black male underground cultures. Unlike Schneemann, who was in part responding to Brakhage's lyrical cinepoetics of his family's bodies by insisting that hers be looked at, these New York women artists choose not to display their own bodies. Instead they foregrounded other culturally marginalized, even disreputable, noir subjects.

Although she rarely got releases, Arbus claimed she developed deep relationships with her subjects—they told her their "secrets" as she clicked away. Unlike Walker Evans, who was "counter-spy" to James Agee's "spy" in *Let Us Now Praise Famous Men*, Arbus relished in the subtle intrigues of street photography. "I can figure myself into any situation. I choose photography projects that are somehow Mata Harish. I'll not risk my life but I'll risk my reputation or my virtue." Arbus's black-edged photographs of "freaks"—Jewish giants at home in the Bronx, identical twins, transvestites, nudists, prowar demonstrators with bad acne—fascinated and repelled the MOMA's audience to its major photography show: New Documents. Esther Bubley had also carried her camera through the streets shooting everyday events with a certain freedom accorded her as a woman: "It has helped particularly with people in the street, the women and children who seem to accept me sooner," she told an interviewer in 1957.[22] Arbus spent hours hanging around the gallery with her thirty images eavesdropping on the remarks of those disgusted by her depictions of outlaws and outsiders. As she said of her work style: "[I]f I stand in front of something, instead of arranging it. I arrange myself."[23] Her arrangement included the gallery space where she could spy on the voyeurs she had created through her own relentless voyeurism.

Clarke's relationship with Jason undercuts her position as filmmaker; but instead of arranging herself, she arranged her camera. Shot on an Auricon camera that needed to be reloaded every ten minutes, Clarke set the camera in one position and filmed Jason Holliday talking for twelve straight hours. Clarke observed "never had anyone [been allowed] to speak for themselves for more than a few minutes at a time" in traditional cinema; thus she gave Jason license to talk and talk, sometimes responding to the prods of her off-screen voice. Ultimately, Clarke does not succeed in unmasking Jason. Instead, he unmasks the very assumptions of cinema vérité; it becomes obvious that his stories about black gay transvestite life are being *performed* for the camera. Most likely they are lies. "For the first time I was able to give up my intense control and allow Jason and the camera to react to each other."[24] Arbus, however, despite her demurral, always maintained control, at least of her shoots, often lying to her subjects to get the pose she wanted. Andy Warhol superstar Viva and feminist Ti-Grace Atkinson both claimed to have been violated by Arbus after she photographed them sprawled naked like ODed junkies for spreads in *New York* and *The London Sunday Times*, respectively.[25] Yet Atkinson had been righteously celebratory of Valerie Solanas's *S.C.U.M. Manifesto* and of her actual shooting of filmmaker Warhol—that celebrity thief deluxe.[26] In their differing excesses, Arbus and Clarke set the stage for feminist ambivalence toward media, exposure, and a politics of celebrity that would mark post-1968 events.

Fourth Reel:

1968 Valerie Solanas, author of the *S.C.U.M. Manifesto*, shoots Andy Warhol

1970 Marie Mencken dies

1971 Diane Arbus commits suicide; a madhouse erupts for possession of her Westbeth studio

Moving private life, fantasy, and obsession into public view and in so doing challenging economic and political structures—through censorship battles, through distribution and exhibition collectives— is the uncanny story of the New American Cinema of the 1960s. Yet, at the same time, the explosion of new filmic forms and images serves paradoxically to reinforce postwar corporate America. As Susan Sontag, riffing on Walter Benjamin and Guy Debord, astutely notes: "A capitalist society requires a culture based on images. . . . Cameras define reality in the two ways essential to the workings of an advanced industrial society: as a spectacle (for masses) and as an object of surveillance (for rulers). The production of images also furnishes a ruling ideology. *Social change is replaced by a change in images*."[27] Sontag was an early champion of the New American Cinema, penning an important analysis of *Flaming Creatures* in 1963; however, by the mid-1970s, she had soured a bit on the radical possibilities of film and photography. In many ways (and Sontag is exemplary, as we'll see later), The Group, its art and its organization, provided a model for radical feminism. Through new forms of political organizing, which included the production of new images— consciousness raising, guerilla theater, all-women's actions and speakouts—women's liberation forged a new movement for social and political change; however, the stumbling block to feminist revolution remained ever in the realm of culture and consciousness (or ideology, or psychology, depending upon to whom one talked). Because, in a capitalist society, social change is replaced by a change in images, altering images—a struggle to find new ways of representing woman to herself, to women collectively, and to men— became central to every aspect of radical action.

"THE PERSONAL IS POLITICAL" (CAROL HANISCH)

In her 1970 "Critique of the Miss America Protest," Carol Hanisch recalls how the action, which launched contemporary radical feminism—the Women's Liberation Movement—into the public eye,

> came out of our group method of analyzing women's oppression by recalling our own experiences. We were watching *Schmearguntz* [sic], a feminist movie, one night at our meeting. The movie had flashes of the Miss America contest in it. I found myself sitting there remembering how I had felt at home with my family watching the pageant as a child, as an adolescent, and a college student. I knew it had evoked powerful feelings. When I proposed the idea to our group, we decided to go around the room with each woman telling how she felt about the pageant. . . . From our communal thinking came the concrete plans for the action.[28]

Hanisch understood the process of consciousness-raising, gleaned from Chinese cadre criticism/self-criticism and speaking bitterness sessions as "a political action," not a therapeutic one. As Kathie Sarachild later noted, "the importance of listening to a woman's feelings was collectively to analyze the situation of women. . . . The idea was not to change the woman. . . . [I]t's male supremacy we want to change."[29] It was out of talk that theory, then action, proceeded to build mass female solidarity.

Hanisch and Sarachild, proponents of the "prowoman line" within radical feminism, sought to support women in their limited choices, even those considered oppressive. Historian Alice Echols contrasts these radical feminists concerned with organizing women as women to those "politicos," who advocated organizing separate women's contingents to antiwar demonstrations. Just as *Schmeerguntz* catalyzed the Miss America action, these too often took their inspi-

FIGURES 41 and 42. Gunvor Nelson and Dorothy Wiley, *Schmeerguntz* (1965). Frame enlargements property of Gunvor Nelson and Dorothy Wiley.

ration from the movies. For instance, "at Florika's suggestion, a number of New York Radical Women members participated in an April 1968 anti-war demonstration as a contingent from NYRW. They dressed like Vietnamese women, handed out leaflets about women's liberation to women only, and ran through the crowd ululating like the Algerian women in Gillo Pontecorvo's 1966 film *The Battle of Algiers.*"[30] Echols relates these two incidents to distinguish between the actions of feminists and politicos. However, these two films—one lyrically documenting two women's uncanny experiences of women's daily life in postwar United States; the other fictionalizing a document about Algerian anticolonialist struggle, featuring militant women setting bombs and amassing in the streets—chart the range of feminist political action in 1968. Public feminist action made tangible "the Society of the Spectacle," in which seeing obscure films, talking about them, demonstrating, and then seeing the political actions eventually broadcast on network TV become steps in mass political organization. All that's needed to complete the picture is New York Newsreel's first all-woman documentary of the all-women Jeannette Rankin Brigade's 1968 action at the Capitol. From critiques of popular culture to celebrations of revolution to documents of women's mobilization, radical feminism and alternative film trailed one another, and each sought to explode the uncanny world of complacent domesticity in the face of the noirish nightmare of violence, assault, and war.

Tellingly, none of these films was part of the dominant film culture of the American 1960s—Hollywood's unraveling studio system and European art cinemas. Arguably, these two film practices, being more pervasive, should have been instrumental in forming a feminist film culture. However, feminist responses to Hollywood and its Other, European art cinema, were not central to the critiques of mass culture mounted by feminists. Despite the edgy rebellion or outright camp typical of 1960s films, which gave them an air of the counter culture, they were not viewed as radical breaks with postwar American pulp even when they came from Europe.[31] Thus they came in for attack for their unreal depictions of women (Jeanne Moreau as the male-identified Catherine in Truffaut's *Jules et Jim* was universally denounced) and for their exploitation of the star system. Yet, poems by lyn lifshin reimagining Marilyn Monroe or Karen Lindsey mourning Jayne Mansfield spoke to the ambivalence feminists felt toward the culture industry's use of female bodies. "Elegy for Jayne Mansfield, July 1967" reads:

> she was a
> sunday news centerfold
> bosoms thrust toward subway-
> rush men leaning on the
> legs of pretty secretaries
> always a bleeding
> divorcé or a beaten child,
> she had a pink voice, and lived in a pink house.
> no hints of a self
> cringing away from sticky headlines
> or an art groping beyond
> barebreasted titters.
>
> we used to have fun laughing at her.
> when she lost her head, the joke turned sick.[32]

The joke turned sick; Jayne Mansfield, Marilyn Monroe, and Miss America tested the limits of radical feminist analyses of culture and its industry.[33] How to come to terms with women who used the system of male supremacy to make it? Hanisch ultimately condemned the Miss America action, with its free-for-all theatrics, admitting slogans such as "Up Against the Wall Miss America" alienated women and blamed those participating in sexist institutions—including marriage—for their self-contributions to an enforced victimization. A "prowoman" line would celebrate women's many subversive responses to her oppression. Thus even Jayne Mansfield needed to be reassessed, perhaps rehabilitated, or, more accurately, the feminist response to Jayne Mansfield needed revising. Solidarity among women required recognition of the underground submerged stream of women's culture within a sexist world, including its most ludicrous and debased extremes.

Ever attentive to the zeitgeist, new stars in updated, hip genre films commercialized dissent, further complicating the relationships among popular culture, public life, and private desire. A smile stretches across the ashen face of platinum-blonde, spit-curled Faye Dunaway as she strokes Warren Beatty's pistol in the opening sequence of *Bonnie and Clyde*. The graphic violence of Arthur Penn's 1967 film came to be seen as a touchstone for the New Left, especially media speculations about it. Bonnie's beret, echoing Che's, was the dress code of the Black Panthers, eventually hitting the fashion pages. *Bonnie and Clyde* retrofitted America's past, showing how the body counts racking up on the nightly news were not aberrations but a key aspect of U.S. history. In one scene, Bonnie sits engrossed in a motion picture theater watching the Busby Berkeley musical *Golddiggers of 1933* for fashion tips. Bosley Crowther of the *New York Times* lambasted the "slap-stick" of *Bonnie and Clyde*, its romance of guns and gangs. His dismissal was mild compared to Page Cook's denunciation in *Films in Review*: "One final word," he appended to his review of the opening night of the Montreal Film Festival, "there is *evil* in the *tone* of the writing, acting, and direction of this film, the calculated effect of which is to incite in the young the delusions that armed robbery and murder are mere 'happenings.' " The period dress and antique cars never for a moment masked the contemporary feel of the images *Bonnie and Clyde* purveyed, as Richard Schickel noted in his *Life* magazine review: "Bonnie and Clyde are the products of the rootlessness of ill-taught youth growing up absurd in a period of historical transition. The parallel between the middle 1930s and the middle 1960s is never too far from the minds of the movie's creators."[34] As Hollywood's studio system increasingly fell apart, independent productions mainstreamed radical critiques of America. *Bonnie and Clyde*'s resurrection of the 1930s, the era of America's Old Left, aestheticized violence by politicizing style according to these mainstream critics.[35] However, young radicals flocked to the film, boosting its flagging attendance after Warner Brothers re-released it in the wake of 1968 assassinations, civil unrest, and Democratic convention police riot.[36]

Film as just such a system of contradictory thought and experience—not merely as a source of negative and positive images—was crucial to at least one feminist theorist. Shulamith Firestone's 1970 manifesto, *The Dialectic of Sex*, found in film the precursor to her ideal postrevolutionary "anti-culture": "the young art of film, based on a true synthesis of the Aesthetic and Technological Modes (As Empiricism itself had been) carried on the vital realistic tradition. . . . [I]t broke down the very division between the artificial and the real, between culture and life itself," she exclaimed ecstatically.[37] Much like Maya Deren, who practiced both critique and art-making, Firestone, an art student at the Chicago Institute of Art during the mid-1960s (where Stan Brakhage would later teach) and "star" of *Shulie*, a cinema vérité documentary about her, saw film as a philosophic system.[38] In this, she paraphrased the conclusion to The Group's "First Statement": "[W]e are not only for the new cinema, we are also for the New Man. . . . [W]e are for art, but not at the expense of life. We don't want false, polished, slick films—we prefer them rough, unpolished, but alive; we don't want rosy films—we want them the color of blood."[39] However, few feminist theorists took up Firestone's line on cinema as prefigurative. Instead, more often they, like Sherry Sonnett Trumbo, asked, "where is the movie that shows us what alternatives and possibilities are open to us as women?" Trumbo noted, "For women, there are very few relevant models offered by movies or the rest of culture that will help ease the fear and pain of liberation."[40] If "A Woman's Place Is in the Oven" rather than behind the camera, how was a feminist film vision to be expressed? In these minor nods toward film criticism, so-called second wave feminists were rehashing debates among Popular Front feminists. Muriel Rukeyser's poem "Movie" skewered the nascent fascism in Hollywood fantasies of female stars: "Spotlight her face her face has no light in it / . . . We focus on the screen: look they tell us / you are a nation of similar whores remember the Maine / remember you have a democracy of champagne— / And slowly the female face kisses the young man, / over his face the twelve-foot female head / the yard-long mouth enlarges and yawns / The End."[41] Like Trumbo, Joy Davidman, film critic for the *New Masses* during the 1940s, challenged the commercial culture and female objectification endemic to Hollywood and America, yet she relished the possibilities mass culture offered radical organizing.

"THE REVOLUTION WILL NOT BE TELEVISED"
(GIL SCOTT-HERON)

If "movies and the rest of culture" offered little of use to feminists, notwithstanding Firestone's attempt to argue otherwise, movies, even alternative cinema, and the rest of culture were still central to maintaining women's oppression. In the "Fourth World Manifesto," Barbara Burris, writing on behalf of her collective, declares:

"A Female culture exists." The emphasis on finding and nurturing that submerged female culture became the genesis of what Alice Echols calls "cultural feminism" because "male culture, which is the dominant culture in every nation, i.e., is synonymous with the national culture, cannot accept a female view of things as expressed by female writers, artists and philosophers."[42] Burris based her conclusions on a dissection of the Algerian revolution's betrayal of National Liberation Front (NLF) women, evidenced in part by Pontecorvo's film *The Battle of Algiers*. She offered a thorough-going critique of Frantz Fanon's emphasis on postcolonial male identity formation through anti-imperialist struggle. Her ideas resonated among black feminists, many of whom had been active in the Black Arts Movement. For instance, Francee Covington writing in Toni Cade's influential 1970 anthology, *The Black Woman*, also uses *The Battle of Algiers* as a source for analyzing the revolutionary potential of U.S. radical movements—antiimperialist, black nationalist, or feminist.[43] Because, as Sontag would argue in "The Third World of Women," "all women live in an 'imperialist' situation in which men are the colonialists and women are the natives, . . . the same basic relations of inferiority and superiority, of powerlessness and power, of cultural underdevelopment and cultural privilege, prevail between men and women in all countries."[44] Thus a film, such as *The Battle of Algiers*, that offered a blueprint for anticolonial struggle, moved from the realm of representation to that of strategic manual. It is a virtual given among all these women that the film is a documentary, because, if film, in general, "broke down the very division between the artificial and the real, between culture and life itself," then this one did so in a powerfully self-conscious way. The impact of the film turned many feminists to documentary to secure the truth of women's lives within a liberated women's cinema.

The collective of documentary filmmakers known as Newsreel updated for a new era of political activism a tradition of destabilizing documentary narratives, stretching from Dziga Vertov's *Man with a Movie Camera* in postrevolutionary Soviet Russia through *Salt of the Earth*, Herbert Biberman's fictional defiance of the blacklist in McCarthyite America. Newsreel's films opened with their trademark film projector and machine-gun staccato, resurrecting the 1930s Film and Photo League's assertion that "the camera is a weapon." In December 1967, the collective announced its birth in the *Village Voice*: "Films made by Newsreel are not to be seen once

FIGURE 43. Gillo Pontecorvo, *The Battle of Algiers* (1968). Museum of Modern Art Film Stills Archive

and forgotten. Once a print goes out, it becomes a tool to be used by others in their own work. . . . We intend to cover demonstrations; to interview figures like LeRoi Jones and [Jim] Garrison; we want to show what is at stake in a housing eviction or in consumer abuses in Harlem; we should provide information on how to deal with the police or on the geography of Chicago."[45] The logic behind Newsreel's perceived need was, in part, "documented" by Haskell Wexler's extraordinary 1969 movie, *Medium Cool*, which follows a television news cameraman as he shoots scenes of Chicago life leading up to the 1968 Democratic convention. *Medium Cool* earned an X-rating (no one under 18 admitted) under the Motion Picture Association of America's newly instituted rating system. A clear move to censor a political film, branding it "pornography," the MPAA appeared to be doing to commercial cinema what the cops had done to underground film a few years earlier and what the television networks were doing to the Vietnam War and domestic resistance almost daily. According to Newsreel: "The news that we feel is significant—any event that suggests the changes and redefinitions taking place in America today, or that underlines the necessity for such changes—has been consistently undermined and suppressed by the media" (*Movie Journal*, 305).

For all its radical form and content—intercutting actual black-and-white documentary footage into the color narrative, improvisational acting, hand-held camera, highly self-reflexive commentary on filmmaking, etc.—*Medium Cool* still featured a man shooting footage of men shooting guns (camera as weapon) and of women at home who may or may not want to be looked at (camera as voyeur). In one scene, Robert Forster has gone to a Southside Chicago apartment to interview a cab driver who found a wallet containing $10,000, turned it in, and then got arrested. As he exits, he is challenged by a black actress who demands he put her on television because "the tube is life," as someone remarks. Delivering images, perhaps the cameraman is obstetrician, but he is nevertheless cut off from real life. The hot everyday life of summer 1968 is antidote to that cool medium, the tube, and it is embodied in the earth mother: a young Vietnam War widow serving canned tomato soup to her teenage son. She challenges Forster to take responsibility for the pictures he takes that end up on her television, invading her life, making her home uncanny, a war zone. But, in Wexler's quotation of Jean-Luc Godard's *Contempt*, she ends up dead in a car smash-up as the two vainly search for her missing boy during the chaos of the convention. The final credits mimic the opening sequence: a passing car slows as someone snaps of photo of the dead couple. The question remained, especially for women, how to "serve the needs of people who want to get hold of news that is relevant to their own activity and thought"? How to film in medium uncool?

The women active in New York Newsreel offered one answer: demand that the white men who were already filmmakers—in effect, the ringleaders of the collective—cede their power by spreading their knowledge to those working in the crew. Rather than lecture the cameraman about his complicity in the violence of the shot, women demanded access to the cameras themselves. They wanted to shoot back. Newsreel collective's female members felt that by making films about black male radicalism, like *Black Panther Party*, the white male filmmakers were either homing in on another's vital revolutionary culture (a form of imperialism), or in making films of *The Columbia Strike* were celebrating their own struggles as if they con-

FIGURE 44. Haskell Wexler, *Medium Cool* (1969). Museum of Modern Art Film Stills Archive

stituted the revolution (another form of imperialism). In one of their first actions, in January 1968, Lynn Phillips and an all-women crew from Newsreel's original thirty members filmed the Jeannette Rankin Brigade, an all-women antiwar organization named for the first woman elected to Congress who voted against U.S. intervention in both world wars, in its attempt to petition Congress to end the war.[46] However, a year later, Christine Choy was filming the Newsreel footage of the Attica prison uprising as a complete novice after Robert Kramer and other founders, including Phillips, had left New York Newsreel.[47] Explaining her early departure, Phillips concluded, "Preciousness and pandering are the Scylla and Charybdis of left culture. Newsreel, to avoid the pandering of 1930s nice-guy sentimentality, lapsed into a muscular kind of French intellectualism; and for all our trashy surface and rough posturing, I think we got as precious as well, Waiting for Godot, or Godard, Waiting for Godard. . . . Besides the women's movement had grown a great deal by then, and there was too much in the feminist critique of the left leadership that was too true and too slow to change."[48]

The slippage between "real life" revolution or struggle—say in Algeria or in Chicago—and filmic ones—say *The Battle of Algiers* or *Medium Cool*—what Phillips called "Waiting for Godard," is precisely what sutured Miss America to revolutionary ululations. That *The Battle of Algiers* recreates the feel of documentary—using techniques *Medium Cool* also mimicked—points to the conventions of truth-telling so important to 1960s political investments in cinema. As Shirley Clarke declared in 1962: "Right now I'm revolting against the conventions of movies. Who says a film has to cost a million dollars and be safe and innocuous enough to satisfy every 12-year-old in America?"[49] Jonas Mekas pointed out that the true documentary work in cinema had been going on in New American Cinema all along. For Mekas, Carolee Schneemann's investigation of her sexuality and her active handling of the film itself offered more real cinema than anything coded as "real," including cinema vérité documentary.[50] Parker Tyler argued that underground films were always "curiously 'documentary' " because they "document the traditional social activity of making life itself into a work of art."[51] According to David James's assessment, "By far the majority of underground films were essentially documentaries of these [homosexual, women's, Bohemian, drug, anti-war] subcultures . . . instances of minority social groups representing themselves." Moreover, "the radical innovation of the underground . . . invent[ed] film as practice rather than as manufacture."[52] Art of life, practice of art, life as art—"the movie equivalent of off Broadway, fresh and experimental and personal" was how Clarke described it. This was *avant la lettre*, the aesthetic flowering of Firestone's dream of "anti-culture," the cinematic dispersion of Hanisch's "personal is political."

"IF YOU'RE GOING TO CHANGE THINGS, YOU'RE GOING TO
MAKE A MESS—EVERY HOUSEWIFE KNOWS THAT!"
(CAROLEE SCHNEEMANN)

Cheap, lightweight equipment and the "cinema of an effortless (as much as it can be) self-expression, which culminated in *Blonde Cobra* and *Flaming Creatures* and 8mm" had made possible a new wave of "women . . . coming to cinema," commented Jonas Mekas in 1963 after viewing new work by Naomi Levine, Storm De Hirsch, and Barbara Rubin. "Now," he declares, "Marie Mencken is no longer alone."[53] In 1966, Marie Mencken, heiress to Maya Deren as mother of the avant-garde, appears as Gerard Malanga's mother in *The Chelsea Girls*. Mencken's career as a filmmaker, like that of her many avant-garde sisters began in collaboration with her husband, Willard Maas.[54] The "istory" of women in art features a litany of wives, lovers, and models tagged on as afterthoughts. For instance, Sheldon Renan concludes his profile of Robert Nelson in the "Gallery of Film-Makers" with the following sentence: "His wife Guvnor [sic] has, with Bill Wiley's wife, Dorothy, made a film called *Schmeerguntz* (1965), which satirizes the modern woman."[55] Both Gunvor and Dorothy, who rarely appear in accounts of underground film history can claim a decent pedigree—the history of modernist women artists is an "istory" of wives and lovers serving as footnotes to greater male visionaries.[56] Jane Brakhage—her body a central image and her camera work a central element of "Brakhage" films—is incorporated within the final title of the films shot in Colorado: "By Brakhage" flickers at the end of *Thigh Line Lyre Triangular* and *Dog Star Man*. These homemade movies of birth and wood chopping are family productions, but celebrating whose personal "metaphors on vision"?

In a 1971 interview with Brenda Richardson, entitled "Women, Wives, Film-Makers," which mocks, but cannot fully escape, the legacy of belittling artists' wives as second-class artists, Nelson and Wiley described the beginning of their collaboration: "Dorothy and I made two little 8mm movies, and Bob went with Bill Wiley, Bob Hudson, and Ron Davis and made *Plastic Haircut*, and that was more like a professional thing—Dorothy and I just fiddled around with little stuff."[57] Four years before, in a conversation recorded in 1967 and transcribed in *Film Culture*, Shirley Clarke and Storm De Hirsch had pointed out that despite being acclaimed filmmakers, "we are both little women" patronized constantly as women artists. Clarke begins their conversation with the tongue-in-cheek question: "Do you think that lady film-makers are mechanically equipped to handle their field?" She compares their status to female trolley drivers in the Soviet Union as the two proceed to circle the woman question in the history of independent cinema.[58] Both of these conversations shy away from declaring women's experimental filmmaking as a form of "women's liberation." Yet each emphasizes the different treatments male and female artists receive from journalists, other artists, and friends. Nelson and Wiley remember bitterly how, after

Schmeerguntz received first prize at the 1966 Ann Arbor Film Festival, male artist friends started speaking to them; Clarke notes that journalists always comment first on her demure appearance.[59]

In this curious diminution of themselves and their work, no matter how resentful, each of these filmmakers calls attention to her difference from her male colleagues, lovers, and husbands. Much as Mexican painter and wife Frida Kahlo had continually referred to herself as "little" compared to her muralist husband Diego Rivera's "giant" presence and art, these women stress the miniature; in so doing, however, they invert its value. Like Esther Bubley, who at 5' 4" started body building after an assignment at a Brooklyn boxing gym because she was so small that she tired from carrying her equipment, they muscled their way into a male domain, then relied on their petite size to get their cinematic results. Standing behind a 35mm camera, as Clarke had, but even holding a smaller 16mm one, offers a way to strap on the phallus and then utterly undo its power by filming the insignificant. In their quests for a tactile, hand-held medium, by the 1970s, Wiley worked exclusively in 8mm and Clarke had turned to video. Were they accepting that they "just fiddled around with little stuff"? Or were they anticipating the image revolution provided by digital cameras?

These pre-Women's Liberation Movement underground cinematic revisions of home movies paved the way for a new radical feminist cinema, but even more daringly, for radical feminism itself. When it screened in 1968, Carolee Schneemann's film *Fuses* got a rave from Mekas as heir(ess) apparent to his pantheon. In production for three years, *Fuses* features long sequences of Schneemann and her lover, James Tenney, having sex as viewed from the point of view of her cat, Kitch. She then scratched the film, baked it in the oven, left it out in the rain, until bodies and film fused. Like Clarke's early film, it too was the object of a censorship battle, which, unlike the cases over films by Anger and Jack Smith (both of which were highly public and theatrical) was unsuccessful in part because of its intensely private disclosure.[60] Private life, in all its trashiness, was what public culture deemed obscene. "With *Schmeerguntz*," notes Nelson, "we wanted to make a 16mm movie, I think. But we had no subject. And one day I was looking at all the gunk in the sink and thought of the contrast between what we do, and what we see that we 'should' be—in ads and things—and that was the idea right from

FIGURES 45 and 46. Carolee Schneemann, *Fuses* (1965). Self-shot color silent 20 minutes. Pacific Film Archive.

there, from the sink."[61] Joyce Weiland's *Rat Life and Diet in North America*—premiering in 1968 at the Jewish Museum—uses close ups of gerbils and cats scurrying amid food left out on her kitchen table to allegorize Canadian and feminist resistance to imperialism, war, and the violence of daily life. Since Maya Deren's *Meshes of the Afternoon* investigated the multiplying uncanniness found within a southern California bungalow, its objects—phonograph, telephone, bread knife, windows, and mirrors—demonically animated as the body of a woman replicates again and again, women's experimental cinema has been imbricated in noir. Like Esther Bubley, Maya Deren was documenting the effects of war. Even domestic spaces are dangerous when the world's skies are filled with bombers; the home no refuge for her or for her refugee husband. She too invented the iconography and thematics of film noir *avant la lettre* as the living room took on a sinister quality of terror in her avant-noir cinema.[62]

Domesticity continued to be the focus of Dorothy Wiley's later 8mm works, such as *Cabbage* (1972), about which she says: "[W]hile watching film, I can abandon myself to the event. I don't find that so easy to do in the kitchen in the morning. I still don't understand that part."[63] Unsettling domestic settings, by turns inviting and erotic and violent and repulsive—domesticity with a vengeance, something Arbus accomplished in her 1963 portraits of New Jersey nudists, making the home into an uncanny place—is part of the complicated interrelationship of photography and image under capitalism, as much an aspect of the publicity of the private as of a "personal politics," which women's film work and feminist politics highlighted.[64] "*Schmeerguntz* is one long raucous belch in the face of the American Home. A society which hides its animal functions beneath a shiny public surface deserves to have such films as *Schmeerguntz* shown everywhere—in every PTA, every Rotary Club, every club in the land. For it is brash enough, brazen enough and funny enough to purge the soul of every harried American married woman," declared Ernest Callenbach in its sole review.[65] Following the leads of Deren and Mencken, Wiley, Nelson, Schneemann, and Weiland domesticated the wars at home and abroad. Personal cinema—home movies of sex and ordinary objects—flowers in women's filmmaking during the 1970s; but it, like *Meshes*, brings the war home. For instance, Chick Strand's 1979 *Soft Fiction* used her girlfriends' weird stories—concluding with a terrifying tale about how, as a young girl, one woman flirted with a Gestapo enabling her family to escape the Nazis—to parody the sincere talking heads of much earnest feminist documentary as it tracked a vaguely noir narrative of a woman escaping her bungalow by train. Homey images eventually became a way to entice women into filmmaking, as Liane Burton explained: "If you can thread a sewing machine, you can thread a projector, and if you can follow a recipe, you can do still photography developing."[66] Yet women reshot underground home movies and documented women's struggles for private audiences—the cognoscenti of the New American Cinema and the committed of the New Left.

"FREE IN THE DUSTY BEAM OF THE PROJECTOR"
(ADRIENNE RICH)

Looking back through Women's Liberation's *Notes* from the First, Second, and Third Years, it becomes clear that if the 1960s marked the emergence of late capitalism, in Ernst Mandel's term, then the long 1968 of feminism and film hints at a brief triumph of the Cultural Revolution. The woman question had been lurking behind Marxism for more than a hundred years, popping its head out at various times only to be pushed back from view. But the late 1960s reorganization of capital and desire opened the floodgates as public space became the site of private conscience, freeing the imagination in Paris and Prague, declaring "Sisterhood is Powerful" in the United States and around the world. "The superstructural movement and play enabled by the transition from one infrastructural or systemic stage of capitalism to another" mitigated, for a time, class-based analyses of social and political change by unleashing "social energies" in the form of new cultural movements, including feminism.[67]

Viewed from today's perspective, in which the distinction between culture, consciousness, and commodity is increasingly elided, the struggles of feminists to "name the system" that oppressed women, as Paul Potter had exhorted the New Left at the 1965 antiwar March on Washington, was exceedingly prescient; Potter later recounted that he had purposely evaded naming the system, capitalism, "because capitalism was for me and my generation an inadequate description of the evils of America—a hollow, dead word tied to the thirties."[68] In part, this explains why guerilla theater actions inspired by film and television became a key form of feminist political organizing. It appeared certain that women's liberation, understood by radical feminists as freedom from men's control, individual men as well as systems of male chauvinism, would never be achieved solely by structural changes in the economic relationships between classes, even sex classes; only a fundamental change in consciousness and in its public expression would accomplish a feminist revolution. After all, like Maya Deren in *Meshes*, Barbara Stanwyck ended up dead, even after admitting she really loved the guy, at the end of both *Double Indemnity* and *The File on Thelma Jordan*. Simply unleashing women's fury at domesticity was not enough.

With its dual struggle against censorship (to gain visibility) and for revolution (to change the world), the work of the underground, both cultural and political, was lodged, in part, within film. Censorship crucially acts as an official refusal to circulate knowledge publicly, by, on the one hand, insisting that the private remain hidden (inhibiting sex), and, on the other, hiding state secrets (waging war), in effect privatizing public information. Politics and culture in the 1960s unraveled and tangled these threads—underground films and Happenings, often public displays of private love and friendship, were raided by the police while the nightly news brought the brutality of state-sponsored death in Vietnam into American living rooms. Thus it makes wacky sense that *Medium Cool* would be given an X-rating by the MPAA; it was deemed pornographic for pointing out how obscene war is. Battling censorship meant forcing a public acknowledgment of this hypocrisy.

If censorship relies on keeping knowledge private, revolution demands the public demonstration of a refusal, bringing the masses into the streets because their solely private existence as individual subjects becomes untenable and they seek power collectively. Women's work in film during the long 1968 united, as radical feminism did, the struggles to fight censorship and make revolution. It located the woman's body—its private spaces and its public consumption—as the uncanny site of a new kind of politics—a politics of the image and of the personal. Fighting censorship meant bringing into view the noirish elements of middle-class women's lives—the vomiting pregnant woman, the sink full of dirty dishes, the shitty diapers, and the images of Miss America—as much as it meant a self-revelation of women's erotic desires. Making revolution meant refuting the culture of images that depended upon the female body and documenting the long history of women's presence yet invisibility in politics by the very mechanisms that had both objectified and ignored women's bodies; it meant celebrating "our bodies ourselves." Exposure, expression, exploitation, excess: the cinema as metaphor for daily life (a theme prevalent in much twentieth-century literature and criticism) became cinema as a design for living—its creation charted in a clunky, curious documentary. Cinema not only documented 1960s movements, however; it actively structured both their politics and poetics. Adrienne Rich's 1970 poem, "Images for Godard" concludes:

> the mind of the poet is the only poem
> the poet is at the movies
>
> dreaming the film-maker's dream but differently
> free in the dark as if asleep
>
> free in the dusty beam of the projector
> the mind of the poet is changing
>
> the moment of change is the only poem[69]

The long 1968 offers a prehistory to feminist film work. First generation feminist films may not have made the revolution; but, through a medium uncool, they did project the moment of change.

Fifth Reel:

"Women's Cinema as Counter Cinema" (Claire Johnston, 1973)

Legend of Maya Deren Project (begun in 1973, first edition appeared in 1988)

Popcorn Venus (Marjorie Rosen, 1973)

Women in Film and Video Conference (Buffalo, New York, 1974)

From Reverence to Rape (Molly Haskell, 1974)

"Visual Pleasure and Narrative Cinema" (Laura Mulvey, 1975)

Women and Film (1975)

Jeanne Dielmann, 23 Quai du Commerce, 1080 Bruxelles (Chantal Akermann, 1975)

Camera Obscura (1977)

Telluride Film Festival—includes Agnes Varda's *L'Opera Mouffe*, Marie Menken's *Orgia*, Nelson and Wiley's *Schmeerguntz*, Anne Severson's *Near the Big Chakra*, and *Fuses* and *Plumb Line* by Schneemann in a program entitled: The Erotic Woman (1977)

Women's Pictures: Feminism and Cinema (Annette Kuhn, 1982)

Women and Film: Both Sides of the Camera (E. Ann Kaplan, 1983)

Thelma and Louise (1991)

1997 Shirley Clarke dies.

CHAPTER 9

MAPPING NOIR

DEAD RECKONING

The Hutchinson River Parkway winds north from the Bronx. Cutting a path through granite hillocks, shadowed by oak and maple and pine, it is a dark somewhat haunted roadway. It is the only federal highway in the United States named for a woman, commemorating the site where Anne Hutchinson, her family, and followers were massacred after they had been banished first from the Massachusetts Bay Colony and then from more religiously tolerant, yet still repressive, Rhode Island. Hutchinson should be considered the first "dark lady" of American political pulp history: a woman who defied her elders—men, both ministers and governors—because she dared to speak openly about her ideas and beliefs. A midwife who herself had sixteen children, Hutchinson began informally recounting Sunday sermons to the women lying in before and after childbirth. Her biblical readings and interpretations drew more and more women, who eventually brought along their husbands as well as their children, until she was running a counter church, preaching her own, not merely recounting others', sermons, declaring her belief in radical predestination. Imprisoned for months while pregnant, she delivered a "monstrous birth" whose death sealed the verdict John Cotton, a supporter of hers, was forced to draw about her—that she was a danger to the community, a heretic to be cast out from the "city on the hill" into the wilderness. Hutchinson's story haunted Nathaniel Hawthorne, whose ancestor Hathorne (Nathaniel adding the letter W as a vague disguise) sat in judgment at the Salem witch trials; she (and her latter-day reincarnation, Margaret Fuller) is the model for defiant Hester Prynne.

The Scarlet Letter, beginning with its long scene in the Custom-House, establishes the basic formula for film noir. Just as almost all of the classic noirs rely on a voice-over narration told from the grave—Mildred Pierce, Al Roberts in *Detour*, Walter Neff in *Double Indemnity*, and, quite literally, Joe Gillis in *Sunset Boulevard*, to name just a few—Hawthorne's tale begins by divulging the story of how the buried story surfaces. The cache of letters and the bizarrely ornamented piece of cloth the narrator finds among the items stored in the attic of the Custom-House where he works a dull office job, the nineteenth-century version of Neff's Pacific All-Risk Insurance Company office. Its secretary pool and its Dictaphones and telephones are merely technological updates of the paper, wood, and charcoal used to record the comings and goings of freight. Paralyzing boredom and routine work mark the daily existence of the men working in offices whether in a Salem Custom-House, a Los Angeles insurance agency, or, like Joe Gillis, a rewrite desk in a Hollywood studio. Each man finds release from his dead-end job in the allure of a diabolical woman.

Barbara Stanwyck may seem a far cry from Hester Prynne, but Billy Wilder (in *Double Indemnity*) and Robert Siodmak (in *The File on Thelma Jordan*) stage her entrance into the plot in practically the same manner that Hester emerges into view in Hawthorne's romance. Framed by the prison door, as her story is framed by that of the Custom-House, Hester appears out of the dark, her mark of disgrace, the scarlet *A*, gleaming in the late-afternoon New England sunshine. Her momentary pause at the door, on view by the spectators mobbing the entrance, offers them a full glimpse of her body and of the small baby she cradles. Reversing the direction Jane Greer comes from when she materializes out of the bright daylight in the doorway of the gloomy Mexican cantina in *Out of the Past*, radiating a pervasive glow into the dark café, Hester leaves behind the dank prison for the light of day; yet those watching her, shrouded in black

FIGURE 47. Sunglasses as Armor. Barbara Stanwyck and Fred McMurray in Jerry's Market in *Double Indemnity* (d. Billy Wilder, 1944).

clothing, present a dark vision. She, like Phyllis Dietrichson or Lizabeth Scott as Coral Chandler in *Dead Reckoning*, an apparition of white light—her blond helmeted hair glowing, her white skin wrapped in a white towel—draws the eye. Walter Neff stares up at Stanwyck as she looks down from the second-floor balcony at him, and we in the audience are pulled into her orbit as well. The camera, like Hawthorne's narrator, forces us to look.

This cinematic spectacle beginning Hester's story is repeated at various moments in the tale—at the marketplace, at the scaffold, at the pulpit, at the minister's window—when visual display and its necessary other, concealment, which is the curse of Arthur Dimmesdale and his townspeople, structure the narrative. Italian critic Sandro Portelli calls *The Scarlet Letter* a grammar of America; American critic Patricia Crain finds it to be America's primer.[1] I prefer the metaphor of the road map. The threads embroidered across Hester's chest provide the contours for what would eventually unfold so daringly in film noir—a framed landscape viewed through headlights and windshield wipers in which women's desires are always open to inspection, suspect precisely because they refuse to be concealed, yet endlessly appearing as an enigma, a problem to be solved, a crime needing punishment. What Hawthorne's map acknowledged was precisely that a representation is all that is necessary because there is no truth to be found either out there or in here. The visually cryptic red markers tell all, if one cares to follow their directions. Secrets are always laid bare, like highway markers announcing each town—Emblem, Wyoming, population 11—along its route. Thus in mapping the paths of America's darkness, Hawthorne outlines how romance—the framed stagy form he insisted best described his work—is essential for uncovering the nation's past politics.

Hawthorne may have borrowed his form and content from the publication of Frederick Douglass's narrative registered in the Clerk's Office of the District Court of Massachusetts in 1845. Douglass too frames his life's story—this time in the form of two testimonials by white men assuring readers of Douglass's legitimacy because the racist ideologies of antebellum America could not accomodate an articulate black writer. William Lloyd Garrison and Wendell Phillips have heard Douglass speak and can verify his words; their reports authenticate his. Douglass begins his tale with an account of witnessing his Aunt Hester's beating by his cruel master, Captain Anthony. Douglass discerns the central facts of his condition as "a witness and a participant" while hiding "terrified and horror-stricken . . . in a closet": "It was the blood-stained gate, the entrance to the hell of slavery, through which I was about to pass. . . . It was a most terrible spectacle." Understanding his impotent complicity in the sexualized racial violence of slavery, and in the peculiar role he now occupies as its witness and narrator, Douglass connects himself and his readers to the visual spectacle of blood and bondage, as well as the erotics of pain and degradation that Hawthorne's Hester also sets into motion. As a young boy, he is dimly aware that his master is overreacting to finding Aunt Hester had disobeyed his orders not to leave his property when she was discovered with (her lover) another slave, Ned Roberts. Douglass notes that Aunt Hester was "a woman of noble form, and graceful proportions, having very few equals, and fewer superiors, in personal appearance, among the colored or white women in our neighborhood." Aunt Hester is a beauty. Frederick, often "awakened at the dawn of day by the most heart-rending shrieks of an own aunt of mine," senses that Captain Anthony seems to take particular relish in torturing her: "[H]e used to tie [her] up to a joist, and whip upon her naked back till she was literally covered with blood." The day Douglass moves from auditor to voyeur, however, that is, the day he stands at the doorway of slavery—its witness and participant—the beating is especially brutal: "Before he commenced whipping Aunt Hester, he took her into the kitchen, and stripped her from neck to waist, leaving her neck, shoulders, and back, entirely naked. He then told her to cross her hands, calling her at the same time a d--d b--h."[2] Tying her hands, he made her stand on a stool stretched out on display before the young boy hiding in the kitchen closet, who watches through the keyhole, waiting his turn. Douglass's Aunt Hester must be degraded by Captain Anthony because of her desirability; he punishes the body her finds so attractive, and does so publicly, as a spectacle performed on the threshold of America's hell. Her bloody back, striped in red—like the lines on a road map—by her master's whip, reappears on Hester Prynne's chest winding amid the red embroidery of her emblem of debasement.

Film noir did not appear—or at least was not named—until French critics got to see the storehouse of embargoed American films after the end of World War II. However, Hawthorne makes clear in Hester's resurrection of Anne Hutchinson—and the hanged Salem witches and perhaps his knowledge of Douglass's aunt as well—that a noir plot underlay the entire history of this continent.[3] The crime story in which a woman figures as bearer of chaos and the resulting trial to ascertain guilt and assess punishment is a narrative that did not begin with European settlers, of course. It goes way back to the Lady Eve (played, naturally, by Barbara Stanwyck). It's a typology in which political history can only be discerned through a framed fictional form. Film noir makes legible a long undercurrent within American political culture—its essential pulpiness, its scandalous dependence on revealing fallen women's crimes with and against their doomed, slightly dimwitted (or at least faint-hearted, remember Dimmesdale) men. Thus we need Barbara Stanwyck to help make sense of Hester Prynne as much as Hester and her riveting *A*, or Aunt Hester and her bloodied back, stand Phyllis in brilliant relief.

We only know Aunt Hester through Douglass's recollections, and Anne Hutchinson through her reported speech recorded at her two trials. Rita Copeland explains how our understanding, even our knowledge, of dissent—until quite recently—is always mediated through a legal and rhetorical system designed to suppress it.[4] While Puritans were a highly literate culture—directly reading the Bible's

229

word was essential to the Reformation—Hutchinson never wrote her readings of text down. What we have is a transcript—a recording in the technology of the time, handwritten probably from notes after the events occured, like the Dictaphone cylinders that Walter Neff keeps filling with his memo to insurance investigator and friend Barton Keyes. Film noir obsessively dwells on devices that mechanically reproduce and transmit the voice—Mike Hammer's telephone answering machine in *Kiss Me Deadly*, Myra Hudson's tape recorder in *Sudden Fear*, the ubiquitous telephones so central to Leona Stevenson in *Sorry, Wrong Number*;[5] or on photography as a record of bodies of evidence—for instance, in *Call Northside 777*, *Pickup on South Street*, and *The File on Thelma Jordan*; or the binoculars attached to a camera, and the tape recorder bugging the telephone in *Pushover*.[6] Thelma Jordan's cinematic punch derives, in part, from identifying Barbara Stanwyck's character as a bleached-blonde prostitute who looks exactly like Phyllis Dietrichson through an old gangland photograph circulating between District Attorney Wendell Corey's office and one from Miami. The scenario mirrors the ship captain's use of an old mug shot to clue Henry Fonda that Stanwyck and her father are gambling hustlers in Preston Sturges's *The Lady Eve*.

The tools of reproduction, faulty as they are, nevertheless enable dissenting and resisting women's voices to be deciphered long after their deaths, but they also may reveal their hidden deceptive pasts. Buried within these forms is a repetitive tale of replication as Anne Hutchinson's monstrous birth grew into Hester Prynne baring her emblazoned breast, whose wild daughter, Pearl, is later revealed to be Daisy Miller glimpsed by Winterbourne kneeling in the enormous oval of the Coliseum before the gigolo Giovanelli, who, like Mrs. Ansley, the "quiet" woman knitting in view of the Coliseum in Edith Wharton's "Roman Fever," begets still another ravishing daughter, Barbara, this time as Phyllis Dietrichson (or Joan Crawford's Mildred Pierce, whose diabolical daughter, Vera, assumes her look and her man), who begets, in the most recent version of a dark lady and her machinery—telephones and (the appropriately named trip-up Linda Tripp's) tape recorders again—Monica Lewinsky.

President Clinton's affair in the lesser oval (office) of the White House played out against the backdrop of this perverse plot. His former lover, Gennifer Flowers mentioned in an interview with

FIGURE 48. The mechanics of noir—visual and audio surveillance. Phil Carey as voyeur and Fred McMurray as auditor in *Pushover* (d. Richard Quine, 1954).

Larry King that as soon as she saw the ubiquitous footage of black-bereted Monica hugging the president, she knew he was involved with the young intern. Monica Lewinsky, revealed Flowers, looked just like her when she, a young reporter at a Little Rock television station, first met Clinton. "Back then, I had dark hair, like his mother," she noted coolly. Thelma Jordan disguised herself by turning into, or returning to, a mousy brunette; the women surrounding Clinton's impeachment—Hillary Rodham Clinton, Paula Corbin Jones, Linda Tripp, Gennifer Flowers, Monica Lewinsky—underwent a series of makeovers, transforming themselves through changing make-up and hair color and styles, weight loss and plastic surgery, into an evolving catalogue of film noir's female types. Each of these women was demonized in highly predictable ways. For instance, in a fundraising letter sent during the 2000 Senate race in New York, the Republican Party described Hillary Clinton with great alliterative flair as "abrasive and annoying, brash and bitter, calculating and scheming, distant and deceitful, polarizing and power-hungry."[7] Without the armor of fiction, it would be practically impossible to make sense of Kenneth Starr's obsessive inquiry into Clinton's personal life, which itself repeats a familiar plot. Roger Chillingworth and Barton Keyes, men who doggedly search out the truth, resisting temptations usually found in the shape of a woman, cannot fathom the ones who cannot stay away—Walter Neff or Cleve Marshall (in *The File on Thelma Jordan*), Arthur Dimmesdale and Bill Clinton as well. Film noir provides the context for understanding the replication of America's dark ladies and the men who fall for them, as well as those who relentlessly seek their exposure. The deep shadows and the glaring light put the shades of gray into high relief.[8] Bill Clinton gleaned the political efficacy of "triangulation" when he stole Republican Party platforms on the sexually loaded and racially coded issues of crime and welfare and refashioned them into his own policy. Douglass viewed these interlocking triangles through a closet door; Hawthorne found them in the moldy papers stuffed in the Custom-House attic; my parents spent Saturday night watching them at the Rialto; I absorbed them on *Million Dollar Movie*; my sons peruse them on the World Wide Web.

DETOUR

I have been arguing for attention to narrative history—to the history of narratives as much as to the narratives of history—found in the trash of America's popular and political cultures. Only a pulp theory can make sense of the strange lineage connecting Monica Lewinsky to Anne Hutchinson; so to conclude, let me take you on a feminist excursion into narrative history, a detour on the road through noir. We begin driving north on the Hutchinson River Parkway heading toward Vermont where poet Anne Stevenson's "family history in letters" (as she subtitled her volume of poetry) was uncovered. *Correspondences*, whose title plays on the varied meanings of the word—epistles back and forth, the harmonious reverberations between one set of objects or representatives and others, sexual intercourse, religious communion—is a saga of two hundred years of New England women's crises over family, work, money, and thwarted dreams of creative expression and sexual desire derived from an actual archival source found in the barn of her family's Vermont farmhouse. Her poems rewrite the letters she found molding there to appear truly authentic by mimicking eighteenth- and nineteenth-century diction and including the archivist's footnotes (in the form of marginalia detailing damage by fire, water, or rodents). As the poems move into and through the twentieth century, various poetic styles are picked up and discarded as first one then another generation of women suffer humiliation at the hands of mothers and lovers, editors and husbands.

The long confessional poem, "From an Asylum: Kathy Chattle to her mother, Ruth Arbeiter," dated May 2, 1954—years before Betty Friedan named the "Feminine Mystique" as the problem that had no name, but only a few years after Olivia de Havilland survived *The Snake Pit*—written by one of the last heirs of the dynasty, is posted from The Good Samaritan Hospital, a mental institution. Once a worker (arbeiter is her maiden name), she is now, as a wife and mother, a slave (chattel), suffering perhaps from "involutional melancholia," like the women Esther Bubley photographed for the *Ladies Home Journal*. The letter offers a litany of middle-class domestic hells: a screaming, colicky baby and cheating, absentee husband leave her a raging new mother perpetually drunk. It concludes with a typical 1950s explanation mounted by the "whitecoats" for why Kathy abandoned her own daughter—"they think you're to blame."[9] Kathy's husband, feeling trapped in "the prison of a family / Baby / shaping him into the / middle class, money-earning / ulcered American Dad," declares her a "slut . . . / [s]lovenly, drunken bitch." Kathy takes off one day on "the first train" into "a wind full of / knife-edged, excitable sunlight. // Walking from Central Station / feeling slenderer, blonder . . ." Her trip to New York—fleeing suburbia for the city streets where she is "Too scared to go to bars. . ." like a femme fatale—sends her "wandering like a schoolgirl from / museum to museum . . ." until she collapses at the Cloisters and ends up "where they've taken my belt and my / wedding ring, where they / specialize in keeping me weeping." Unable to transform from the "nice girl" she was raised to be into a femme noire, Kathy ends up installed in psychological melodrama (65–70). However, Stevenson's family history concludes with a 1972 letter from this same woman, now renamed after her divorce and an expatriate writer, to her estranged father: "It is a poem I can't continue. / It is America I can't contain" (88). Moving away from the enclosure of domestic space, she discovers the nation itself is as constricting. These private episodes of loss cannot contain the nation; yet they are precisely the stuff of 1970s feminist revisions of American political discourse. During the Vietnam War, the noir vision of domestic hell lurking within the middle-class family extends to the political realm to include the gunk in the kitchen sink.

The tradition of Marxist-feminist criticism argues for the importance of analyzing both social and literary texts as complementary, interruptive, and, sometimes, competing narratives, suggesting that literary scholarship must never forget social relations.[10] How could it? Even the most personal confessions, those that "can't continue . . . can't contain," failing at Whitman's democratic "I am large. I contain multitudes" seek other voices, reveal whole nations, in caches of secret and hidden documents that are the heart of contemporary feminist historical inquiry. We write literary history not to escape or forget the troubling geography in which the clipping or the letter or the drawing now dwells, but precisely to detail this climate as well as its earlier one. Situating a book in history or fancying literature from history—doing both kinds of literary history—reveals the past and so enables a close reading of the pulpy present.

When Stevenson came upon the cache of family letters in the early 1970s, women's historians were busily reinventing the discipline of history to include and understand such private forms as the diary or letter as legitimate data—seen then as a window on that supposedly separate sphere of woman: private life. Recently, Felicity Nussbaum has argued that the construction of the private self in those diaries and letters is preeminently a public and political act enabling Enlightenment subjectivity, and so empire and capitalist accumulation—the big stuff of politics and economics. At a time when feminist historians find the public/private split useless, is it any wonder that feminist novelists, like Hawthorne a century and a half ago, pick up history—that no longer exclusive realm of public truth—for their fiction?; or more accurately, turn again to historical fiction to argue contemporary political issues?

BELOVED ARROGANCE AND VINDICATION

Three late twentieth-century novels by American women—Toni Morrison's *Beloved* (1987), Frances Sherwood's *Vindication* (1993), and Joanna Scott's *Arrogance* (1990)—take their subjects from historical figures and incidents in order to circulate feminist political theory within contemporary popular culture.[11] These books, as literary histories, allow us to think about why writing historical narratives or narrating writerly histories offers us a politics for and a history of the present. They put forth a pulp theory of this present trashy era. These works are all dilettante's histories—works by those "lovers of the fine arts," those "refusers of a profession," rank "amateurs," "parasites," to quote from some of the citations found in the *Oxford English Dictionary*. Novelists are really counterfeit dilettantes (the true ones being artists or musicians and their fans), which makes them even more likely to tell the truth than those in the profession of truth-telling: "I'm suspicious about the nature of history or biography, and what really happened and what didn't happen," says Frances Sherwood. "The biographers might rely on Mary's letters, but have you ever written a letter that was a lie? I have."[12] Critics severely chastised each author—even as they praised each for her poetic erudition—for wholesale "fiction-mongering," lying, tampering with the historical record, such as it is, then meddling in the politically correct.[13] The controversies surrounding these novels point to the uneasiness with which we approach those transgressors of boundaries—be they poets, dilettantes, femmes fatales, or feminists.

Toni Morrison took what had been a footnote in histories of the slave community—Margaret Garner's murder of her child (which she found in Angela Davis's citation of Herbert Aptheker's offhanded remark published in a Communist Party USA journal during the cold war years)—as the center of her massive novel about the secret heart of the nation—slavery and racism—and spun pages and pages of sensuous descriptions of clothing, food, work, tools, and instruments of torture.[14] Certain critics faulted her for not leaving these "unspeakable things unspoken."[15] When Morrison tapped the mind of the enslaved mother, she provided a counterhistory from Davis's footnote to the gap in Frederick Douglass's narrative (one of the sources for *Beloved*) about his mother's absence: "I do not recollect of ever seeing my mother by the light of day. She was with me in the night. She would lie down with me, and get me to sleep, but long before I waked she was gone. Very little communication ever took place between us. . . . Never having enjoyed, to any considerable extent, her soothing presence, her tender and watchful care, I received the tidings of her death with much the same emotions I should have probably felt at the death of a stranger."[16] Morrison lets us see a woman who worked from sun to sun then walked miles to sleep briefly with her son. She lets us know that a mother's love can go unrecognized. The tree on Sethe's back, scars left from the horrendous beating she endured as a slave, grow out of his Aunt Hester's whippings; they are her darker scarlet letter. Morrison was savaged, much as Zora Neale Hurston had been during the 1930s, for staging a minstrel show in prose, pandering to the sensational desires of a mass white public—in this case, a white feminist one.

Beloved focuses on "what a woman suffers as a slave," motherhood, and maternity, the emotions, but also the legalities, of blood bonds, ownership, and parental rights, and the racial history of reproduction and property rights, in short, the gothic residue of racialist sexuality.[17] The novel links the history of American racism and the legacy of slavery to contemporary debates on abortion, welfare, and teen pregnancy, which have galvanized the New Right in its backlash against the movements for liberation among African Americans and other racial minorities, and among women and gays of all races. Morrison's novel investigates questions about legitimate and illegitimate mothering, about the work of the reproductive body in the political economy of America, about the discomfort female sexuality elicits within patriarchal culture. Its presentism, its conscious "design to placate sentimental feminist ideology," and its (critical and theoretical) controversies left it open to political attack. Critic Stanley Crouch denounced its "melodrama" and its "biblical grandeur." Because its supernatural elements moved it out of the realm of history into that of fantasy, Crouch likened Morrison's politics and poetics to those of "P. T. Barnum."[18]

Lest it appear that only critics at *The New Republic* express outrage that a novelist tampers with history, Margaret Forster, the feminist biographer of Daphne Du Maurier, revealed a surprisingly similar panic a few years later about Frances Sherwood's *Vindication*. Frances Sherwood's stunning 1993 novel so provoked its *New York Times Book Review* critic that she felt compelled to warn readers that the story of Mary Wollstonecraft being told by Sherwood in this novel was not factually verifiable. But truth is not really what was at issue. In her biography *Love, Anarchy and Emma Goldman*, Candace Falk revealed that the 1970s feminist heroine had been the love slave of Ben Reitman. Doing the work that feminist historians do, Falk had discovered a cache of letters between the anarchist and the hobo in the archives of the Bancroft Library at UC Berkeley. These same sources from private life—diaries and letters—have been the means feminist historians use to place women as a subject in history. However, it seemed from the response to Falk's research that they only attain value if they reinforce positive images about women. With few exceptions, Falk's disclosure about Goldman's "sexual slavery" (the title of Kathy Barry's 1978 book), coming as it did at the height of the feminist sex wars, were met with outrage by feminists.

Unlike Falk, whose facts debunked a kind of feminist heroine worship seeking to align the personal with the political, Sherwood's crime was to embellish the scanty facts and question why we think personal life corresponds to political ideology and action at all. Damned if you do, damned if you don't. Forster's concerns revolve around three distressing scenes in Sherwood's novel: Wollstonecraft's slippage into madness after her break-up with Henry Fusili; her pleasure as a s/m bottom; and her abuse of her first-born daughter, Fanny. None of these incidents, asserts Forster, could possibly have occurred: "Mary Wollstonecraft? Whipped? It's just as likely that she would have snatched the whip and turned it on him," she declares in a huff.[19] That Sherwood's novel takes liberties, if you will, with Wollstonecraft's life and art (Mary Wollstonecraft was after all not only a historian, political theorist, and journalist but a novelist herself) in order to discuss what the reviewer for the *Library Journal* notes as "so many trendy topics—child abuse, mental illness, homosexuality, and drug addiction—without departing from the basic facts" is precisely what makes the novel convincing as a literary history.[20] And, if one takes seriously complaints about biographies and their failure to bring their subjects to life, it is clear that only novelists might be able to animate "the indirect author/hero of this mess."[21]

What else is historiography but a continual revision? Forster's sense that history is cheapened when called to serve the present as if it has sold itself like some bar maid is akin to Crouch's anger at Morrison's appeal to the "ideology . . . [of] the black woman as the most scorned and rebuked of victims." In her own justification of the liberties taken with literary decorum, however, Wollstonecraft argued "I have rather endeavoured to pourtray [sic] passions than manners. . . . I could have made the incidents more dramatic [but] would have sacrificed my main object, the desire of exhibiting the misery and oppression, peculiar to women, that arise out of the partial laws and customs of society. In the invention of the *story*, this view *restrained* my fancy; and the *history* ought to be considered, as of woman, than of an individual."[22] Wollstonecraft's last piece of writing fails as a novel, according to critic Moira Ferguson, because it returns to her treatise on education, coming full circle to reproduce the effect of a political exhortation; in other words, it is not about a character but about a class, womankind.[23] For Wollstonecraft, however, the novel served as a pedagogical tool, another vehicle by which she could traffic in the political arguments of her day. (This is precisely the strategy Caroline Slade employed a century and a half later; see chapter 6.) The reviewer for London's *New Statesman and Society* ultimately champions Wollstonecraft's didactic fiction over Sherwood's fabulation: "If we are Wollstonecraft, then she is us, and the conclusion is somehow much more presumptuous than the premise."[24] But why must this be so? Both authors narrate a feminism that complicates the picture of woman's story and history by depicting women as victims, or, more dangerously, exonerating them as victimizers, or, more damning still, suggesting that they may be both at the same time, constructing, as reviewer Fletcher calls it, "a feminist continuous present." By participating in contemporary political debates through literary history, Sherwood embraces Wollstonecraft's (and indeed feminism's) best history, but the slippage among genres so common in the eighteenth century is highly questionable these days.

Vindication airs many of the dark corners of this continuous contradiction, such as, the noncongruence between ideology and desire as played out in the feminist sex debates of the 1980s. Until the publication of books by Nadine Strossen, Sally Tisdale, and Katha Pollitt, Sherwood's novel was one of the few mainstream publications to push a so-called prosex line.[25] The feminist antiporn argument received wide attention in the mass-marketed form of Andrea Dworkin's tome, *Intercourse*; it was mainstreamed by feminist slicks like *Ms.* and rarefied by the academic legal credentials of Catherine MacKinnon.[26] However, the feminist anticensorship and prosex arguments circulated in work by Pat Califia, Alice Echols, Suzie Bright, and Carol Vance only within small presses and little magazines—Cleis Press, Monthly Review Press, *On Our Backs*.[27] *Vindi-cation* is a history of the present dressed up, in perfect period costume, as a historical fiction from the eighteenth century. If *Vindica-tion* is a history of the present, then of course Wollstonecraft is us. Yet foremothers' names are not to be sullied; women's history celebrates remarkable and exceptional women. To suggest that an Amazon such as Wollstonecraft may have harbored a less-than-PC set of desires is troubling within a backlash world. Sherwood's Wollstonecraft took her cues from the controversies about pornography, s/m, butch/femme, engaging, or rather rupturing, American academic feminism during the 1980s and from 1940s femme fatales.

Joanna Scott's 1990 novel pivots on Viennese artist Egon Schiele's twenty-four day prison sentence in 1912 for "disseminating indecent drawings and endangering public morality." These charges were the only ones to stick after he was accused of abducting a young peasant girl who had posed for his life drawings of nude girls masturbating and embracing.[28] Schiele's case, tried in the village of Neulengbach, was no cause célèbre in prewar Austria, but Scott effectively distills the events preceding and following his arrest to elaborate her rococo meditation on his obsessive artistic genius. The novel is narrated retrospectively by the young girl but relies often on the voice of Schiele's new model and lover. Taking these few weeks as the central instance in the artist's short life, Scott composes a novel that explores the political history of fin-de-siècle Vienna and, of course, anticipates American millennial concerns as well.

As in the other examples, Scott stretches a footnote into a full-length alternative history of the artist and his city.[29] Art historians usually hurry over the "tragic time" of Schiele's imprisonment, minimizing and even dismissing the grim and clearly political poetry screaming from his self-portraits made in his cell.[30] Intent on viewing Schiele as "one of the most normal" people whose life "was relatively eventless," critics declare in no way was he a "rebel"; rather he was only concerned with his art, which figurative and erotic, to be sure, is really just abstraction because the images are not fixed spatially. They float without orientation to ground.[31] However, as curator James Demetrios has implied, precisely because these works are aberrations in Schiele's career—they are dated, titled, and the figures do appear in spatial contexts—they should be seen as significant; they interrupt the more purely formalist considerations dominating art history, in general, and Schiele criticism in particular.[32] These twelve charcoal, pencil, and watercolor studies of the artist curled under thin blankets on his bare cot are captioned with such inflammatory titles as "To Confine the Artist Is A CRIME, It MEANS MURDERING UNBORN LIFE" or "For My Art I Will Gladly Endure to the END." Schiele's melodramatic *cri du coeur* anticipated a history of censorship within European nations, from Hitler's Germany to Stalin's Soviet Union, that destroyed works and lives. However, his more local, seemingly less political, trial and imprisonment has even more in common with recent events in the United States.

Again, Scott's exaggerated literary history provides a device for probing the present. Like Sherwood, she pushes fiction into an argument with biography. Scott, too, was chastised by critics, who could not fault the novel's "sensuous, provocative patterns" detailed through "rich experiences, intriguing perceptions." Yet she failed to "bring either Schiele or his art to life" being "more . . . a treatise than a novel, it's often bulky with exposition, and perilously short on active characters and dramatic scenes."[33] Of course, because Scott chooses to focus on the trial and imprisonment of the artist for pornography, one can hardly miss her very contemporary references to arts' funding and censorship controversies circulating around the Cincinnati Art Musuem's exhibit of Robert Mapplethorpe's photography, Andre Serranos's "Piss Christ," performance artists Karen Finley, Holly Hughes, and the rest of the NEA Four, and other cases that figured so prominently in the sexual hysteria of the Reagan/Bush years. Less well known perhaps was the case of Jacqueline Livingston, a photographer who was fired from her Cornell University job after complaints surfaced about a series of nude photographic portraits she took of her father-in-law, then husband, and son. What caused the ruckus was a sequence of images of her young son masturbating; these were interpreted to be child pornography. Other cases—such as the furor over Sally Mann's book of photographs about her children, or Jock Sturges's investigation by the FBI after lab technicians claimed his nude images of his and friends' children trafficked in child pornography—were less well publicized than the case of the NEA Four but are even more chilling in their implications. Feminist artists and curators, such as Connie Samaras, Carol Jacobson, and Carole Vance, have repeatedly demonstrated—in their work, their writings, and most particularly in their struggle to present others' work—that there are large and dangerous unintended consequences to feminist challenges to pornography.[34] Those most interested in policing degrading images enable the state to determine deviance, which includes even feminists. Art and female desire suffer in the name of protection. But anyone who had been watching film noirs already knew this.

CORRESPONDENCES

Even if critics have had a rough time recognizing the singular contributions of these women's literary histories, I hope I have made it clear that the novels borrow from a feminist literary tradition operative since Wollstonecraft. Like the femme fatale, feminist literary history emerges on the threshold between the enigma and the stereotype, the unwritten and the rewritten.[35] Like Walter Benjamin's "Angel of History," this angle on history ever looks over its shoulders even as it plants itself firmly in the present, only to be blown forward by the storms of complaint. Anne Stevenson's verse history reimagined America from the perspective of those just barely outside its center—middle-class WASP women—and returns the novel to its epistolary origins, even as she pushed poetic diction into everyday vernacular. The many women who write most of these letters are shown to be willful, contemptible, self-involved, racist, pathetic, anguished; they speak of money, violence, war, civil unrest, madness, sex, children, and poetry, tracing how families produce and reproduce themselves. In short, they survey all the debates raging among feminists during the late 1960s and 1970s.

For two hundred years, the work of feminism has been, in part, to peer into the recesses of private life, to locate it within public and political culture. Unraveling family and, by extension, social history through the discovered sack of letters hanging like the Moor's shriveled head at which the young Orlando jousts his make-believe lance in the chilly attic of his ancestral home formed Josephine Herbst's 1930s Trexler trilogy.[36] Herbst's one-hundred-year saga of her family's struggle to achieve and maintain middle-class stability developed from the stories Herbst heard her mother tell during long hours spent hiding in storm shelters against the tornadoes of western Iowa. Her mother's stories, retold by Anne Trexler, were kept alive through her words, but their veracity depended on the "bags of old letters hanging from the rafter like beheaded corpses as if the written works of the dead somehow pledged the family to immortality."[37] Letters in the attic, mildewed and moth-eaten, like the moldy packet found in Hawthorne's Custom-House, keep memory and history alive. They legitimate the secret history of any family lucky enough to possess a house, eventually becoming the sources for subsequent social histories once their location has been discovered and their secrets deposited in the archives for future generations of scholars to peruse. The novelist has privileged access to this source of family immortality, of history—her letters may even be among those saved. Herbst obliquely makes this point by including excerpts of her own reportage, often written in the form of letters to *The New Masses* from various sites of struggle: foreclosed farms and dairy cooperatives in the Midwest; sugarcane workers' soviets in Realengo, Cuba; the anti-Nazi underground in Berlin. These documentary narratives shore up the literary history of postbellum America encapsulated in the Trexler saga.

As Woolf and Herbst knew, stealing the words of one's forebears provides fodder for exactly the kind of story most fitting for pulp modernist narrative. Hart Crane reveals a secret affair in his poem, "My Grandmother's Love Letters," which were "pressed so long / Into a corner of the roof / That they are brown and soft, / And liable to melt as snow."[38] Discovered, we learn from his biographer, in the secret hideout Crane found for his boyhood masturbation, they let us in on the author's desires more than his grandmother's. Crane's discovery of his grandmother's secret literary history, "hung by an invisible white hair," then rummaged in the family archives of the attic, updates an American Gothic convention—revealing the secret of the purloined letter or the Custom-House.[39] Nathanael West's *Miss Lonelyhearts* trafficked in the sad, absurd letters sent to his desk by those lacking the stability of a house with an attic, those on the margins of a commodified world of canned emotion, in search of hope and advice from the all-knowing soothing voice of a dissipated, alienated journalist. Anne Stevenson, like Herbst and West, shifted the modernist focus from the secret reader of (scarlet) letters to the social saga they narrated, returning to Hawthorne's romance, turning private dispatch into political diatribe. The racial and sexual inversions connecting Anne Hutchinson to Aunt Hester in *The Scarlet Letter*, on the one hand, or Stevenson's Kathy Chattle to Morrison's Sethe, on the other, crisscross the map of noir. Esther Bubley's bus trip west through Ohio then south through Kentucky reversed the direction the pregnant Sethe took after she escaped bondage at Sweet Home. Perhaps Bubley's Greyhound passed the train hurtling Cross Damon east to Penn Station where he might have glimpsed Lutie Johnson waiting on the platform enroute to Chicago. The forces that banished the pious Anne Hutchinson from the city on the hill were different from those that sent Bubley, a Russian-Jewish girl from the heartland of Superior, Wisconsin, to New York and Washington, D.C., three hundred years later, but they were not that different: a restless, rebellious desire spurred by the darkness lurking within themselves and their landscapes. They followed the map of the hundreds of film noirs from the postwar years and the thousands of photographs from the Depression decade, as well as the many novels and poems that echo them, as they strayed off the highway and found the detour toward the political truth of pulp fiction, which charts, in black and white and noir, America's pulp modernism.

NOTES

INTRODUCTION: ON PULP MODERNISM

1. Simone de Beauvoir, *America Day by Day*, trans. Carol Cosman (Berkeley: University of California Press, 1999), 113.

2. Theodor Adorno, *Minima Moralia: Reflections from Damaged Life*, trans. E. F. N. Jephcott (1974; reprint, London: Verso, 1984), 48.

3. Mary McCarthy, "Mlle. Gulliver en Amerique," in *On the Contrary: Articles of Belief, 1946–1961* (New York: Farrar, Strauss, Cudahy, 1962), 24–31.

4. As this book was going to press, the Twin Towers of the World Trade Center were destroyed by two hijacked airplanes killing thousands and transforming the New York skyline. De Beauvoir's prescience about the aftermath of World War II was horribly fulfilled.

5. Nelson Algren, *Chicago: City on the Make* (Sausalito, Calif.: Contact Books, 1961), 105.

6. Richard Severo, "Jane Greer, 76, Film Noir Star Who Returned to Do a Remake," *New York Times*, August 28, 2001, A17. In her obituary, Jane Greer, co-star with Robert Mitchum in *Out of the Past*, is quoted as replying to her son, when he told her she was the "Queen of Film Noir," that she really didn't know what film noir was.

7. Quoted in C. L. R. James, *American Civilization*, ed. Anna Grimshaw and Keith Hart (Oxford: Basil Blackwell, 1993), 130.

8. See Nino Frank, "A New Kind of Police Drama: The Criminal Adventure" (1946) and "Americans Are Also Making *Noir* Films" (1946), in Alain Silver and James Ursini, eds., *Film Noir Reader* 2, 15–24 (New York: Limelight Editions, 1999).

9. Quoted in Jane Jacobs, *The Death and Life of Great American Cities* (New York: Vintage, 1961), 310.

10. Ann Douglas, *The Feminization of American Culture* (New York: Knopf, 1977), argues that with the rise of sentimental female fiction in the mid-nineteenth century, American intellectuals were forced to resort to a rhetoric of cheap emotions to effect political change. Andreas Huyssen, "Mass Culture

as Woman," *After the Great Divide: Modernism, Mass Culture, Postmodernism* (Bloomington: Indiana University Press, 1986), argues that a virile modernist poetics raged against the decadence of a feminized popular realm.

11. For a new assessment of the many vernancular modernisms found in mid-century America, see Jani Scandura and Michael Thurston, eds., *Modernism, Inc.: Body, Memory, Capital* (New York: New York University Press, 2001).

12. Michael Szalay, *New Deal Modernism: American Literature and The Invention of The Welfare State* (Durham: Duke University Press, 2000); Saverio Giovacchino, *Hollywood Modernism: Film and Politics in the Age of the New Deal* (Philadelphia: Temple University Press, 2001); Jani Scandura and Michael Thirston, eds. *Modernism, Inc.: Body, Memory Capital* (New York: New York University Press, 2001) refer to "vernacular modernism," as does Paul Buhle among others; Cary Nelson discusses the modernism "we have wanted to forget" in *Revolutionary Memory: Recovering the Poetry of the American Left* (New York: Routledge, 2001); Marshall Berman speaks of "low" and "street" modernism in *All That is Solid Melts into Air: The Experience of Modernity* (New York: Penguin, 1988). Houston A. Baker, Jr., *Modernsim and the Harlem Renaissance* (Chicago: University of Chicago Press, 1987) outlines an "Afro-American modernism." In his address to the 2001 Modernist Studies Association convention, Ramon Saldívar identified a "transnational modernism" in the poetry of Americo Paredes.

13. Kenneth Fearing, "C Stands for Civilization," *Collected Poems of Kenneth Fearing* (1940), New York: AMS Press, 1977, p. 101. All further references appear in the text.

14. For a discussion of Fearing's use of advertising slogans, see Rita Barnard, *The Great Depression and the Culture of Abdundance: Kenneth Fearing, Nathanael West, and Mass Culture in the 1930s* (Cambridge: Cambridge University Press, 1995), esp, chapter 5.

15. Klaus Theweleit, *Male Fantasies, vol. 1.: Women, Floods, Bodies, History* Trans. Stephen Conway (Minneapolis: University of Minnesota Press, 1987).

16. Gilles Deleuze, *Coldness and Cruelty*, in *Masochism* (New York: Zone Books, 1991), 72.

17. Adorno, *Minima Moralia* , 218.

18. See Laurence Miller, "Evidence for a British *Film Noir* Cycle," *Film Criticism* 16 no. 2 (1991): 42–51, which lists 331 films made between 1940 and 1959; Tony Williams, "British *Film Noir*," in Alain Silver and James Ursini, eds., *Film Noir Reader 2* (New York: Limelight Editions, 1999), 243–70, also lists hundreds of films and stresses the interplay between American directors, actors, and writers and their British counterparts to suggest that there is both a distinctive British version, and to argue that it had an impact on American film as much as it borrowed from it.

19. For an extended analysis of the markings of race and ethnicity in this film, see E. Ann Kaplan, " 'The Dark Continent of Film Noir': Race, Displacement and Metaphor in Tourneur's *Cat People* (1942) and Welles's *The Lady from Shanghai* (1948)," in E. Ann Kaplan, ed. *Women in Film Noir*, 2nd ed. (London: British Film Institute, 1998), 183–201.

20. Rosita Forbes, *Women Called Wild* (New York: E. P. Dutton, Inc., 1937). The final chapter of her book, which follows female slaves and prostitutes and communists and soldiers around the world, concludes with the stories of a fox woman from Central America and a hyena woman from Abyssinia. Bram Dijkstra, *Evil Sisters: The Threat of Female Sexuality and the Cult of Manhood* (New York: Alfred Knopf, 1996), details how the "endless procession of gigantic spiders, vampires, cats, tentacled monsters, snake-bedecked women, women with (or better yet, turning into) wolves, black panthers, gorillas, bats, cobras, and whatever other gaping-mouthed predators . . . were to become the most lasting cultural heritage of turn-of-the-century biological 'science' " (146). He uses the *Amazing Stories* cover from October 1949 to illuminate how "the biology of female reversion [was] revealed by pulp" (caption, 147).

21. Charlotte Nekola, "Ida Lupino," *Dream House: A Memoir* (New York: W. W. Norton, 1993), 89–92.

22. This catalog could go on and on, an ever-proliferating list of neo-retro-noir films, novels, photographs, fashion, neighborhoods, etc. See, among many such examples, William L. Hamilton, "Style Noir," *New York Times*, September 15, 1997, B1, 6; Peter Marks, "As It Turns Artistic, A Noirish Enclave Steps Into the Light," *New York Times*, October 10, 1997, B1, 26 [about Dumbo in Brooklyn]; Constance C. R. White, "Why Coy Can Sizzle Hotter Than Brazen," *New York Times*, November 5, 1997, A23, which describes designer John Bartlett's "noir-inspired tomato-red leather coat" for "vixens." The year 1997 marked the fiftieth anniversary of the Hollywood blacklist; a commemoration held at the Academy of Motion Picture Arts and Sciences was organized by the industry's unions. Shunned by studio executives, it ended in a noir fashion: "A sad footnote to the evening was the death of the 82-year-old screenwriter Paul Jarrico, another blacklist victim, whose car ran off the road when he was on his way home," reported Bernard Weinraub, " At the Movies," *New York Times*, October 31, 1997, 11. For the twentieth anniversary of Roman Polanski's "renovating" the genre in *Chinatown*, see Jim Shepard, "Jolting Noir With a Shot of Nihilism," *New York Times*, February 9, 1999, Arts and Leisure, 24. Spike Lee's noirish resurrection of the 1977 Son of Sam summer, *Summer of Sam*, used an advertisement splashing the tabloid headlines from the *Daily News* across a full page of the Arts and Leisure section of the *New York Times*, May 2, 1999, 31. A Turner Classic Movies channel film noir series featuring less–well known noir films provided the occasion for Bernard Weinraub to gather four surviving femme fatales showcased in this series to remi-

nisce about their screen personae. "They're Gorgeous, Mysterious and Ready to Make a Sap Out of You," *New York Times*, August 23, 1999, B1, 5. In 1999, the Oscars were disrupted by supporters of Abraham Polonsky and other black-listed directors protesting the unanimous decision of the Academy of Motion Picture Arts and Sciences presentation of an honorary Oscar to Elia Kazan, see Bernard Weinraub, "Early Oscars Go to Coburn, Dench, and 'Shakespeare'," *New York Times*, March 22, 1999, B1, 3.

23. Janet Maslin, "The Rewards of Obsessing About Film," *New York Times*, April 14, 2001, A20.

24. Michael Pye noted that the protagonist "is also, noticeably, a film creature. She's in dark glasses, with a classy car and perfect makeup, a mouth like a red gash—like every thieving, conniving woman in a film noir. Like, say Janet Leigh in the start of *Psycho*. Her wig comes off, to shocking effect, in sexual fights, just like Connie Towers (remember?) in *The Naked Kiss*. "Serial Mom," *New York Times Book Review*, April 10, 1999, 29. The month before, Ed McBain described the formula for the "2 or 3 cents a word" private eye story: "I always started a P.I. story with a blonde wearing a tight shiny dress. When she crossed her legs, you saw rib-topped silk stockings and garters taut against milky white flesh, boy." "She Was Blond. She Was in Trouble. And She Paid 3 Cents a Word.," *New York Times*, March 29, 1999, B1, 3. However, commenting on the "explosion in the ethnicity of the detectives," Martin Arnold notes "the ranks of the new-breed fictional detective include gay teachers, a lesbian restaurant owner, a document examiner, psychologists, a forensic anthropologist, a quadriplegic police criminologist, a sports agent, an Egyptologist. . . . In short, all have professions. They don't have to depend on a sexy woman slipping them a pair of greasy Ben Franklins." "Making Books," *New York Times*, April 15, 1999, B3.

25. Nicholas Christopher, *Somewhere in the Night: Film Noir and the American City* (New York: Free Press, 1997), insists with the French critics that film noir is "*a way of seeing the world*" (63; emphasis in original). He dissects the interconnections among the cell-like rooms of each apartment building, every office building in the modern city, and the bridges, cars, trains traversing them and linking them that reveal the inner workings of an alienating yet all-pervasive postwar capitalism. Eddie Muller, *Dark City: The Lost World of Film Noir* (New York: St. Martins. 1998), places the films and their audiences within this wild imaginary landscape. He understands that all film noirs, no matter where they are set, are about this doomed place.

I. ALREADY FRAMED: ESTHER BUBLEY INVENTS NOIR

1. See Giuliana Bruno, *Streetwalking on a Ruined Map: Cultural Theory and the City Films of Elvira Notari* (Princeton: Princeton University Press,

1993), for a discussion of the role urban movies—both as sites and as sights, that is, both the theater spaces themselves and the images that were shown there—played in unleashing urban Italian women from the constraints of the home.

2. Esther Bubley, United States Office of War Information Negative #LC22132-D. All citations from the Esther Bubley Collection of the FSA/OWI photographs in the Library of Congress.

3. Andrea Fisher, *Let Us Now Praise Famous Women: Women Photographers for the U.S. Government, 1935 to 1944* (London: Pandora, 1987), 105.

4. Bubley, OWI Negative #LC21005-E.

5. Bubley, OWI Negative #LC21016-E

6. Bubley, OWI Negative #LC21021-E.

7. Cornell Woolrich [William Irish], *I Married a Dead Man* (1948) (New York: Penguin Books, 1982), 19. The novel was made into the 1950 noir melodrama starring Barbara Stanwyck, *No Man of Her Own.* (Like *Raw Deal*, it was one of the rare examples, *Mildred Pierce* being another maternal noir that also starts with a woman's [Joan Crawford] recollections, to feature a female voice-over narration).

8. OWI Negative #LC38314-E. Esther Bubley's caption.

9. Naremore deconstructs the famous sex scene in *Out of the Past*, which is encoded through actions that reposition a lamp and the door, suggesting that "the codes of erotic lighting have an affinity with the codes of mystery lighting." He goes on: "After drying Kathie's [Jane Greer] hair with a towel, Jeff [Robert Mitchum] passionately embraces her and tosses the towel across the lamp, which pitches over in a gust of wind from the open doorway." Then the camera shifts outside the cabin returning as Jeff's silhouette looms up from the dark to shut the door. James Naremore, *More Than Night: Film Noir in Its Contexts* (Berkeley: University of California Press, 1998), 182.

10. These are all images from OWI negative nos. 32333–32353, specifically, 32340-E, 32334-E, 32351-E, and 32342-E.

11. See Miles Barth, ed., *Weegee's World* (New York: International Century of Photography/ Boston: Bulfinch Press, 1997), for information on Weegee.

12. See, for instance, Eunice Fuller Barnard, "College Girl: 1932–33," *Scribner's Magazine* 94 (January 1933): 51. For more on the educated, professional woman's image during the 1930s, see Laura Hapke, *Daughters of the Great Depression: Women, Work, and Fiction in the American 1930s* (Athens: University of Georgia Press, 1995), ch. 6.

13. In "Kiss the City Goodbye," *Lusitania* 7 (Spring 1996): 56–66, and "City of Fear: Defensive Dispersal and the End of Film Noir," *Any* 18 (1997): 14–18, Edward Dimendberg argues that these two zones of film noir imagi-

nation are differentiated not only spatially but temporally as well when the road became significant with postwar suburbanization and highway subsidies; however, many early and classic film noirs—*Detour* and *Out of the Past*, among them—are located in the movement from one zone to the other, anticipating the zigzagging back and forth between the old neighborhood and the new by the embourgeoisment of the white ethnic working class throughout the 1950s and '60s.

14. Minneapolis College of Art and Design Calendar of Events, Special Commencement Edition, May 1998, n.p.

15. From a handwritten biographical résumé in her working notebook of 1965. Uncataloged papers, Esther Bubley estate. Jean Bubley, executor.

16. Rosita Forbes, *Women Called Wild* (New York: E. P. Dutton & Co., Inc., 1938). The volume is illustrated with incredible woodcuts by Isobel R. Beard.

17. Two novels from the late 1930s—Bessie Breuer's *The Daughter* (New York: Simon and Schuster, 1938) and Leane Zugsmith's *A Time to Remember* (New York: Random House, 1936)—consider the emerging conflicts building within young Jewish women who have been provided with an education and are trying to Americanize themselves. Zugsmith's novel, which addressed family conflicts arising when daughters, rather than fathers, found work, was based on the League of Women Shoppers' support for the newly organized shopgirls at Orbach's. Breuer's novel focused on an alienated teenager whose divorced mother is too preoccupied to notice that her daughter's growing suicidal depression stemmed only when the girl meets up with striking fisherman and farmworkers in Florida. Both link a crisis in lower-middle-class Jewish life to the economic crisis facing the nation during the Depression. Part of what unsettles these young women is the ways in which they must enter the workforce despite family conflicts about the resulting freedom. Zugsmith's Aline Weinstein and Breuer's daughter test out sexual and political autonomy opened up for middle-class Jewish girls by the Left; they meet Gentile men with whom they have relationships, and they join political groups antithetical to their parents' limited political involvements. Moreover, middle-class possibilities of shopping, white-collar work, and travel have dislodged them from ghetto or community ties, secured by religion, labor unions, and family. Only the Left offers a replacement for these. By the 1940s, Communist Party membership was almost 50 percent female, and with almost 50 percent of the Party being Jewish, this became a space of Jewish female circulation. Bubley's upper Midwestern Jewish background is reflected back at her in the mirrors of the girls in rooming houses, with one, Pearl Ginsburg, clearly a radical, who has refused to pay her rent increase. See Paula Rabinowitz, *Labor and Desire; Women's Revolutionary Fiction in Depression America* (Chapel Hill: University of

North Carolina Press, 1991), and "Not Sappho, Sacco: Women, Art and Movement in the 1930s," *Intellectual History Newsletter* 19 (1997): 15–18; Laura Hapke, *Daughters of the Great Depression: Women, Work, and Fiction in the American 1930s* (Athens: University of Georgia Press, 1995).

18. Simone de Beauvoir, *America Day by Day*, trans. Carol Cosman (Berkeley: University of California Press, 1999), 165.

19. Unpublished typescript excerpts of a transcription of an interview by Tony Van Witsen of NBC, November 4, 1984, p. 6. Esther Bubley estate.

20. "Life in a Waiting Room," Photograph from series with text about the "entire story of bus transportation . . . made for the Standard Oil Co. of New Jersey." Esther Bubley estate. The series won first prize in the Picture Sequence category of the annual competition sponsored by the Encyclopaedia Brittanica Book of the Year and the University of Missouri School of Journalism.

21. Katherine Dieckmann, "Photography: A Nation of Zombies," *Art in America* 77 (November 1989): 55–57.

22. Bubley, OWI Negative #LC37670-E (Chicago, Ill., Sept. 1943).

23. Bubley, OWI Negative #LC37932-E. Bubley's caption reads: "A girl getting off the Macon bound Greyhound bus in Georgia. Passengers can get off at any place they wish along the road." September, 1943.

24. Bubley, OWI Negative #LC37468-E "A gas station on the road between Columbus and Cincinnati, Ohio, which is now used as a home. It is only one of many which are so converted." September, 1943.

25. Bubley, OWI Negative #LC37684-E (Chicago, Ill., Sept. 1943).

26. In a 1956 diary entry logging a job for Pepsi International (between Managua and Mexico City), she lists the following images: "air travel, passengers, baggage, cargo, behind scenes, different kinds of country, drinking (Pepsi), eating, embarking, disembarking, meeting and greeting, leave taking, reservations." Esther Bubley estate.

27. Caption for OWI Negative #37430, Esther Bubley Bus Trip, September 1943. This list runs down two pages and includes various brand names as modifiers– "Barbasol shaving cream," "Lux soap," as well as explanations for "ammonia inhalant (in case you get sleepy at night)," and "witness pad (for accidents)." Typescript, 5-6; Esther Bubley collection. In the typescript entitled "Bus Driver and Family," Bubley narrates the stories of the drivers and of the passengers in greater detail. This packet of materials included bus schedules and advertisements, as well as a detailed twenty-page description of the driver and passengers, featuring the recount of "Us on a Bus."

28. See note 26.

29. Bubley, OWI Negative #LC36894-E

30. de Beauvoir, *America*, 165.

31. 1948 diary/workbook. Esther Bubley estate.

32. Joan Younger, "What *Is* Mental Illness?" *Ladies Home Journal* 64 (April 1949): 36–37, 234. Follow-up articles by Joan Younger urged consideration of "Public Enemy # One: Mental Illness" and called for solutions in "Psychiatry Needs You," showing the necessary work of psychiatric nurses.

33. There are two boxes of photographs from "Mental Hospitals" in the Esther Bubley estate.

34. This picture won a prize in an exhibit at the University of Missouri. It became a standard image in psychiatry textbooks.

35. The *DSM-I* (1950) called this depression "involutional psychotic reaction." The *DSM-II* (1968) defines involutional melancholia as a "disorder . . . characterized by worry, anxiety, agitation, and severe insomnia. Feelings of guilt and somatic preoccupations are frequently present and may be of delusional proportions." In 1969, Francis J. Braceland was reporting on "Changes in the Treatment of Involutional Melancholia," in *Hospital and Community Psychiatry* 20 (May 1969): 136–40, and touting the improvements found in patients undergoing the "safeguards" in electroshock that aided recovery, where previous uses of endocrine replacement therapy had been unsuccessful on the women diagnosed. He describes those he encountered in the 1930s as follows: "Their child-bearing period was over; their children were grown, their husbands busy; their early dreams and desires were not to be fulfilled; their sexual life, if it ever was interesting, was waning. The future held little for them but old age and loneliness. To those who had traded upon their physical attractiveness, it was an especially distressing time. It was an era when women hated and resented middle-age and the menopause, and their anxiety and hostility could be expressed only against themselves. It was a period, too, when women were not as emancipated as they are today. They seemed to age more quickly in the culture of the 1930s, and what the future held had little charm for them" (29). However, a decade later, when the next *DSM* was in preparation, Margaret Weissman was unmasking "The Myth of Involutional Melacholia" in the pages of *Journal of American Medicine* 242 (August 24–31, 1979): 742–44. Her research set off a slew of investigations questioning "Is There an Involutional Melancholia?," which noted that by the end of the Second World War, the "place of involutional melancholia seemed well assured." P. Pichot and C. Pull, in *Comprehensive Psychiatry* 22 (January/February 1981): 2–10; yet a decade after feminism, it had disappeared.

36. *The Story of Serpasil* (Summit, N.J.: Ciba Pharmaceutical Products, Inc., 1955). This promotional brochure is in the Esther Bubley estate and can be found in the University of Minnesota Biomedical Library.

37. Esther Bubley, "Research for November *Profile of Youth* for 1949 *Ladies Home Journal*, p. 3. Esther Bubley estate.

38. Title of the photo essay done for OWI. Esther Bubley Collection.

39. "Working School Girl," "Teen-Age Poison," "Teen-Age Cruelty," *Ladies Home Journal* (November 1949): 62–66.

40. Journal entry, Feb. 18 (n.d. [1950?]). Rome, Italy. Esther Bubley estate. In this entry, Bubley notes that she has discovered her "ancestors." "I have joined the human race. It is like finding ones [sic] family at last."

41. Telephone conversation with Sally Forbes, Bubley's assistant, September 29, 1999.

2. DOMESTIC LABOR: FILM NOIR, PROLETARIAN LITERATURE, AND BLACK WOMEN'S FICTION

1. James Naremore, *More Than Night: Film Noir in Its Contexts* (Berkeley: University of California Press, 1998), 240–41. Naremore connects this to Norman Mailer's "White Negro" and the emergence of a critique of racism within Hollywood cinema in the wake of the Second World War.

2. Walter Benjamin, "The Work of Art in the Age of Mechanical Reproduction," in Hannah Arendt, ed., *Illuminations*, trans. Harry Zohn (New York: Schocken Books, 1969), 220.

3. Benjamin, "The Work of Art," 223–34.

4. Speaking of the 1940s', " 'woman's film' (or more accurately, the 'white woman's film')," Mary Ann Doane's notes: "When black women are present [in the 'woman's film'], they are the ground rather than the figure; often they are made to merge with the diegesis. They inhabit the textual sidelines, primarily as servants." *Femmes Fatales: Feminism, Film Theory, Psychoanalysis* (New York: Routledge, 1991), 232–33.

5. Fanny Hurst's novel *Imitation of Life* (1933) was immediately turned into a film by John Stahl (1934), then revived in 1959 by Douglas Sirk. It has served as a nodal point for much feminist theorizing on race, identity, and sexuality. See Mary Ann Doane, "Dark Continents: Epistemologies of Racial and Sexual Difference in Psychoanalysis and Cinema, in *Femmes Fatales*, 209–48; Marian Heung, " 'What's the Matter with Sara Jane?': Daughters and Mothers in Douglas Sirk's *Imitation of Life*," *Cinema Journal* 26, no. 3 (Spring 1987): 21–43; Sandy Flitterman-Lewis, "*Imitation(s) of Life*: The Black Woman's Double Determination as Troubling 'Other',"*Literature and Psychology* 34, no. 4 (1988): 44–57; Lauren Berlant, "National Brands/National Body: *Imitation of Life*," in Hortense Spillers, ed., *Comparative American Identities: Race, Sex, and Nationality in the Modern Text* (New York: Routledge, 1991), 110–40.

6. The whole question of what the "Left" was during this period is up for grabs; however, James Smethurst describes the nexus of intellectuals, writers, and organizations in Chicago that nurtured Gwendolyn Brooks as the "CPUSA subculture" of Chicago; he notes that Ann Petry wrote for "the Left-influenced newspaper," *People's Voice*. He cites a 1950 *Phylon*,

review of "New Poets," where Margaret Walker called Brooks a "forties" writer. James Smethurst, *The New Red Negro: The Literary Left and American American Poetry, 1930–1946* (New York: Oxford University Press, 1999), 58, 41, 179. See also William J. Maxwell, *New Negro, Old Left: African-American Writing and Communism Between the Wars* (New York: Columbia University Press, 1999), 2.

7. For a materialist reading of American naturalism, see June Howard, *Form and History in American Naturalism* (Chapel Hill: University of North Carolina Press, 1985); for a reading of *Cat People* as a racial allegory, see E. Ann Kaplan, "The 'Dark Continent' of Film Noir: Race, Displacement and Metaphor in Tourneur's *Cat People* (1942) and Welles's *The Lady from Shanghai* (1948)." In E. Ann Kaplan, ed., *Women in Film Noir*, 2nd ed. (London: British Film Institute, 1998), 183–201.

8. Alan Wald, *Writing From the Left: New Essays on Radical Culture and Politics* (London: Verso, 1994), and Michael Denning, *The Cultural Front: The Laboring of American Culture* (London: Verso, 1996), have different perspectives on this subject; but both agree that limiting cultural radicalism to the novels written during the 1930s [as Barbara Foley, *Radical Representations: Politics and Form in U.S. Proletarian Fiction, 1929–1941* (Durham, N.C.: Duke University Press, 1993); Robert Shulman, *The Power of Political Art: The 1930s Literary Left Reconsidered* (Chapel Hill: University of North Carolina Press, 2000); and many others, myself included, have done], skews the cultural vision of American radicalism by connecting it firmly to an established genre and a conventional period. When I was thinking through the difference gender made on the proletarian novel in *Labor and Desire: Women's Revolutionary Fiction in Depression America* (Chapel Hill: University of North Carolina Press, 1991), I limited my investigations to the years between Agnes Smedley's *Daughter of Earth* (1929) and Mary McCarthy's *The Company She Keeps* (1941), including works by Tillie Olsen and Meridel Le Sueur that had been completed during the 1930s but never published until the 1970s; however, I excluded Margaret Walker's *Jubilee* because she spent more than twenty years writing it. By delimiting the subject as I had— trying to read the novels produced in direct response to the pronouncements of literary radicals, like Michael Gold and Philip Rahv—I had contributed to another form of what I criticized them and their subsequent literary historians and critics of doing. Just as they failed to see women's literary radicalism, because gender and sexuality reconfigured the form and content of proletarian culture, by limiting my study to a period and a genre, I failed to see how black nationalism and feminism further revised proletarian literature.

9. But, as I will show in chapter 3, Richard Wright's 1953 answer to *Invisible Man, The Outsider*, is a postwar work.

10. Grace Hutchins, *Women Who Work* (1934), summarized the double burden of the working-class woman as follows: "[O]n top of a long day's work in the home, the working mother goes out for another stretch of five or six hours' work, scrubbing and cleaning floors and stairs and toilets. . . . " in Charlotte Nekola and Paula Rabinowitz, eds., *Writing Red: An Anthology of American Women Writers, 1930–1940* (New York: The Feminist Press, 1987), 339.

11. Mel Watkins, "Gwendolyn Brooks, 83, Passionate Poet, Dies," *New York Times*, December 5, 2000, C22. " 'I wrote about what I saw and heard in the street,' Ms. Brooks once said. 'I lived in a small second-floor apartment at the corner, and I could look first on one side and then the other. There was my material.' " The Bronzeville poems were recommended to the editors of Harper & Row by Richard Wright, who admired her ability to capture "the pathos of petty destinies, the whimper of the wounded, the tiny incidents that plague the lives of the desperately poor, and the problems of common prejudice." Watkins notes that "Ms. Brooks wrote a novel, *Maud Martha*, which received scant consideration when it was published in 1953. [It] was overshadowed by her achievements as a poet and invidiously compared with Richard Wright's *Native Son* and Ralph Ellison's *Invisible Man*, epic novels with clear-cut socio-political themes."

12. Belle Traub, "Discovered: A Modern Slave Block!" *The Negro Liberator* (June 15, 1935), quoted in Mary Battenfeld, "The World Problem is a Personal Problem: Women Document the 1930s," which analyzes this article. (Paper delivered at American Studies Association, New Orleans 1988.)

13. Ella Baker and Marvel Cooke, "The Bronx Slave Market," *The Crisis* 42 (November 1935): 330–31, 340.

14. Louise Mitchell, "Slave Markets Typify Exploitation of Domestic," *The Daily Worker* (May 5, 1940). Reprinted in Gerda Lerner, ed., *Black Women in White America: A Documentary History* (New York: Vintage Books, 1973), 229–31.

15. Barker and Cooke, "Bronx Slave Market," 331. Two years later, Marvel Cooke described the efforts of domestics to organize the Domestic Workers' Union and win uniform contracts. Marvel Cooke, "Modern Slaves," *The Amsterdam News* (October 16, 1937), in Lerner, *Black Women in White America*, 232–34.

16. Marita Bonner Occomy, "One True Love," in Joyce Flynn and Joyce Occomy Stricklin, *Frye Street and Environs: The Collected Works of Marita Bonner* (1941; reprint, Boston: Beacon Press, 1987), 219–27. Originally published in *Opportunity*, this story of the futility of black female struggles for education may have been an impetus for Brooks's character, Hattie's, bitter assessment of night school.

17. Gwendolyn Brooks, *Blacks* (Chicago: Third World Press, 1994), 52.

All further citations to Brooks's works come from this collection and appear in the body of the text.

18. Jacqueline Jones, *Labor of Love, Labor of Sorrow: Black Women, Work and the Family from Slavery to the Present* (New York: Vintage Books, 1985), 220.

19. "Harlem Crime," *The Crisis* 46 (December 1939): 366, 377–78.

20. Ann Petry, *The Street* (Boston: Houghton Mifflin, 1946), 41, 45. All further references from this edition appear in the body of the text.

21. Chester Himes, *The Quality of Hurt* (New York: Paragon House, 1972), 28.

22. Ibid., 18–19. Frederick Douglass, *Narrative of the Life of Frederick Douglass, An American Slave, Written by Himself* (1845; reprint, Garden City, N.Y.: Dolphin Books, 1963), 3.

23. Doc and Lou reported in the *Daily Worker* that it was "Not Sunny for Girl Slaves in 'Sunny' Florida," who worked fifteen-hour days as waitresses for $5 and picked up "a little extra on the side" from a "man friend" (January 4, 1929): 4. Waiting tables, as a public form of domestic service, thus is directly linked to prostitution; it is through the restaurant that the woman finds her clients. Another issue of the *Daily Worker* features two articles headlined: "Scrub Women Slave While World Sleeps; Wages Miserable" and "In Chicago, Waitresses Slave 70 Hour Week as Union Officials Fail Them" (March 13, 1929): 4. Again these women are defined as slaves because they serve and scrub, like domestics, in public places.

24. *Daily Worker* (September 23, 1929): 3.

25. Bessie Smith, "Washerwoman's Blues," 1928. *Empty Bed Blues* (Columbia G30450).

26. Phyllis Palmer, *Domesticity and Dirt: Housewives and Domestic Servants in the United States, 1920–1945* (Philadelphia: Temple University Press, 1989), 6.

27. In her discussion of the NBC/PBS series *I'll Fly Away*, Cheryl Johnson makes clear the necessary distinction between the iconography and history of the black mammy and that of the black maid. She shows how actress Regina Taylor resists the ideological pull of the racist image of the mammy by appearing as a "beautiful woman" who has her own family, narrates her own story, and participates as an activist in the civil rights movement of the 1950s. Cheryl Johnson, "A Restless Domesticity: Feminizing the Black Domestic in *I'll Fly Away*," After the American Century Conference, Oregon State University, April 19–21, 2001, forthcoming in *Wide Angle*.

28. David R. Roediger, *The Wages of Whiteness: Race and the Making of the American Working Class* (London: Verso, 1991), p. 85.

29. See Paula Rabinowitz, *Labor and Desire*, esp. 34–58; Elizabeth Faue, *Community of Suffering and Struggle: Women, Men and the Labor Move-*

ment in Minneapolis, 1915–1945 (Chapel Hill: University of North Carolina Press, 1991), esp. 69–99; Barbara Melosh, *Engendering Culture: Manhood and Womanhood in New Deal Public Art and Theater* (Washington, D.C.: Smithsonian Institute Press, 1991), esp. 15–32. On the connections between masculinity and interracial solidarity, see William J. Maxwell, *New Negro, Old Left*, esp. ch. 4.

30. Fannie Austin, "The Negro Working Women," *The Daily Worker* 2 (May 1930): 4 (emphases added).

31. Roediger explains that in Republican rhetoric this term allied artisans, small manufacturers, craftsmen, as well as mechanics, workingmen, and tradesmen against "the parasitic designs of bankers, undeserving paupers, monopolists, aristocrats and corporations," as well as slaves. See *The Wages of Whiteness*, 50–55.

32. Katherine Q. Seelye, " 'Working Families' Becomes a Theme Meant to Attract Female Voters," *New York Times*, August 22, 2000, A18. The phrase was meant to appeal to the "waitress mom," but it seemed to resonate well with more professional women—teachers and day care licensers are the two interviewed in the article—who also called themselves "working class."

33. The lyrics to Florence Reece's "Which Side Are You On?"can be found in Charlotte Nekola and Paula Rabinowitz, eds., *Writing Red*, 182–83.

34. "Domestic Workers Too Must Organize and Fight," by a Worker Correspondent to the "Working Woman Special" *The Daily Worker*, March 2, 1931, Sec. 2, p. 8, exhorts houseworkers, maids, chambermaids, day workers and live-ins to "build a union of domestic workers to defend our interests." By the time the United States entered the Second World War and better-paying jobs opened up in various industries for black women, notes Jacqueline Jones, Baltimore newspapers were trumpeting that "The Whip Changes Hands," as black domestics organized to raise wages and improve working conditions. In the South, "mysterious 'Eleanor Clubs' (named for the notorious busybody of a First Lady)—groups of black women who colluded to withhold their labor from the job market"—demanded concessions from white employers (*Labor of Love, Labor of Sorrow*, 237).

35. Trudier Harris, *From Mammies to Militants: Domestics in Black American Literature* (Philadelphia: Temple University Press, 1982), 14.

36. See Nancy Armstrong, *Desire and Domestic Fiction: A Political History of the Novel* (New York: Oxford University Press, 1987); Terry Eagleton, *The Rape of Clarissa: Writing, Sexuality and Class Struggle in Samuel Richardson* (Minneapolis: University of Minnesota Press, 1982), among other critical histories of the novel.

37. For some examples of interracial women's alliances during the 1930s, see Mollie V. Lewis, "Negro Women in Steel"; Mary Heaton Vorse, "Hard-

Boiled;" Myra Page, "Leave Them Meters Be!" and "Water!," in Nekola and Rabinowitz, eds., *Writing Red*, 276–78, 291–98; Lauren Gilfillan, *I Went to Pit College* (New York: Viking, 1934); *Union Maids* (d. Julia Reichert, Miles Mogeluscu, and James Klein, 1976).

38. See Doane's analysis of the complicated "act" that Sarah Jane performs, in "Dark Continents" in *Femmes Fatales*, 237–38.

39. In its first issue, *Ebony* interviewed black stars about these roles; Butterfly McQueen complained about being still being relegated to the maid, Lottie, in *Mildred Pierce*. "*Mildred Pierce*" *Ebony* I (January 1946): 30.

40. James M. Cain, *Mildred Pierce* (1941; reprint, New York: Penguin Books, 1946), 50.

41. Doane argues that "pretense, ontology, and the visible real" are "the core of its [the maternal melodrama] discourse." Moreover, "blacks are insistently *there*, never central, but an important component of the discourse, of its reality-effect" ("Dark Continents" in *Femmes Fatales*, 235, 239).

42. Langston Hughes, "Madam's Past History," in Arnold Rampersad and David Roessel, eds., *The Collected Poems of Langston Hughes* (New York: Alfred Knopf, 1995), 301. In *The New Red Negro*, 106, 172–75, Smethurst argues that the Madam series may have been written in response to Brooks's "Hattie Scott" poems, which he claims were a response to Richard Wright's *Native Son*, 247, n. 8. See also Bill Mullen, *Popular Fronts: Chicago and African-American Cultural Politics, 1935–1946* (Urbana: University of Illinois Press, 1999), 167–76.

43. [Dorothy] Myra Page, *Gathering Storm: A Novel of the Black Belt* (London: Martin Lawrence, 1932), 122. For a discussion of the interracial dynamics between women in this and other white women's proletarian novels from the early 1930s, see Susan Sowinska, "Writing Across the Color Line: White Women Writers and the 'Negro Question' in the Gastonia Novels," in Bill Mullen and Sherry Linkon, eds., *Radical Revisions: Rereading 1930s Culture* (Urbana: University of Illinois Press, 1996), 120–43.

44. In "Madam's Calling Cards," instead Alberta K. Johnson "had some cards printed." (Rampersad and Roessel, eds., *The Collected Poems of Langston Hughes*, 301).

45. Fannie Hurst, *Imitation of Life* (1933; reprint, New York: Permabooks, 1959), 77.

46. See any number of feminist readings of film noir, but especially relevant is Mary Ann Doane, "*Gilda*: Epistemology as Striptease," in *Femmes Fatales*, 92–118.

47. Gwendolyn Brooks, *Maud Martha* (1953), reprinted in *Blacks*, 141–321.

48. Smethurst notes in particular "at the hairdresser's," the section of the multipart poem about domestic worker "Hattie Scott," who "Got Madam

C. J. Walker's first. /Got Poro Grower next. / Ain't none of 'em worked with me, Min" (Brooks, *A Street in Bronzeville*, in *Blacks*, 53).

49. Ramona Lowe, "The Woman in the Window," in Nekola and Rabinowitz, eds., *Writing Red*, 79–83, (emphasis in original). Langston Hughes's "Madam and Her Madam" deatils the tense "love and theft," as Eric Lott called minstrelsy, in the exchange characterizing white women's misguided relationship to black women. It, like Ramona Lowe's story, takes a damning and ironic view of Fannie Hurst's fantasy (Rampersad, 285).

50. Roediger, *Wages of Whiteness*. Lauren Berlant, "Race, Gender, and Nation in *The Color Purple*," *Critical Inquiry* 14 (Summer 1988): 831–59, notes that Sofia's refusal to accept the mayor's wife's offer to her that she work as her maid, with her vocal "Hell no!" represents the first time Celie imagines rebellion to the rule of racial oppression. That ultimately Sofia lands in prison for this refusal, and is then further punished by being paroled into service as the mayor's maid suggests just how imbricated the state is with the private family (843).

51. Michael Denning, *The Cultural Front*, 60–62.

52. For a contemporary history of black migration, which means black men and their labor power, see Arna Bontemps and Jack Conroy, *They Seek a City* (Garden City, N.Y.: Doubleday, Doran and Co., Inc, 1945).

53. Doane, "Dark Continents" in *Femmes Fatales*, 241.

3. DOUBLE CROSS: WRI(GH)TING AS *The Outsider*

1. See Alain Bergala, "Weegee and Film Noir," trans. Alexandra Bonfante-Warren, in Miles Barth, ed., *Weegee's World*, (New York: International Center of Photography/Boston: Bullfinch Press, 1997), 69–77.

2. David Madden, *Proletarian Writers of the Thirties* and *Tough Guy Writers of the Thirties* (Carbondale: Southern Illinois University Press, 1968). By the 1950s, during the height of McCarthyism, many literary radicals had turned exclusively to popular genres. For instance, Ed Lacy's *Lead with Your Left* (New York: Harper and Bros., 1957), a crime novel set in New York, refers not too subtly to the author's political leanings. See Alan Wald, *Exiles from a Future Time* (Chapel Hill: University of North Carolina Press, 2002), for a detailed account of the mass cultural turn made by many writers affiliated with the Popular Front.

3. Georgia O'Keeffe, *Georgia O'Keeffe* (New York: Viking Press, 1976), n.p. Commentary to plate #58.

4. For only one example: In the scene in *The Outsider*, where Cross Damon kills both Gil Blount, the communist, and "Herr Herndon," the fascist landlord, Wright employs cinematic conventions from many film noirs—the darkened angled stairway (from *The Big Clock*), the fight in a

cramped apartment lit only by the flickering flames of a smoldering fire (from *Out of the Past*), the sounds of blows landing mixed with the tinkling of broken glass (from *The Lady from Shanghai*), a phone left dangling off the hook (from *Detour*), the bloody corpses left on the rug (from *Mildred Pierce*), the bloody weapons wiped with a handkerchief (from *Lady in the Lake*). Richard Wirght, *The Outsider* (1953; reprint New York: Perennial Library, 1965), pp. 223–28. All further references to this edition appear in the text.

5. See Dick Hebdige, *Subculture: The Meaning of Style* (London: Methuen, 1979); and Angela McRobbie, "Gender and Subculture," in Stuart Hall and Tony Jefferson, eds., *Resistance Through Rituals: Youth Subcultures in Postwar Britain* (Birmingham: Center for Cultural Studies, 1975).

6. All this seems far removed from race relations, but seeing enough of the films, it jumps out at you, so that the glaring lack of scholarship on it is bizarre. Manthia Diawara, "*Noir* by *Noirs:* Toward a New Realism in Black Cinema," in Joan Copjec, ed., *Shades of Noir* (London: Verso, 1993), 261–78, looks at movies made from Chester Himes' *Rage in Harlem* and focuses on the black revisions of the genre. A few critics have looked at the new black gangsta films as a third flowering of the style, but only a few critics have explored noir's racial codings. See also Mary Ann Doane, *Femmes Fatales: Feminism, Film, Theory, Psychoanalysis* (New York: Routledge, 1991); Eric Lott, "The Whiteness of Film Noir," *American Literary History* 9 (1997): 542–66; E. Ann Kaplan, ed., *Women in Film Noir*, new edition (London: British Film Institute, 1998); James Naremore, *More Than Night: Film Noir in Its Contexts* (Berkeley: University of California Press, 1998); Jonathan Munby, *Public Enemies, Public Heroes: Screening the Gangster from Little Caesar to Touch of Evil* (Chicago: University of Chicago Press, 1999).

7. "Roots and Branches," unpublished typescript (foreword to *Eight Men*), 5. Quoted in Michel Fabre, *The World of Richard Wright* (Jackson: University Press of Mississippi, 1985), 71.

8. Fabre, "From Tabloid to Myth" and "The Man who Killed a Shadow," in *The World of Richard Wirght*, 93–121.

9. For information on Wright's direct quotations from the *Tribune*, see Fabre, *World*, 65; and on the tradition of Chicago crime fiction derived from newspaper accounts, see Nelson Algren, *Chicago: City on the Make* (Sausalito, Calif.: Contact Press, 1961), 21–22. Margaret Walker, *How I Wrote Jubilee and Other Essays on Life and Literature* (New York: The Feminist Press, 1990), 33–49, tells of her aiding Wright's *Native Son*.

10. Yale Collection of American Literature (YCAL), Beinecke Manuscript and Rare Book Library, Richard Wright Papers, Box 95, Folder 1255, Horace Cayton, letter to Richard Wright, around August 29 or 30 [1945?]. Hereafter refered to as "Wright Papers."

11. See Richard Wright's "A Blueprint for Negro Writing," *New Challenge* 2 (Fall 1937): 58–65, on the importance of inventing an African-American realism. Wright's criticism of Zora Neale Hurston's 1934 novel, *Their Eyes Were Watching God,* turned on its use of folksy dialect, which, he felt pandered to white audiences used to viewing black culture through the distorted lens of the "minstrel show." Richard Wright, "Between Laughter and Tears," *New Masses* (October 5, 1937): 22, 25.

12. Michel Fabre, *The Unfinished Quest of Richard Wright* (New York: William Morrow and Co., 1973), 316

13. See Wright Papers, Box 53, Folder 639: Milton Rugof, *Herald Tribune,* Sunday, March 22, 1953, 4, calls it "sheer melodrama, a compost of sex and crime—lurid." An unidentified March 22, 1953, review by Carter Brooke Jones in the "Richard Wright Scrapbook" declares: "*The Outsider* is a melodrama. . . . It's almost as if Henry James took over a plot devised by Mickey Spillane." Lewis Vogler of the *San Francisco Chronicle,* April 5, 1953, called it "a full-scale ideological melodrama." The *New Yorker,* March 28, 1953, coins a neologism, "melodramative," to describe the novel. Granville Hicks's front-page Sunday *New York Times Book Review,* March 22, 1953, notes "*The Outsider* is both a melodrama and novel of ideas." Rey L. Gillespie of the *Cleveland Plain Dealer,* April 19, 1953, states simply: "[T]he climax is melodrama involving the Communists." Even the Clarksdale, Mississippi, *Press-Register* weighed in commenting on the book's noir-like jacket: "*The Outsider* is a gripping, melodramatic story of violence and psychology that has the shocking effect of shattered glass—which is, incidentally, symbolized by a solarized cover design." Arna Bontemps sums it all up in the *Saturday Review,* March 28, 1953, when he asserts that "Richard Wright's mind has always run to melodrama."

14. Wright Papers, "Richard Wright Scrapbook," Box 50, Folder 653. Jones, unidentified review in note 13. Melvin Altshuler in the *Washington Post,* March 22, 1953, declares: "If Mickey Spillane were to rewrite *The Outsider,* even he—with his formula that nothing succeeds so well as excess—would not tax credulity as much as Wright has." James N. Rhea writing in the Providence, Rhode Island, *Journal* condemns "*The Outsider* [a]s the worst novel I have ever read. . . . Without the intellectual and symbolic trappings, it might have been a corking good Mickely Spillane sort of thriller."

15. Wright Papers, Box 53, Folder 639. Rhea review in note 14. Herman Kogan called it a "cops-and-robbers story," in *Chicago Sun and Times,* March 22, 1953; while *Jet,* March 26, 1953, decried it as a "whodunit."

16. James Naremore, *More Than Night: Film Noir in Its Contexts* (Berkeley: University of California Press, 1998), 45

17. Wright Papers, Box 53, Folder 639. *Jet,* March 26, 1953.

18. Wright Papers, Box 97, File 1314. Ralph Ellison, letter to Ellen Wright, March 26, 1952.

19. John F. Callahan notes Ellison's debt to Wright for sparking his literary career after Wright, coeditor of *New Challenge*, asked the younger man to review a novel for the Fall 1937 issue. " 'On the basis of this review,' Ellison recalled, 'Wright suggested that I try a short story, which I did.' " Wright accepted the story about riding the rails, it was set into galley proofs, but bumped for space. *New Challenge* then failed. John F. Callahan, introduction to Ralph Ellison, *Flying Home and Other Stories* (New York: Random House, 1996), x.

20. Wright Papers, Box 97, File 1314. Ralph Elison, letter to Richard Wright, January 21, 1953. He even includes a sales figure around 15,000.

21. Wright Papers, Box 97, File 1314 [p.41]. Ralph Ellison, letter to Richard Wright, February 1, 1948.

22. Ibid.

23. Ralph Ellison, "The Seer and the Seen," in *Shadow & Act* (New York: Signet, 1966), 112.

24. See Ellison letter dated February 1, 1948, in note 21.

25. Ellison letter dated January 21, 1953, in note 20.

26. Wright Papers, Box 53, Folder 639. March 30, 1953, and placed in the Richard Wright Scrapbook unsourced.

27. Wright Papers, Box 52, Folder 637. "Biographical Remarks."

28. Wright Papers, Box 52, Folder 636, "Introductory Section," n.d. In a typescript of this statement, Wright details how after 1946, when he and his family traveled to France, "a lull set in," during which he was sorting out his personal philosophy after leaving both the country and communism. He explains, "Elementary honesty prompts me to testify that the basic reality of our world—its meaninglessness, its poverty, its wars, its oppressions!—that once compelled me to be a Communist has not altered; indeed, the sickness of our time has not waned but waxed." Wright Papers, Box 52, Folder 637, Typescript 1,1952–53.

29. Wright Papers, Box 52, Folder 631. Early draft, n.d. In notes to himself about the court martial incident, Wright outlines the plot of *Cornering a Man*, which begins with "Negro in Army," tracks his increasing isolation from "order," and concludes with his "Disappearance." Other titles that Wright considered early on included "Cross: a novel," and "Man Upside Down: a novel." As late as August 7, 1952, Wright's editor at Harper's, Jack Fischer, offered these alternative titles: "A man Called Damon"; "The man with Two Names"; "The Victim"; "Man of Violence"; "Second Chance"; "A Name from a Grave"; "Man in Trouble."

30. Wright Papers, Box 105, Folder 1589. Letter to Richard Wright, March 19, 1948.

31. Dashiell Hammett, *The Maltese Falcon* (1929; reprint New York: Pocket Books, Inc., 1945), 200.

32. Richard Wright, *The Outsider* (1953; reprint, New York: Perennial, 1965), 130.

33. Ibid. See Joan Copjec, "The Phenomenal Nonphenomenal: Private Space in *Film Noir*," in Joan Copjec, ed., *Shades of Noir* (London: Verso, 1993), 167–97, for a discussion of "the detective function" played by Barton Keyes in *Double Indemnity* and his use of statistics and numbers to confound bureaucracies even as he feeds their murderous enterprise (171). Ely Houston clearly owes much to Edward G. Robinson's savory performance of this role.

34. For a discussion of knowledge and how "it changes the *impossible* into the *prohibited*" in film noir, see Slavoj Žižek, " 'The Thing That Thinks': The Kantian Background of the *Noir* Subject," in Joan Copjec, ed., *Shades of Noir*, 199–226.

35. W. E. B. Du Bois, *The Souls of Black Folk* (1903; reprint, New York: Vintage Books, 1990) 42.

36. The book-jacket cover illustration implies the connections between the novel and film noir; it looks just like a movie title: A black solarized photograph of a shattered pane of glass (a bullet-smashed windshield?) on the front; Wright's somber face matching it against the black background on the back. See Figure 28.

37. Wright Papers, Box 93, Folder 1167. Nelson Algren, letter to Richard Wirght, March 12, 1940, pp. 1–3.

38. Wright Papers, Box 98, Folder 1354. Richard Wright, typescript draft of letter to Mike Gold [1940?], pp. 5–6, 7.

39. Ibid., p. 10.

40. The same year, Vera Caspary, whose novel about a working-class girl who "passes" herself off as high class, *Laura*, would become one of the important film noirs of the 1940s, published *The White Girl* (New York: Grosset and Dunlap, 1929), a novel about light-skinned Solaria Cox, who "passes" for white in Chicago. Caspary, like Larsen, is concerned with the ways passing and criminality (or at least guilt) intertwine with desire. After being revealed as having "got nigger blood in your veins," she begins to unravel psychologically (161). "She thought of a spot on the hem of her white moiré dress and of a colored man in Chicago, and of a little boy with coppery brown curls, then she opened her eyes and she saw a rectangle of pale yellow light shining on the floor, and she heard the horns of lonely taxicabs querulously wailing" (171). A few years later, another Jewish woman writer of melodrama, Fannie Hurst, patron of Zora Neale Hurston, published her passing novel, *Imitation of Life*. Clearly, for these Jewish left-wing (or at least left-leaning) women, the story of African-American women pass-

ing offered a cogent metaphor for their own struggles to assimilate. Like many left-wing Jewish writers, actors, and composers—Guy Endore (*Babouk*), Elie Seigmeister, Al Jolson—racial cross-dressing served as a way to assert one's Americanness without assuming the mantle of racist "whiteness" and to challenge Hitler's anti-Semitism without calling attention to one's Jewishness. See Alan Wald's discussions of this in *Writing From the Left: New Essays on Radical Culture and Politics* (London: Verso, 1994); Susan Gubar, *Racechanges: White Skin, Black Face in America* (New York: Oxford University Press, 1997); Michael Rogin, *Blackface, White Noise: Jewish Immigrants in the Hollywood Melting Pot* (Berkeley: University of California Press, 1996). That this is a theme with enduring power is clear from Philip Roth's 2000 PEN/Faulkner Award-winning novel, *The Human Stain*, in which its protagonist is a light-skinned black classics professor who passes as a Jew.

41. Perhaps one of the most damning jibes at *The Outsider* occurred because of this repeated phrase. A September 26, 1953, *New Yorker* "No comment" passage features quotations mentioning "woman as body of woman," from pages 22, 26, 27, 39, 47, 85, 128, 217, concluding: "about time, too." Wright Papers, Box 53, Folder 639.

42. *The Outsider* plays with the lists of alliterative words Wright was constantly scribbling as he worked through the novel. One dated June 12–22, 1947, for a draft entitled "Cross Damon: The Age of Man," reads as follows: "Dread, Despair, Delirium, Deliverance, Destiny, Damnation, Dream, Decision, Death, Defeat, Damnation, Doubt." Wright Papers, Box 48, Folder 606.

43. See Caren Irr, *The Suburb of Dissent* (Durham: Duke University Press, 1998), ch. 5, and Barbara Foley, *Radical Representations* (Durham: Duke University Press, 1994), ch. 5, for excellent analyses of the ways in which Wright inverts and twists the proletarian novel plot to deal with racial conflicts.

44. Wright Papers, Box 48, Folder 601, ms. p. 158 [?]. This synopsis offers the story of both Cora in James M. Cain's *The Postman Always Rings Twice* and Gloria in Horace McCoy's *They Shoot Horses, Don't They?*

45. See Harold T. McCarthy, *The Expatriate Experience: American Novelists and the Idea of America* (Rutherford, N.J.: Fairleigh Dickinson University Press, 1974), 185, on Wright's reliance on newspaper clippings to write *The Outsider*.

46. Nicholas Christopher, *Somewhere in the Night: Film Noir and the American City* (New York: Free Press, 1997), 163–65, highlights the "wholesale political corruption, graft, and racketeering—with cities so sick as to be on the verge of moral implosion," notable in *The Racket* (1951) and *The Street with No Name* (1948), as a "hyperbolic" Baudelairean "hyperreality."

47. Many noir screenwriters were active in the CPUSA and the Screen

Writers Guild—Daniel Mainwaring, Clifford Odets, Dashiell Hammett, Ben Maddow, among them. See Otto Friedrich, *City of Nets: A Portrait of Hollywood in the 1940's* (New York: Harper and Row, 1986), 72–82, who links the Screen Writer's Guild to film noir through Hammett's Sam Spade. Many left-wing writers turned to writing detective and other genre fiction under pseudonyms in 1940s and '50s after McCarthyite blacklists were instituted. See Alan Wald, *Writing from the Left* (London: Verso, 1994), for an account of the process by which writers in the CPUSA moved into genre fiction after the 1930s. David Madden notes in his introduction to *Proletarian Writers of the Thirties* (Carbondale: Southern Illinois University Press, 1968) that he got the idea for the anthology after putting together a collection on *Tough Guy Writers of the Thirties* because of the similarities in names and styles among the authors.

48. Nelson Algren, *Chicago: City on the Make*, 22.

49. Mark Naison, *Communists in Harlem During the Depression* (New York: Grove Press, 1983), 300.

50. Wright Papers, Box 98, Folder 1354. Richard Wright, typescript draft of letter to Mike Gold [1940?], p. 9.

4. BLANC NOIR: RURAL PULP AND DOCUMENTARY MODERNISM

1. The 2000 census shows a marked reverse for many cities as their populations grew dramatically in the wake of the massive immigration during the 1990s. New York's population, for instance, tops eight million again; however, in most large cities now, whites constitute a minority, with Hispanics and Asian immigrants representing the largest percentage of growth, thus sealing the image of the urban center as a foreign zone. Lenny Bruce's routines about how everyone in New York was Jewish but no one in Minneapolis could be, even if her name were Rabinowitz, and Woody Allen's 1977 film, *Annie Hall*, clearly satirize but also perpetuate this urban/rural, ethnic/white bread cultural divide.

2. As I completed the final copyediting on this book, nineteen men hijacked four commercial jets, which were used to damage the Pentagon and destroy the Twin Towers of New York's World Trade Center, killing thousands. It now becomes clear that the international face of the United States is, as it has always been, New York City and Washington, D.C. The meaning of the Oklahoma City bombing, as an act of *domestic* terrorism, becomes even clearer. In fact, the slow response of President George W. Bush to New York's plight suggests just how difficult it is for post-1960s political leaders to acknowledge the totality of America. The outpouring of support from the nation to New Yorkers will perhaps revise the paradigm I am outlining in this chapter.

3. Sarah Boxer, "How the Other Half Defies Its Image," *New York Times*, News of the Week in Review, April 30, 1995, 6.

4. In his June 4, 1995, column for the *New York Times Sunday Magazine*, "Who's John Doe," William Safire provides an etymology of the word, "heartland," that makes clear its connection to both militaristic and folk discourses.

5. Russell Baker, "Not Quite Paradise," *New York Times*, May 2, 1995, A17, reminds his readers that this was the same place that was home to the rural gangsters of 1930s fame—John Dillinger, Bonnie and Clyde, Pretty Boy Floyd, and before them the site of Andrew Jackson's deadly Indian wars. In his remarks, Baker echoes Nelson Algren's assessment of Bonnie and Clyde: "They were outcasts of the cotton frontier. They were children of the wilderness whose wilderness had been razed; who came to maturity in the hardest of times. Clyde might have survived to a sad old age by chopping cotton. Bonnie might have knocked about as a sharecropper's wife or a prostitute until worn out by hard use. The two chose, instead, to give everyone a run for their lives. And, having once committed themselves, made a run which verged upon the uncanny." Nelson Algren, introduction to *The True Story of Bonnie and Clyde*, ed. Jan I. Fortune (New York: New American Library, 1968), 16–17. Since the bombing, revisited six years later through the closed-circuit televised coverage of Timothy McVeigh's execution in another heartland locale, Terre Haute, Indiana, the nation has witnessed a series of brutal school shootings by teenagers. In each case—Colombine High School in suburban Denver, Santana High School in suburban San Diego, an elementary school in Paducah, Kentucky, and so on—the refrain echoes that already heard: "This sort of thing doesn't happen here." The meaning is clear: we're white, middle-class, church-goers, who moved out of the city to protect our children from the dangers of the inner city—guns, drugs, gangs—the violent milieu of a minority underclass.

6. Jonathan Munby argues for continuity among 1930s gangster films and the German expressionist cinema of the preceding decades (made by many of the same directors) and film noirs of the 1940s and 1950s (many of whose directors were also German refugees). He points to the sounds of urban culture as distinctly ethnic and anticorporate as the reasons for instituting the censorship of the Hays Production Code and shows how this earlier code paved the way for the HUAC hearings' blacklist in the postwar era. Munby finds many links between the earlier and later period, effectively countering traditional film histories that speak of noir style as aberrant. Moreover, he argues, classic Hollywood genre films, far from being rigidly determined to solidify an oppressive corporate regime, remain far more open to subversive play than formalist film critics would usually allow.

266

Jonathan Munby, *Public Enemies, Public Heroes: Screening the Gangster from Little Caesar to Touch of Evil* (Chicago: University of Chicago Press, 1999).

7. See Abigail Solomon-Godeau, *Photography on the Dock*, (Minneapolis: University of Minnesota Press, 1992), on the various editions of Engels's book and the changing uses of visuals within each text. According to Solomon-Godeau, within a few decades visual aids were essential to the construction of knowledge about urban industrial plight. Nancy Armstrong details the cultural work of city photography in Britain, *Fiction in the Age of Photography: The Legacy of British Realism* (Cambridge, Mass.: Harvard University Press, 1999).

8. See Alan Wald, *Writing from the Left* (London: Verso, 1994), on the continuities between 1930s literary radicalism and later popular genre fiction and film. For the interconnections between proletarian and tough-guy writing in the 1930s, see David Madden, ed., *Proletarian Writers of the Thirties* and *Tough Guy Writers of the Thirties* (Carbondale, Ill.: Southern Illinois University Press, 1968; 1967). For technological connections between 1930s genre films and later film noir, see the Public Broadcasting Service series, *American Cinema*, especially the segment on film noir.

9. Patricia Zimmermann links images of Albanian refugees from the Kosovo War to Lange's portrait in "Matrices of War: Digitality and Destruction," paper presented at "After the American Century" Conference, Oregon State University, April 19, 2001.

10. However, virtually all recent advertising and prime-time TV, from *Cops* to *Hill St. Blues* to *Homicide* to Nike and EPT (Early Pregnancy Testing) ads to MTV music videos, rely on documentary techniques, especially those established by cinema vérité; infomercials which seamlessly blend the rhetoric of testimonial common to both documentary and advertisement rely on the talking head. So-called reality television depends on product placement and the ubiquity of surveillance cameras to secure its verisimilitude. Raymond Williams, *Television: Technology and Cultural Form* (New York: Methuen, 1975), has pointed out that television's "flow" blurs any differences between one image and another—scan lines resembling a mantra (as Nam June Paik has shown in such works as *TV Buddha*), indiscriminately filled with one thing or another, blend into a seamless whole.

11. See Margaret Walker's reminiscences of Richard Wright in *How I Wrote Jubilee and Other Essays on Life and Literature* (New York: Feminist Press, 1990), 33–49.

12. Noted in Hope Hale Davis's memoir, *Great Day Coming: A Memoir of the 1930s* (South Royalton, Vt.: Steerforth Press, 1994), 326–27. Nelson Algren wonders whether Bonnie Parker's devotion to Clyde Barrow occured because she was "acting out a *True Confessions* epic that could end

no other way than in death beside her dying lover." In Jan Fortune, *True Story of Bonnie and Clyde*, 14.

13. See Paula Rabinowitz, *Labor and Desire: Women's Revolutionary Fiction in Depression America* (Chapel Hill: University of North Carolina Press, 1991), 194, note 52, which quotes from a letter to the editors of *New Masses*. Minnesota Historical Society, Meridel Le Sueur papers, Miscellaneous Correspondences, 1940–1961. Folder 6. Henry Cheney, letter to Meridel le Sueur. Thanks to Julia Mickenberg for bringing this to my attention.

14. Kenneth Burke explains how this rhetorical move instills a sense of identification between the powerful and their followers in *A Rhetoric of Motives* (New York: Prentice Hall, 1950). See also James Agee and Walker Evans, *Let Us Now Praise Famous Men* (1941; reprint, Boston: Houghton Mifflin, 1980), 115, where Agee with biting irony uses FDR's words as the epigraph for the section entitled "Money."

15. See Raymond Williams, *The Country and the City* (London: Paladin, 1975), 23. I am indebted to Susan Kollin for pointing out how the interconnections between modernism's dependence on the distinctions between pulp and documentary are related to the older divisions of rural from urban.

16. Quoted in Milton Meltzer, *Dorothea Lange: A Photographer's Life* (New York: Farrar, Strauss and Giroux, 1978), 161–62.

17. For a detailed analysis of the form and content of this genre, see John Roger Puckett, *Five Photo-Textual Documentaries for the Great Depression* (Ann Arbor, University of Michigan Press, 1984).

18. For an anatomy of this dualism, see chapter 1, "Sunshine or *Noir*," Mike Davis, *City of Quartz: Excavating the Future in Los Angeles* (1990; reprint, New York: Random House, 1992), 15–98.

19. Quoted in Jack Hurley, *Portrait of a Decade: Roy Stryker and the Development of Documentary Photography in the Thirties* (Baton Rouge, La.: Louisiana State University Press, 1972), 70. For a discussion of the change in Stryker's mandate to the FSA photographers as a triumph of the corporate state, see Terry Smith, *Making the Modern: Industry, Art and Design in America*, (Chicago: University of Chicago Press, 1993), especially chapter 7.

20. These documentary images followed such negative literary portrayals of the hypocrisy of rural America, as Sinclair Lewis's *Babbitt* and *Main Street* or Willa Cather's disturbingly erotic visions of prairie life. But by the 1930s, modernist sensibility had turned middlebrow and was redeeming the very places skewered a decade before. Of course, a facet of American identity since the Puritans, who were performing an "errand into the wilderness," has been precisely the intense ambivalence elicited by the new world's vast open space, appearing uninhabited and untamed.

5. MELODRAMA/MALE DRAMA: THE SENTIMENTAL CONTRACT OF
AMERICAN LABOR FILMS

1. Tillie Lerner, "The Strike," *Partisan Review* 1 (November 1936). Reprinted in Charlotte Nekola and Paula Rabinowitz, eds., *Writing Red: An Anthology of American Women Writers, 1930–1940* (New York: The Feminist Press, 1987), 245.

2. Florence Reece, "Which Side Are You On?," in Nekola and Rabinowitz, *Writing Red*, 182.

3. See Ruth McKenney, *Industrial Valley* (1939; reprint, Ithaca: Cornell University Press, 1992; Martha Gellhorn, *The Trouble I've Seen* (New York: William Morrow, 1936); Lallah Davidson, *South of Joplin* (New York: W. W. Norton, 1939); and selections in *Writing Red*.

4. Lauren Gilfillan, *I Went to Pit College* (New York: Literary Guild, 1934). For a detailed discussion of this book, see Paula Rabinowitz, *Labor and Desire: Women's Revolutionary Fiction in Depression America* (Chapel Hill: University of North Carolina Press, 1991), chapter 4.

5. Georg Lukács, "Reportage or Portrayal?" [1932] in Rodney Livingstone, ed., *Essays on Realism*, trans. David Fernbach (Cambridge, Mass.: MIT Press, 1981), 49.

6. Claudia L. Johnson, *Equivocal Beings: Politics, Gender and Sentimentality in the 1790s: Wollstonecraft, Radcliffe, Burney, Austen* (Chicago: University of Chicago Press, 1995), 2.

7. See Raymond Williams, *Culture and Society: 1780–1950* (1953; reprint, New York: Columbia University Press, 1983), 3–12.

8. Lukács, "Reportage or Portrayal?," 50.

9. On the complicated refusal of femininity in the rejection by modernism of sentimentality, see Rey Chow, *Women and Chinese Modernity: The Politics of Reading Between East and West* (Minneapolis: University of Minnesota Press, 1991), and Suzanne Clark, *Sentimental Modernism: Women Writers and the Revolution of the Word* (Bloomington: Indiana University Press, 1991). On the gendered iconography of the Left, see Rebecca Zurier, *Art for the Masses: A Radical Magazine and its Graphics, 1911–1917* (Philadelphia: Temple University Press, 1988); Barbara Melosh, *Engendering Culture: Manhood and Womanhood in New Deal Theater and Art* (Washington, D.C.: Smithsonian Institute Press, 1991); Elizabeth Faue, *Community of Suffering and Struggle: Men, Women and Labor in Minneapolis, 1915–1945* (Chapel Hill: University of North Carolina Press, 1991).

10. For critical analyses of melodrama as a debased form that allowed marginalized peoples, especially women and the working class, a popular platform for resistance within generic and social containment, see Martha

Vicinus, "Helpless and Unfriended: Nineteenth-Century Domestic Melodrama," *New Literary History* 13 (Autumn 1981); Jackie Byars, *All That Hollywood Allows: Re-Reading Gender in 1950s Melodrama* (Chapel Hill: University of North Carolina Press, 1991); Christine Gledhill, "The Melodramatic Field: An Investigation," in *Home Is Where the Heart Is: Studies in Melodrama and the Woman's Film* (London: British Film Institute, 1987); Lynn Hunt, *The Family Romance of the French Revolution* (Berkeley: University of California Press, 1992); Ien Ang, *Watching Dallas: Soap Opera and the Melodramatic Imagination* (London: Routledge, 1989); Michael Denning *Mechanic Accents: Dime Novels and Working-Class Culture in America* (London: Verso, 1987). The standard theoretical work on the mechanics of melodrama is Peter Brooks, *The Melodramatic Imagination: Balzac, Henry James, Melodrama and the Mode of Excess* (New Haven, Conn.: Yale University Press, 1976).

11. Lewis W. Hine, *Men At Work: Photographic Studies of Modern Men and Machines* (1932) (New York: Dover Publications, Inc., 1977).

12. Terry Smith, *Making the Modern: Industry, Art and Design in America* (Chicago: University of Chicago Press, 1993), analyzes the way in which 1930s celebrations of machines enabled the rise of a corporate state. See also Michael Szalay, *New Deal Modernism: American Literature and the Invention of the Welfare State* (Durham, N.C.: Duke University Press, 2000). Left-wing filmmakers, such as Leo Hurwitz, however, celebrated the "machine itself, as an instrument for the transformation of labor and material into what people need." Michael and Jill Klein, "Native Land: An Interview with Leo Hurwitz," *Cineaste* 6 (1974): 7. The aesthetics of streamlining, Raymond Loewy, one of its most creative designers, told *Life*, meant "that society could be industrialized without becoming ugly." Quoted in Jane N. Law, "Designing the Dream," in Fania Weingartner, ed., *Streamlining America*, (Dearborn, Mich.: Henry Ford Museum and Greenfield Village, 1986), 21.

13. See Joan W. Scott's critique of Gareth Stedman Jones's reading of the Chartist's political claims in *The Language of Class* in *Gender and the Politics of History* (New York: Columbia University Press, 1988); Elizabeth Faue, *Community of Suffering and Struggle* on women's organizing during the 1930s Minneapolis Truckers' Strike, and Rabinowitz, *Labor and Desire* on the gendered iconography of class in proletarian novels of the 1930s.

14. Hugo Gellert, *Karl Marx's "Capital" in Lithographs* (New York: Ray Long and Richard Smith, 1934).

15. But there is some truth to it. In an interview with Carol Brightman, "Mary, Still Contrary," *The Nation* (May 19, 1984): 611–20, Mary McCarthy describes the faces of the men in the Gdansk shipyard as familiar, like those of the workers in this country she watched picket the great industries during her youth in the 1930s; their supple muscles and slender figures assuming the

heroic poses Hine pictured. "Those young workers [in Solidarity]," she says, "I've never seen such handsome men. . . . You know, we haven't had a worker in this country that looked like that in fifty years." The bodies of 1930s American workers photographed by Hine have Renaissance proportions in stark contrast to the physiques of late twentieth-century workers pictured by Milton Rogovin, in Rogovin and Michael Frisch, *Portraits in Steel* (Ithaca, N.Y.: Cornell University Press, 1993). However, "brawny, heroic, manly men . . . are back," as heroes since September 11, 2001, according to Patricia Leigh Brown, "Heavy Lifting Required: The Return of Manly Men," *New York Times*, News of the Week in Review (October 28, 2001), 5. Brown quotes "conservative social critic" Camille Paglia's echo of Mary McCarthy: "I can't help noticing how robustly, dreamily masculine the faces of the firefighters are. These are working-class men, stoical, patriotic."

16. See Harriet Arnow, *The Dollmaker* (1954; reprint, New York: Avon Books, 1972). This story had been a staple of 1930s proletarian fiction. The many novels about the Gastonia, North Carolina, strike centered on the transition from folk culture to a culture of capitalist exploitation and the especially difficult time women, as repositories of family lore and tradition, had adjusting to the changes. See Joseph Urgo, "Proletarian Literature and Feminism: The Gastonia Novels and Feminist Protest," *Minnesota Review* 24 (Spring 1985): 64–84.

17. While the Corporation for Public Broadcasting has been a primary funder for many documentaries, including those investigating class relations in America, its audience is decidedly middle class. In *Pets or Meat*, Moore may have been working out a certain ambivalence toward PBS, which funded his films but which does not "bring the working class of this country into its network. . . . [T]hey don't ever seem to speak to people like us." Jay Bobbin, "Moore Moves 'Nation' to Fox," Glens Falls *Post-Star*, July 20, 1995, D8.

18. Speaking of *TV Nation*, Moore comments, "[I]t's very bizarre and rare that a group of people such as me and my friends would be able to come from Flint, Mich., and have a network TV show." Bobbin, D8.

19. Paul Arthur, "Jargons of Authenticity (Three American Moments)," in Michael Renov, ed., *Theorizing Documentary* (New York: Routledge, 1993), 104.

20. This is Douglas Wixson's name for those Midwestern proletariat authors, such as Jack Conroy, who came out of the working class, see *The Worker-Writer in the Midwest* (Urbana: University of Illinois Press, 1993). In the late 1920s, Mike Gold's editorials in the *New Masses* often called for a new movement of worker-correspondents to "Tell us your story . . . in the form of a letter. . . . Write as you talk. Write." Michael Gold, "A Letter to Workers' Art Groups," *New Masses* 5 (September 1929): 16.

21. In *Industrial Valley*, her reportage novel about the United Rubber-workers Union strike in Akron, Ohio, McKenney remarks on the geography of the company town in which the heights are reserved for the ruling families, with managers situated midway between them and the vast working-class neighborhoods spread around the plants in the valley.

22. Walter R. Baranger, "On Line, Management Also on Picket Line," *New York Times*, July 24, 1995, D6. This tactic has been employed as well by cyberspace corporations: "a section on Amazon[.com]'s internal Web site gives supervisors antiunion material to pass on to employees" and alerts managers of tell-tale warning signs that a union is trying to organize. Be wary of " 'hushed conversations when you approach which have not occurred before' and 'small group huddles breaking up in silence on the approach of the supervisor.' " Steven Greenhouse, "Amazon.com Is Using the Web to Block Union's Effort to Organize," *New York Times*, November 29, 2000, C1–2. At the same time, however, organizing efforts have been carried out in cyberspace. In 1996, the University Faculty Alliance and the AAUP at the University of Minnesota successfully fought a Board of Regents' effort to revise the tenure code by effectively using e-mail to communicate with the more than three thousand faculty members.

23. See Ben Hamper, *Rivethead: Tales from the Assembly Line* (New York: Warner Books, 1992), for a full accounting of Hamper's fascinating gendering of mental illnesses. Thanks to Carol Mason for bringing this to my attention. The effects of unemployment are among the most devastating chronicles of work life in late twentieth-century America. The stories of displaced workers are full of alcoholism, depression, suicide, abuse, and so forth. The alienation of labor Marx detailed seems even more exacerbated by the loss of self accompanying loss of work. See the interviews in *Portraits of Steel* conducted by oral historian Michael Frisch for moving accounts of the psychic wreckage caused by plant closures.

24. Jay Bobbin, columnist for the Tribune Media Services, quotes Moore's remarks on "one of a series of really wonderful ironies" that his television show, *TV Nation*, which often scrutinized corporate America, aired in 1994 on NBC, moved in 1995 to Fox, owned by international media tycoon, Rupert Murdoch, CEO of the News Corporation, which owns Fox among many other tabloids. Glens Falls *Post-Star* July 20, 1995, D8.

25. "Warner Acquires 'Roger' Docu for World Distribution," *Variety* 337 (November 1, 1989): 12.

26. See Chester Burger, "What Michael Didn't Say About Roger," *Public Relations Journal* 46 (April 1990): 40–42; Susan Duffy, "The Real Villain in *Roger & Me*? Big Business," *Business Week* (January 8, 1990): 42–45; David C. Smith, "Michael & Roger: GM Critic's Film Makes No Pretense at Fairness," *Ward's Auto World* 25 (November 1989): 5.

27. See Carl Plantinga, "Roger and History and Irony and Me," *Michigan Academician* 24 (Spring 1992): 511–20; and Carley Cohan and Gary Crowdus, "Reflections on *Roger & Me*, Michael Moore and His Critics," *Cineaste* 17: 4 (1990): 25–30.

28. This controversy was played out in the pages of the *New York Times* among other widely read national media venues and took on new life after it was learned that the film was not nominated for an academy award: on January 19, 1990, D. P. Levin reported that "Maker of Documentary That Attacks GM Alienates His Allies," C12; then on February 1, 1990, Richard Bernstein asked "*Roger & Me*: Documentary? Satire? Or Both?," C20; on March 2, 1990, D. Bensman contributed an op-ed piece stating: "*Roger & Me*: Narrow, Simplistic, Wrong," A33; on March 26, 1990, V. J. Dimidjian responded in a letter to the editor, "*Roger & Me*," A16. In the midst of this, *Newsweek* asked "Will GM Retaliate?" (February 26, 1990): 4.

29. Bobbin, "Moore Moves 'Nation' to Fox," D8.

30. In *The Family Romance of the French Revolution* (Berkeley: University of California Press, 1993), historian Lynn Hunt argues that melodrama was a key factor in the decision to behead royalty because this popular theatrical form securely differentiated between the righteous and evil ones, and applauded ridding the stage of evil power. Moore is hardly advocating Roger's death; but his ability to collapse the situation into a struggle between himself and his adversary—richer, more powerful, more deceitful—recalls this plot.

31. Of course, the title *American Dream* refers to the post–World War II promise, which film noir undercuts and exposes, made to the white working class of a home, a car, a stable job, and so forth earned at the expense of militant unions and through the build-up of a militarized federal budget. But I also think that because of the way the film portrays family conflicts, it is not entirely wrong to sit Freud before this dream and put his analytic powers to work.

32. Earl Browder, *The People's Front* (New York: International Publishers, 1938), 56, 235.

33. For a devastating critique of the vestiges of Popular Front culture lurking within left-wing expressions of solidarity with the working class, see Jesse Lemisch, "I Dreamed I Saw MTV Last Night," *The Nation* (October 18, 1986): cover, 374–76.

34. Anthony McCall and Andrew Tyndal, "Sixteen Working Statements," *Millennium Film Journal* 1 (Spring/Summer 1978), 36. See also Noel King, "Recent 'Political' Documentary: Notes on *Union Maids* and *Harlan County, USA*," *Screen* 22, no. 2 (1981): 7–18.

35. Peter Rachleff, review of *American Dream*, *The Oral History Review* 20 (Spring/Fall 1992): 94–96.

36. Peter Rachleff, *Hardpressed in the Heartland* (Boston: South End Press, 1993), details the history of the UFCW in Austin, as well as offers a completely different picture of the effects of the P-9 strike for the U.S. labor movement. A labor historian at Macalester College in St. Paul, Minnesota, Rachleff was instrumental in establishing the Twin Cities Support for P-9. Rachleff alerted me to the footage stored in Wisconsin's archives. (Personal communication, April 21, 1996). Tim Leland, business agent for the building trades union in Minnesota, voiced a great deal of criticism of the P-9ers, echoing Andersen that the strike was hopelessly doomed and thus resulted in hundreds of Hormel workers in Austin and Owatonna, Minn., losing their jobs. (Personal interview, November 10, 1994)

37. Rachleff's book is one of the two; the other is Hardy Green, *On Strike at Hormel: The Struggle for a Democratic Labor Movement* (Philadelphia: Temple University Press, 1990).

38. See Wini Breines, *Community and Organization in the New Left, 1962–1968: The Great Refusal* (New York: Praeger; South Hadley, Mass.: J. F. Bergin, 1982), on the 1960s movements' adoption of this model for organizing. I will take this up at length in chapter 8.

39. Robert Markley, "Sentimentality as Performance: Shaftesbury, Sterne and the Theatrics of Virtue," in Felicity Nussbaum and Laura Brown , eds., *The New Eighteenth Century* (New York: Methuen, 1987), 211–12.

40. James Agee and Walker Evans, *Let Us Now Praise Famous Men* (Boston: Houghton-Mifflin, 1941).

6. NOT "JUST THE FACTS, MA'AM":
SOCIAL WORKERS AS PRIVATE EYES

1. Horace McCoy, *They Shoot Horses, Don't They?* (New York: Simon and Schuster, 1935), 126, 128. All further citations appear in the text. McCoy's novel, a tour-de-force of noir images about Hollywood's lowlife, precursor by four years to both Nathanael West's *The Day of the Locusts* and Raymond Chandler's *The Big Sleep*, is framed by the blaring sentence of the court, broken into thirteen chapters, concluding with the exhortation that the narrator will be "executed and put to death." As in many noir narratives, a retrospective voice from the grave recounts the crime that inexorably followed the regular guy's descent into the underworld because of his fatal encounter with a woman.

2. Kevin Brownlow, *The Parade's Gone By* (New York: Ballantine, 1968), includes a long interview with Joseph Henabery, assistant director of *Intolerance*, in which he describes how, *The Mother and the Law*, this "little, cheap, quickie picture," evolved from a "potboiler"and "tearjerker" into the monumental saga *Intolerance* (55–56).

3. In her 1932 reportage, "Women on the Breadlines," Meridel Le Sueur comments that there really isn't a name, a category, much less an agency that can address the plight of single impoverished women. *New Masses* 7 (January 1932): 5–6; reprinted in Elaine Hedges, ed., *Ripening* (Old Westbury, N.Y.: Feminist Press, 1982), 137–43. See also, Ruth E. Bowles, "A Social Worker Looks at Black Bottom," *Crisis* (July 1930): 211–13, about black women waiting on Cincinnati street corners for day work as maids, and night work as prostitutes, after their men have left them.

4. See Burton Bledstein, *The Culture of Professionalism* (New York: W. W. Norton, 1976); Julia Swindells, *Victorian Writing and Working Women* (Minneapolis: University of Minnesota Press, 1985); Linda Gordon, *Heroes of Their Own Lives* (New York: Viking, 1988); Denise Riley, *Am I That Name?: Feminism and the Category of "Women" in History* (Minneapolis: University of Minnesota Press, 1988); Carolyn Steedman, *Childhood, Culture and Class in Britain* (New Brunswick, N.J.: Rutgers University Press, 1990); Carolyn Steedman, *Past Tenses: Essays on Writing, Autobiography and History* (London: Rivers Oram Press, 1992), on the interlocking relationship between the professionalization of middle-class women and the pathologizing of poor women in the United States and Britain, especially during the late nineteenth and early twentieth centuries.

5. Muriel Rukeyser, "Book of the Dead," *U.S. 1* (New York: Covici Friede, 1938), 15. All further citations appear in the text. For an analysis of this "modernist poem as a radical document," see Robert Shulman, *The Power of Political Art: The 1930s Literary Left Reconsidered* (Chapel Hill: University of North Carolina Press, 2000), chapter 6.

6. Clinch Calkins, *Some Folks Won't Work* (New York: Harcourt, Brace and Co., 1930), for what may be the first book-length example of popularizing American social workers' case studies through fiction. Of course, true crime sensations had been staples of dime novels. Steedman's essays on working-class girls' narratives in *Past Tenses* links them to the rise of public investigations of poverty.

7. Caroline Slade, *Sterile Sun* (New York: Vanguard Pres, 1936). All references appear in the text.

8. I am using Swindells's discussion of professionalism, which relies on Geoff Esland, "Professions and Professionalism," in Geoff Esland and Graeme Salaman, eds., *The Politics of Work and Occupations* (Milton Keyes: Open University Press, 1980), 216, an analysis of how the professional classes emerged in the nineteenth century as " 'reality definers' and organizers of dominant thought from their position in the division of labor" (Swindell, 4).

9. Linda Gordon, *Heroes*, 245–47. Further references appear in the text.

10. Carolyn Steedman, *Landscape for a Good Woman: A Story of Two Lives* (New Brunswick, N.J.: Rutgers University Press, 1987), 6, describes how

personal narratives (especially by those outside of the mainstream) construct "resolutely social" political theory.

11. Gordon, *Heroes*, 215–18, discusses how child protection services defined young poor girls' "sexual deliquency." Susan Rubin Suleiman, *Authoritarian Fictions: The Ideological Novel as a Literary Genre* (New York: Columbia University Press, 1983), claims the hallmark of "authoritarian fiction," such as Slade's, is its redundant didacticism.

12. In "Narrate or Describe?" Georg Lukács outlines the differences between realism (which allows the representation of totality through social narratives [good]) and naturalism (which sinks to pornographic descriptions of psychological states [bad]). Arthur D. Kahn, ed. and trans., *Writer and Critic and Other Essays* (New York: Grosset and Dunlap, 1970). Unfortunately, at least to my mind, Slade seems to have moved from description to narration in her 1940s novels. Caroline Slade, *Margaret* (New York: Vanguard Press, 1946), published after the War, participates in the democratization of social problems, making it a novel of significance for all mothers, whereas Slade's first novel was directed to an audience of professionals. For a comprehensive analysis of the expansion of progressive parenting during this period, see Julia Mickenberg, "Educating Dissent: Children's Literature and the Left," Ph.D. diss., University of Minnesota, 2000.

13. Caroline Slade, *The Triumph of Willie Pond* (New York: Vanguard Press, 1940), 25.

14. Martha Gellhorn, "Ruby," from *The Trouble I've Seen*, in *The Collected Novellas of Martha Gellhorn* (1936; reprint, New York: Knopf, 1993).

15. Rachel Swarns, "Welfare as We Know It Goes Incognito," *New York Times*, News of the Week in Review (July 5, 1998), 1, rehearses the history of welfare "reform." In Slade's second novel, *The Triumph of Willie Pond*, Willie Pond, the laid-off tubercular WPA ditch digger, eventually commits suicide in order to "provide" for his family, which can only receive ADC (the predecessor to AFDC) in his absence, once he is deemed an able-bodied (though still unemployed) worker after recovering from TB in a state-run sanatorium. In short, Slade foresaw the contradictory history of welfare by noting its corrosive effect on the family, its band-aid solutions to structural unemployment, and its nightmarish bureaucracy.

16. Slade's novels were part of a subgenre of 1930s radical novels featuring social workers; I discuss these in the context of "women's revolutionary fiction," in Paula Rabinowitz, *Labor and Desire: Women's Revolutionary Fiction in Depression America* (Chapel Hill: University of North Carolina Press, 1991), 92. Records show Slade, second cousin to Walker Evans, to have been a member of the League of American Writers in 1936. (Thanks to Alan Wald and Theodore Crane for these bits of biographical information.)

17. See jacket blurb on the back cover of Caroline Slade, *Margaret* (New York: Vanguard, 1946).

18. Luella R. North, review of *Sterile Sun*, *The Survey* (November 1936): 352. Gellhorn's novel was written while she was a guest of Eleanor Roosevelt at the White House.

19. William Dane, review of *Miss Bailey Says*, *Social Work Today* (June 1934): 21.

20. Gertrude Springer, review of *The Triumph of Willie Pond*, *Survey Midmonthly* (June 1940): 212.

21. Gertrude Springer, review of *Lilly Crackell*, *Survey Midmonthly* (August 1943): 223.

22. Frank C. Bancroft, review of *The Triumph of Willie Pond*, *Social Work Today* (November 1940): 29.

23. Jacket blurb, back cover, *Margaret*.

24. For a comparison of Chandler's narratives to *Ulysses*, see Fredric Jameson, "The Synoptic Chandler," in Joan Copjec, ed., *Shades of Noir* (London: Verso, 1993), 33–34. *Ulysses* was listed first of the top one hundred twentieth-century novels in English by the Modern Library.

25. Josephine Herbst, "Ignorance Among the Living Dead," *New Masses* (January 1929): 4. A similar point is made by Herbst in her short memoir, "Yesterday's Road," *New American Review* 3 (1968): 84–104.

26. Josephine Herbst tells the story in "A Year of Disgrace," *Noble Savage* 3 (1961); reprinted in Josephine Herbst, *The Starched Blue Sky of Spain and Other Memoirs* (Boston: Northeastern University Press, 1991), 53–98. My copy of Slade's novel, a signed first edition owned by Martha H. Gro, her back-slanting signature barely edging the cover, was found in an upstate New York used bookstore; I had read reviews of the novel years ago but was never able to track it down from libraries. See Cathy N. Davidson, *Revolution and the Word: The Rise of the Novel in America* (New York: Oxford University Press, 1985), 5–10, for an ethnography of the book and the importance of scrutinizing the object itself.

27. Gertrude Springer, *Ask Miss Bailey*, *The Midmonthly Survey Pamphlets*, Series II, 1933, 25. Miss Bailey's solution, empathizing with Carrie, was to send a younger woman social worker with a pair of donated silk stockings to the home.

28. Raymond Chandler, *The Big Sleep* (1939), in *The Raymond Chandler Omnibus* (New York: Knopf, 1964).

29. Gertrude Springer, *Ask Miss Bailey*, *The Midmonthly Survey Pamphlet*, Series I, 1933, 6–7. Gordon, *Heroes*, explains how providing food, clothing, and shelter had both positive and negative impact on child neglect cases.

30. Ann Petry, *The Street* (Boston: Houghton Mifflin, 1946), 389. Further references appear in the text.

31. Unfortunately, this story is still on-going. Pam Belluck reports that Catherine Ferguson, public defender for the seven-year-old Chicago boy falsely accused of murdering Ryan Harris with an eight-year-old accomplice, noted that parents in the black community were resigned to having the police and other authorities remove their children: "In a white middle-class community, parents would have broken down the door and said, 'Let me in there!' " "Murder Chrages Dropped Against 2 Boys in Chicago," *New York Times*, September 5, 1998, A1, 10.

32. Marita Bonner, "The Whipping" (1935), in Charlotte Nekola and Paula Rabinowitz, eds., *Writing Red: An Anthology of Women Writers, 1930–1940* (New York: Feminist Press, 1987), 75. Further references in text.

33. Gertrude Springer, *Ask Miss Bailey*, Series II, 1933, 29.

34. During the summer of 1998, another scandal about the welfare system in New York City exploded as, first, three children were discovered to have been sexually abused by their parents and relatives in Brooklyn after they were returned from foster care to their home, and then, a two-year-old boy was found starving and locked away in a dark room left on a urine-stained mattress while in foster care. In both cases, it appears that caseworkers neglected to inspect the homes and actually see the children for themselves. Visual inspection is essential to child protection.

35. For an explanation of how Oscar Lewis's thesis about the culture of poverty contributed to the Johnson administration's Great Society, see Diana Pearce, "Welfare Is Not *for* Women: Why the War on Poverty Cannot Conquer the Feminization of Poverty," in Linda Gordon, ed., *Women, the State and Welfare* (Madison: University of Wisconsin Press, 1990), 265–79.

36. Louis L. Bennett, "Problems of Homecoming," *Survey Midmonthy* (September 1944): 246–48. Some "problems" noted by the director of Veterans' Service Center in New York included "family difficulties," "education and jobs," "housing," and "emotional disturbance and instability."

37. Raymond Chandler's original screenplay revealed Buzz as the amnesiac murderer, but the U.S. Navy objected to this depiction of a veteran and insisted on a rewrite. See Alain Silver and Elizabeth Ward, *Film Noir: An Encyclopedic Reference to the American Style*, 3rd ed. (Woodstock, N.Y.: Overlook Press, 1992), 36–37; and James Naremore, *More Than Night: Film Noir in Its Contexts* (Berkeley: University of California Press, 1998), 107–14.

38. In fact, the trumpeting of this problem itself became a problem, forcing Sallie Bright, executive secretary for the National Publicity Council for Health and Welfare Services, to exhort everyone, especially social workers and journalists, to "Stop Calling Them Problems," *Survey Midmonthly* (May 1945): 139–40

39. *Social Work Today* (January 1938): 26.

40. Editorial, *Social Work Today* (June–July 1940): 5–6.

41. *Social Work Today* (October 1940): 11–12.

42. *Social Work Today* (February 1942): 30.

43. *Social Work Today* (January 1941): 12.

44. Caroline Slade, *Lilly Crackell* (New York: Vanguard, 1943), 602.

45. This is Fritz Redl's term in "Zoot Suits: An Interpretation," *Survey Midmonthly* (October 1943): 259.

46. Slade, *Lilly Crackell*, 602.

47. Eliot Ness, "Sex Delinquency as a Social Hazard," *Proceedings of 1944 National Conference of Social Workers*, 279.

48. Slade, *Lilly Crackell*, 602.

49. Ethel L. Ginsburg, "The Case Worker in a Veterans' Service Center," *Survey Midmonthly* (May 1945): 126.

50. "Study Says Welfare Changes Made the Poorest Worse Off," *New York Times*, August 23, 1999: A13.

51. For more on this history, see Theda Skocpol, *Protecting Soldiers and Mothers: The Political Origins of Social Policy in the United States* (Cambridge, Mass.: The Belknap Press, 1992), especially chapters 8 and 9; Barbara J. Nelson, "The Origins of the Two-Channel Welfare State," in Linda Gordon, ed., *Women, the State, and Welfare*, 123–51.

52. Johnnie Tillmon, "Welfare Is a Women's Issue," in Rosalyn Baxandall, Linda Gordon, and Susan Reverby, eds., *America's Working Women: A Documentary History—1600 to the Present* (New York: Vintage, 1976), 355–58.

53. Lest one forget the currency of this connection, see Dan Barry, "Police Used Brothel So Often, Madam Got Worried," *New York Times*, July 18, 1998, A1, 10.

54. Karen Tice, *Tales of Wayward Girls and Immoral Women: Case Records and the Professionalization of Social Work* (Urbana: University of Illinois Press, 1998); and Beverly Stadum, *Poor Women and Their Families: Hardworking Charity Cases, 1900–1930* (Albany: State University of New York Press, 1992), present feminist readings of early twentieth-century case histories about poor girls and women. The pages of *The Survey* and *Social Worker Today* turn from a concern with male unemployment and female prostitution during the Depression to the plight of those facing war mobilization (and later, demobilization) during the 1940s.

55. I have not read Caroline Slade's *Job's House* but have located a copy in the New York State Library in Albany.

56. Carolyn Steedman, *Landscape for a Good Woman: A Story of Two Lives* (New Brunswick, N.J.: Rutgers University Press), 2.

7. BARBARA STANWYCK'S ANKLET

1. Jacques Derrida, *The Truth in Painting*, trans. Geoff Bennington and Ian McLeod (Chicago: University of Chicago Press, 1987), 381.

2. "A pair of shoes is more easily treated as a *utility* than a single shoe or two shoes which aren't a pair. The pair inhibits at least, if it does not prevent, the 'fetishizing' movement; it rivets things to use, to 'normal' use; it shoes better and makes things walk according to the law." He goes on to question what either Heidegger or Schapiro would have done with "a painting with only one shoe, especially a single high heel as in Magritte's *La Lune* or Lindner's *The Shoe*. Would they have been able to produce . . .?" Derrida, *Truth in Painting*, 332–33.

3. "Shoes. Dream shoes. Shoes to power the imagination. We sat spellbound before *Mildred Pierce*. Our eyes followed her feet . . . her shoes. . . . Inevitably black, they featured three-inch talons, a slightly raised platform, and a delicate strap encircling the ankle. Her shoes were a sign—but of what?" ask Shari Benstock and Suzanne Ferriss in the introduction to their collection, *On Fashion* (New Brunswick, N.J.: Rutgers University Press, 1994), 1.

4. Thanks to Cora Leland for bringing this term to my attention, which comes from the interdiction against sandals outlined in the dress code governing employees at Arthur Andersen and other accounting firms in the United States. See Colin McDowell, *Manolo Blahnik* (New York: Harper-Collins, 2000), who quotes Blahnik as confirming that "the first two cracks" of toe cleavage is a "very important part of the sexuality of the shoe." Quoted in Penelope Green, "Fall Reading, From Head to Toe," *New York Times*, September 4, 2000, B10.

5. Derrida, *Truth in Painting*, 269. Sigmund Freud, "On Dreams," trans. James Strachey, *Standard Edition of the Complete Psychological Works of Sigmund Freud*, vol. 5: 633–86. Hereafter noted as *SE*.

6. Wendy Lesser, "Stanwyck," in *His Other Half: Men Looking at Women through Art* (Cambridge, Mass.: Harvard University Press, 1991), 225–61.

7. Farah Jasmine Griffin, "Style Heritage," *Harpers Bazaar* (October 2001): 176–78.

8. Sigmund Freud, "Fetishism," *SE*, vol. 21, 152–53.

9. Freud, "Fetishism," *SE*, vol. 21, 156.

10. Freud, "Three Essays on Sexuality," *SE*, vol. 7, 154, fn 2 [added 1920].

11. Freud, "Three Essays," *SE*, vol. 7, 153.

12. Freud, "Three Essays," *SE*, vol. 7, 155, (emphasis in original).

13. Gilles Deleuze, *Coldness and Cruelty*, in *Masochism* (New York: Zone Books, 1991), 31.

14. Victor Turner, *The Forest of Symbols: Aspects of Ndembu Ritual* (Ithaca, N.Y.: Cornell University Press, 1967), 28, 29, 30.

15. Samuel Beckett, *Waiting for Godot* (New York: Grove Press, 1954), 44.

16. The picture appears in Astrid Proll, ed., *Baader-Meinhof: Pictures on the Run, '67–'77* (Zurich and New York: Scalo, 1998), 35. Thanks to Christina White for bringing it to my attention. Its caption reads in English: "Rudi Dutschke's shoe in Kurfurstendam shortly after shots had been fired by a right-wing assailant, 11th April 1968."

17. On the "ideological" and historical differences between these two men, see Derrida, *Truth in Painting*, 281. Martin Heidegger, "The Origin of the Work of Art," in *Poetry, Language, Thought*, trans. Albert Hofstadter (New York: Harper and Row, 1971), 15–87. Meyer Schapiro, "The Still Life as a Personal Object—A Note on Heidegger and Van Gogh," in Marianne L. Simmel, ed., *The Reach of Mind: Essays in Memory of Kurt Goldstein* (New York: Springer Publishing, Colo., 1968), 203–09. Derrida's long essay on this "debate" appears in "Restitutions," in *The Truth in Painting*. It became the jumping off point for Fredric Jameson's *Postmodernism: Or, The Cultural Logic of Late Capitalism* (Durham, N.C.: Duke University Press, 1991), 6–11, as well as other less widely read texts; see below.

18. Karl Marx, *Capital: A Critique of Political Economy*, vol. 1, trans. Samuel Moore and Edward Aveling, (1887; reprint New York: International Publishers, 1967), 72, 74.

19. Marx, *Capital*, vol. 1, 76, 72 (emphasis added).

20. Walter Benjamin, *The Arcades Project*, trans. Howard Eiland and Kevin McLauglin (Cambridge, Mass.: Belknap Press of Harvard University Press, 1999), 662.

21. Emile Durkheim, *The Elementary Forms of the Religious Life*, trans., Joseph Ward Swain (1915; reprint, New York: The Free Press, 1969), 203.

22. For critiques of these sentiments, see a cryptic set of questions by Derrida: "What if Heidegger were already questioning beyond this already coded thematics? What if he were also wary of the concept of fetishism according to Marx or according to Freud? And what if he wanted to take the whole of this problem up again, and the whole question of the thing in truth which exercises the notion of fetishism?" (334). See also, the analysis of "the rhetoric of iconoclasm," in W. J. T Mitchell, *Iconology: Image, Text, Ideology* (Chicago: University of Chicago Press, 1986), 151–208.

23. Benjamin, *Arcades*, 669.

24. Walter Benjamin, "Unpacking My Library," in Hannah Arendt, ed., *Illuminations*, trans. Harry Zohn (New York: Schocken, 1968), 59–67.

25. Susan Stewart, *On Longing: Narratives of the Minature, the Gigantic, the Souvenir, the Collection* (Durham, N.C.: Duke University Press, 1993), 151.

26. Douglas Mao, *Solid Objects: Modernism and the Test of Production* (Princeton: Princeton University Press, 1998), 4.

27. Virginia Woolf, *Orlando: A Biography* (1928; reprint, Hammondsworth: Penguin Books, 1942), 212.

28. Walter Benjamin, *Arcades*, 594.

29. Roland Barthes, *Mythologies*, trans. Annette Lavers (New York: Hill and Wang, 1972), 39.

30. James Agee and Walker Evans, *Let Us Now Praise Famous Men* (Boston: Houghton Mifflin, 1941), 262–63.

31. Gertrude Jobes, *Dictionary of Mythology, Folklore and Symbols*, vol. 2 (New York: Scarecrow Press, 1961–1962), 1440.

32. Quoted in Jean Chevalier and Alain Gheerbrat, *A Dictionary of Symbols*, trans. John Bruckman-Brown. (Oxford: Blackwell, 1994), 876.

33. Joseph J. Kockelman, *Heidegger on Art and Art Works* (Dordrecht: Martinus Nijhoff Publishers, 1985), 127.

34. Schapiro, "Still Life," in Simmel, *The Reach of Mind*, 206.

35. See Otto Poggeler, "Heidegger on Art," in Karsten Harries and Christoph Jamme, eds., *Martin Heidegger: Politics, Art, and Technology* (New York: Holmes and Meier, 1994), 106–24.

36. Art Spiegelman, *Maus II: A Survivor's Tale: And Here My Troubles Began* (New York: Pantheon, 1991), 60–63.

37. Marjorie Garber, *Vested Interests: Cross-Dressing and Cultural Anxiety* (New York: HarperCollins, 1993), 44–45, cites *Information for the Female-to-Male Crossdresser and Transsexual*, which relies on John T. Molloy's note that "for the small man . . . the best shoes are traditional wingtip" and on Nancy Friday's *My Secret Garden* mention of female transvestites' interest in "wingtip shoes," to suggest that wingtips were part of the "imitation man look."

38. Agee and Evans, *Let Us Now Praise Famous Men*, 258.

39. Elin Schoen Brockman, "A Woman's Power Tool: High Heels," *New York Times*, March 5, 2000. In response, Deborah L. Rhode commented on the bizarre spectacle of powerful women lawyers mincing around in their "thigh-high stiletto-heeled boots" and other "footwear that maims" in an op-ed piece, "Step, Wince, Step, Wince," *New York Times*, October 18, 2000, A31.

40. Advertisement for pierresilber.com in *New York Times*.

41. Michael Wilson, *Salt of the Earth*, screenplay 1953, (Old Westbury, N.Y.: The Feminist Press, 1978), 61.

42. Erwin Panowsky defines iconography as the study of "the subject matter or meaning of works of art," *Studies in Iconology: Humanistic Themes in the Art of the Renaissance* (New York: Harper and Row, 1962), 3. In his rumination on the "theory of imagery," W. J. T. Mitchell notes: "We can

never understand a picture unless we grasp the ways in which it shows what cannot be seen." *Iconology: Image, Text, Ideology* (Chicago: University of Chicago Press, 1986), 39.

43. See "The Family of Little Feet," "Chanclas," and "A House of My Own," in Sandra Cisneros, *The House on Mango Street* (1984; reprint, New York: Vintage, 1991) 39–42, 46–48, 108.

44. The discovery of the bloody size-12 Bruno Magli shoeprints left on Nicole Simpson's walkway became only the most recent spectacular example of this. The search to identify the tread was undertaken by a Japanese firm specializing in shoe print recognition at crime scenes. The fact that only a few hundred pairs of this size existed worldwide and O. J. Simpson owned one of them, however, was not sufficient evidence to convict.

45. Leslie Kaufman, "A Walk on the Wild Side Stirs the Shoe Industry," *New York Times*, July 9, 2000, 3:1,8, notes that in the United States, women's shoe sales have been remarkably consistent since the end of World War II. During the 1990s, despite the consumer boom, women's shoe sales have grown steadily at only 1.8 percent per year, consistent with figures from the 1940s, excluding a spike during the 1980s when athletic footwear became popular.

46. See Carolyn Steedman, "Landscape for a Good Woman," in *Past Tenses: Essays on Writing, Autobiography and History* (London: Rivers Oram Press, 1992), 21–40. See also her book of the same title.

47. Charlotte Nekola, "Good Mothers, Bad Daughters," in *Dream House: A Memoir* (New York: W. W. Norton, 1993), 42–56.

48. C. L. R. James, *American Civilization*, ed. Anna Grimshaw and Keith Hart (New York: Blackwell, 1993), 131.

8. MEDIUM UNCOOL: AVANT-GARDE FILM AND UNCANNY FEMINISM

1. Sigmund Freud, "The 'Uncanny'" (1919), *On Creativity and the Unconscious* (New York: Harper Torchbook, 1958), 122–61.

2. "For structures of feeling can be defined as social experiences *in solution* . . ." Raymond Williams, *Marxism and Literature* (Oxford: Oxford University Press, 1977), 133 (emphasis in original).

3. Fredric Jameson, "Periodizing the '60s," in Sohnya Sayers et al. eds., *The Sixties Without Apology* (Minneapolis: University of Minnesota Press, 1984), 208.

4. For an excellent detailed account of France and film and 1968, but one that says nothing about women, much less feminism, see Sylvia Harvey, *May '68 and Film Culture* (London: British Film Institute, 1978).

5. Jay Boyer, "You Will Never Read the Novel You Might Like To," Sohnya Sayres et al., eds., *The Sixties Without Apology*, 309–10. Even when a

work of fiction appears about the New Left, such as Alix Kates Shulman's *Burning Questions*, it does so in the form of a nonfictional memoir, complete with a treatise on the history of radical women's autobiographies. Novels about Vietnam—such as Philip Caputo's *Rumor of War* or Tim O'Brien's *The Things They Carried*—are read as nonfiction memoir. In many ways, the legacy of Vietnam narratives is the memoir. For a discussion of how trauma informs genre, see Julia Bleakney, "Reproducing the Vietnam War: Bodies, Places, Memories," Ph.D. preliminary examination, English Department, University of Minnesota, November 2000.

6. Todd Gitlin, *The Sixties: Years of Hope, Days of Rage* (New York: Bantam, 1987), 242–43.

7. Gitlin, *The Sixties*, 243.

8. Henry Abelove, "Some Speculations on the History of Sexual Intercourse During the Long Eighteenth Century in England," *Genders* 6 (November 1989): 125–30.

9. Raymond Williams, *The Country and the City* (London: Paladin Press, 1975), describes this problem.

10. Roland Barthes, *Camera Lucida: Reflections on Photography*, trans. Richard Howard (New York: Hill and Wang, 1981), 98

11. Patricia Zimmermann, *Reel Families: A Social History of Amateur Film* (Bloomington: Indiana University Press, 1995). Freud notes that, "Many people experience the feeling [of the uncanny] in the highest degree in relation to death and dead bodies, to the return of the dead, and to spirits and ghosts." ("The 'Uncanny'," 149).

12. "The First Statement of the New American Cinema Group," *Film Culture* 22–23 (Summer 1961): 130–31.

13. Quoted in Lawrence Van Gelder, "Shirley Clarke Is Dead at 77; Maker of Oscar-Winning Film," *New York Times*, September 26, 1997, C19.

14. Stan Brakhage, letter to Dolores Daniels, *Film Culture* 40 (Spring 1966): 73–75.

15. Stan Brakhage, "Defense of the 'Amateur' Filmmaker," *Filmmakers Newsletter* (Summer 1971): 20

16. "An Interview with Kenneth Anger, Conducted by *Spider Magazine*," *Film Culture* 40 (Spring 1966): 68.

17. Carolee Schneemann, *More Than Meat Joy: Complete Performance Works and Selected Writings*, ed. Bruce McPherson (New York: Documentext, 1979), 122–27.

18. "Vietnam a Vegetable Culture Which Leaves No Garbage," notes about "Snows" in Schneemann, *More Than Meat*, 120.

19. Schneemann, "Naked Action Lecture," in *More Than Meat*, 180. The performance happened on June 27, 1968.

20. Schneemann, "Istory of a Girl Pornographer," in *More Than Meat*, 192.

21. Quoted in Van Gelder, "Shirley Clarke Is Dead at 77."

22. Don Langer, "Tips on Photography," *New York Herald Tribune*, September 29, 1957, 4:7.

23. Both Arbus quotations are from an interview with Ann Ray in *Newsweek*; quoted in Patricia Bosworth, *Diane Arbus: A Biography* (New York: Knopf, 1984), 248.

24. John Wakeman, *World Film Directors, Vol. 2, 1945–1985,* "Shirley Clarke," (New York: H. W. Wilson Company, 1988), 222.

25. See Patricia Bosworth, *Diane Arbus,* for more juicy details, 261–64, 295–98.

26. Ti-Grace Atkinson, "On Violence in the Women's Movement," *Amazon Odyssey* (New York: Links Books, 1974), 198.

27. Susan Sontag, *On Photography* (New York: Farrar, Strauss and Giroux, 1977), 178 (emphasis added).

28. Carol Hanisch, "Critique of the Miss America Protest," in *Notes From the Second Year: Women's Liberation* (New York: New York Radical Women, 1970), 86–87.

29. Quoted in Alice Echols, *Daring to Be Bad: Radical Feminism in America, 1967–1975* (Minneapolis: University of Minnesota Press, 1989), 86-7.

30. Echols, *Daring to Be Bad,* 86.

31. Ethan Morder, *Medium Cool: The Movies of the 1960s* (New York: Knopf, 1990), 287, delves into a history of 1960s Hollywood's "own apocalypse."

32. Robin Morgan, ed., *Sisterhood Is Powerful: An Anthology of Writings from the Women's Liberation Movement* (New York: Vintage, 1970), 496. Reprinted from *Women: A Journal of Liberation* (1970).

33. Gloria Steinem and George Barris, *Marilyn* (New York: New American Library, 1986).

34. Crowther's review appeared in *New York Times,* August 14, 1967; Schickel's in *Life,* October 13, 1967. All reprinted in John Cawelti, ed., *Focus on Bonnie and Clyde* (Englewood Cliffs, N.J.: Prentice Hall, 1973), 22–25.

35. Violence, and its almost slapstick visualization, propelled the renaissance of the genre film: *Bonnie & Clyde* updated the late 1930s rural gangster film; *Butch Cassidy & the Sundance Kid* cashed in on the western Sergio Leone had already restored; and with *Rosemary's Baby*, Roman Polanski resurrected an eerily contemporary monster movie. But the genres had been feminized; Faye Dunaway, Claudia Cardinale, and Mia Farrow figure centrally in these films.

36. Peter Biskind, *Easy Riders, Raging Bulls: How the Sex, Drugs and*

Rock 'n' Roll Generation Saved Hollywood (New York: Simon and Schuster, 1998), 46.

37. Shulamith Firestone, *The Dialectic of Sex: The Case for Feminist Revolution* (New York: Bantam, 1970), 188.

38. This 1967 film, *Shulie*, by Jerry Blumenthal, Sheppard Ferguson, James Leahy, and Allan Rettig was "adapted" as a "shot-by-shot, line-by-line recreation" in 1997 by Elisabeth Subrin. Director's notes. Program notes for "Fakes/Remakes: Stretching the Truth," Walker Art Center, Minneapolis, Minnesota, March 20, 1999.

39. "First Statement," *Film Culture* 22–23, 133.

40. Sherry Sonnett Trumbo, "A Woman's Place Is in the Oven," in *Notes from the Third Year: Women's Liberation* (New York: New York Radical Women, 1971), 91. Reprinted from the *New York Times*.

41. Muriel Rukeyser, *Theory of Flight* (New Haven, Conn.: Yale University Press, 1935), 87. See Rebecca Hill, "Fosterites and Feminists, Or 1950s Ultra-Leftists and the Invention of AmeriKKKa," *New Left Review* (1998), argues that these critiques of Hollywood are central to left-wing feminism in the postwar years and so offer a continuity between the two periods.

42. Barbara Burris, "Fourth World Manifesto," *Notes from the Third Year*, 109.

43. Francee Covington, "Are the Revolutionary Techniques Employed in *The Battle of Algiers* Applicable to Harlem?" in Toni Cade, ed., *The Black Woman: An Anthology* (New York: Signet, 1970), 244–54.

44. Susan Sontag, "The Third World of Women," *Partisan Review* 60 (1973): 180–206.

45. Newsreel Manifesto was reprinted by Mekas in his January 25, 1968, *Village Voice* column. Reprinted in Mekas, *Movie Journal: The Rise of a New American Cinema, 1959–1971* (New York: Collier Books, 1972), 305–6.

46. Charlotte Bunch, *Passionate Politics: Feminist Theory in Action, Essays 1968–1986* (New York: St. Martin's Press, 1987), 5–6; Echols, *Daring to Be Bad*, 54–59, describes these actions.

47. David James, *Allegories of Cinema: American Film in the Sixties* (Princeton: Princeton University Press, 1991), 217.

48. David Talbot and Barbara Zheutlin, *Creative Differences: Profiles of Hollywood Dissidents* (Boston: South End Press, 1978), 362. Ironically, both Kramer and Phillips, who also parted ways, became interested in narrative forms: Kramer, who died in 1998, made a number of feature-length narrative films with European financing, among them *Milestones*, which traced the demise of the 1960s New Left; Phillips moved into soap opera, seeing it as a popular female form whose never-ending story-line appeared to undo classic Hollywood cinema and mobilize a female mass audience. She and friends produced an alternative radio soap opera, "Winds of Change," in St.

Louis; eventually, she became a scriptwriter for the satirical television soap, *Mary Hartman, Mary Hartman*.

49. Quoted in Van Gelder, "Shirley Clarke Is Dead at 77."

50. Nancy Ellen Dowd, "Popular Conventions," provides a devastating critique of *Battle of Algiers*'s "cloying" fakery in *Film Quarterly* 22, no. 3 (Spring 1969). David James forcefully makes this point in his *Allegories of Cinema*, especially in the chapter on Brakhage.

51. Parker Tyler, *Underground Film: A Critical History* (New York: Grove Press, 1969), 69.

52. James, *Allegories*, 119–120.

53. Mekas, *Movie Journal*, 89–90.

54. Maya Deren made her first film with her husband, director and cinematographer Alexander Hammid; Chick Strand started Canyon Cinema with her filmmaker husband, Bruce Baillie; filmmaker Freude Bartlett was married to videographer Scott Bartlett; Emily Breer and Robert Breer both made films, and so forth.

55. Sheldon Renan, *An Introduction to the American Underground Film* (New York: E. P. Dutton, 1967), 174.

56. With the exception of the *Film Quarterly* review and interview and Renan's off-hand remark, I can find no mention of this germinal film in any accounts of underground, experimental, expanded, or avant-garde cinema, until a brief quotation of the Callenbach review in Wheeler Winston Dixon, *The Exploding Eye: A Re-Visionary History of 1960s American Experimental Cinema* (Albany: State University of New York Press, 1997). Even Patricia Mellencamp's *Indiscretions*, whose subtitle is: "Avant-garde Film, Video and Feminism" (Bloomington: Indiana University Press, 1990), fails to mention this momentous event. Of the mini-industry of memoirs and histories about the 1960s, only Alice Echols's careful recreation of those "Daring to Be Bad" mentions this film.

57. Brenda Richardson, "Women, Wives, Film-Makers: An Interview with Gunvor Nelson and Dorothy Wiley," *Film Quarterly* 25, no. 1 (Fall 1971): 34–41.

58. Shirley Clarke and Storm De Hirsch, "A Conversation," *Film Culture* 46 (Autumn 1967), 44–54 (published October 1968).

59. Richardson, "Women, Wives, Film-Makers," 36; Clarke and De Hirsch, "A Conversation," 50.

60. Kate Haug, "Femme Experimentale: Interviews with Carolee Schneemann, Barbara Hammer, and Chick Strand," *Wide Angle* 20 (January 1998): 1–19, reprints a letter from Adrienne Mancia on Museum of Modern Art stationery, dated August 1968, in which she "regret[s] that Carolee Schneemann's film, FUSES, is confronted with problems of censorship" (18).

61. Richardson, "Women, Wives, Film-Makers," 35.

62. In 1978, J. Hoberman noted that "*Meshes* seems less related to European surrealism than to the Freudian flashbacks and sinister living-rooms that typify Hollywood's wartime 'noir' films. Located in some hilly L.A. suburb, the house where Deren's erotic, violent fantasy was filmed might be around the corner from Barbara Stanwyck's place in *Double Indemnity*." J. Hoberman, "The Maya Mystique," *The Village Voice* 23, no. 20 (May 15, 1978): 54. However, Deren's 1943 film, like Esther Bubley's photographs, predates almost all film noirs. Repeating Hoberman, critic Lauren Rabinovitz notes that "*Meshes of the Afternoon* adopts the dominant visual vocabulary associated with the emerging *film noir*—high contrast lighting, extreme camera angles, character point-of-view shots—but displaces it onto a narrative of a woman subject contending with her own fragmentation and disequilibrium." Lauren Rabinovitz, *Plots of Resistance: Women, Power and Politics in the New York Avant-garde Cinema, 1943–71* (Urbana: University of Illinois Press, 1991), p. 56.

63. *Canyon Cinema Catalogue #6* (1988), 247.

64. The phrase is taken from Sara Evans' book of the same name.

65. Ernest Callenbach, review of *Schmeerguntz, Film Quarterly* 19, no. 4 (Summer 1966): 67.

66. "Filmmaking," *The Second Wave* 2, no. 3 (1973): 32, transcript of a 1972 interview with Maureen McCue on Boston's public radio station, WBUR.

67. Fredric Jameson, "Periodizing the '60s," in *The Sixties Without Apology*, 208.

68. Paul Potter, *A Name for Ourselves*, quoted in Gitlin, *The Sixties*, 185. However, as David Bernstein, who was also present at the speech, suggests, underlying this sensibility were two others directly related to the productivity of censorship for revolution: McCarthyism had successfully indoctrinated even those radicals most critical of it into suspicion of anything that smacked of communism, on the one hand; and "the system" was at the same time tacitly understood by everyone who heard this phrase to be capitalism. Thus self-censorship served, paradoxically, to open up new metaphors and movements (personal communication).

69. Adrienne Rich, *Poems: Selected and New, 1950–1974* (New York: W. W. Norton, 1975), 169–172. Reprinted from *The Will to Change* (New York: W. W. Norton, 1971).

9. MAPPING NOIR

1. Personal communication with Sandro Portelli; Patricia Crain, *The Story of A: The Alphabetization of America from the New England Primer to The Scarlet Letter* (Stanford: Stanford University Press, 2000).

2. Frederick Douglass, *The Narrative of the Life of Frederick Douglass, An American Slave, Written by Himself* (1845; reprint, Garden City, N.Y.: Dolphin Books, 1963), 7–9.

3. We might ask, with Shelley Fisher Fishkin, "Was Hester Black?" It is quite possible, given her somewhat abolitionist sentiments, that Nathaniel's wife, Sophia, had read Douglass's narrative. See Fishkin, *Was Huck Black?: Mark Twain and African-American Voices* (New York: Oxford University Press, 1994) and arguments by critic Viola Sachs that Herman Melville's Ishmael is based on a black sailor as well. Lecture delivered at Terza Università degli Studi di Roma (Spring 2000).

4. See "Introduction," Rita Copeland, ed., *Criticism and Dissent in the Middle Ages* (Cambridge: Cambridge University Press, 1996).

5. J. P. Telotte notes that the "tangled networks" of the telephone are suggestive of the "anxious atmosphere that seems to surround every effort at speaking in the noir world." *Voices in the Dark: The Narrative Patterns of Film Noir* (Urbana: University of Illinois Press, 1989), 74.

6. For new research into film noir, the law, and the state, see the work-in-progress of Nancy West, Zoë Druick, and Helen Lennon.

7. Quoted in John M. Broder, "The Devil and Political Fund-raising," *New York Times*, News of the Week in Review, December 10, 2000, 4.

8. In a series of brilliant op-ed pieces, which netted her the Pulitzer Prize, Maureen Dowd understood this better than anybody else during the long impeachment saga: See, for example, "The 16th Minute," *New York Times*, September 1, 1999, A23, which details the afterlife of Monica Lewinsky's fortunes selling purses "with names resplendent of Hester Prynne," like "Garden Patch" on the World Wide Web; and "Pulp Nonfiction," *New York Times*, News of the Week in Review, September 13, 1998, 21, which reads Kenneth Starr's report as a "445-page Harold Robbins novel," and likens Monica Lewinsky's role in the narrative to "a stereotype, Monica became the raging, vengeful Glenn Close character in *Fatal Attraction*." In a post-Clinton recycling of the noir imaginary, Dowd revealed that she had learned that President George W. Bush's nickname for her is "The Cobra." "I Have a Nickname!!!" *New York Times*, April 29, 2001, 4:11.

9. Anne Stevenson, *Correspondences* (Middletown, Conn.: Wesleyan University Press, 1974), 70. Further citations appear in the text.

10. See June Howard, "Towards a Marxist-Feminist Cultural Analysis," *Minnesota Review* 20 (Spring 1983): 77–92, and Deborah Rosenfelt and Judith Lowder Newton, "Introduction: Toward a Materialist-Feminist Criticism," in Rosenfelt and Newton, eds., *Feminist Criticism and Social Change: Sex, Class, and Race in Literature and Culture* (New York: Metheun, 1985), for two examples from the mid-1980s.

11. I do not want to imply that only women novelists are engaged in dil-

letante historiography. Clearly, so are E. L. Doctorow (*Ragtime* and *The Book of Daniel*), Gore Vidal (*Hollywood, Burr* and the America cycle), Don DeLillo (*Libra, Underworld*), Robert Coover (*The Public Burning*), to name just a few. "The force of history," as DeLillo puts it, is the province of fiction. However, the works I consider seem to be doing more than the already mammoth task of setting the writer's "pleasure, his eros, his creative delight in language and his sense of self-preservation against the vast and uniform Death that history tends to fashion as its most enduring work" (Don DeLillo, "The Power of History," *The New York Times Magazine* [September 7, 1997]: 60–63). They are allowing the psychological expansiveness of fiction not only to reanimate the past but to intervene in the present.

12. Diane Prenatt, "Interview with Frances Sherwood," *Belles Lettres: A Review of Books by Women* 10 (Spring 1995): 22–26.

13. According to Marc Penka, Emerson condemned Hawthorne's "fiction-mongering" as unworthy of the philosophical questions with which he was concerned. " 'The Deep Taint of His Nature': Uncanny Allegory and Mr. Hawthorne's Gothic," Ph.D. diss., University of Minnesota, 2001.

14. Davis quotes Herbert Aptheker's passing comment that "[O]ne may better understand now a Margaret Garner, fugitive slave, who, when trapped near Cincinnati, killed her own daughter and tried to kill herself. She rejoiced that the girl was dead—'now she would never know what a woman suffers as a slave'—and pleaded to be tried for murder. I will go singing to the gallows rather than be returned to slavery.' " Angela Davis, *Women, Race and Class* (New York: Random House, 1981), 21; Herbert Aptheker, "The Negro Woman," in *Masses and Mainstream* 11 (February 1948): 12.

15. Toni Morrison, "Unspeakable Things Unspoken: The Afro-American Presence in American Literature," *Michigan Quarterly Review* 28 (Winter 1989): 1–34.

16. Frederick Douglass, *Narrative*, 2.

17. The vexed and strange interrelationship of fiction and history within slave women's literary cultures includes as well the research by Jean Fagin Yellin into Harriet Jacobs's *Incidents in the Life of a Slave Girl, Written by Herself*, which authorized it as a genuine slave narrative, not merely the sentimental fiction of Lydia Child as it had been presumed to be by literary historians. Because the conventions of the sentimental novel were more clearly recognizable within Jacobs's narrative than within that of Douglass (though his tale relies on virtually every coding of the sentimental, also), her story was viewed with suspicion by generations of scholars. Hers is surely a bizarre, even gothic, story; but the tale seemed fantastic in part because it conformed so accurately to popular narrative forms.

18. Stanley Crouch "Aunt Medea," review of *Beloved*, *The New Republic* 19 (October 1987): 38–48. See also Marilyn Judith Atlas, "Toni Morrison's *Beloved* and the Reviewers," for a comprehensive reading of the various responses to the novel. *Midwestern Miscellany* 18 (1990): 45–57.

19. Margaret Forster, "This Is Sort of Your Life, Mary Wollstonecraft," *New York Times Book Review* (July 11, 1993): 21.

20. Edward B. St. John, review of *Vindication*, *Library Journal* 118 (March 15, 1993): 109.

21. Stendhal writing of the scandal surrounding the Baron de Pontalba's attempted murder of his daughter-in-law and his subsequent suicide, quoted in Angeline Goreau, "A Spectacular Mess of a Marriage," (review of *Intimate Enemies: The Two Worlds of the Baroness de Pontalba* by Christina Vella) *New York Times Book Review* (August 31, 1997): 6–7. Goreau concludes her favorable review of the biography by longing "for a novelist who could explore the intricate workings of motivation, who could trace the see-sawings of power and control, who could ask the tricky question of who the 'author' of this family's story finally was" (7).

22. Mary Wollstonecraft, *Maria, or The Wrongs of Women*, "Author's Preface," (1798; reprint, New York: W. W. Norton, 1975), 7 (emphasis added).

23. See Moira Ferguson's introduction to Wollstonecraft, *Maria*, especially p. 20.

24. Loraine Fletcher, review of *Vindication*, *New Statesman and Society* 6 (June 4, 1993): 40.

25. Katha Pollitt, *Reasonable Creatures: Essays on Women and Feminism* (New York: Knopf, 1994); Sallie Tisdale, *Talk Dirty to Me: An Intimate Philosophy of Sex* (New York: Doubleday, 1994); Nadine Strossen, *Defending Pornography: Free Speech, Sex and the Fight for Women's Rights* (New York: Scribners, 1995). All reviewed in *The Nation* (February 20, 1996).

26. Andrea Dworkin, *Pornography: Men Possessing Women* (New York: Putnam, 1981), and *Intercourse* (New York: Free Press, 1987); "Is One Woman's Sexuality Another Woman's Pornography?" *Ms.* [Special Issue] (April 1985).

27. The 1980s sex debates were often far more vicious than the relatively balanced term, "debate," would suggest. Some of the decade's key texts promoting the "prosex line" include: Angela Carter, *The Sadeian Woman and the Ideology of Pornography*, (New York: Pantheon, 1978); *Heresies* #12 "Sex Issue"(1981); *Diary of a Conference on Sexuality*, "The Scholar and the Feminist," Barnard Women's Center, 1982; Sue Cartledge and Joanna Ryan, *Sex & Love: New Thoughts on Old Contradictions* (London: The Women's Press, 1983); Ann Snitow, Christine Stansell, and Sharon Thompson, eds., *Powers of Desire: The Politics of Sexuality* (New York: Monthly Review Press, 1983); Car-

ole Vance, ed., *Pleasure and Danger: Exploring Female Sexuality* (Boston and London: Routledge and Kegan Paul, 1984); Jane Root, *Pictures of Women: Sexuality* (London: Pandora Press, 1984); Varda Burstyn, ed., *Women Against Censorship* (Vancouver and Toronto: Douglas & McIntyre, 1985); Joan Nestle, *A Restricted Country* (Ithaca, N.Y.: Firebrand Books, 1987). See Paula Rabinowitz, "Ethnographies of Women: *Soft Fiction* and Feminist Theory," in *They Must Be Represented: The Politics of Documentary* (London: Verso, 1994), 157–75, for an account of the ways in which the sex debates played out in women's experimental films. More mainstream conservative/libertarian 1990s reinventions include Camille Paglia, *Sex, Art and American Culture: Essays* (New York: Vintage, 1992) and *Vamps and Tramps: New Essays* (New York: Vintage, 1994); Katie Roiphe, *The Morning After: Sex, Fear, and Feminism* (Boston: Back Bay Books, 1993).

28. Erwin Mitsch, *The Art of Egon Schiele*, trans. W. Keith Haughan (London: Phaidon Press, 1975), 34–35.

29. Michiko Kakutani's predictably less-than-enthusiastic review was entitled "Portrait of a Tortured Artist in a Tortured City," *New York Times*, July 27, 1990, C25.

30. A rare critical essay on his prison work is Alessandra Comini, "Egon Schiele in Prison," *Albertina-Studien* 4 (1974): 123–37. All of the images are reproduced in Erwin Mitsch, *Egon Schiele in der Albertina* (Graphische Sammlung Albertina, 1990).

31. Serge Sabarsky, *Egon Schiele* (New York: Rizzoli, 1985), 8–9.

32. James T. Demetrios, *Egon Schiele and the Human Form: Drawings and Watercolors* (Des Moines, Iowa: Des Moines Art Center, 1971). After describing Schiele's coded inscriptions, however, Demetrios makes a point of not including any of the prison images in the show. It is not clear why, but the show's title stresses "form."

33. *Times* reviewers on both sides of the Atlantic concurred in their estimations of the novel. Scott Bradfield, "Onan and Egon," *New York Times Book Review* (August 19, 1990): 14, said the first and third things quoted in this sentence. Neil Taylor, review of *Arrogance*, *Times Literary Supplement* (July 26, 1991): 20, said the second.

34. Constance Samaras and Carol Jacobson detail these and other cases, such as Jacobson's first-amendment fight with the University of Michigan Law School over its censorship of an exhibition, "Porn'Im'Agery," she curated, and explore their effects in a special issue of *The New York University Law School Law Review* 38, nos. 1 and 2 [on "The Sex Panic: Women, Censorship, and Pornography"] (1995).

35. During the late 1980s, feminists retreated from earlier assumptions "distinguishing" public from private. Nancy Armstrong and Joan Scott jointly swept away any logical reasons for retaining them. Each laid bare the

underlying assumptions shoring up women's literature, one the one hand, women's history, on the other. With feminist literary critics such as Felicity Nussbaum arguing that the private expressions of self by eighteenth-century bourgeois women through diaries and autobiographies helped codify middle-class subjectivity, and feminist social historians such as Linda Gordon claiming the working-class home as a central site of state formation through the organization of social welfare programs, it is difficult to see just where the private ends and the public begins, or vice versa. Nussbaum, *The Autobiographical Subject: Gender and Ideology in Eighteenth-Century England* (Baltimore: Johns Hopkins Unviersity Press, 1989); Gordon, *Heroes of Their Own Lives: The Politics and History of Family Violence* (New York: Viking, 1998).

36. Woolf's 1928 novel, *Orlando: A Biography*, takes as its subject the slippage between fiction and biography as it traces the 300-odd-year life span of its eponymous wealthy boy-man-woman writer-hero. With its central concerns of tracing the political effects of gender, race, and class on the bodies of individuals, *Orlando* was the gold standard for materialist-feminist British literary history.

37. *Pity Is Not Enough*, *The Executioner Waits*, and *Rope of Gold* are the titles of the three Josephine Herbst novels that never actually appeared as a trilogy until Warner Books reissued them together in 1985. Herbst, *Rope of Gold*, (1939; reprint, New York: The Feminist Press, 1984), 169.

38. The poem appeared in Crane's 1926 volume, *White Buildings*. Hart Crane, "My Grandmother's Love Letters," in *The Collected Poems of Hart Crane* (New York: Liveright, 1933), 65. The poem goes on to ask "Are your fingers long enough to play / Old keys that are but echoes?" John Eugene Unterecker, *Voyager: A Life of Hart Crane* (New York: Farrar Strauss and Giroux, 1969), reads this poem in light of Crane's boyhood sexuality.

39. As noted above, "discovered" documents offer a source for American revisionist historiography in *The Scarlet Letter*. Hawthorne rethinks, in light of Republican failures, his family's and his nation's sordid past through Hester Prynne's tale. This tradition is particularly important to African-American women's literary tradition: from Harriet Jacobs waging guerrilla warfare against her master from her attic enclosure by writing a series of letters posted secretly from afar to Rita Dove narrating her grandparents' lives through lyrics culled from family letters, diaries and mementos in *Thomas and Beulah* (Pittsburgh: Carnegie-Mellon University Press, 1987).

INDEX

Adams, Ansel, 116
Adorno, Theodor, 1, 10–11, 178, 201
AFL-CIO, 133
African-American authors, 20
African Americans, 5, 61
Agee, James, 119, 141, 204; and mixed genres, 83; on objects, 48; on rural poverty, 109; on shoes, 181–82, 184, 186–87
Aid to Dependent Children (ADC), 146, 161, 163
Aid to Families with Dependent Children (AFDC), 163–64
Akermann, Chantal, 196
Aldrich, Robert, 12, 186
Algren, Nelson, 1, 3, 5, 91–92
Amazing Stories, 12
America Day by Day (de Beauvoir), 2
American Dream (Kopple), 20, 126, 131–41
American landscape, 228; Adorno on 1; de Beauvoir on, 43; in film noir, 14, 16, 243. *See also* City; Heartland; Rural
Andersen, Hans Christian, 189
Andersen, Lewie, 133, 136, 138
Anderson, Benedict, 16–17
Anger, Kenneth, 200–201, 218
Annals of the American Association of Political and Social Sciences, 160
Ann Arbor Film Festival, 218
Aptheker, Herbert, 235
Arbus, Diane, 82, 202–205, 220
Arcades Project, The (Benjamin), 180
Archer, Bill, 164
Arden, Eve, 73
Armstrong, Nancy, 123
Arnow, Harriet, 129
Arrogance (Scott), 234, 239–40
Arzner, Dorothy, 119, 197
Astor, Mary, 19
Atkinson, Ti-Grace, 204–205
Avant-garde film, 22, 193. *See also* Experimental film; New American Cinema

Baker, Ella, 65, 70, 75, 78
Bakhtin, Mikhail, 17
Ball, Lucille, 119
Barclay, Gwen, 160
Barnard, Rita, 7
Barry, Kathy, 237
Barthes, Roland, 176, 181, 198
Barton Fink (Coen), 32
Basic Instinct (Verhoeven), 111
Battle of Algiers, The (Pontecorvo), 208, 212, 216

Battle of Chile, The (Guzman), 139
Beard, Isobel, 13
Beatty, Warren, 209
Beloved (Morrison), 234–37
Bendix, William, 159
"Benito Cereno" (Melville), 93
Benjamin, Walter, 1, 17, 205, 241; on aura, 61; on ownership, 177–81
Bennett, Joan, 76
Berkeley, Busby, 119, 210
Berlant, Lauren, 79
Berry, Abner, 88
Best Years of Our Lives, The, 3
Bezzerides, A. I., 102, 112
Biberman, Herbert, 187, 212
Big Clock, The (Fearing), 7
Big Combo, The (Lewis), 27, 112
Big Heat, The (Lang), 8, 27, 32, 34
Big Sleep, The (Chandler), 155
Black Boy (Wright), 91
Black Mask, 93
Black Metropolis (Wright), 91
Black Panther Party (Newsreel), 214
Black Panthers, 210
Black Woman, The (Cade), 212
Blodgett, Ruth, 151, 154
Blond Venus (Von Sternberg), 78
Blood Simple (Coen), 42, 107
Blue Dahlia, The (Marshall), 159
Bluest Eye, The (Morrison), 64
B-movies, 4, 8, 59, 173; and left-wing writers, 17, 97. *See also* Film noir
Body and Soul (Rossen), 112
Bogart, Humphrey, 2, 9–10, 18, 144
Bonner, Marita, 66, 157–58
Bonnie and Clyde (Penn), 210
Book-of-the-Month Club News, 151
Bourke-White, Margaret, 54, 109, 120; in *Life*, 21, 33, 42, 118. *See also* Women photographers

Boxer, Sarah, 106
Boyer, Jay, 194
Brakhage, Jane, 217
Brakhage, Stan, 198–99, 201, 203, 211
Breuer, Bessie, 250n17
Bright, Suzie, 238
British noir, 174
Brooks, Gwendolyn, 19, 66; *Maud Martha*, 63, 76, 80
Browder, Earl, 134
Brown, William Wells, 93
Bruno, Giuliana, 28
Bubley, Esther, 82, 220, 243; bus trip, 45–54, 191; in *Ladies Home Journal*, 54–59, 233; as OWI photographer, 19, 28, 42–44; on street photography, 204, 218; in Washington, D. C., 9, 30, 32–39. *See also* Women photographers
Burke, Edmund, 123, 125
Burke, Kenneth, 114
Burns, Ben, 88
Burris, Barbara, 211–12
Burton, Liane, 221
Bush, George W., 114–15

Cabbage (Wiley), 220
Cade, Toni, 212
Caged (Cromwell), 174
Cagney, Jimmy, 99
Cain, James M., 4, 72, 91, 96
Califia, Pat, 238
Callenbach, Ernest, 220
Call Northside 777 (Hathaway), 230
Camera Lucida (Barthes), 176
Canned Heat, 115
Canyon Cinema, 197
Capital (Marx), 126, 186
Capone, Al, 99
Capote, Truman, 107
Carver, Lily, 27

Caseworker reports, 148–49

Caspary, Vera, 263*n*40

Cat People (Tourneur), 11, 26, 64, 173

Cayton, Horace, 85–86

Censorship, 218, 222, 266*n*6, 288*n*68

Chandler, Raymond, 4, 155, 165

Chaplin, Charles, 130, 171, 180

Chelsea Girls, The (Warhol), 217

Chesler, Phyllis, 197

Chestnutt, Charles, 93

Chicago, 68; in African-American literature, 66, 93, 97; Nelson Algren on, 1, 3, 5; Esther Bubley photographs of, 46

Chicago Defender, The, 76

Chinatown (Polanski), 16, 84

Choy, Christine, 215

Cinema vérité, 202, 204, 211

Cisneros, Sandra, 188, 191

Cities, American, 2. *See also* Chicago; Los Angeles; New York; San Francisco

City, 3, 94, 101, 118–19

Clarissa (Richardson), 71

Clarke, Shirley, 216–18, 199; *The Connection*, 196, 202; *Portrait of Jason*, 203–205

Clinton, Bill, 158, 230–32

Clinton, Hillary Rodham, 231

Clotel (Brown), 93

Cobbett, William, 124, 126

Coen, Ethan and Joel, 20, 32, 42, 107

Collins, Marjory, 28–29

Columbia Strike, The (Newreel), 214

Communist Party of the United States (CPUSA), 8, 85; and African Americans, 20, 65, 88–89; Hitler-Stalin Pact, 160; in

The Outsider, 92, 96; and women, 250*n*17

Connection, The (Clarke), 202

Conroy, Jack, 130

Conte, Richard, 27

Contempt (Godard), 214

Cook, Elisha, Jr., 26

Cook, Page, 210

Cooke, Marvel, 70, 75, 78

Cool World, A (Clarke), 202

Cooper, Gary, 189

Coover, Robert, 197

Copeland, Rita, 229

Coppola, Francis Ford, 99

Corey, Wendell, 90, 94, 231

Corporate Campaign, 133, 136, 138

Correspondences (Stevenson), 232–34

Cotton, John, 226

Covington, Francee, 212

Crabbe, George, 114

Crain, Patricia, 227

Crane, Hart, 242

Crane, Stephen, 64

Crawford, Joan, 25, 72, 78–79, 230

Crime, 16, 33, 147, 229

Crimson Kimono, The (Fuller), 84

Crisis, 65

Criss Cross (Siodmak), 99

Crouch, Stanley, 236–37

Crowther, Bosley, 210

Daily Worker, The, 129, 153; on African-American writers, 88, 92; on domestic labor, 65, 68–69

Dali, Salvador, 6–7

Dance, Girl, Dance (Arzner), 119

Dark City (Dieterle), 96

Dassin, Jules, 105

Daughter, The (Breuer), 250*n*17

Davidman, Joy, 211

Davidson, Cathy, 123

Davis, Angela, 235
Davis, Ben, 92
Davis, Hope Hale, 113
Dead Reckoning (Cromwell), 9, 227
Dead Reckoning (Fearing), 7
de Beauvoir, Simone, 1–3, 43–44, 50–51
Debord, Guy, 205
de Havilland, Olivia, 78, 233
De Hirsch, Storm, 217
Deindustrialization, 126, 129, 136
Delano, Jack, 119
Deleuze, Gilles , 10, 176
Delon, Alain, 33, 63
Demetrios, James, 239
Denning, Michael, 6, 64, 79
Depression, The, 6, 18, 94; photography during, 19–20, 42, 106, 110; social welfare during, 158, 160–61
Deren, Maya, 211, 217, 222; domestic uncanny, 9, 196, 220, 288*n*62
Derrida, Jacques, 172, 177
Detective novels, 4, 82, 179; and Richard Wright, 85–86, 91
Detectives, 18, 21, 95; as investigators, 142–43, 147, 155–56; in film noir, 60, 63. *See also* Private eye
Detour (Ulmer), 4, 39, 171, 226; Ann Savage in, 25, 74
Detroit Free Press, The, 129
Detroit News, The, 129
Devil in a Blue Dress (Franklin), 84
Dialectic of Sex (Firestone), 210
Dial M for Murder (Hitchcock), 15
Dickens, Charles, 109
Dickens, Hazel, 133
Dietrich, Marlene, 78, 189
Documentary, 22, 203, 109, 112
Documentary film, 221; *The Battle of Algiers* and, 212, 216; Kopple's films, 131–41; about labor, 121; Lorentz's films, 115–16; *Roger & Me*, 126–31
Documentary photography, 105–106, 117, 124
Dog Star Man (Brakhage), 217
Doliner, Henry, 160
Dollmaker, The (Arnow), 129
Domesticity, 22, 56, 220
Domestic labor, 65, 67–68
Domestic labor debates, 63
Domestic workers, 70
Dos Passos, John, 98
Double Indemnity (Wilder), 4, 94, 132; femme fatale in, 30, 36; Barbara Stanwyck in, 25, 84, 90, 222, 226–27; Barbara Stanwyck's footwear in, 142, 172, 191
Douglas, Ann, 6
Douglas, Kirk, 25
Douglass, Frederick, 68, 122, 235; on sexual violence in slavery, 228–30, 232
Dowd, Maureen, 289*n*8
Dragnet, 167
Dream House (Nekola), 190
Du Bois, W. E. B., 90
Du Maurier, Daphne, 236
Dunaway, Faye, 209
Dutschke, Rudi, 176
Dworkin, Andrea, 238

Echols, Alice, 206, 208, 212, 238
El Greco, 54
Eliot, T. S., 8
Ellison, Ralph, 20, 85; *Invisible Man*, 83, 87–89, 94–95
Ellroy, James, 16
Enciclopedia delle Donne, 54
Engels, Friedrich, 109
Evans, Walker, 54, 118, 171; *Let Us Now Praise Famous Men*, 48,

119–20, 181–82, 204; photographs of shoes, 184, 186
Experimental film and women, 217–20

Fabre, Michel, 85–86
Falk, Candace, 236–37
Fargo (Coen), 20, 107–108, 131
Farm Security Administration (FSA), 5, 20, 42, 111; Dorothea Lange, 106–107, 113, 115–17; Lange's "Migrant Mother," 110, 119. *See also* Resettlement Administration
Farm Security Administration/ Office of War Information (OWI), 19, 28, 44, 48–49. *See also* Office of War Information (OWI)
Farrell, James T., 91, 153–54
Faurer, Louis, 28–29
Fearing, Kenneth, 6–8, 98
Federal Emergency Relief Administration, 152
Federal Housing Authority, 162
Federal Security Agency, 161–62
Female literary tradition, 241–42
Female sexuality, 8, 26, 145, 166. *See also* Lesbians
Feminism, 212, 221–23, 235; and avant-garde film, 193, 205, 208–209; sex debates, 238–39; and welfare, 164. *See also* Women's Liberation
Feminist film culture, 195–97, 211, 218–21
Feminist literary history, 234
Femme fatale, 6, 18, 59, 124, 233; and black women, 61–63, 95–97, 73–74, 79–80; and sexuality, 26–29, 143, 172. *See also* Femme noire

Femme noire, 63–64
Ferguson, Moira, 238
Fetishism, 10, 175–76, 178, 180
File on Thelma Jordan, The (Siodmak), 9, 94, 222, 232; Barbara Stanwyck in, 25, 90, 226, 230
Film Culture, 199–200
Film-Makers' Co-op, 197
Film noir, 2, 132, 226; and the city, 118–19; as context, 14, 231–32; and documentary, 112; and proletarian culture, 63–64, 141; and race, 79–80, 84, 91; veterans in, 165. *See also* B-movies
Film noir iconography, 39, 55, 259n4. *See also* Icons; Objects
Film and Photo League, 39, 212
Finley, Karen, 240
Firestone, Shulamith, 210, 216
Fisher, Andrea, 28, 46
Fitzgerald, Ella, 67
Flaherty, Robert, 125
Flaming Creatures (Smith), 205
Flint Voice, The, 130
Florika, 208
Flowers, Gennifer, 230
Fonda, Henry, 173
Forbes, Rosita, 12–13, 43
Force of Evil (Polonsky), 98, 102, 112
Ford, Glenn, 32, 142
Ford, James, 100
Ford, John, 145
Forster, Margaret, 236
Forster, Robert, 214
Frames, 228
Frank, Robert, 82
Freud, Sigmund, 12, 171; on fetishism, 175–76, 178, 180; on shoes, 173; on the uncanny, 193
Friedan, Betty, 233
From Reverence to Rape (Haskell), 196

Fuller, Samuel, 27, 175, 187, 196
Fuses (Schneemann), 218–19
Fusili, Henry, 237

Gangster films, 6, 10, 18, 36, 144
Gangsters, 67, 84, 99; C. L. R.
    James on, 9–10; in film noir,
    95–96, 101
Gardner, Ava, 142
Gardner, Erle Stanley, 165
Garner, Margaret, 235
Garrison, William Lloyd, 228
Gathering Storm (Page), 75, 78
Gelber, Jack, 196
Gellert, Hugo, 8, 120, 126–28,
    185–86
Gellhorn, Martha, 21, 42, 150–52,
    156
GI Bill of Rights, 158, 162, 191. *See
    also* Servicemen's Readjustment
    Act of 1944
Gilda (Vidor), 3, 96, 101, 142
Gilfillan, Lauren (Harriet Wood-
    bridge), 122, 140
Gilman, Charlotte Perkins, 63
GIs, 42, 165. *See also* Veterans
Gish, Lillian, 39
Gitlin, Todd, 194–96
Godard, Jean-Luc, 214–15, 223
Godfather, The (Coppola), 36, 99
Gold, Mike, 8, 92, 102
Golddiggers of 1933, The (LeRoy),
    210
Goldman, Emma, 237
Gold Rush, The (Chaplin), 2, 180
Gone with the Wind (Fleming), 78
Gordon, Linda, 148, 150
Gore, Al, 70
Grahame, Gloria, 25; in *The Big
    Heat*, 8, 27, 32, 34
Gramsci, Antonio, 194
Granger, Farley, 186

Grapes of Wrath, The (Ford), 119
Grapes of Wrath, The (Steinbeck),
    113
Greed (Von Stroheim), 2
Green, Hardy, 136, 139
Greene, Graham, 87
Greer, Jane: in *Out of the Past*, 9,
    19, 25, 96, 226
Griffin, Farah Jasmine, 174
Griffith, D. W., 39, 133, 145
Griswold v. Connecticut, 196
Group, The, 205, 211
Gruber, Ruth, 43
Gun Crazy (Lewis), 112

Halevy, Leon, 181
Hammett, Dashiell, 4, 91
Hamper, Ben, 130
Hanisch, Carol, 206, 209
Happenings, 201, 222
Hard-Pressed in the Heartland
    (Rachleff), 135
Harlan County, USA (Kopple), 131,
    133–36, 139–41
Harris, Trudier, 71
Haskell, Molly, 196
Hawthorne, Nathaniel, 226–29,
    232–34, 242–43
Hays code, 173
Hayworth, Rita, 4, 96, 142
Heartland, 114, 116, 131; as imag-
    ined landscape, 107–108, 266n5.
    See also Rural
Hebdige, Dick, 83
Heidegger, Martin, 171–72, 177, 181,
    184
Henle, Jim, 154
Henricksen, Leonardo, 140
Herbst, Josephine, 129, 154, 241–42
Herndon, Angel, 100
Herrmann, John, 154
Hersey, John, 16

Hicks, Granville, 87
High Sierra (Walsh), 10
Himes, Chester, 68, 88, 102
Hine, Lewis, 124–25
Hiroshima (Hersey), 16
Hitchcock, Alfred, 55, 95, 186
Hitler-Stalin Pact, 160
Holiday, Billie, 61, 67
Holliday, Jason, 204
Hollywood, 9, 15, 197, 208; and documentary, 113, 117, 120
Hollywood Babylon (Anger), 201
Hormel, Jay, 133
Horne, Lena, 67
House on Mango Street, The (Cisneros), 188
House Un-American Activities Committee (HUAC), 4, 16–17
Hughes, Holly, 240
Hughes, Langston, 74, 76
Hurst, Fannie, 19, 72, 75
Hurston, Zora Neale, 236
Hurwitz, Leo, 115
Huston, John, 18
Hutchinson, Anne, 225–26, 229–30, 242–43
Huyssen, Andreas, 6

Icons, 30, 36, 172. *See also* Objects
If He Hollers, Let Him Go (Himes), 102
I Married a Dead Man (Woolrich), 32, 95
Imitation of Life (Hurst), 19, 64, 79; black and white women in, 72, 75, 78
In Cold Blood (Capote), 107
Intercourse (Dworkin), 238
International Congress on Dialectics of Liberation, 201
International Labor Defense (ILD), 92, 100

Interstate Highway Act of 1956, 158, 163
Intolerance (Griffith), 145
Invisible Man (Ellison), 20, 64, 83, 87
Involutional melancholia, 54, 233, 252*n*35
I Went to Pit College (Gilfillan), 122

Jackson, Jesse, 132
Jacobs, Jane, 3
Jacobson, Carol, 240
James, C. L. R., 9–12, 191
James, David, 216
Jane Eyre (Brontë), 71
Jeanne Dielmann, 23 Quai du Commerce, 1080 Bruxelles (Akermann), 196
Jeannette Rankin Brigade, 208, 215
Jeffords, Susan, 159
Jerome, V. J., 100
Jet, 87–88
Jim Crow, 80, 93, 97; in women's photographs, 44, 52
Jobes, Gertrude, 183
Job's House (Slade), 147
Johnson, Claudia, 123
Johnson, Lyndon, 164
Jones, Jacqueline, 67–68
Jones, Paula Corbin, 231
Joyce, James, 154
Jubilee (Walker), 64
Jules et Jim (Truffaut), 208

Kahlo, Frida, 218
Keillor, Garrison, 16, 131
Keinholz, Ed and Nancy, 32
Khrushchev, Nikita, 186
Killers, The (Siodmak), 32, 99, 142
King, Larry, 231
Kiss the Blood Off My Hands (Foster), 52

Kiss Me Deadly (Aldrich), 12, 27, 186, 230

Kockelman, Joseph, 184

Kopple, Barbara, 126, 131–41

Korsch, Karl, 177

Kramer, Robert, 215

Kustom Kar Kommando (Anger), 200

Labor, 184, 186

Lacy, Ed, 102

Ladd, Alan, 159

Ladies Home Journal, 43, 52, 233; Bubley's assignments for, 54–56, 59

Lady Eve, The (Sturges), 173, 230

Lady in the Lake (Montgomery), 3

Lady from Shanghai, The (Welles), 52

Lake, Veronica, 159

Lancaster, Burt, 32, 142

Lange, Dorothea, 42, 54, 115, 118; at FSA, 106–107, 110, 113, 119–20, 183; theory of documentary, 116–17

Larsen, Nella, 92

Late capitalism, 221

Laura (Preminger), 95

Lead with Your Left (Lacy), 102

Leigh, Vivien, 78

Lemisch, Jesse, 134

Le samourai (Melville), 33, 63

Lesbians, 30, 147, 151

Lesser, Wendy, 173

Lesy, Michael, 107

Let Us Now Praise Famous Men (Agee and Evans), 48, 83, 141, 204

Lewinsky, Monica, 18, 230–31

Lewis, H. H., 8, 126

Lewis, Joseph H., 27, 112

Life, 4, 43, 111, 117; Margaret Bourke-White in, 21, 33, 42

lifshin, lyn, 208

Lilly Crackell (Slade), 147, 153, 162, 165

Lindsey, Karen, 208–209

Literary history, 289*n*11

Literary radicalism, 6, 254*n*8. *See also* Proletarian literature

Little Caesar, 144

Livingston, Jacqueline, 240

Local P-9, 131–41

Lorentz, Pare, 115

Los Angeles, 5

Lost Weekend, The (Wilder), 3

Louisiana Story (Flaherty), 125

Love, Anarchy and Emma Goldman (Falk), 236–37

Lowe, Ramona, 79

Luce, Henry, 10

Lukács, Georg, 123

Lupino, Ida, 10, 15, 18, 80, 197; in *Road House*, 19, 73, 173

Maas, Willard, 217

MacKinnon, Catherine, 238

Maddow, Ben, 98

Maggie, Girl of the Streets (Crane), 64

Maids: in literature, 68, 75; in film noir, 60, 62–64, 72, 74. *See also* Domestic worker

Maltese Falcon, The (Hammett), 89

Maltese Falcon, The (Huston), 18, 143

Man with a Movie Camera (Vertov), 131, 212

Mann, Sally, 240

Mansfield, Jane, 208–209

Mao, Douglas, 179–80

Mao Zedong, 111–12

Mapplethorpe, Robert, 240

Marcantonio, Vito, 147

Margaret (Slade), 147, 149, 151

Markley, Robert, 137

Marquand, John, 54

Marx, Karl, 126; on commodity fetishism, 177–78, 180; in Hugo Gellert's book, 126–27, 171, 185–86; on rural life, 107

Masculinity: instability of, 184, 186; of the working class, 20, 69, 126, 138, 201, 270n15; affect of WWII on, 162. *See also* Working stiff, GIs, Veterans

Masochism, 11

Mass culture, 6, 211

Maud Martha (Brooks), 63–64, 76–77, 80

Maus (Spiegelman), 185

Mayhew, Henry, 109

McCarthy, Mary, 2

McCarthyism, 8, 187

McDormand, Frances, 108

McMurray, Fred, 25, 84, 142, 172–73

McQueen, Butterfly, 72, 78

McRae, Joel, 186

McRobbie, Angela, 83

Mechanical reproduction, tools for, 230–31

Medium Cool (Wexler), 213–17, 222

Meeker, Ralph, 186

Mekas, Jonas, 198–99, 216, 218

Melish, John Howard, 154

Melodrama, 11, 18; and domesticity, 62–63, 71, 233; in *The Outsider*, 85–87, 261n13; and working-class militancy, 124, 130, 133, 138

Melodrama, noir, 52, 74

Melodrama, racial, 20

Melville, Herman, 93, 95, 125

Melville, Jean-Pierre, 33, 63

Mencken, Marie, 197, 216–17

Men at Work (Hine), 124

Meshes of the Afternoon (Deren), 9, 196, 220, 222

Metalious, Grace, 196

Midmonthly Survey, 153

"Migrant Mother" (Lange), 19, 110, 119, 141

Mildred Pierce (Cain), 19, 79

Mildred Pierce (Curtiz), 72–73, 79

Miles, Vera, 55

Million Dollar Movie, 14, 232

Miss America, 197, 216, 222

Miss America protest, 195, 206, 209

Miss Lonelyhearts (West), 32, 242

Mitchell, Juliet, 196

Mitchell, Louise, 66

Mitchell, Thomas, 145

Mitchum, Robert, 25

Moby-Dick (Melville), 125

Modernism, pulp, 97, 100; American, 2, 4, 6, 10; and documentary, 112; female, 39

Modernism, vernacular, 6

Monroe, Marilyn, 208–209

Moore, Michael, 126, 129–31

Moreau, Jeanne, 208

More Than Night (Naremore), 14

Morocco (Von Sternberg), 189

Morrison, Toni, 64, 84, 234–37

Moses, Robert, 5

Mother and the Law, The (Griffith), 145

Motion Picture Association of America (MPAA), 213, 222

Moynihan, Daniel Patrick, 158, 164

Mrs. Party's House (Slade), 147, 165

Mulvey, Laura, 196

Muni, Paul, 99

Murder Is My Business (Weegee), 39

Museum of Modern Art (MOMA), 202, 204

Musketeers of Pig Alley, The (Griffith), 39

My Dark Places (Ellroy), 16

My Fair Lady (Lerner and Loewe), 125

Naison, Mark, 100

Naked City (Dassin), 82

Naked Kiss, The (Fuller), 27, 196; leather in 175, 187, 192

Nana (Zola), 82

Naremore, James, 14, 60, 87

Nation, Carrie, 145

National Conference of Social Workers, 161

National Endowment for the Arts, 111, 240

Native Son (Wright), 85–86, 91, 96, 113

Neal, Tom, 25, 33, 171

Negulesco, Jean, 73

Nekola, Charlotte, 15, 190

Nelson, Gunvor, 196–97, 217–18

Nelson, Robert, 217

Neo-retro-noir, 22, 247*n*22

Ness, Eliot, 161

New American Cinema, 199, 205, 221

New American Cinema Group (The Group), 199, 202. *See also* Group, The

New Day Films, 197

New Deal, 5, 111, 115–16, 160

New Left, 194, 196–97, 210, 221

New Masses, The, 7–8, 65, 120, 154, 211

New Republic, The, 236

Newsreel, 197, 208, 212–15

New York, 3, 70, 265*nn*1, 2

New York Film Festival, 202

New York Radical Women, 208

New Yorker, The, 158

Night and the City (Dassin), 4, 105

Night and Fog (Resnais), 177

Nixon, Robert, 85

Noir America, 2

Noir effect, 16, 42

No Man of Her Own (Leisen), 28, 32, 95

Nussbaum, Felicity, 234

Oates, Joyce Carol (Rosamond Smith), 16

Objects, 21; in Bubley's photographs, 49–51; in film noir, 15, 39, 171–72, 220; theories about, 11, 175–80. *See also* Icons

Odets, Clifford, 98

Office of Defense Health and Welfare Service, 161

Office of War Information (OWI), 56, 191; Esther Bubley at, 9, 19, 28, 42–43

O'Hara, Maureen, 119

O'Keeffe, Georgia, 83

Olsen, Tillie Lerner, 121

Ophuls, Max, 62

Opportunity, 79

Ottley, Roy, 88

Out of the Past (Tourneur), 4, 9, 19, 25, 99; black woman in, 60; detective in, 143–44; femme fatale in, 95–96, 226; telephone in, 39

Outsider, The (Wright), 19, 20, 142; as a film noir, 83–102

Page, Myra, 75

Palance, Jack, 25

Palmer, Phyllis, 69, 75

Parker, Eleanor, 174

Passing (Larsen), 92–94

Passing stories, 263*n*40

Pedicord Apt. (Keinholz), 32

Penn, Arthur, 210

People's Front, The (Browder), 134

Performance, 201, 204

Petry, Ann, 19, 63, 71, 156–58

Peyton Place (Metalious), 196

Phantom Lady (Siodmak), 26, 30, 74; shoes in, 174, 192

Phillips, Lynn, 215–16

Phillips, Wendell, 228

Photography, 20, 198

Pickup on South Street (Fuller), 230

Plessy v. Ferguson, 93

Plow That Broke the Plains, The (Lorentz), 115

PM, 21, 82

Poe, Edgar Allan, 85, 90

Polanski, Roman, 16

Pollitt, Katha, 238

Polonsky, Abraham, 98, 112

Pontecorvo, Gillo, 208

Popular Front, 17, 79, 109; and popular culture, 76, 11–12, 134–35

Portelli, Sandro, 227

Portrait of Jason (Clarke), 202–204

Postman Always Rings Twice, The (Garnett), 9

Private eye, 143, 156

Proletarian culture, 6, 20

Proletarian literature, 63–64, 113

Prostitutes, 67–68, 96, 147–50

Prostitution, 20, 72, 74; in fiction, 165–67

Psychoanalysis and Feminism (Mitchell), 196

Public Enemy, The (Wellman), 144

Pudd'nhead Wilson (Twain), 93

Pulp: in fiction, 18, 71, 82, 86; in narrative, 30; in theory, 235

Pulp Fiction (Tarantino), 15

Pulp magazines, 89

Pulp modernism. *See* Modernism, pulp

Pushover (Quine), 230

Rachleff, Peter, 135–37, 139–41

Racism, 85, 236; in CPUSA, 98–100

Raines, Ella, 30, 74, 174

Rat Life and Diet in North America (Weiland), 220

Raw Deal (Mann), 52

Reader's Digest, 158

Reagan, Ronald, 130, 132, 158

Reckless Moment, The (Ophuls), 62, 75–76

Redbook, 43

Red Harvest (Hammett), 91

Reece, Florence, 70, 121–22

Reitman, Ben, 237

Renan, Sheldon, 217

Reportage, 83, 121–22, 146, 242

Resettlement Administration (RA), 107

Resnais, Alain, 176

Revueltas, Rosaura, 187

Reynolds, Paul, 89

Rich, Adrienne, 223

Richardson, Brenda, 217

River, The (Lorentz), 116

Rivera, Diego, 218

Road House (Negulesco), 19, 73–74, 173

Robinson, Edward G., 2, 84, 99

Robinson Crusoe (Defoe), 178

Rodgers, Ray, 133, 136, 138

Rodriguez, Joseph, 106

Roediger, David, 69, 79

Roger & Me (Moore), 20, 126–31

Roman noir, 7, 83

Roosevelt, Eleanor, 54

Roosevelt, Franklin D., 114–15

Rope of Gold (Herbst), 129

Rossen, Robert, 112

Rossetti, Christina, 12

Rosskam, Edwin, 113

Rukeyser, Muriel, 146, 211

Rural, 114–15, 120, 141, 186

Salt of the Earth (Biberman), 187–88, 212

Samaras, Connie, 240

San Francisco, 2, 85, 115–16

Sarachild, Kathie, 206

Sarris, Andrew, 15

Savage, Ann, 25, 33, 74

Scarface (Hawks), 144

Scarlet Letter, The (Hawthorne), 226–29, 232

Schapiro, Meyer, 177

Schickel, Richard, 210

Schiele, Egon, 239–40

Schmeerguntz (Nelson and Wiley), 196, 206–207, 217–18, 220

Schneemann, Carolee, 197, 201–203, 216, 218–19

Scorpio Rising (Anger), 200–201

Scott, Joanna, 234, 239–40

Scott, Lizbeth, 9, 25, 96, 228

S.C.U.M. Manifesto (Solanas), 205

Sentimentality, 18; in American culture, 10, 290*n*17; history of 122–26; and labor 133, 186

Serenade (Cain), 91

Serranos, Andre, 240

Servicemen's Readjustment Act, 162

Servier, Jean, 184

Sexuality, 61, 73, 237–40. *See also* Female sexuality; Lesbians

Sex and violence, 2. *See also* Crime

Sherwood, Frances, 234–40

Shoes: as commodities, 177–80; in film noir, 172–75, 186–92; in philosophy, 171–74, 183–86; as symbols, 171–77

Shore, Dinah, 5

Shulie (Blumenthal, Ferguson, Leahy, Rettig), 211

Silence of the Lambs, The (Demme), 111

Silver, Alain, 11

Simon, Carly, 15

Simon, Simone, 26, 173

Simpson, O. J., 15, 283*n*44

Sinatra, Nancy, 189

Siodmak, Robert, 226

Slade, Caroline, 21, 238; novels by, 146–55, 161–62, 165–67

Slesinger, Tess, 119

Smethurst, James, 76–77

Smith, Bessie, 67–69

Smith, Jack, 198, 218

Smith, Roger, 129–30

Smith, Susan, 15

Snake Pit, The (Litwak), 233

Social Protection Program, 161

Social Security Act of 1935, 158–59

Social workers, 21, 143, 147; in fiction, 150–62, 165–67

Social Work Today, 153, 160

Soft Fiction (Strand), 220

Solanas, Valerie, 205

Sontag, Susan, 205, 212

Sorry, Wrong Number (Litwak), 39, 230

Spiegelman, Art, 185

Springer, Gertrude, 153

Stagecoach (Ford), 145

Stanwyck, Barbara, 4, 191; *Double Indemnity*, 25, 84, 142, 172–73, 222, 226–28; *The File on Thelma Jordan*, 9, 25, 90, 222, 226; *The Lady Eve*, 173, 229–30; *No Man of Her Own*, 28, 32, 95

Starr, Kenneth, 232

Starr Bright Will Be With You Soon (Smith), 16

Steedman, Carolyn, 167, 190

Steinbeck, John, 113

Steiner, Ralph, 115

Sterile Sun (Slade), 146, 148–49, 152, 154–55

Stevenson, Anne, 232–34, 241–43

Stewart, Susan, 179

Stieglitz, Alfred, 39

Stott, William, 112

Strand, Chick, 220

Strand, Paul, 115

Strangers on a Train (Hitchcock), 95, 186

Street, The (Petry), 19, 63–64, 67, 156

Street in Bronzeville, A (Brooks), 66

Strong, Anna Louise, 43

Strossen, Nadine, 238

Stryker, Roy, 19; at FSA, 119; at OWI, 28, 42, 50–51

Studs Lonigan (Farrell), 91

Sturges, Jock, 240

Sturges, Preston, 173, 186

Sudden Fear (Miller), 25, 230

Sullivan's Travels (Sturges), 186

Sunset Boulevard (Wilder), 226

Survey, The, 152–53

Svilova, Yelizaveta, 131

Swendenborg, Emanuel, 183

Tarantino, Quentin, 15

Tate, Sharon, 16

Taylor, Paul Schuster, 107

Television, 18

Tennessee Valley Authority (TVA), 116

Tenney, James, 218

Theory of the Leisure Class, The (Veblen), 124

Theweleit, Klaus, 8

They Live by Night (Ray), 52

They Shoot Horses, Don't They? (McCoy), 144, 148

Thieves' Highway (Dassin), 102, 112

Thieves' Market (Bezzerides), 102, 112

Thigh Line Lyre Triangular (Brakhage), 217

Tompkins, Jane, 123

Tillmon, Johnnie, 164

Time to Remember, A (Zugsmith), 250n17

Tisdale, Sally, 238

Tombes, Andrew, Jr., 30, 174

Too Late for Tears (Haskin), 25, 96

Touch of Evil (Welles), 84

Tourneur, Jacques, 11, 60, 64, 173

Towers, Constance, 175, 187–88

Towne, Robert, 16

Traub, Belle, 65

Trevor, Claire, 145

Trials, 16–17, 229

Trilling, Diana, 153

Tripp, Linda, 230

Triumph of Willie Pond, The (Slade), 147, 149–50, 153

Trouble I've Seen, The (Gellhorn), 150

True Stories, 113

Trumbo, Sherry Sonnett, 211

Tucker's People (Wolfert), 98, 102, 112

Tugwell, Rexford G., 5

Turner, Lana, 9

Turner, Victor, 176

Twain, Mark, 93

12 Million Black Voices (Wright), 64, 91, 113

Twin Cities Support for P-9, 136

Tyler, Parker, 216

U.S. 1 (Rukeyser), 146–47

Ulysses (Joyce), 154

Uncanny, 9, 12, 193, 220

United Food and Commercial Workers (UFCW), 131–41

United Mine Workers, 134, 141

United States Army, Information and Education Division, 159

Updike, John, 16

Vance, Carole, 240

Van Gogh, Vincent, 171, 174, 182, 184–86; *Les Soulieres*, 178

Vanguard Press, 154

Van Witsen, Tony, 44

Veblen, Thorsten, 124

Vertov, Dziga, 131, 212

Veterans, 4, 8, 89, 158–59, 162–65. *See also* GIs

Vietnam War, 16, 234; and film, 194, 201, 213, 222

Village Voice, The, 212

Vindication (Sherwood), 234

Violence, 285n35

Viva Superstar, 204

Vogue, 42

Voyeurism, 204

Waiting for Godot (Beckett), 176

Wald, Alan, 6, 64

Walker, Margaret, 64, 85, 113

Walker, Robert, 186

Wallace, Henry A., 164

Wallace, Jean, 27

Ward, Elizabeth, 11

Warhol, Andy, 204–205

War on Poverty, 164

Washington, Booker T., 90

Webster, Harvey Curtus, 87

Weegee (Arthur Fellig), 21, 33, 82

Weiland, Joyce, 220

Welfare, 157–59, 163, 278n34

Wellstone, Paul, 134

West, Nathanael, 32, 242

Wexler, Haskell, 213–15

Wharton, Edith, 230

White Girl, The (Caspary), 263n40

Wilde, Cornel, 173

Wilder, Billy, 226

Wiley, Dorothy, 196, 217–18

Williams, Aubry, 160

Williams, Frances, 75

Williams, Raymond, 114, 123–24, 194

Williams, William Carlos, 109

Winter, Ella, 43

Wolcott, Marion Post, 19, 44, 52

Wolfert, Ira, 98, 102, 112

Wollstonecraft, Mary, 236–39

Woman's Film, The (Newsreel), 197

Women Called Wild (Forbes), 13, 43

Women and Economics (Gilman), 63

Women and Madness (Chesler), 197

Women Make Movies, 196–97

Women photographers, 42

Women's Liberation Movement, 194, 218, 221–23. *See also* Feminism

Women's literary tradition, 19, 241

Woolf, Virginia, 180, 242

Woolrich, Cornell, 32–33, 95

Working stiff, 124, 141

Works Progress/Projects Administration (WPA), 107, 113, 160

World War I, 6, 16

World War II: in African-American literature, 80, 89; and film noir, 12, 17–18, 159; and welfare, 158–63; women's work and 27, 58, 68

Wright, Ellen, 87

Wright, Richard, 2, 61, 76; *12 Million Black Voices*, 64, 91, 113; *Black Boy*, 91; *Black Metropolis*, 91; *Native Son*, 83, 91, 113; *The Outsider*, 19, 83–87, 89–90, 92–102

Wrong Man, The (Hitchcock), 55

Yield to the Night (Tompson), 174

You Have Seen Their Faces (Caldwell and Bourke-White), 109

Younger, Joan, 55

Zola, Emile, 82

Zoot suit, 83, 161

Zugsmith, Leane, 250n17